Biopharmaceutics and Pharmacokinetics

Second Edition

Biopharmaceutics and Pharmacokinetics

Second Edition

V. Venkateswarlu

M.Pharm., Ph.D., PDF (USA)

Senior Director,
Dr. Reddy's Laboratories Ltd.,
Hyderabad.

Formerly Associate Professor,
University College of Pharmaceutical Sciences,
Kakatiya University, Warangal, Andhra Pradesh.

Pharma Med PRESS
An Imprint of
Pharma Book Syndicate

PharmaMed Press
An imprint of Pharma Book Syndicate

A unit of BSP Books Pvt. Ltd.

4-4-309/316, Giriraj Lane,
Sultan Bazar, Hyderabad - 500 095.

Published by

PharmaMed Press

An imprint of Pharma Book Syndicate

A unit of BSP Books Pvt. Ltd.

4-4-309/316, Giriraj Lane, Sultan Bazar, Hyderabad - 500 095.
Phone: 040-23445605, 23445688; Fax: 91+40-23445611
E-mail: info@pharmamedpress.com

ISBN : 978-93-52300-53-2 (HB)

Dedicated to

My Mother, Rosamma

and

My Wife, Veeramma

Preface to Second Edition

I am thankful to the students and faculty of all the colleges for their continuous support and providing insights on each topic in depth during this decade of my book. First edition is originated from my several years of teaching and research experience in academics.

I have moved from academics to industry and started using the principles of Biopharmaceutics and Pharmacokinetics in formulation development in wide range of dosage forms and designs. I am thankful to Dr. Reddy's Laboratories for creating Center of Excellence in Biostudies (COE-Bio) and providing a unique opportunity to build the team. Untiring efforts of my team members over last five years has given greater insight into the practical applications of Biopharmaceutics and Pharmacokinetics in biosuccess.

I felt that it is the time to share the practical knowledge gained by me and my team to the other scientists. Second edition is revised by the members of COE-Bio of Dr. Reddy's Laboratories Ltd. and edited by me.

I am thankful to Mr. K. B. Sankara Rao, Head of IPDO and Dr. Reddy's Laboratories Ltd., for giving me an opportunity to head COE-Bio and to revise the first edition with the knowledge gained for the last five years.

- V. Venkateswarlu

Contributors

Dr. Deepika Aggarwal, MPharma, PhD
Manager
Dr. Reddy's Lab. Ltd
Bachupally, Hyderabad

(*Chapters : 3, 4, 10 and 11*)

Dr. Naveen Ahuja Khurana, MPharma, PhD
Asst. Manager
Dr. Reddy's Lab. Ltd
Bachupally, Hyderabad

(*Chapters : 5, 6, 7 and 8*)

Bhupesh Pratap, MS (Pharmacology)
Asst. Manager
Dr. Reddy's Lab. Ltd
Bachupally, Hyderabad

(*Chapters : 1, 2, 9, 12 and 13*)

UNIVERSITY COLLEGE OF PHARMACEUTICAL SCIENCES
KAKATIYA UNIVERSITY, WARANGAL - 506 009 (A.P.) INDIA

Prof. (Dr.) Y. Madhusudan Rao
M. Pharm., Ph.D.

Grams : KAKATIYA
Fax : 0870 - 2453508, 2432699
Ph: Off. : 2432699, Res. : 2570543
2438001 - 5 Extn. : 304
e-mail : ymrao123@yahoo.com

FOREWORD TO FIRST EDITION

The study of Biopharmaceutics and Pharmacokinetics is an essential and important part of pharmaceutical education. The selection of a proper dosage form, route of administration and dosage regimen for successful therapy depends mostly on the knowledge acquired from this subject.

Dr. V. Venkateswarlu has done a commendable job in writing a book titled 'Biopharmaceutics and Pharmacokinetics' in a simple and lucid way. The students at undergraduate and graduate level will find it very useful. He has covered the various chapters of Biopharmaceutics like factors affecting absorption, bioavailability, metabolism and pharmacokinetics like compartmental, non-compartmental, non-linear in a very simple way. The question bank given at the end of chapters and worked out problems are two important contributions which will be of great help to students. Inclusion of essential statistical treatments is also given in an easy way.

I congratulate Dr. Venkateswarlu for his excellent piece of work in writing this text. This book will be useful for students of pharmacy at different levels. In my opinion this will be to the satisfaction of pharmacy student at large.

(PROF. Y. MADHUSUDAN RAO)

Preface to First Edition

This book deals with the basics of the two disciplines of biopharmaceutics and pharmacokinetics. Different factors such as biological, physiochemical and formulation that influence the therapeutic efficacy of a drug are covered in biopharmaceutics. The absorption, distribution, metabolism and excretion of drugs are studied under this subject.

Pharmacokinetics is a study of the time course of drug absorption, distribution, metabolism and excretion. It also concerns with the relationship of these processes to the intensity and time course of pharmacological (therapeutic and toxicological) effects of drugs and chemicals. From its inception in 1937 with the classic papers of Torsten Teorell (International Archives of Pharmacodynamics,1937), pharmacokinetics has evolved at an incredible rate.

At the elementary level, pharmacokinetics is a tool to optimise the design of biological experiments with drugs and chemicals. It has become increasingly important in the design and development of new drugs and in the reassessment of old drugs. Clinical applications of pharmacokinetics have resulted in improvement in drug utilization and direct benefits to the physicians and patients.

The students have to learn the basics of biopharmaceutics and pharmacokinetics to understand the various procedures and advances in drug design, product development, therapeutic drug monitoring, etc. The pharmacokinetics part of this book covers the fundamentals of one compartment open model, multi-compartmental pharmacokinetics. One compartment open model is presented in an elaborate manner to make the students familiar with various aspects of pharmacokinetics. Mathematical equation are developed using simple integration and differentiation methods to enable the students to understand the concepts easily. Practice problems are provided where necessary, and a question bank is included at the end of each chapter to help the students more. Extreme care has been exercised to present the concepts in a simple way.

Every biological scientist should have knowledge in statistics in order to assess the significance of the results of his experiments. Hence, a chapter on biostatistics with practice problems is included in the book.

I have made an humble attempt to present the subject in a lucid manner and have taken all humanly possible care to avoid mistakes. Still any mistake found in this book by the readers may please be brought to my notice, for improvement.

I thank my colleagues, friends and family members for their help and encouragement. I am specially grateful to Prof. Y. Madhusudan Rao for his foreword to the book.

- V. Venkateswarlu

Contents

CHAPTER 3

Drug Distribution

CHAPTER 4

Drug Elimination

Chapter 6

One Compartment Open Model

Chapter 7

Multi-Compartment Models

CHAPTER 8
Multiple-Dose Regimens

CHAPTER 9
Non-linear Pharmacokinetics

CHAPTER 10
Non-compartmental Pharmacokinetics

Chapter 11

Bioavailability and Bioequivalence

Chapter 12
Biostatistics

Chapter 13
In vitro Dissolution Testing

1

Introduction to Biopharmaceutics

1.1 Introduction

The therapeutic response of a drug is normally dependent on an adequate concentration of the drug being achieved and then maintained at the site or sites of action of the drug. In the case of systemically acting drugs it is generally accepted for clinical purposes that a dynamic equilibrium exists between the concentration of drug in blood and the concentration of drug at its site(s) of action. It means that a linear relationship exists between the drug level in blood and drug concentration at the site of action. Therefore, drug concentration at the site of action can be predicted from blood concentration of drug.

Strictly, the concentration of drug in plasma water (i.e., protein free plasma) is a more accurate index of drug concentration at the site(s) of action than is the concentration of drug in whole plasma since a drug may often bind in a reversible manner to plasma protein. Only drug that is unbound (which is free and is dissolved in plasma water) can pass out of the plasma through the capillary endothelium and reach other body fluids and tissues and finally to its site(s) of action. However, to measure the concentration of an unbound drug in plasma water requires more complex and sensitive assay methods than to measure the total concentration of both unbound and bound drug in plasma.

However, it should be realized that this simplification may not always be valid. Indeed one should not draw inferences about the clinical effects of a drug from its plasma concentration until it has been established that the two are consistently correlated. The concentration of a drug in plasma depends on numerous factors. These includes the

1. relative amount of an administered dose that enters the systemic circulation (bioavailability)
2. the rate and extent of absorption
3. the rate and extent of distribution of the drug between the systemic circulation and other tissues and fluids
4. the rate of elimination of the drug from the body.

Fig. 1.1 shows the factors that influences the concentration of drug in blood. In case of I.V. bolus, the total dose of the drug administered reaches the circulation immediately. Where it undergoes the processes of protein binding, distribution, metabolism, renal excretion and elimination by all possible routes. After reaching the systemic circulation, the drug reaches its site(s) of action by the process of distribution, elicits its pharmacological action as long as the drug concentration in blood is above the minimum therapeutic level.

In case of extravascular administration of a drug in suitable dosage form, additional factors such as release of drug from dosage form and absorption of drug from the site of administration influences the concentration of drug in blood.

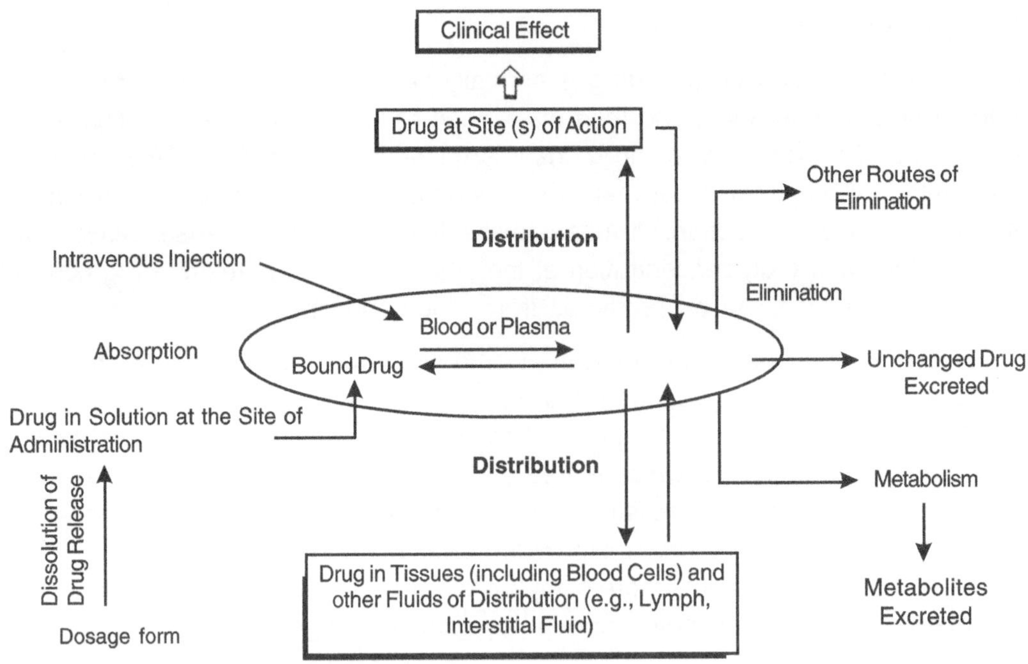

Fig. 1.1 Schematic Representation of Drug Absorption, Distribution and Elimination.

It follows that there are two aspects of drug absorption that are important in clinical practice, namely, the rate of absorption and the extent of absorption. Simply because a certain dose of a drug is being administered to a patient, there is no guarantee (except for intravenous administration) that all of that dose will reach the systemic circulation. The fraction of an administered dose of the drug that reaches the systemic circulation in unchanged form is known as **bioavailable dose**. The relative amount of an administered dose of a particular drug that reaches the systemic circulation intact and the rate at which this occurs is known as **bioavailability**. Bioavailability is thus concerned with the rate and extent at which the intact form of a particular drug appears in the systemic circulation following extravascular administration of the drug. The bioavailability exhibited by a drug is thus very important in determining whether a therapeutically effective concentration is achieved at the site(s) of action or not.

Hence, according to the definition of bioavailability, an administered dose of a particular drug in an oral dosage form will be 100% bioavailable only if the drug is completely released from the dosage form into the solution in the gastrointestinal fluids. The released drug must also be completely stable in the solution in the gastrointestinal fluids and all the drug must pass through the gastrointestinal barrier into the mesenteric circulation without being metabolized. Finally, the entire absorbed drug must pass into the systemic circulation without being metabolized on passing through liver. Thus any factor which adversely effects either the release of the drug from the dosage form, its dissolution in the gastrointestinal fluids, its stability in the gastrointestinal fluids, its permeation through and stability in the gastrointestinal barrier or its stability in the hepatic portal circulation will influence the bioavailability exhibited by that drug from the dosage form in which it was administered.

1.2 The Concept of Biopharmaceutics

Many factors have been found to influence the time course of a drug in the plasma and thereby its concentration at the site(s) of action. These include the foods eaten by the patient, the effect of the disease state on drug absorption, the age of the patient, the site(s) of absorption of the administered drug, co-administration of other drugs, the physical and chemical properties of the administered drug, the type of dosage form, the composition and method of manufacture of the dosage form and the size of dose and frequency of administration of the dosage form. Thus, a given drug may exhibit differences in its bioavailability if-

1. it is administered in the same type of dosage form by different routes, e.g., an aqueous solution of a given drug administered by the intramuscular and oral routes of administration.
2. it is given by the same route of administration but in different dosage forms, e.g., an emulsion, suspension and tablet administered by peroral route.
3. it is given by the same route of administration and in the same dosage form, but formulation and methods of manufacture of the dosage form are different, e.g. different formulations of an aqueous suspension of a given drug administered by the peroral route.

The variability by a drug in bioavailability from different formulations of the same type of dosage form or from different types of dosage forms etc., can cause the patient to be under or over medicated. The result may be a therapeutic failure or serious adverse effects, particularly in the case of drugs that have a narrow therapeutic indices.

The entry of a drug into the systemic circulation following its administration usually involves :

1. the release of the drug from its dosage form into a solution in the biological fluids at the absorption site, and
2. the movement of the dissolved drug across the biological membranes into the systemic circulation.

The study of the various factors that can affect aforesaid processes and the application of this knowledge to obtain the expected therapeutic effect from a drug product when it is used by a patient is known as *biopharmaceutics*.

2

Absorption of Drugs from Gastrointestinal Tract

2.1 Introduction

The absorption process is developed in the biological system for getting required organic and inorganic chemicals (nutrients) into the systemic circulation to maintain life. Drugs are absorbed into the systemic circulation by the same processes that are meant for the absorption of nutrients. A majority of drugs are administered orally and vast majority of orally administered drugs are intended to be absorbed from the gastrointestinal tract. The study of absorption of drugs from the GIT enables us to understand the mechanisms of absorption.

In order to understand the numerous factors that can potentially influence the rate and extent of appearance of an intact drug into the systemic circulation, a schematic illustration of the steps involved in the release and gastrointestinal absorption of a drug from tablet is presented in Fig. 2.1. It is evident from this figure that the rate and extent of appearance of the intact drug into the systemic circulation depends on a succession of rate processes.

2.2 Rate-Limiting Step in Bioavailability

The slowest step in the series of rate processes that controls the overall rate and extent of appearance of intact drug in the systemic circulation is called **the rate-limiting step**. The particular rate-limiting step may vary from drug to drug. Thus for a drug which exhibits a very poor aqueous solubility, the rate at which the drug dissolves in the gastrointestinal fluids is often the slowest step and therefore exhibits a rate-limiting effect on the drug bioavailability. In contrast, for a drug having a high aqueous solubility its dissolution rate will be rapid and the rate at which the drug crosses the gastrointestinal membrane will be the rate-limiting step.

Other potential rate-limiting steps includes

1. the rate of release of the drug from the dosage form (especially important in the case of controlled release dosage forms)
2. the rate at which the stomach empties the drug into the small intestine (gastric emptying rate)
3. the rate at which drug is metabolized by the enzymes in the intestinal mucosal cells during its passage into the mesenteric blood vessels
4. the rate of metabolism of the drug during its initial passage through the liver (e.g. first pass effect).

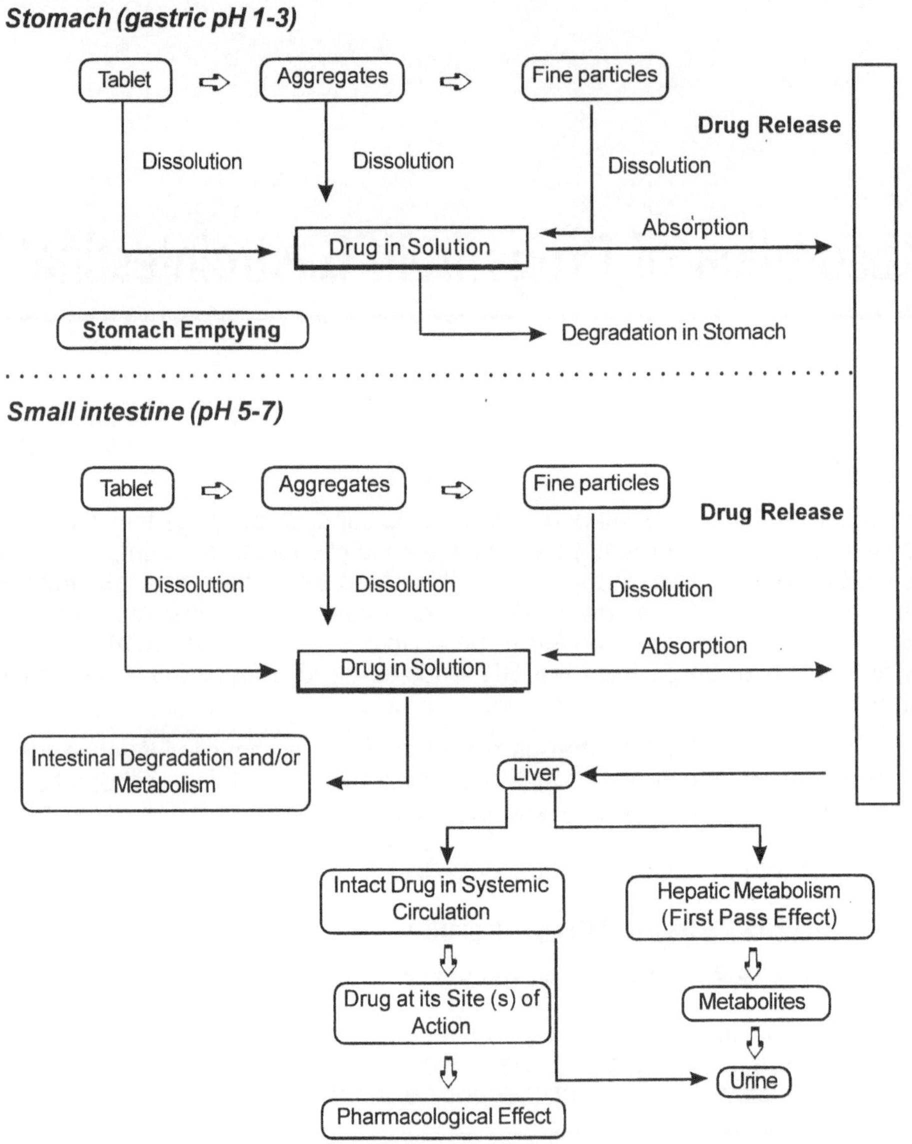

Fig. 2.1 Schematic illustration of steps involved in the appearance of an intact drug in the system circulation following peroral admistration of a tablet.

2.3 Anatomical and Physiological Considerations of the Gastrointestinal Tract (GIT)

The gastrointestinal tract (GIT) is a highly specialized region of the body whose primary functions involves the processes of secretion, digestion and absorption. Since all nutrients needed by the body, with the exception of oxygen, must first be ingested orally, processed by the GIT, and then made available for absorption into the blood stream, the GIT represents an important barrier and interface with the environment.

Fig. 2.2 illustrate the gross functional anatomy of the GIT. The liver, gallbladder, and pancreas, although not part of the gut, have been included since these organs secrete materials vital to the digestive and certain absorptive functions of the gut. The lengths of various regions of the GIT (mean values)are presented in Table 2.1. The small intestine, comprising the duodenum, jejunum and ileum, represents more than 60% of the length of the GIT, which is consistent with its primary digestive and absorptive functions. In addition to the daily food and fluid intake, the GIT and associated organs secrete about 8 liters of fluids per day. Of this total, between 100 and 200 ml of stool water is lost per day, indicating an efficient absorption of water throughout the tract.

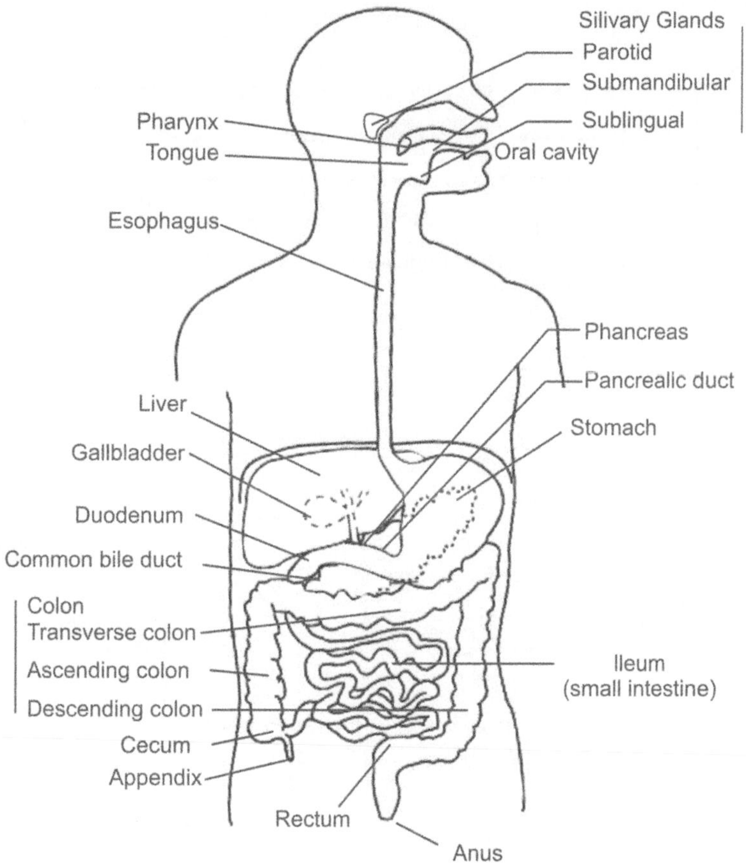

Fig. 2.2 The gross functional anatomy of the GIT.

Table 2.1 Lengths of Various Regions of the Human Gastrointestinal Tract

Region	Mean length (Cm)
Over all length	550-650
Duodenum	25-40
Jejunum	150-200
Ileum	250-300
Colon	120-160

2.3.1 Common Anatomical Features of GIT

A common anatomical feature of the entire GIT is its four concentric layers. Beginning with the luminal surface, these are the mucosa, submucosa, muscularis external and serosa (Fig. 2.3). The three outer layers are similar throughout most of the tract; however, the mucosa has distinctive structural and functional characteristics at different regions of the GIT and is most important with respect to the absorption of drugs from the lumen of the gastrointestinal tract.

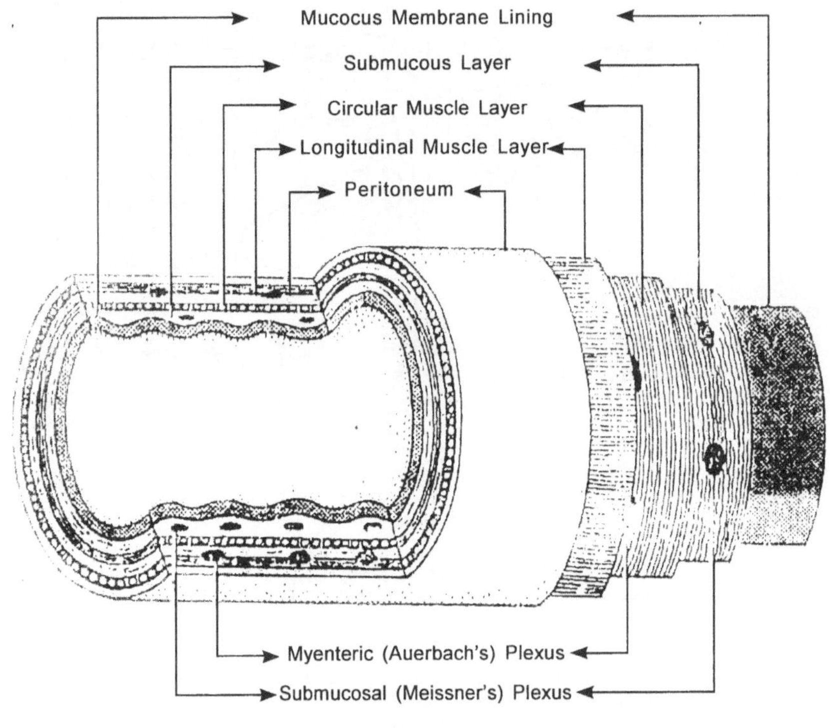

Fig. 2.3 Common Anatomical Features of the GIT.

The mucosa is the innermost layer of the gastrointestinal tract that is surrounding the lumen and is divided into

1. *Epithelium* or epithelial comprises of a single layer of columnar and some specialized secretory cells. Of these cells only the columnar cells are concerned with absorption.
2. *Lamina propia* lies between the basement membrane and the muscularis mucosa, which contains connective tissue, blood and lymph vessels that carry the absorbed materials into the general circulation.
3. *Muscularis mucosa* which is a relatively thin layer of muscle fibres. These mucosae are highly specialized in each organ of the gastrointestinal tract, facing a low pH in the stomach, absorbing a multitude of different substances in the small intestine, and also absorbing specific quantities of water in the large intestine. Reflecting the varying needs of these organs, the structure of the mucosa can consist of invaginations of secretory glands (e.g., gastric pits), or it can be folded in order to increase surface area (examples include villi and plicae circulares).

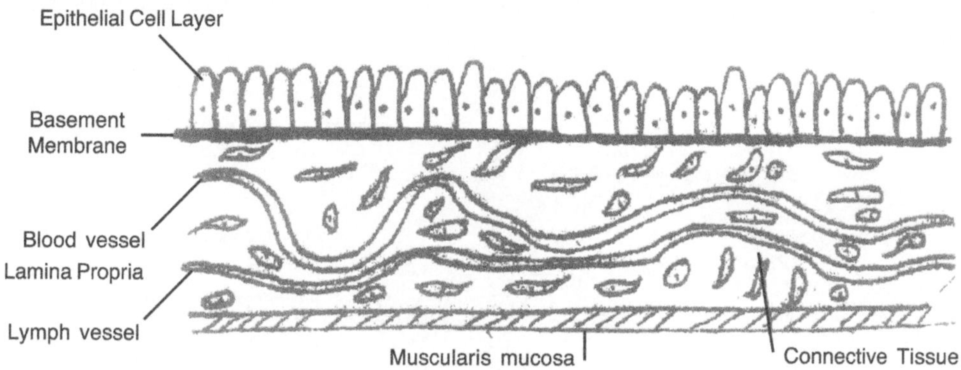

Fig. 2.4 Anatomical Details of Mucosa.

The submucosa consists of a dense irregular layer of connective tissue with large blood vessels, lymphatics and nerves branching into the mucosa and muscularis. It contains Meissner's plexus, an enteric nervous plexus, situated on the inner surface of the muscularis external.

Muscularis external consists of an inner circular layer (which prevents the food from going backwards) and a longitudinal outer muscular layer (which shortens the tract). The coordinated contractions between these layers lead to peristalsis and propels the bolus through the GI tract. Between the two muscle layers are the myenteric or Auerbach's plexus.

Adventitia consists of several layers of epithelium. When the adventitia is facing the mesentery or peritoneal fold, the adventitia is covered by a mesothelium supported by a thin connective tissue layer, together forming a serosa, or serous membrane.

2.3.2 Stomach

After oral ingestion, materials are presented to the stomach, whose primary functions are storage, mixing, and reducing all components to a slurry with the aid of gastric secretions and then emptying these contents in a controlled manner into the upper small intestine (duodenum). Complex neural, muscular and hormonal processes accomplish all of these functions.

Anatomically, the stomach has classically been divided into following parts:

1. Cardia where the contents of the esophagus empty into the stomach
2. Fundus formed by the upper curvature of the organ.
3. Corpus body the main, central region.
4. Antrum (or pyloric part), the lower section of the organ that facilitates emptying the contents into the small intestine.

Although there are no sharp distinctions among these regions, the proximal stomach, made up of the fundus and body, serves as reservoir for ingested material and the distal region (antrum) is the major site of mixing motions and acts as a pump to accomplish gastric emptying. The fundus and body regions of the stomach have relatively the little tone in their muscular wall, and as a result these regions can distend to accommodate a meal of up to 1 liter.

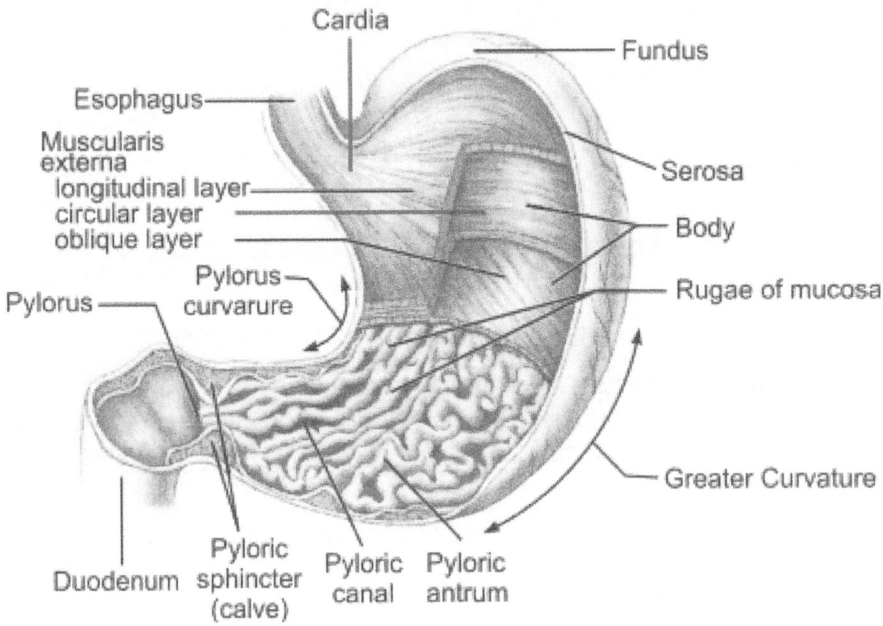

Fig. 2.5 The gross functional anatomy of the stomach.

An epithelial layer of columnar cells and the surface mucous cells line the mucosal surface of the stomach. Along this surface are many tubular invaginations, referred to as gastric pits, at the bottom of which are found specialized secretory cells. These secretory cells form part of an extensive network of gastric glands which produce and secrete about 2 liters of gastric fluid daily. Covering the epithelium cell surface is a layer of mucus 1.0

to 1.5 mm thick. This material, made up primarily of mucopolysaccharides, provides a protective lubricating coat for the cell lining.

Sub-mucosa layer lies over the mucosa and consists of fibrous connective tissue, separating the mucosa from the next layer and contain *Meissner's plexus.*

Over the sub-mucosa, the *muscularis external* is present and has three layers of smooth muscle instead of two as generally present in the other GIT part.

- ***Inner oblique layer:*** This layer is specific for stomach and not seen in other parts of the digestive system. This layer is creates the motion that churns and physically breaks down the food.
- ***Middle circular layer:*** this layer is mainly present in the pyloric region and is consisting of a thick circular muscular wall which is normally tonically constricted forming pyloric sphincter, which controls the movement of chyme into the duodenum.
- ***Outer longitudinal layer:*** Auerbach's plexus is found between this layer and the middle circular layer.

In the stomach the mucosal folds increase the total surface area over that afforded by a flat smooth lining. Although the stomach does not function primarily as an absorption organ, its excellent blood supply and the fact that a drug can potentially reside in the stomach from 30 minutes up to several hours in contact with a reasonably large epithelial surface provide conditions that are conducive to the absorption of certain drugs, e.g. weak acidic drugs.

2.3.3 Small Intestine

The small intestine, comprising the duodenum, jejunum, and ileum has a unique surface structure making it ideally suited for its primary role of digestion and absorption. The small intestine is the most important site for drug absorption in the GIT. The outstanding anatomical feature of the small intestine is tremendous large epithelial surface area through which drug absorption can take place. Fig. 2.6 shows the anatomical features that enhanced the surface area for absorption. This large epithelial surface area results from the existence of Kerkrings, Villi and Microvilli.

1. Kerkrings: These are the folds in the intestinal mucosa.
2. Villi: Villi are finger like projections which arise from the entire mucosal surface (including the folds of Kerkrings) of the small intestine. Villi range in length from 0.5 to 1.5 mm and these are estimated to be 10-40 villi per square millimeter of the intestinal mucosa. Each villus is covered by a single continuous layer of the epithelium, which is primarily made up of the columnar absorption cells and the mucus-secreting goblet cells. In terms of absorption from the small intestine, the columnar cells are extremely important, since it is the anatomical structure of the apical surface of each columnar cell (i.e. the cell surface facing the intestinal lumen), which further increases the epithelial surface area of the small intestine that is available for drug absorption.
3. Microvilli: The apical surface of each cell consists of numerous minute slender projections, approximately 1 μm long, known as microvilli. Microvilli appears to be microtubular projections of the apical cell membrane of each columnar cell. There are 700 to 1000 microvilli per columnar cell.

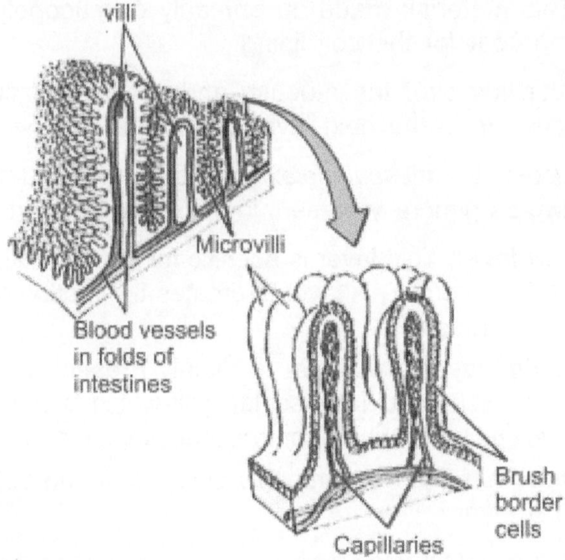

Fig. 2.6 Anatomical features of the small intestine, accounting for its large surface area.

The microvilli together with the villi and folds of Kerkrings are estimated to increase the surface area available for absorption by 600 times that which would be available if the inner surface of the small intestine was flat.

The microvilli region is also been referred to as the striated border. This is one region where the process of absorption is initiated. In close contact with the microvilli is a coating of fine filaments composed of weakly acidic sulfated mucopolysaccharides. This coating is known as the glycocalyx. In addition to the glycocalyx, there are two further layers of material between the microvilli and the luminal contents of the small intestine. They are

1. A layer of protective mucus secreted by the goblet cells
2. The so-called un-stirred aqueous layer.

Fig. 2.7. shows the absorption of a drug from the lumen of the intestine into the blood via villi which involves the passage of the drug through several barriers and regions. Thus drug molecules in the lumen of the small intestine must first diffuse through the unstirred aqueous layer, the mucus layer and the gllycocalyx in order to reach the microvilli, i.e., the apical cell membrane of the columnar cell. The apical cell membrane of each epithelial cell lining the gastrointestinal tract appears to be tightly bound to that of the adjacent epithelial cells. This so-called 'tight junction' between the cell membranes of the adjacent epithelial cells acts as a barrier to the intercellular passage of drug molecules from the intestinal lumen to the lamina propria. Thus, a drug molecule must cross the apical cell membrane into the interior of a columnar cell. After diffusing through the fluids within this cell, a drug molecule must cross the basal cell membrane of the columnar cell. On emerging from the columnar cell, the molecule must cross the underlying basement membrane into the lamina propria. Finally, after diffusing through the tissue region of the lamina propria, drug molecules must cross the endothelium of one of the blood capillaries present in this region. Drug molecules would then be carried away in the blood to the systemic circulation via the blood stream of the capillary network in the villi. However, it is possible that the absorption of highly lipid-soluble drugs, particularly if administered in an oily vehicle, may occur via fat absorption pathways. In such cases, drug removal from the villi would involve the central lacteal and the lymphatic circulation.

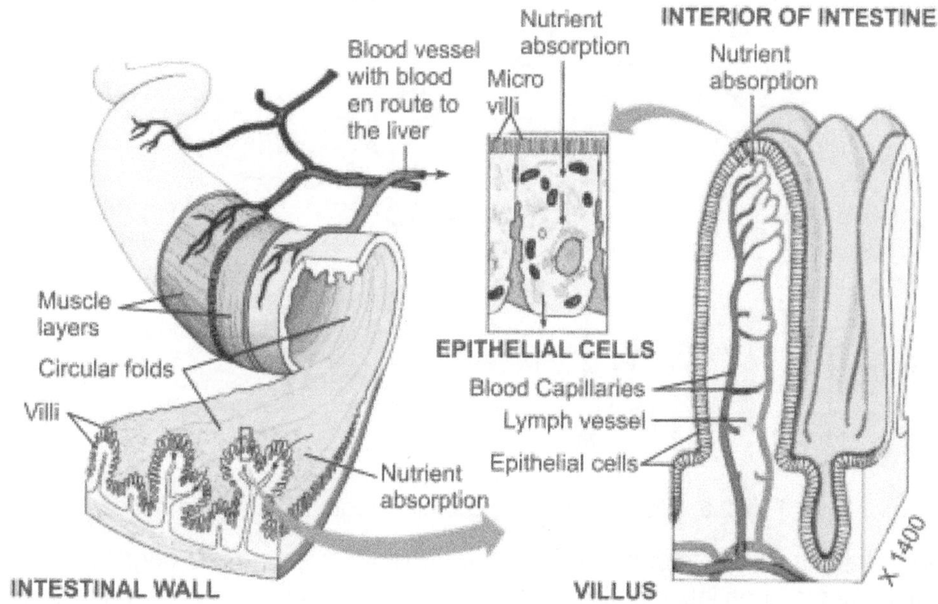

Fig. 2.7 Diagrammatic representation of Intestinal wall and pathway of drug absorption in intestinal lumen.

Although the above description of drug absorption refers specifically to the small intestine, absorption from other areas of GIT would also involve the passage of drug through similar barriers and regions.

2.3.4 Large Intestine

The large intestine, the last part of GIT, often referred to as the colon has two primary functions:

1. absorption of water and electrolytes, and
2. storage and elimination of fecal matter.

The large intestine, which has a greater diameter than the small intestine, is connected to the later at the ileocecal junction. The wall of the ileum at this point has a thickened muscular coat called the ileocecal sphincter which forms the ileocecal valve, the principal function of which is to prevent the back flow of fecal matter from the colon into the small intestine. From a functional point of view, the large intestine may be divided into two parts:

1. The proximal half, concerned primarily with absorption which includes the cecum, ascending colon, and portions of the transverse colon

2. The distal half, concerned primarily with storage and mass movement of fecal matter, which includes part of the transverse and descending colon, the rectum, and anal regions, terminating at the internal anal sphincter.

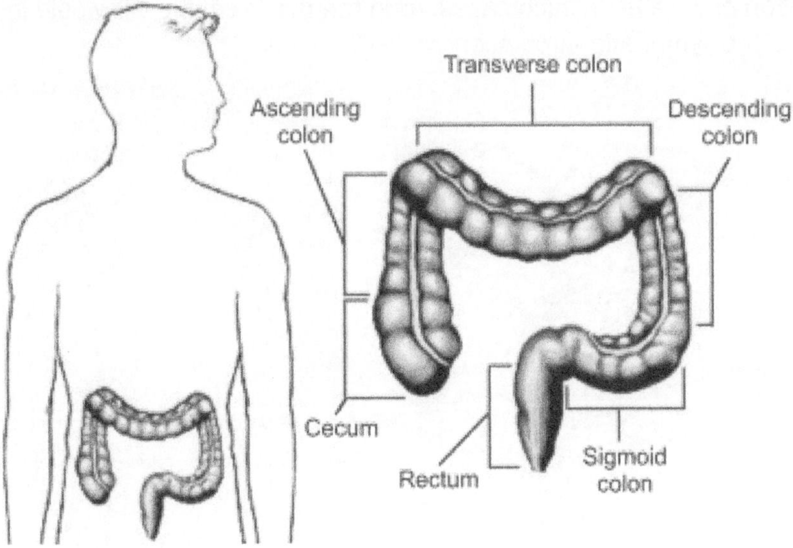

Fig. 2.8 Diagram of the anatomical region of Large intestine.

Structurally, the large intestine is similar to the small intestine, although the luminal surface epithelium of the large intestine lacks villi. The muscularis mucosa, as in the small intestine, consists of inner circular and outer longitudinal layers.

The large intestine serves as a site for the absorption of the drug that has not been completely absorbed in the more proximal regions of the GIT. i.e., the stomach and the small intestine. Incomplete drug absorption in the more proximal regions may be due to the physicochemical properties of the drug itself (e.g. very low aqueous solubility and dissolution rate) or as a result of the intended slow release of the drug from a prolonged/ sustained/controlled release dosage form. In general if a large proportion of an orally administered dose of a drug reaches the large intestine, it is likely that the drug will exhibit a poor bioavailability.

2.3.5 Nature of the Cell Membrane

A drug molecule must pass through several cell membranes, intracellular fluid, and extracellular fluid to reach the general circulation. For absorption into the cell, a drug must traverse the cell membrane. Membranes are major structures in cells, surrounding the entire cell (plasma membrane) and acting as a boundary between the cell and the interstitial fluid. In addition, membranes enclose the most of the cell organelles (e.g. the mitochondrion membrane, nuclear membrane). Functionally, membranes act as a selective barrier to the passage of molecules. Cell membranes act as **semipermeable membranes**, because water, some selected small molecules, lipid soluble molecules pass through them easily, while highly charged molecules and large molecules do not.

The transmembrane movement of drugs is influenced by the composition and structure of the cell membranes. Cell membranes are generally thin, approximately 70 to 100 A° in thickness. Cell membranes are primarily composed of phospholipids with inter-dispersed carbohydrates and integral protein groups in the form of a bilayer. Two types of proteins occur in the cell membrane, the **integral proteins** that protrude all the way through the membrane and the **peripheral proteins** that are attached only to the surface of the membrane and do not penetrate. Many of the integral proteins provide structural **channels** (or **pores**) through which water-soluble substances, especially the ions, can diffuse between the extracellular and intracellular fluids. However, these proteins have selective properties that cause preferential diffusion of some substances more than others. Some of the integral proteins act as **carrier proteins** for transporting substances against the concentration gradient, which is called an **active transport**. Still others act as **enzymes**.

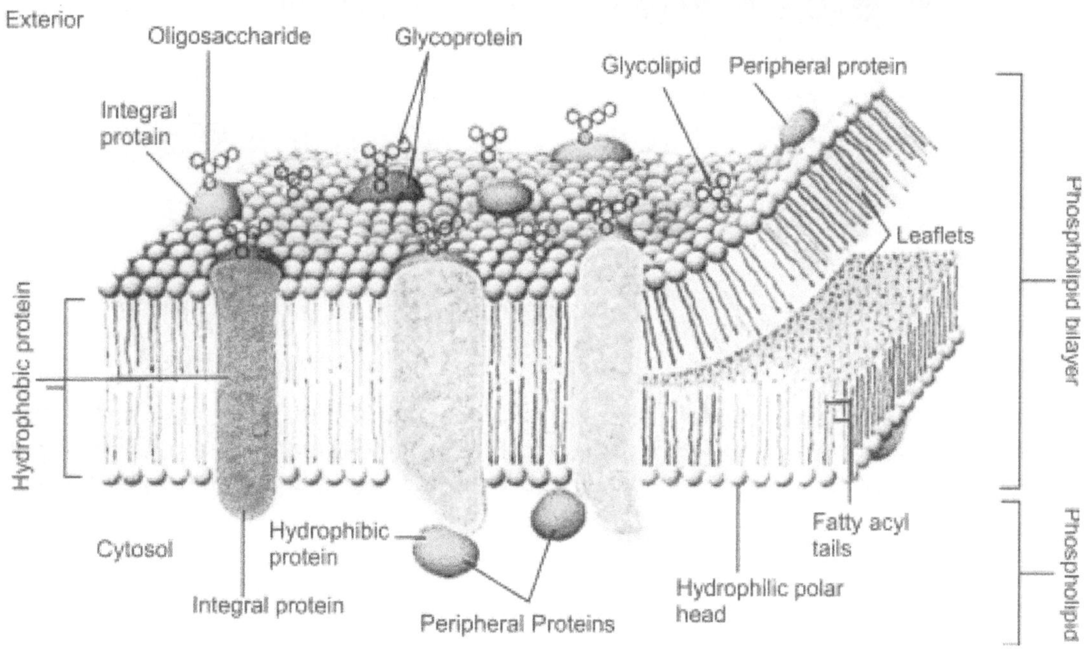

Fig. 2.9 General structure of a cell membrane.

The peripheral proteins occur either entirely or almost on the inside of the membrane, and they are normally attached to one of the integral proteins. These peripheral proteins function almost entirely as enzymes.

The membrane carbohydrates occur almost invariably in combination with proteins and lipids in the form of **glycoproteins** and **glycolipids**. In fact the most of the integral proteins are glycoproteins, and about one tenth of the lipid molecules are glycolipids. The "glyco" portion of these molecules almost invariably protrude to the out side of the cell, dangling outward from the cell surface. Many other carbohydrate compounds, called proteoglycans, which are mainly carbohydrate substances bound together by small protein cores, are often loosely attached to the outer surface of the cell as well. Thus, the entire surface of the cell often has a loose carbohydrate coat called the *glycocalyx*.

There are several theories as to the structure of the cell membrane. One **lipid bilayer or unit membrane** theory, originally proposed by Davson and Danielle, considers the cell membrane to be composed of two layers of phospholipids between the two surface layers of proteins, with the hydrophilic 'head' groups of the phospholipids facing the protein layers and the hydrophobic "tail" groups of the phospholipids aligned in the interior. The lipid bilayer theory explains the observation that lipid-soluble drugs tend to penetrate the cell membranes more easily than the polar molecules. However, the bilayer cell membrane structure does not account for the diffusion of water, low-molecular-weight molecules such as urea, and certain charged ions.

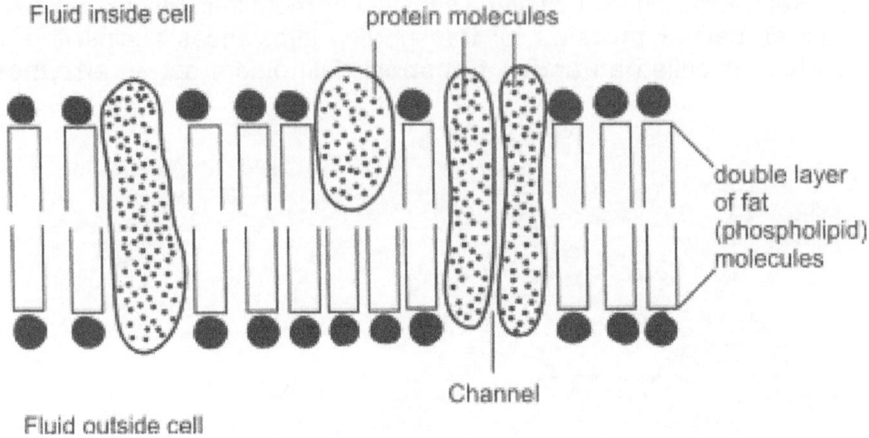

Fig. 2.10 Cell membrane according to lipid bilayer theory.

Another **fluid mosaic model**, proposed by Singer and Nicolson, explains the transcellular diffusion of polar molecules. According to this model, the cell membrane consists of globular proteins embedded in a dynamic fluid, lipid bilayer matrix (Fig 2.11). These proteins provide

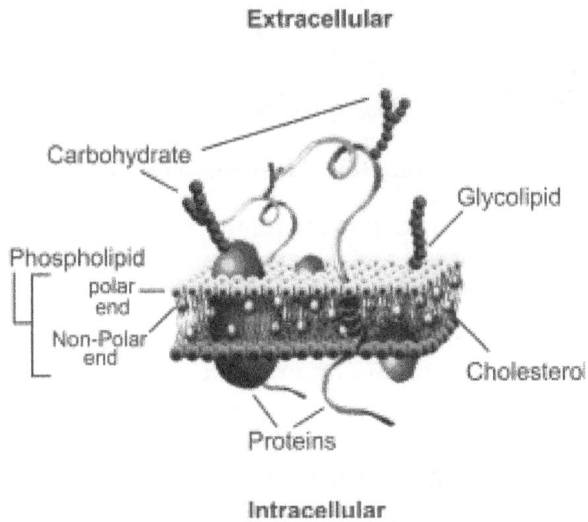

Fig. 2.11 Cell membrane according to Fluid mosaic theory.

a pathway for selective transfer of certain polar molecules and charged ions through the lipid barrier. As shown in Fig. 2.11, transmembrane proteins are inter-dispersed throughout the membrane. Two types of pores of about 10 nm and 50 to 70 nm were inferred to be present in membranes based on capillary membrane transport studies. These small pores provide a channel through which water, ions (e.g. Na^+, K^+ and Cl^-) and urea may move across the membrane. Other proteins embedded in the membrane do not cross the entire membrane. Some surface glycoproteins perform important functions as biologic or drug receptors.

2.3.6 Pathways of Drug Absorption

Once the drug is present in GI fluids in the form of a solution, it has the potential to be absorbed. Whether the drug is in absorbable form or not depends on the physicochemical properties of drug (i.e. its inherent absorbability), and on the properties of environment around it (e.g. pH, the presence of interfering materials, and the local properties of the absorbing membrane). Suppose that there are no interfering materials that affect its absorption, then the drug molecule must diffuse from GI fluids to the absorbing membrane surface. The most appropriate definition of drug absorption is the penetration of the drug across the intestinal membrane and its appearance in unchanged form in the blood draining from the GIT. Two important points should be considered about this definition:

1. It is often assumed that drug disappearance from the GI fluids represent absorption. This is true only if the disappearance from the gut represent appearance in the blood stream. This is often not the case, for example, if the drug degrades in GI fluids or if it is metabolized within the intestinal cells.
2. The term intestinal "membrane" is rather misleading since this "membrane" is not a unicellular structure but really a number of unicellular membranes parallel to one another. Thus, for a drug molecule to reach the blood it must penetrate the mucous layer and glycocalyx covering the GI lumen, the apical cell surface, the fluids within the cell, the basal membrane, the basement membrane, the tissue region of the lamina propria, the external capillary membrane, the cytoplasm of the capillary cell, and finally the inner capillary membrane.

   For a drug molecule to be absorbed from the GIT and gain access to the systemic circulation it must effectively penetrate all the regions of the intestine just cited. Once the drug is in solution, there are three important factors that govern the process of absorption:

   1. The physicochemical properties of the drug molecule,
   2. The properties and components of the GI fluids, and
   3. The nature of the absorbing membrane.

   These points are discussed in detail in the following sections. Let us assume that the drug molecule has penetrated most of the barriers in the intestine and has reached the lamina propria region. Once the drug molecule is in this region, it may either diffuse through the blood stream or penetrate the central lacteal and reach the lymph. Fig. 2.9. depicts the organization of blood capillaries and lymph vessels in the villi. Most drugs, if not all, reach the systemic circulation via the blood stream of the capillary network in the villi.

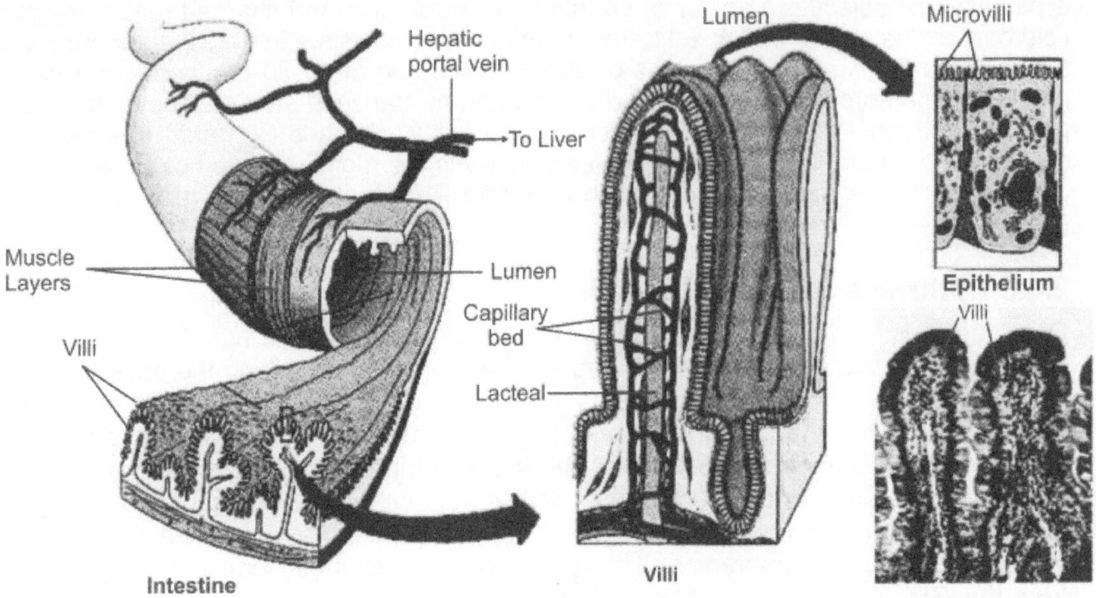

Fig. 2.12 (A) A magnified view of Villi in Small Intestine.

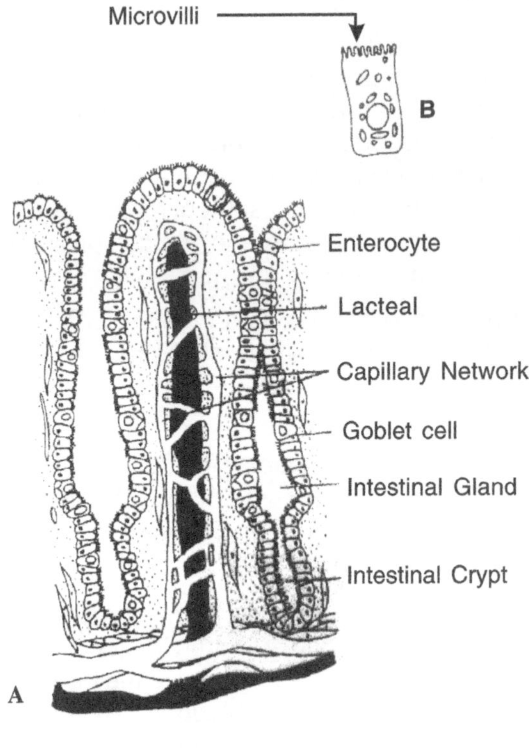

Fig. 2.12 (B) Enterocyte showing micro villi.

The reason for this dominance over lymphatic route is because of the fact that the villi are highly and rapidly perfused by the blood stream. The blood flow rate to the GIT in humans is approximately 500 to 1000 times greater than lymph flow. Thus, although the lymphatic system is a potential route for drug removal from the intestine, it will account for only a small fraction of the total amount of drug absorbed. Although the capillary and lymphatic vessels are rather permeable to most low-molecular-weight and lipid-soluble compounds, the capillary membrane represents a more substantial barrier than the central lacteal to the penetration of a very large molecule or a combination of molecules. Therefore, triglycerides are transported in the form of chylomicron (about 0.5 um in diameter) by the lymphatic route into the systemic circulation.

2.4 Mechanisms of Drug Absorption

It is apparent from the pathways of drug transport that absorption of a drug from the lumen of the GIT into blood involves the passage of drug molecules across several cellular membranes and fluid regions within the mucosa, i.e. the gastrointestinal/blood barrier. The epithelium lining the GIT is considered to constitute the main cellular barrier to the absorption of drugs from the GIT. The drug molecules in GI fluids must cross the unstirred aqueous layer, mucus layer and glycocalyx to reach the apical cell membrane. The passage of drug molecules through this membrane is achieved by several mechanisms. They are

- Passive Diffusion
- Active Transport or Carrier Mediated Transport
- Facilitated Diffusion
- Ion-Pair Formation
- Convective Transport or Pore Transport
- Vesicular Transport or Pinocytosis

2.4.1 Passive Diffusion

In this process the apical cell membrane of a columnar absorption cell plays a passive role and does not participate actively in the transport process. The rate of drug transport is determined by

1. The physicochemical properties of the drug
2. The nature of the membrane and the concentration gradient of the drug across the membrane. The process of passive diffusion initially involves partition of a drug between the aqueous fluid in the GIT
3. The lipoidal-like cell membrane of the lining epithelium.

The drug in solution in the membrane then diffuses across the membrane followed by a second partition of drug between the membrane and the aqueous fluids within the columnar absorption cells. The drug would cross the other cell membranes in the gastrointestinal/blood barrier by this sequence of steps and thus would eventually enter the blood of the capillary network in the lamina propria.

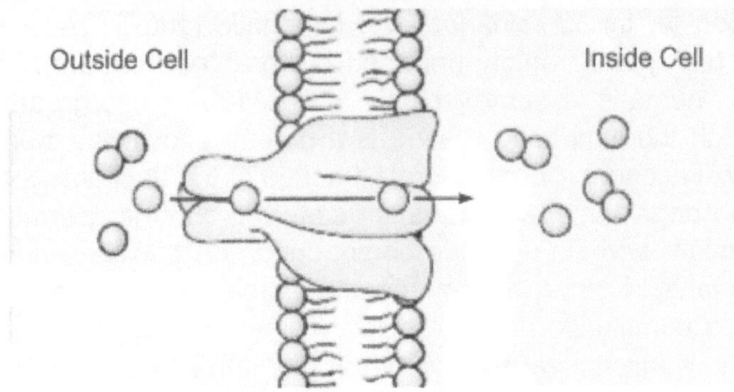

Fig. 2.13 Passive diffusion.

If we consider that the cell membranes and fluid regions making up the gastrointestinal/ blood barrier could be represented by a single 'membrane', then the stages involved in the gastrointestinal absorption of a drug by passive diffusion could be represented by the simple model shown in Fig 2.14.

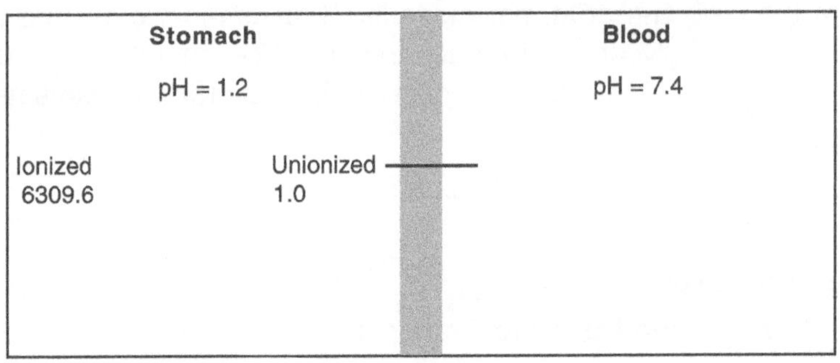

Fig. 2.14 Schematic representation of the equilibrium distribution of aminopyrine (pKa 5.0) between the stomach and the blood.

A passive diffusion is the process by which molecules spontaneously diffuse from a region of higher concentration to a region of lower concentration. This process is passive because no external energy is expended. In Fig. 2.14, drug molecules move forward and back across a membrane. If the two sides have the same drug concentration, forward-moving molecules will be balanced by molecules moving back, resulting in no net transfer of the drug. When the left side is higher in concentration, at any given time, the number of forward-moving drug molecules will be higher than the number of backward-moving molecules and the net result would be a transfer of molecules to the right side, as indicated by the solid arrow.

Passive diffusion of drugs across the gastrointestinal/blood barrier can often be described mathematically by **Fick's law of diffusion**. Accordingly the rate of appearance of a drug in the blood, i.e. rate of absorption of the drug is given by,

$$dx/dt = \frac{DA}{h} (K_1 \, Cg - K_2 \, Cb) \qquad .....(2.1)$$

Where:

dx/dt = the rate of appearance of drug in the blood at the site of absorption

D = the effective diffusion coefficient of the drug in the gastrointestinal 'membrane'

A = the surface area of the gastrointestinal 'membrane' available for absorption by passive diffusion

K_1 = the apparent partition coefficient of the drug between the gastrointestinal 'membrane' and the GI fluids

Cg = the concentration of drug in solution in the GI fluids at the site of absorption

K_2 = the apparent partition coefficient of the drug between the gastrointestinal 'membrane' and the blood

Cb = the concentration of the drug in the blood at the site absorption

h = the thickness of the gastrointestinal 'membrane'

According to equation 2.1, the rate of drug absorption is directly proportional to the diffusion coefficient (D), the surface area available for absorption (A), the concentration gradient (K_1 Cg - K_2 Cb) and inversely proportional to the thickness of the gastrointestinal membrane (h). In order to be absorbed from the GIT by passive diffusion, a drug molecule should have sufficient solubility in the GI membrane and then it should exhibit sufficient solubility for the blood such that it can partition readily out of the 'membrane' phase into the blood. Drug on entering the blood in the capillary network in the lamina propria will be carried away from the site of absorption by the rapidly circulating gastrointestinal blood supply and will become diluted by:

1. distribution in a large volume of blood, i.e. the systemic circulation,
2. distribution into body tissue and other fluids of distribution, and
3. by metabolism and excretion.

In addition, the protein in the blood may bind the drug molecules and there by lower the concentration of 'free' (diffusable) drug in the blood. Consequently, the blood acts as a 'sink' for the absorbed drug and ensures that the concentration of the drug in the blood at the site of absorption is low in relation to the concentration of drug in solution at the absorption site, i.e. Cg >> Cb. The 'sink' conditions provided by the systemic circulation ensures that a large concentration gradient is maintained across the gastrointestinal 'membrane' during the absorption process. The passive absorption process is driven solely by the concentration gradient of the diffusable species of the drug which exists across the gastrointestinal/blood barrier. Under such conditions K_1 Cg >> K_2 Cb and thus (K_1 Cg - K_2 Cb) approximates to K_1 Cg, and equation 2.1 may be written in the form given below:

$$dx/dt = \frac{DA}{h}(K_1\ Cg) \qquad .....(2.2)$$

For a given drug and 'membrane' under specified conditions, D, A, K_1 and h may be regarded as constants which can be incorporated into a combined constant known as the permeability constant, P. Hence, equation 2.2 becomes the following.

$$dx/dt = P\ Cg \qquad ....(2.3)$$

Where

$$P = \frac{DA}{h} K_1 \qquad .....(2.4)$$

Equation 2.3 is an expression for a first order kinetic process and indicates that the rate of passive drug absorption will be proportional to the concentration of the absorbable drug in solution in the GI fluids at the site of absorption.

It is assumed that the drug in aqueous solution on each side of the gastrointestinal/blood barrier (Fig. 2.10) exists entirely in the form of a single absorbable species which exhibited definite partition coefficients for distribution between:

1. the aqueous GI fluids and the lipid 'membrane', and
2. the blood and the lipid 'membrane'.

However, many drugs have both lipophilic and hydrophilic chemical substituents. Those drugs that are more lipid-soluble tend to traverse the cell membranes more easily than less lipid-soluble or more water-soluble molecules. For drugs that act as weak electrolytes, such as weak acids and bases, the extent of ionization influences the rate of drug transport. The ionized species of the drug contains a charge and is more water-soluble than the unionized species of the drug, which is more lipid-soluble. The extent of ionization of a weak electrolyte will depend on both the dissociation constant of the drug (i.e. its pKa value) and the pH of the medium in which the drug is dissolved. Thus, the rate of passive absorption of a weak electrolyte drug is related to the fraction of the total drug that exists in the unionized form in solution in the GI fluids at the site of absorption. This fraction is determined by the pKa of drug and the pH of its aqueous environment in accordance with the **Henderson-Hasselbalch** equation for weak acids and bases. The influence of pH of the GI fluids on the absorption of drug molecules from the GIT form the basis of the pH-partition hypothesis.

2.4.2 Active Transport or Carrier Mediated Transport

Most drugs are absorbed from the gastrointestinal tract by passive diffusion. However, a few lipid-insoluble drugs (such as 5-fluorouracil) and many substances of nutritional interest are absorbed by an active transport mechanism. In contrast to passive diffusion, active transport involves active participation by the apical cell membrane of the columnar absorption cell (and presumably also by the membranes consisting the gastrointestinal/blood barrier) in the gastrointestinal absorption of a drug.

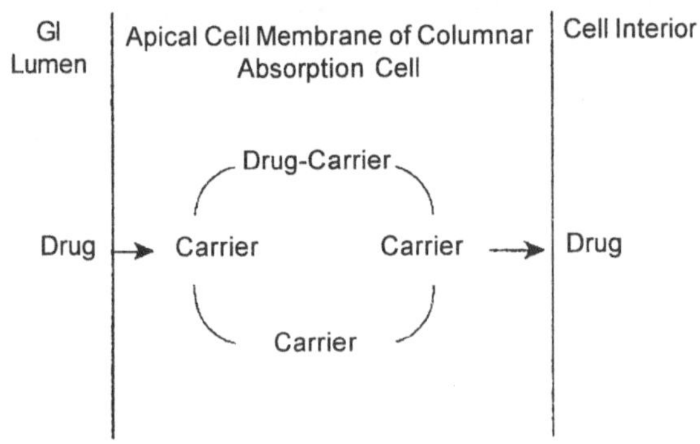

Fig. 2.15 Active transport of a drug across a cell membrane.

A 'carrier' which may be an enzyme or some other component of the cell membrane is responsible for the active transport of nutrients and drugs. The carrier-mediated transport system is basically developed for the absorption of nutrients or other chemicals, which are required for the maintenance of life of the living systems. However, a drug molecule, which structurally resembles a natural substrate that is actively transported is likely to be actively transported by the same carrier mechanism.

Fig. 2.16 An example of this type of active transport is the sodium-potassium pump (Figure 5-15 in your textbook), which consists of a membrane protein that uses ATP to pump Na^+ (sodium) out of the cell and K^+ (potassium) into the cell. These unbalanced accumulations of Na^+ and K^+ are needed for proper nerve functioning. The carrier (now free) returns to its initial position in the surface of the cell membrane. It is now ready to transport another molecule or ion.

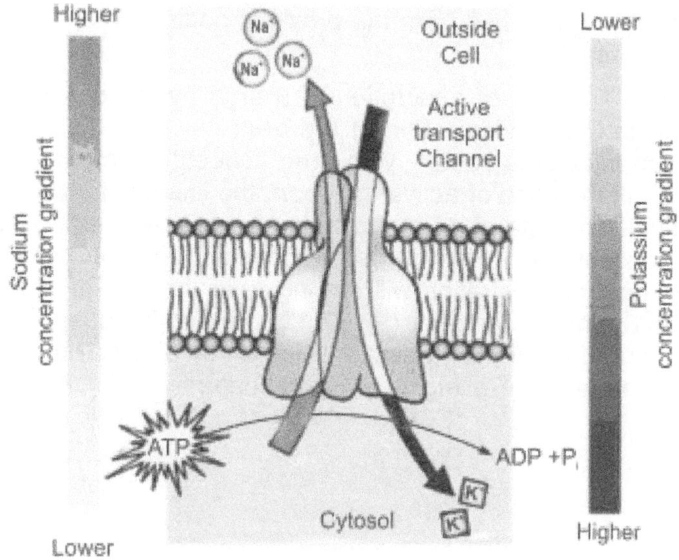

Fig. 2.16 Active transport by Sodium Potassium Pump.

Many nutrients such as sugars and amino acids are transported across the gastrointestinal 'membrane' by an active transport process. Vitamins such as thiamine, nicotinic acid, riboflavin and pyridoxine require an active transport system. The anticancer drug 5-fluorouracil, methyldopa and nicotinamide are absorbed by active transport. Active transport also plays an important role in the renal and biliary secretion of many drugs and metabolites.

The characteristic features of the active transport or carrier-mediated transport are:

1. **Transportation against concentration gradient :** An active transport is characterized by the transport of the drug against a concentration gradient- that is, from the regions of low concentrations to the regions of high concentrations. Therefore an active transport is an *energy consuming* absorption process. In the case of the gastrointestinal absorption of drugs, drug transport occurs from the GIT to the blood and the concentration of drug in GI fluids is always higher than that of blood. The carrier system is generally a 'one-way' transport system. However, in the case of nutrients, the concentration of some nutrient in GI fluids is less than that of blood. The active transport of nutrients is against the concentration gradient.

2. **Selectivity :** There appears to be several carrier-mediated active transport systems in the small intestine. Each carrier system is highly selective with respect to the chemical structure of the substances whom it transports. Thus if a drug structurally resembles a natural substrate which is actively transported then that drug is likely to be transported by the same carrier mechanism. The drug levodopa shows structural similarity with the amino acids tyrosine and phenylalanine. Therefore levodopa is transported by that carrier system which transport the amino acids, tyrosine and phenylalanine.
3. **Specific Location in GIT :** Each carrier system is generally concentrated in a specific segment of the GIT. The substance which is transported by that carrier will thus be absorbed preferentially in the location of the highest carrier density. For example, more riboflavin is absorbed from the proximal portion of the small intestine than the other part of intestine.
4. **Saturability :** The rate of absorption of a drug by the passive diffusion is directly proportional to the concentration of the drug in the GI fluids. Therefore, the rate of absorption increases linearly with drug concentration in the GI fluids as shown in Fig. 2.12. In the case of active transport, the linearity between drug concentration in the GI fluids and rate of drug absorption is observed at a low drug concentration. At higher concentrations, the carrier mechanism becomes saturated and a further increase in drug concentration will not increase the rate of absorption, i.e. the rate of absorption remains constant (Fig. 2.12). This is because of the fact that only a certain amount of carrier is available in the surface of cell membrane which will be completely saturated at a higher drug concentration.

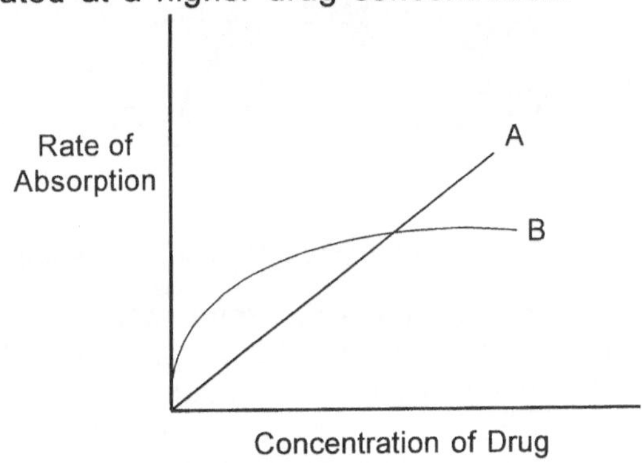

Fig. 2.17 Relation between drug concentration at the absorption site and rate of absorption by passive diffusion (line A) and active transport (curve B).

5. **Competitive Inhibition :** Each carrier-mediated system is specific for a chemical structure. Drugs of similar structure may compete for binding sites on the carrier. Therefore, competitive inhibition of absorption of a drug by other drug or nutrient which have a structural similarity, is observed.

2.4.2.1 Rate of Absorption in Carrier-Mediated Transport

The number of apparent carriers in the intestinal membrane is limited. Therefore, the rate of carrier-mediated transport must be described by **Michaelis-Menten equation**.

$$\text{Absorption rate} = \frac{V_{max}\,Cg}{Km + Cg} \qquad .....(2.5)$$

Where Cg is the drug concentration at the absorption site, Vmax is the maximum velocity of the absorption process and is a constant for a given drug. Km is called Michaelis-Menten constant. At a low drug concentration, such that Km >> Cg,

$$\text{Absorption rate} = \frac{V_{max}\,Cg}{Km} \qquad .....(2.6)$$

Therefore, under these conditions absorption process follows the first-order kinetics and a linear relationship is observed between drug concentration and rate of drug absorption. As the concentration of drug molecules increases, the linearity between the drug concentration and rate of absorption diminishes. When Cg >> Km,

$$\text{Absorption rate} = \frac{V_{max}\,Cg}{Cg} \qquad .....(2.7)$$

It means that the active transport system is saturated and a constant absorption rate is observed beyond a certain drug concentration (Fig. 2.12).

2.4.3 Facilitated Diffusion

Facilitated diffusion is also a carrier -mediated transport system. I.e. a carrier molecule is involved in the transport. The difference between an active transport and facilitated diffusion is that the active transport can transport drug molecules against a concentration gradient, while the facilitated diffusion can not transport drug molecules against a concentration gradient. Therefore, facilitated diffusion does not require an energy input. The drug molecules move along with the concentration gradient which is the driving force in this process. However, because facilitated diffusion is carrier -mediated, it shows all other characters of an active transport such as structure selectivity, saturability, competitive inhibition by the structurally related compounds, and a specific location in GIT. In terms of drug absorption, a facilitated diffusion seems to play a very minor role.

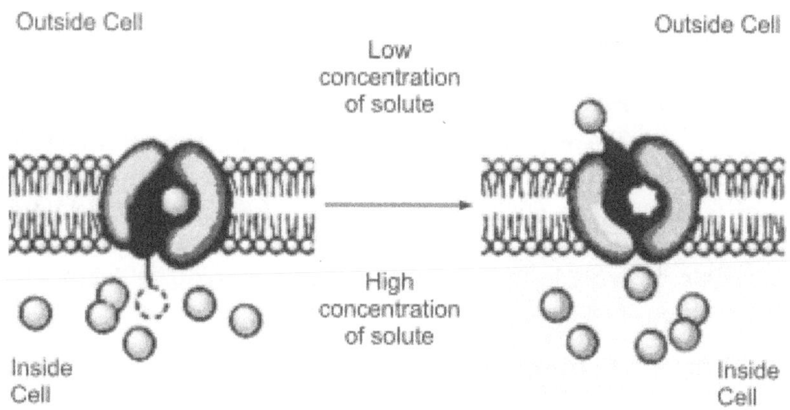

Fig. 2.18 Facilitated Diffusion.

2.4.4 Ion-Pair Formation

Strong electrolyte drugs such as quaternary ammonium compounds and tetracyclines are ionized over the entire gastrointestinal pH. Therefore, the ionized form of the drug can not partition directly into the lipoidal cell membrane. Further, the size of these ionized forms is too large to pass through the aqueous filled pores or channels that exist in the cell membrane. However, the interaction of such drug ions with the oppositely charged endogenous organic ions leads to the formation of an ion pair whose overall charge is neutral. This neutral complex (i.e. ion-pair) diffuses more easily across the lipoidal cell membrane due to its lipid solubility. The drugs propranolol and quinine show a good absorption when paired with oleic acid and hexylsalicylate, respectively.

2.4.5 Convective Transport or Pore Transport

Very small molecules such as water, urea and low molecular weight sugars and organic electrolytes are able to cross the cell membranes rapidly as if there is no barrier for their passage. This observation is explained with the help of the aqueous filled pores or channels assumed to be present in a cell membrane. The effective radius of these channels has been estimated to be of the order of 0.4 nm. As a result of molecular size limitations, this mechanism of absorption appears to be of minor importance with respect to the gastrointestinal absorption of large water-soluble drug molecules or ions. However, convective absorption is involved in the renal excretion of drugs and the uptake of drugs into the liver.

2.4.6 Vesicular Transport or Pinocytosis

Pinocytosis or vesicular transport is the process of engulfing particles or dissolved materials by the cell. The mechanism is comparable to phagocytosis and involves invagination of the material by the apical cell membrane of the columnar absorption cells lining the gastrointestinal tract to form vacuoles containing the material. These vacuoles then cross the columnar absorption cells. This mechanism of the absorption process appears to be of little importance for drugs but is important for the absorption of macromolecules such as proteins. Vesicular transport is the proposed process for the absorption of orally administered Sabin Polio Vaccine and various large proteins.

2.5 Factors Governing Gastrointestinal Drug Absorption

2.5.1 Physiological Factors

A drug must be in a solution before it can be absorbed from the GIT. The rate of drug release/dissolution can under certain conditions be the rate-controlling step in the appearance of a drug in the systemic circulation. Therefore, physiological factors that influence the drug release and dissolution from the dosage form are also considered wherever applicable. In order to understand various physiological factors that can influence the absorption of drug, it is assumed that the drug is in solution in appropriate GI fluids.

2.5.1.1 Site of Absorption and Surface Area Available for Absorption

The biological environments and the areas of membrane available for absorption in the stomach, the small intestine and the large intestine are quite different and these differences give rise to variations in the rate and extent of absorption of a drug from these anatomical regions.

The presence of folds in the mucosa, villi and microvilli are responsible for the small intestine having the largest effective surface area available for absorption. Consequently, the small intestine is the region of maximum absorption for a majority of drugs, even though the pH of the intestinal fluid does not provide optimum conditions for the absorption of certain drugs, e.g., weak acidic drugs. In addition to its large absorptive surface area, the small intestine is the most important region for carrier-mediated drug absorption, i.e. the small intestine is the location of the highest 'carrier' density.

In contrast to the small intestine, the absorptive surface areas of the stomach and the large intestine are relatively small, since neither of these regions possesses villi or microvilli. Despite the relatively small absorptive surface area available in the stomach, certain drugs (e.g. weak acidic drugs in solution which are in a unionized form) are absorbed in this region. It should be noted that following oral administration of a drug in solution a major part of the stomach's absorptive area will be immediately in contact with the dissolved drug and, provided that the intrinsic physicochemical properties of the drug allow permeation of the gastrointestinal/ blood barrier, a good absorption may occur. However, because the absorptive surface area in the stomach is so small compared to that in the small intestine, the rate and the extent of absorption of a given drug from the stomach will, in most cases, be less than from that of the small intestine. The large intestine functions as an absorptive site for drugs that are so slowly absorbed that a significant portion of the administered dose passes through the stomach and small intestine unabsorbed. In addition, the large intestine is important for the absorption of some drugs such as sulphasalazine, which must be degraded by the bacterial flora in this region before absorption can occur.

2.5.1.2 Components and Properties of GI Fluids

The characteristics of the aqueous GI fluid to which a drug product is exposed will exert an important influence on what happens to that dosage form in the GIT and on the pattern of absorption.

One important property of GI fluids is pH, which varies considerably along the length of the tract. There is a considerable **intersubject variation** in gastrointestinal pH depending upon such factors as:

1. General health of the individual,
2. Presence of localized disease conditions (e.g. gastric and duodenal ulcers) along the GIT,
3. Types and amount of food ingested, and
4. Drug therapy.

In the case of drug therapy, anticholinergic drugs inhibit or reduce gastric secretion and the oral administration of antacids usually elevates gastric pH for a short period of time.

The gastric fluids are highly acidic, usually ranging from pH 1 to 3.5. There appears to be a diurnal cycle of gastric acidity, the fluids being more acidic at night and fluctuating during the day, primarily in response to food ingestion. The gastric fluid pH generally increases when food is ingested and then slowly decreases over the next several hours.

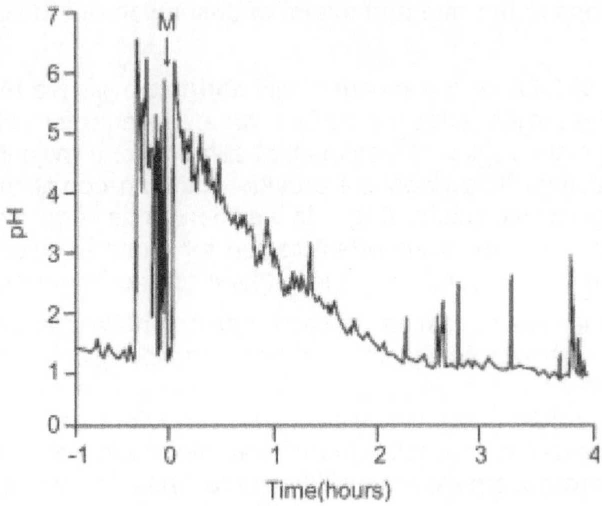

Fig. 2.19 Typical pH profile in the stomach Meal admnistration is indicated by the letter M.

An abrupt change in pH is encountered when moving from the stomach to the small intestine. Pancreatic secretions have a high concentration of bicarbonate, which neutralizes gastric fluid entering the duodenum and thus helps to regulate the pH of fluids in the upper intestinal region. Neutralization of gastric fluids in the duodenum is important to avoid damage to the intestinal epithelium, prevent inactivation of pancreatic enzymes, and prevent precipitation of bile acids, which are poorly soluble in acid pH. The pH of intestinal fluids gradually increases when moving in the distal direction, ranging from 5.7 in the pylorus to 7.7 in the proximal jejunum. The fluid in the large intestine is generally considered to have a pH of about 8.

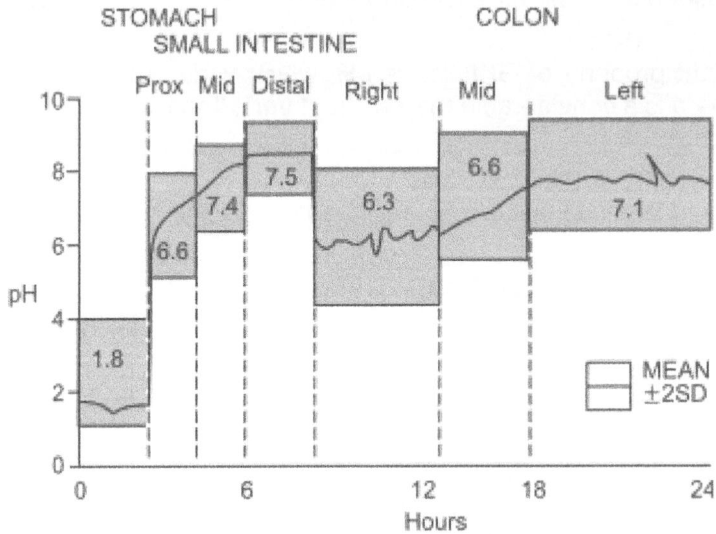

Fig. 2.20 Range of gastrointestinal pH profiles along the GI tract in normal subjects.

pH in the small intestine in healthy humans in the fasted and fed state		
Site	**Average pH, asted state**	**Average pH, fed state**
mid-distal	4.9	5.2
Duodenum	6.1	5.4
	6.3	5.1
Jejunum	4.4 - 6.5	5.2 - 6.0
	6.6	6.2
Ileum	6.5	6.8 - 7.8
	6.8 - 8.0 (range)	6.8 - 8.0
	7.4	7.5

The rate of dissolution of a drug from a dosage form depends on the solubility of the drug in GI fluids. GI fluid pH decides the solubility of the drug since most of the drugs are either weak acids or bases. Weak acidic drugs dissolve most readily in alkaline media, and therefore will have a greater rate of dissolution in the intestinal fluids compared to gastric fluids. Basic drugs will dissolve most readily in acidic solutions, and thus the dissolution rate will be greater in gastric fluids compared to the intestinal fluids.

Since dissolution is a prerequisite step to absorption and is often the rate-limiting step, especially for poorly water soluble drugs, pH will exert a major influence on the overall absorption process. Since the major site of drug absorption is the small intestine, it would be seem that poorly soluble basic drugs must first dissolve in the acidic gastric fluids in order to be well absorbed from the intestine, as the dissolution rate in the intestinal fluid will be low.

Another way by which the gastrointestinal pH can influence drug absorption is in the case of drugs that exhibit a limited chemical stability in either acidic **(e.g.. *Proton pump inhibitors*)** or alkaline environments. Since the rate and extent of degradation is directly dependent on the concentration of drug in solution, an attempt is often made to retard dissolution in the fluid where degradation is observed. There are preparations of various salts or esters of drugs (e.g. erythromycin) that do not dissolve in a gastric fluid and thus are not degraded but dissolve in the intestinal fluid prior to absorption.

Gastrointestinal pH may influence the absorption of drugs by influencing the degree of ionization of drugs in the GI fluids. In general the unionized form of a drug in solution will be absorbed faster than the ionized form of the drug at any particular site along the GIT. This effect of the gastrointestinal pH on drug absorption is discussed under pH-Partition hypothesis.

In addition to the pH considerations, the GI fluids contain various materials which have been shown to influence absorption, particularly bile salts, enzymes, and mucin. Bile salts, which are highly surface active may enhance the rate and/or the extent of absorption of poorly water soluble drugs by increasing the rate of dissolution in the GI fluids (e.g. griseofulvin). Bile salts may also reduce drug absorption (e.g. neomycin and kanamycin) through the formation of water-insoluble and non-absorbable complexes. Since the intestinal fluids contain large concentrations of various enzymes needed for digestion of food, it is reasonable to expect certain of these enzymes to act on a number of drugs. Pancreatic enzymes hydrolyze chloremphenicol palmitate. Pancreatin and trypsin are able to deacetylate N-acetylated drugs and mucosal esterases appear to attack various esters of penicillin. **Mucin** a viscous mucopolysaccharide that lines and protects the intestinal epithelium, has been thought to bind certain drugs non-specifically (e.g. quaternary ammonium compounds) and thereby prevent or reduce absorption. This behavior may particularly account for the erratic and incomplete absorption of these charged compounds. Mucin may also represent a barrier to drug diffusion prior to reaching the intestinal membrane.

2.5.1.3 Gastric Emptying

Since most drugs are best absorbed from the small intestine, any factor that tends to delay movement of a drug from the stomach to the small intestine will influence the rate (and probably the extent) of absorption and therefore the time needed to achieve maximal plasma concentrations and pharmacological response. The effectiveness by which drugs can be delivered through the gastrointestinal tract is influenced by a number of key physiological variables including

(a) Transit time of preparations through each of the major intestinal segments

(b) The reciprocal of transit, the residence time of delivery systems in the various gut segments

(c) influences acting on the delivery system in each compartment, including physical disintegration, intraluminal digestion, mucosal uptake, biotransformation and absorption.

As a result, gastric emptying may represent a limiting factor in drug absorption in addition to rate of dissolution or inherent absorbability of drug. Gastric emptying is quantified by one of several measurements, including emptying time, emptying half-time ($t_{50\%}$), and emptying rate.

Emptying time is the time required for the stomach to empty the total initial stomach contents. **Emptying half-time** is the time it takes for the stomach to empty one-half of its initial contents. **Emptying rate** is a measure of the speed of emptying. Emptying time and emptying rate are inversely related.

Gastric emptying appears to be an exponential process. Standard low bulk meals and liquids are transferred from the stomach into the duodenum in an apparent first order rate process, i.e. the rate of gastric emptying is proportional to the volume of the material remaining in the stomach. As a result, plots of log volumes remaining in the stomach versus time will provide a straight-line relationship. This relationship is not strictly linear at early and later times of stomach emptying process. A linear relationship between the square root of the volume remaining in the stomach versus time has been observed.

The relationships between gastrointestinal physiology and drug delivery will be addressed under the following subheadings

(a) Esophageal transit: Human oesophagus is around 25 cm in length and to move 10 ml liquid bolus from the mouth to the stomach takes less than 15 seconds, even when the individual is supine but may take even upto a minute in case of impaired oesophageal peristalsis, as occurs in many elderly patient. Solids move much more slowly along the oesophagus than do liquids, and abnormal transit of solid medications in the oesophagus has important clinical implications as several medications are well known to produce mucosal injury when they lodge in the oesophagus

(b) Gastric emptying: Gastric emptying plays a very important role in determining the amount of drug absorbed. Proper appreciation of the role that gastric emptying plays in the delivery of drugs requires an understanding of gastrointestinal motor function during fasting and after meals.

Stomach motility under fasting or interdigestive state:

In healthy humans, the contractile movements of the gastrointestinal tract during fasting are known to comprise phase I (silent state, no contraction), phase II (random, irregular contraction), and phase III (frequent, regular contraction). Among these stages, phase III has been termed as the **Interdigestive migrating motor complex** (IMMC). It is made up of a group of contractile waves that migrate from the proximal to the distal part of GIT successively over a constant period, characterized by an interval of 100 to 150 minutes during fasting in normal subjects.

Fasted Pattern of Motility: The motility pattern (i.e. inter digestive myoelectric cycle or migrating myoelectric complex (MMC) of the stomach has four different phases (Fig 2.21). Each phase lasts for a different period of time and possesses different contraction strength. The following is a schematic representation of four contraction phases.

- **Phase I** (basal state) is a period without any motor activity, except for occasional contractions and lasts for 40-60 min with rare contractions.
- **Phase II** (pre burst state) lasts for a similar period of time with increasing contraction strength and frequency (up to 40 millimeter Hg) with intermittent action potential and contractions. As the phase progresses the intensity and frequency also increases gradually.
- **Phase III** (burst state) lasts for 4-6 min with the highest contraction strength (up to 80 millimeter Hg), which is necessary to empty large indigestible particles (e.g., en enteric-coated tablet) from the stomach. It includes intense and regular contractions for short period. It is also known as the housekeeper wave. It is this Phase 3 contraction that empties digest food and deliver chyme to the intestine for indigestible solids from the stomach.
- **Phase IV** is a transition period between phase III and phase I, typically last for 15-30 min. The whole cycle is repeated approximately every 2 hours until a formal meal time.

During fasting condition, the gastric emptying of solutions and suspensions of fine drug particles (liquids especially those that are close to isotonicity =280 mOsm/kg) is generally much faster and less variable than that of solid dosage forms, including larger granules.

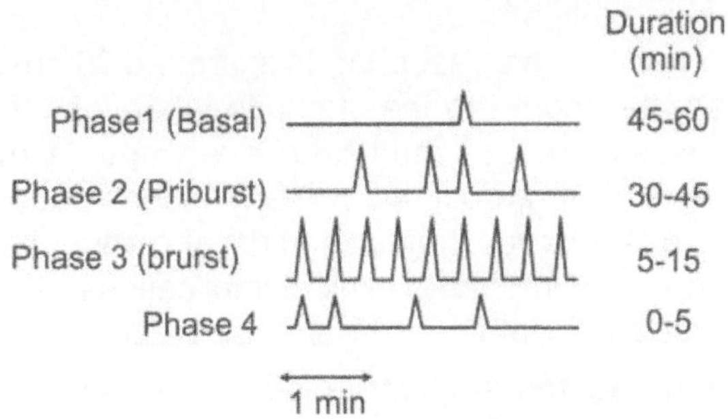

Fig. 2.21 Showing various phases of MMC.

Gastric Residence Time and Emptying Rate for Various Dosage Forms

1. **Non-disintegrating monolithic dosage forms**: In fasting conditions, the GRT of non-disintegrating monolithic dosage forms (coated tablets, matrix tablets, osmotic tablets, hydrophilic matrix capsules...) is highly variable process (all or none) and totally unpredictable (**10 to 120 minutes**). Dosage form units with a diameter of more than 7.5 mm are reported to have an increased GRT compared with those with a diameter of 9.9 mm. The tablets were probably treated as indigestible solids, and since the volunteers were fasted at the time of administration, subsequent gastric emptying of the tablets was probably due to phase III of the MMC. If the tablets were administered just before a 'housekeeper wave', then they would be rapidly emptied from the stomach. However, if they were administered just after phase III activity then it is probable that the tablets would not be emptied until the next 'housekeeper wave' occurred some 2 h later.
2. **Capsules**: Normally capsules emptied from stomach in 60-90 min (initially capsules float in the stomach and then slowly settle down in stomach)
3. **Solutions**: The gastro duodenal pressure produced by the slow, sustained contraction of the proximal stomach controlled the emptying of the solutions. (20-60 min depending upon concentration)
4. **Suspensions:** 20-50 min depending upon concentration
5. **Pellets:** GRT is a function of dosage form buoyancy that is dependent on the density. In fasting conditions, pellets are rapidly emptied from the stomach as a bolus. Particles of different densities ranging from 0.5 to 2.9 g/cm3, empty in a similar manner. The lack of influence of density on stomach emptying agrees with Davis et al., 1986, who observed in humans who were in the fasted state that there is no difference between the rate of gastric emptying of floating and nonfloating (0.96 or 1.96 g/CM3) single unit dosage forms. We suggest that in the interdigestive state, particles of different densities are mixed and entrapped in gastric mucous. Thus the dispersion of individual particles is limited. The particles of various densities rather than float or sink in a

limited gastric fluid volume in the stomach are held loosely together in a mass and emptied with mucous during the late phase II of the MMC.

(a) **Light pellets**- showed the typical pattern of slow emptying following a lag phase (30-75 min, because light pellet generally float in the fluid content and start to empty only when the fluid level in the stomach decreases.) and stay around 90-150 min in jejunum, 60-120 min in ileum and around 20 hrs in colon)

(b) **Intermediate density Pellets**: intermediate density started to empty from the stomach at about 20 min. Emptying was initially rapid, but was soon interrupted by the ingestion of food.

(c) **Heavy Pellet:** Emptying of the heaviest pellets followed a two-stage process. Approximately one-third of the pellets emptied rapidly after an initial lag period, the emptying then being delayed for a second more prolonged lag period. The remainder of the pellets then emptied rapidly and completely (60-300 min.)

6. **Large single-unit matrix delivery systems:** Stagnation of large single-unit matrix delivery systems is often observed at the ileocaecal region. This phenomenon is highly variable (1-12 h) and unpredictable. It never happens with multiple-unit dosage forms
7. **Shape of dosage form** – Tetrahedron and ring shaped devices with a flexural modulus of 48 and 22.5 kilo pounds per square inch (KSI) are reported to have better GRT $\approx$ 90% to 100% retention at 24 hours compared with other shapes
8. **Single or multiple unit formulation** – multiple unit formulations show a more predictable release profile and insignificant impairing of performance due to failure of units, allow co-administration of units with different release profiles or containing incompatible substances and permit a larger margin of safety against dosage form failure compared with single unit dosage forms;

Stomach Motility under Fed State: After consuming a classical solid meal, the interdigestive pattern is replaced by a long period of irregular contractile activity with no apparent rhythm. Initially there is a delay time of 20 to 30 minutes in which there is negligible gastric emptying which is followed by a phase in which the rate of emptying is roughly linear. In contrast, liquids are generally transported out of the stomach at an exponential rate. The rate of gastric emptying is strongly influenced by both volume and composition of gastric contents, which makes considerable sense.

Fed Pattern of Motility: The motility pattern of the stomach during fed state is completely different that at the fasted state. There are no distinctive phases. The contraction has moderate strength in the range of 15-20 millimeter Hg. There are two types of contraction: peristaltic contraction and cystolic contraction. These two contraction patterns are coordinated to achieve the diminution of the size of the stomach by mixing and grinding. The systolic contraction is mainly the result of circular muscle contraction, whereas the peristaltic contraction is mainly the result of longitudinal contraction (Fig. 2.22).

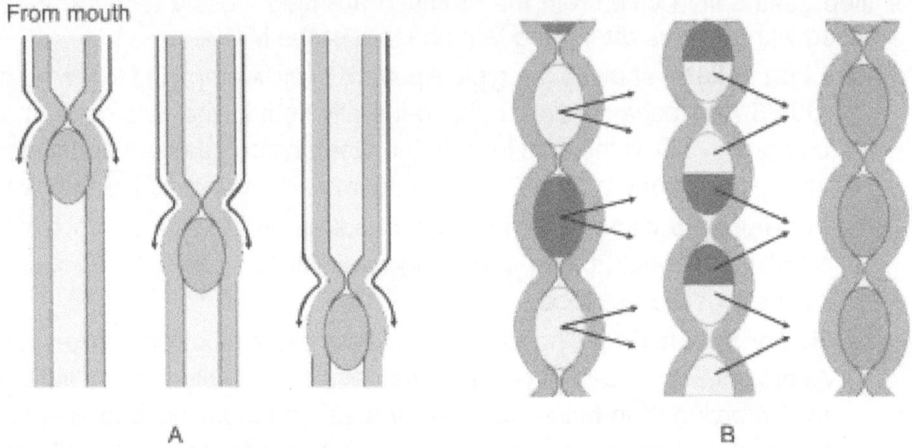

Fig 2.22 (A) Peristaltic contraction (result of longitudinal contraction); (B) cystolic contraction: result of circular muscle contraction.

Factors Affecting Fed State Motility

1. *Fat:* An increase in the fat content decreases the emptying rate.
2. *Carbohydrate:* An increase in the sugar content decreases the emptying rate.
3. *Protein:* An increase in the protein content decreases the emptying rate.
4. *Amount of food:* An increase in the amount of food taken decreases the emptying rate.
5. *Physical form:* An increase in the solid content of the food decreases the emptying rate.
6. *Acidic content:* An increase in the? acidic content decreases the emptying rate. This is because acid has to be neutralized by pancreatic juices, duodenal juices and intestinal secretion after it is emptied.
7. *Hormonal factor:* Progesterone increase GI transit time, and decreases esophageal sphinction tone. This is the main reason some pregnant woman have higher vomiting potential.
8. *Posture:* Stomach contents are emptied faster when standing up than lying down. This posture effect may explain why bed-stricken patients tend to have poor appetites.
9. *Dosage form factor:* Many other factors also influence the gastric emptying rate, which are responsible for observed intersubject variations in bioavailability. Factors promoting gastric emptying include
   1. Hunger
   2. Anxiety
   3. The patient's body posture (i.e. lying on the right side)
   4. Alkaline buffer solution
   5. The intake of liquids

6. Cold food
7. Diseases such as hyperthyroidism
8. Drugs such as metoclopramide (a potent antiemetic, which is thought to act by direct stimulation of cholinergic neurons), particularly when gastric emptying is unusually slow.

Gastric emptying is retarded by

1. Fatty foods
2. High bulk (viscous) diet
3. High concentration of electrolytes or hydrogen ions (acidic solutions)
4. Mental depression
5. Lying on the left side
6. Diseases such as gastric ulcers, pyloric stenosis, gastroenteritis, hypothyroidism
7. Drugs such as anticholinergics, tricyclic antidepressants, narcotic analgesics, aluminium hydroxide and alcohol.

As a general rule, drugs should be ingested on an empty stomach with a glass of water to provide optimal conditions for dissolution and absorption. This rule is particularly important for those drugs unstable in gastric fluids (e.g. penicillin and erythromycin), enteric-coated dosage forms, and those compounds best absorbed in the lower portion of the intestine (e.g. vitamin B_{12}). There are exceptions to this general rule. These exceptions include drugs that are irritating to the stomach (e.g. phenylbutazone, nirtrofurantoin), those compounds absorbed in the proximal portion of the small intestine by a specialized mechanism (e.g. riboflavin), and those compounds where the presence of certain food constituents are known to enhance absorption (e.g. griseofulvin absorption is enhanced in the presence of fatty food).

While any increased gastric emptying rate will probably increase the rate (and possibly the extent) of absorption of drugs best absorbed from the small intestine from rapidly dissolving dosage forms, the converse may be true in other circumstances. For example, if the dosage form must first be exposed to the acidic gastric fluids to initiate disintegration or dissolution, rapid emptying may reduce the rate and extent of absorption. Similarly, if the drug dissolves slowly from the dosage forms, a shortened residence time in the stomach may reduce the extent of dissolution and absorption. Hence, a decrease in gastric emptying rate(i.e. increased gastric residence time) would permit a longer time in which dissolution of such a drug could occur in the more favorable acidic pH conditions of stomach.

Small Bowel Transit: From the stomach, enters the small intestine where it comes in contact with an environment which is entirely different from that of the stomach. Since the small intestine is the primary site of drug absorption, the longer the residence time in this region the greater is the possibility of complete absorption, provided that the drug is stable in the intestinal fluid and does not react with the components of intestinal fluid to form insoluble or unabsorbable complex.

Coordinated contractions of Intestinal smooth muscle participate in several ways to facilitate digestion and absorption in the small intestine as foodstuffs are mixed with digestive enzymes from the pancreas and bile salts from the biliary system; nutrient molecules in the lumen are constantly dispersed, allowing them to contact the epithelium where enzymatic digestion is completed and absorption occurs and besides chyme is moved down the digestive tube, making way for the next load and also eliminating indigestible, perhaps toxic substances.

In humans, there are two types of intestinal movements

1. **Propulsion:** The propulsive movements primarily determine the intestinal transit rate and thus the residence time of a drug or dosage form in the small intestine. The principal type of propulsive motility, seen particularly in the esophagus and small intestine, is peristalsis, a ring of muscle contraction which appears on the oral side of a bolus of ingesta and moves toward the anus, propelling the contents of the lumen in that direction; as the ring moves, the muscle on the other side of the distended area relaxes, facilitating smooth passage of the bolus.

   (a) **Peristalsis:** occurs only after most nutrients have been absorbed. Generally, it requires about 2 hours for undigested material to arrive at the ileocecal valve. Each peristaltic wave initiated in the duodenum begin to sweep slowly along the small intestines, moves around 10-70 cm before dying out. Each successive wave is initiated a bit more distally, and this pattern of peristaltic activity, migrating mobility complex, continues until the undigested food is moved to the ileum a 2 hour trip. The gastro-ileal reflex causes the ileocecal sphincter to relax.

   (b) **Mixing:** If ingested materials were simply propelled through the digestive tube, it will not be getting digested and absorbed, because the digestive enzymes would not be adequately mixed with the ingesta and the bulk of the ingesta would not come in contact with the epithelial cells that absorb nutrients. Mixing movements of the small intestine bring the gut contents, in which the drug is present, into intimate contact with the surface epithelium and thereby provide a larger effective surface area for absorption. The villi contract during this process result in a "milking" action so that lymph flows from the central lacteal into the lymphatic system. These mixing movements will improve drug absorption for two reasons: (a) by increasing the dissolution rate and (b) by increasing the contact area between the drug and epithelial membrane.

   The interdigestive period is seen between meals, when the lumen is largely devoid of contents. During such times, so-called housekeeping contractions propagate from the stomach through the entire small intestine, sweeping it clear of debris. This complex pattern of motility is also known as the migrating motor complex and is the cause of "growling".

   The time of residenceis important since it will decide the amount of time the dosage form has for dissolution and for drug absorption. The greater the intestinal motility, the shorter the residence time and the less time there is for dissolution and absorption of drugs to occur. Peristaltic waves propel intestinal contents down the tract at about 1 to 2 cm/sec. Therefore, it takes 3 to 10 hours to move a meal in the form of chyme along the entire length of the small intestine.

Intestinal Residence Time and Emptying for Various Dosage Forms

1. **Non-disintegrating monolithic dosage forms**: In fasting conditions, the IRT of non-disintegrating monolithic dosage forms (coated tablets, matrix tablets, osmotic tablets, hydrophilic matrix capsules...) is highly variable process (all or none) and totally unpredictable (**120 to 300 minutes**).
2. **Capsules**: Normally capsules emptied from stomach in 60-90 min (initially capsules float in the stomach and then slowly settle down in stomach) and move to duodenum and generally get dissolve till then.
3. **Solutions**: The gastro duodenal pressure produced by the slow, sustained contraction of the proximal stomach controlled the emptying of the solutions. (158-234 min depending upon concentration)
4. **Suspensions:** 120-150 min depending upon concentration
5. **Pellets:** IRT is a function of dosage form buoyancy that is dependent on the density. In fasting conditions, pellets are rapidly emptied from the stomach as a bolus and reach in intestine where they remain for a long period.
   (a) **Light pellets:** showed the typical pattern of slow emptying following a lag phase (30-75 min, because light pellet generally float in the fluid content and start to empty only when the fluid level in the stomach decreases.) and stay around 90-150 min in jejunum, 60-120 min in ileum and around 20 hrs in colon)
   (b) **Intermediate density Pellets:** intermediate density started to empty from the stomach at about 20 min. Emptying was initially rapid, but was soon interrupted by the ingestion of food and stay around 50-120 min in jejunum, 60-120 min in ileum and around 15 hrs in colon).
   (c) **Heavy Pellet:** Emptying of the heaviest pellets followed a two-stage process. Approximately one-third of the pellets emptied rapidly after an initial lag period, the emptying then being delayed for a second more prolonged lag period. The remainder of the pellets then emptied rapidly and completely (60-300 min) and then slowly get removed from intestine.
6. **Large single-unit matrix delivery systems:** Stagnation of large single-unit matrix delivery systems is often observed at the ileocaecal region. This phenomenon is highly variable (1-12 h) and unpredictable. It never happens with multiple-unit dosage forms.
7. **Single or multiple unit formulation:** multiple unit formulations show a more predictable release profile and insignificant impairing of performance due to failure of units, allow co-administration of units with different release profiles or containing incompatible substances and permit a larger margin of safety against dosage form failure compared with single unit dosage form.

Intestinal motility is most important for:

1. Those dosage forms which release the drug slowly (e.g. sustained release/controlled release/ prolonged release products),
2. Enteric-coated dosage forms which release drug only when they reach the small intestine,
3. The drugs which dissolve slowly in the intestinal fluid and
4. Drugs which are absorbed only in certain regions of the small intestine. For e.g. riboflavin is absorbed by carrier-mediated transport in the proximal regions of the small intestine.

There are a variety of factors that will influence intestinal motility and thereby influence drug absorption. The degree of physical activity, age, disease state, and emotional condition of a patient may increase or decrease the intestinal motility. Other drugs taken concurrently may affect GI motility and thus indirectly affect the rate and extent of availability of a particular drug. Such changes in GI motility may increase, decrease, or have no effect on the extent of availability of the drug from an oral dosage form.

Drug absorption from the colon is likely to be quite slow in comparison to the small intestine because of the smaller effective surface area available for absorption. Drugs that are most likely to be presented to the colon for absorption are those present in dosage forms which release drug slowly (e.g. sustained release or enteric-coated tablets) or which have dissolved incompletely higher in the tract.

(a) **Ileocolonic Transit:** The junction between the small and large bowel represents an ecological and physiological transition of considerable biological importance. In the stomach and small intestine, food residue and endogenous secretions are exposed to an essentially sterile environment through which their transit can be measured in hours. On entering the large intestine, contents encounter a rich bacterial flora and transit through the large intestine can be as long as several days.Some evidence exists that the most distal segments of small intestine (terminal ileum) can store residue between meals and that the eating of a subsequent meal stimulates the emptying of ileal contents into the colon. Contents pass from the distal ileum into the colon as boluses, separated by periods during which flow may be more like a steady trickle, Perhaps 50% or more of total colonic filling occurs as a series of boluses.

The movement of liquids and small solids has been compared and is not greatly different. Little or no information is available on the movement of larger solids through the ileocolonic junction. In addition, it is now well established that the presence of dietary residues in the ileum, particularly fat and carbohydrate, can stimulate mechanisms whereby gastric emptying and transit through the upper small intestine are slowed ("ileal brake").

(b) **Colonic and Rectal Transit:** Colonic and rectal motility and transit plays important role in case of sustained or controlled release or targeted drug delivery to the colon. Colonic motility is described by irregular contractile activity occupying less than 50 % of the total time during the interdigestive phase but increasing in frequency and amplitude shortly after a meal is taken. In addition, the circadian rhythm of colonic motility is also important, with contractile activity reducing to virtually zero at night.Colonic delivery of drugs must take into account the variable transit from mouth to caecum, which we know is mostly influenced by gastric emptying, but also an unpredictable and variable delay in transit across the ileo caecal valve, which will further influence caecal entry times of delayed release dosage forms. Another major factor is the wide differences in movement across the colon and considerations of differential colonic movement between liquids and solid forms, especially in the case of large single units such as a pharmaceutical dosage forms. For example, mean caecal to anal transit time is approximately 36 hours in white caucasians on a mixed "western" diet. This may vary considerably if diet is high in fibre or constipation is a problem. By comparison, colo anal transit may be as short as 2 3 hours in diarrhoeal or inflammatory bowel conditions or > 100 hours in pathological constipation. This variability in transit makes for difficulties in the accurate placement of topically acting drugs to the colon, especially when delivered by the oral route.

2.5.1.4 Blood Flow to the GIT

The entire GIT is highly vascularized and therefore well perfused by the blood stream. The splanchnic circulation, which perfuses the GIT, receives 28% of cardiac output, and this flow drains into the portal vein and then goes to the liver prior to reaching the systemic circulation. Since the liver is the most important organ in the body for drug metabolism and metabolizes some drugs rapidly, there is a possibility that a large fraction of the dose will never reach the systemic circulation because of the hepatic metabolism during absorption. This phenomenon is known as the "first-pass effect", responsible for a decreased bioavailability of certain drugs.

The dependence of intestinal absorption of drugs on the blood flow rate changes from the blood flow, independent to blood flow limited as the absorbability of the substances increases. Therefore, absorption will be independent of the blood flow for those drugs that are poorly permeable. Intestinal blood flow may be the rate-limiting step in the absorption of drugs that can readily penetrate the intestinal membrane and in the absorption of drug molecules that are small enough to easily penetrate the aqueous pores in the membrane. However, relatively large deviation from the normal mesenteric blood flow rate is required to produce an important change in the absorption rate. In general, the rate of drug absorption will be unaffected by any normal variability in mesenteric blood flow because the blood flow is rarely the rate-limiting step in the absorption process. Ordinarily, changes in mesenteric blood flow that result from disease or drug effects must be substantial and sustained to significantly influence drug absorption.

2.5.2 Physicochemical Factors

The absorption and hence the bioavailability of a drug is influenced by many of its physicochemical properties. A detailed study of these properties enables the product designer to formulate the drug in a most suitable form.

2.5.2.1 Oil/Water Partition Coefficient (Lipid Solubility)

The primary physicochemical properties of a drug influencing its passive absorption into and across biological membranes are

1. oil/water partition coefficient (Ko/w)

2. extent of ionization in the biological fluids (determined by its pKa value)
3. pH of the fluid in which it is dissolved, and its molecular weight or volume.

The cell surface of the biological membranes, including those lining the entire GIT, is lipid in nature. Therefore, the general rule is that the higher the lipid solubility of the drug, the greater is the permeability of a drug molecule through the biological membrane (i.e. the oil/water coefficient or lipid solubility of drugs and their absorption rates are linearly related). There are two classes of exceptions to this general rule. They are, (1) highly branched compounds penetrate the membranes more slowly than would be expected based on their Ko/w values, and (2) smaller polar molecules penetrate the membranes more readily than would be expected based on their Ko/w values. The reason for the first exception is that branched compounds must disrupt the local lipid structure of the membrane and will encounter a greater steric hindrance than a straight chain molecule. This effect with a branched compound is not adequately reflected in simple aqueous-lipid partitioning studies (i.e. in the Ko/w values). The explanation for observed deviations in the case of small polar molecules rapid membrane penetration is that cell membranes, although lipid in nature, are not continuous but interrupted by small water-filled channels or pores; such membranes are best described as being lipid-sieve membranes. As a result, small polar molecules pass through the aqueous "pores" readily.

2.5.2.2 Drug Dissociation Constant and Gastrointestinal pH

Most drug molecules are either weak acids or bases which will be ionized to an extent determined by the compounds pKa (pKa is the negative logarithm of the dissociation constant of a drug) and the pH of the biological fluid in which it is dissolved. The importance of ionization in drug absorption is based on the observation that the unionized form of the drug has a greater Ko/w than the ionized form, and since Ko/w is a prime determinant of membrane penetration, ionization would be expected to influence absorption. The interrelationship between the degree of ionization of weak electrolyte drug (which is determined by its dissociation constant and the pH at the absorption site) and the extent of drug absorption is embodied in the pH-partition hypothesis of drug absorption.

The pH-Partition Hypothesis

The pH-partition theory (given by Brodie et al.) of drug absorption is based on the assumption that the gastrointestinal/blood barrier acts as a lipid barrier towards weak electrolyte drugs which are absorbed by passive diffusion. The gastrointestinal/blood barrier is permeable to the non-ionized form of a weak acidic or basic drug but impermeable to the ionized form. Consequently, according to the pH-partition hypothesis, the absorption of a weak electrolyte drug will be determined chiefly by the extent to which the drug exists in its unionized form at the site of absorption.

Thus according to this, the process of absorption is governed by

1. The dissociation constant of the drug (pKa)
2. The lipid solubility or Ko/w of unionized drug
3. pH at absorption site

The extent to which a weak acidic or basic drug ionizes in solution in GIT fluids or blood may be calculated using the appropriate form of the Henderson-Hasselbalch equation.

For a weak acidic drug having a single ionisable group, the following equation is used.

$$pH - pKa = \log \frac{[\text{ionized}]}{[\text{unionized}]} \qquad .....(2.8a)$$

$$\text{Percent drug ionized} = \frac{10^{(pH-Pka)}}{1+10^{(pH-pKa)}} \times 100 \qquad .....(2.8b)$$

Where [unionized] and [ionized] are the respective concentrations of the non-ionized and ionized forms of the weak acidic drug, which are in equilibrium in solution. pH refer to the pH of the environment in which both forms of the weak acidic drug are in equilibrium i.e. pH of the GI fluids or the blood.

For a weak basic drug having single ionizable group, the analogous equation is

$$pKa - pH = \log \frac{[\text{ionized}]}{[\text{unionized}]} \qquad .....(2.9a)$$

$$\text{Percent drug ionized} = \frac{10^{(pka-PH)}}{1+10^{(pka-PH)}} \times 100 \qquad .....(2.9b)$$

Absorption of a Weak Acidic Drug

In order to understand the absorption of weak acidic drugs from GIT, let us consider the absorption of salicylic acid. Consider the distribution of salicylic acid having a pKa of 3.0 between the blood and gastric fluid. For the purpose of calculation assume that the pH of gastric fluid is 1.2 and the pH of blood is 7.4. Equation 2.8 (a) may be used to calculate the relative amounts of ionized and unionized forms of salicylic acid that are in equilibrium in solution in the gastric fluid or blood.

In gastric fluid, pH =1.2

$$pH - pKa = \log \frac{[\text{ionized}]}{[\text{unionized}]}$$

$$1.2 - 3.0 = \log \frac{[\text{ionized}]}{[\text{unionized}]}$$

Therefore, $\frac{[\text{ionized}]}{[\text{unionized}]} = \text{antilog}(-1.8) = 0.016$

It means the ratio of the concentrations of the ionized and unionized forms of salicylic acid is 0.016 : 1, respectively. A great portion (98.4%) of the drug in solution in the gastric fluid exists in the unionized form i.e. absorbable form. Therefore, this drug is absorbed rapidly from gastric fluids and enters the blood. In the blood, the drug will experience a pH of 7.4. The extent of ionization of the drug in the blood may be calculated using equation 2.8 a as follows:

$$pH - pKa = \log \frac{[\text{ionized}]}{[\text{unionized}]}$$

$$7.4 - 3.0 = \log \frac{[\text{ionized}]}{[\text{unionized}]}$$

Therefore, $$\frac{[\text{ionized}]}{[\text{unionized}]} = \text{antilog } (4.4) = 25119$$

Thus, the ratio of the concentrations of the ionized and unionized forms of a weak acidic drug in solution in the blood is 25119 : 1, respectively. It is evident that the weak acidic drug, once present in the blood, will exist almost entirely (99.996%) in its ionized form. It means only 0.004% of the drug is in unionized form in the blood. Thus, irrespective of the sink conditions provided by the systemic circulation to the absorbed drug, the concentration gradient is maintained towards the blood. Hence, there will not be any tendency for the weak acidic drug in the blood to be absorbed back into the stomach.

Let us assume that the stomach and blood are two compartments separated by the gastrointestinal/blood barrier. The barrier is permeable only to unionized form of the drug and thus, there exists an equilibrium between the concentration of unionized form of the drug in the stomach and that in the blood. The ionized form of the drug in the stomach and the blood are in equilibrium with the unionized form in each compartment. The equilibrium distribution of the weak acidic drug (e.g. salicylic acid, pKa 3.0) between gastric fluid (pH 1.2) and blood (pH 7.4) may be represented as shown in Fig. 2.23.

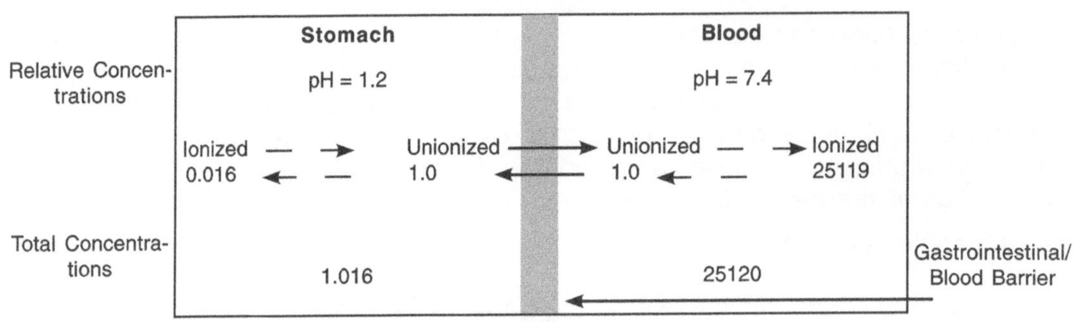

Fig. 2.23 Schematic representation of the equilibrium distribution of salicyclic acid (pKa 3.0) between the stomach and the blood.

The total equilibrium concentration of salicylic acid (a weak acidic drug) is approximately 25000 times greater in the blood than in the stomach. Hence, according to the pH-partition hypothesis, weak acidic drugs which exist predominantly in the unionized form at gastric pH are well absorbed from the stomach.

Absorption of Weak Basic Drug

Let us now consider the distribution of a weak basic drug, aminopyrine (pKa 5.0) between the gastric fluids (pH 1.2) and the blood (pH 7.4). The appropriate equation for the calculation of relative concentrations of the ionized and unionized forms of aminopyrine at pH 1.2 and 7.4 is,

$$\text{pKa} - \text{pH} = \log \frac{[\text{ionized}]}{[\text{unionized}]}$$

The relative equilibrium concentrations of ionized and unionized forms of aminopyrine in the gastric fluid compartment and the blood compartment are in the ratio of 6310.6 and 1.004, respectively (Fig. 2.14). At equilibrium, the total concentration of the weak basic drug in the stomach is approximately 6300 times greater than that in the blood. Thus according to the pH-partition hypothesis, drugs, which are predominantly ionized at gastric pH are poorly absorbed from the stomach. In calculating the distribution of a typical weak acidic drug and a typical weak basic drug between the stomach and blood, it has been assumed that an equilibrium distribution is attained. In practice such an equilibrium will rarely (if any) is achieved, since, the stomach and blood are not closed or static compartments. The drug is removed from the stomach into the intestine by normal contractions of the stomach. The drug, which enters the blood, is removed from the site of absorption by the circulation of the blood and is removed from the blood by distribution into tissues, by glomerular filtration, and by metabolism.

Drugs	pKa	pH/site of absorption
Very weak acidic drugs (pKa>8)		Drug will remain unionized at all pH values; and absorbed along the length of GIT
e.g.		
Pentobarbitol	8.1	
Hexobarbitol	8.2	
Phenytoin	8.3	
Moderately weak acidic drugs (pKa 2.5-7.5)		Drug will be unionized in gastric pH and ionized in intestinal pH; absorption is mainly from stomach and upper part of GIT
e.g.		
Cloxaclin	2.7	
Aspirin	3.5	
Phenylbutazone	4.5	
Strong Acid drugs (pKa <2.5)		Ionize at all pH, poorly absorbed from GIT
e.g.		
Disodium Cromoglycate	2.0	
Very weak basic drugs (pKa<5)		Drug will remain unionized at all pH values; and absorbed along the length of GIT
e.g.		
Theophylline	0.7	
Diazepam	3.7	
Moderately weak basic drugs (pKa 5-11)		Ionized at gastric pH, relatively unionized at intestinal pH; better absorbed from intestine
e.g.		
Heroine	6.6	
Amitryptyline	9.4	
Strong Basic drugs (pKa>11)		Ionize at all pH, poorly absorbed from GIT
e.g.		
Guanethidine	11.7	

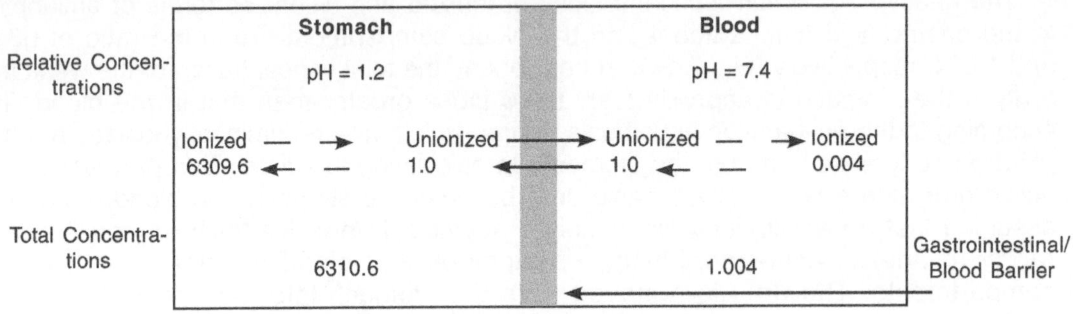

Fig. 2.24 Schematic representation of the equilibrium distribution of aminopyrine (pKa 5.0) between the stomach and the blood.

Limitations of the pH-Partition Hypothesis

According to the pH-partition hypothesis, acidic drugs should best be absorbed from acidic solutions where pH < pKa, while basic drugs would best be absorbed from alkaline solutions where pH > pKa. This general principle is supported by the observations that acidic drugs are better absorbed at acidic pH and basic drugs at basic pH from stomach, where surface area and other factors other than pH are constant.

However, some deviations from pH-partition hypothesis were observed. Some compounds (e.g. salicylic acid) which are essentially completely ionized in the buffer solutions were rapidly absorbed. To explain these exceptions its suggested that there exist a 'virtual membrane pH" on the surface of the absorbing membrane (about 5.3), different from the bulk pH of the buffer solution. This pH determines the fraction of unionized form of drug and hence dictates the absorption pattern. Although there may indeed be an effective pH at the immediate surface of the intestinal membrane, different from the pH of solutions bathing the lumen, there is overwhelming experimental evidence indicating that many drugs in the ionic form are well absorbed. At the same pH (i.e. pH 6), acidic and basic drugs are more rapidly absorbed from the intestine compared to the stomach. This is by virtue of the larger intestinal surface area but not because of "virtual membrane pH". If all other conditions were the same, the unionized form of a drug in solution would be more readily absorbed than the ionized form. However, conditions along the GIT are not uniform and hence most drugs, whether ionized or unionized (i.e. regardless of pH), are best absorbed from the small intestine as a result of the large surface area of this region.

A further illustration that the absorption of a drug from the gastrointestinal tract is not solely dependent on the drug being unionized is provided by the observation that a number of drugs are poorly absorbed from certain areas of the GIT despite the fact that their unionized forms predominate in such areas. For instance, barbitone (pKa 7.8), which is almost totally unionized at the gastric pH, is only poorly absorbed from the stomach. However, thiopentone which has a similar pKa value (pKa 7.6) is much better absorbed from the stomach than the barbitone. The reason for this difference is that the absorption of drugs is also affected by the lipid solubility exhibited by the unionized forms. Thus the unionized form of thipentone, being more lipid soluble than the unionized form of barbitone, exhibits its a greater affinity for the gastrointestinal membrane and is thus better absorbed from the stomach.

A further observation which can not be explained by the pH-partition hypothesis is that certain drugs (e.g. quaternary ammonium compounds and tetracyclines) are absorbed readily despite being ionized over the entire pH range of the GIT.

To summarize, the pH-partition hypothesis provides a useful guide in predicting general trends in drug absorption and it remains as an extremely useful concept. There are numerous examples illustrating the general relationship among pH, pKa and drug absorption developed in this hypothesis. The primary limitation of this concept is the assumption that only unionized drug is absorbed, when in fact the ionized species of some compounds can be absorbed, albeit at a slower rate. There is also the presence of unstirred water layers at the epithelial membrane surface, which can alter the rate of drug diffusion. Further more, the hypothesis is based on data obtained from a drug in solution. In a practical sense, there are other considerations, which are more likely to govern the pattern of drug absorption and these include dissolution rate from solid dosage forms, the large intestinal surface area, and the relative residence times of the drug in different parts of the GIT. In general, drug absorption in humans takes place primarily from the small intestine regardless of whether a drug is a weak acid or base.

2.5.3 Dissolution

The dosage forms administered by the oral route are mainly either a solution, or suspension, tablet or hard gelatin capsules. The drug in solution form is available for absorption as soon as it uniformly distributes in fluid of the stomach. Some times a drug in solution when administered may precipitate in the fluids of the stomach due to a change in pH, in which case the fine precipitate should again dissolve in the fluids of the stomach. The drug particles of a suspension must undergo dissolution so that the drug is in solution for absorption. In case of tablet or capsule dosage forms, they should first undergo disintegration to release aggregates or granules and then deaggregation into fine particles. The dissolution of a drug takes place from a dosage form as such, aggregates or granules and fine particles. A drug in solution is absorbed through the gastric mucosa and reaches systemic circulation (Fig. 2.15). Stomach emptying causes the emptying of the drug in solution, fine particles, aggregates and even the dosage form into the small intestine which undergo dissolution as explained above.

It can be seen from the Fig. 2.15 that the dissolution of a drug from the fine particles determines the rate at which the drug comes into solution and thereby the absorption of the drug.

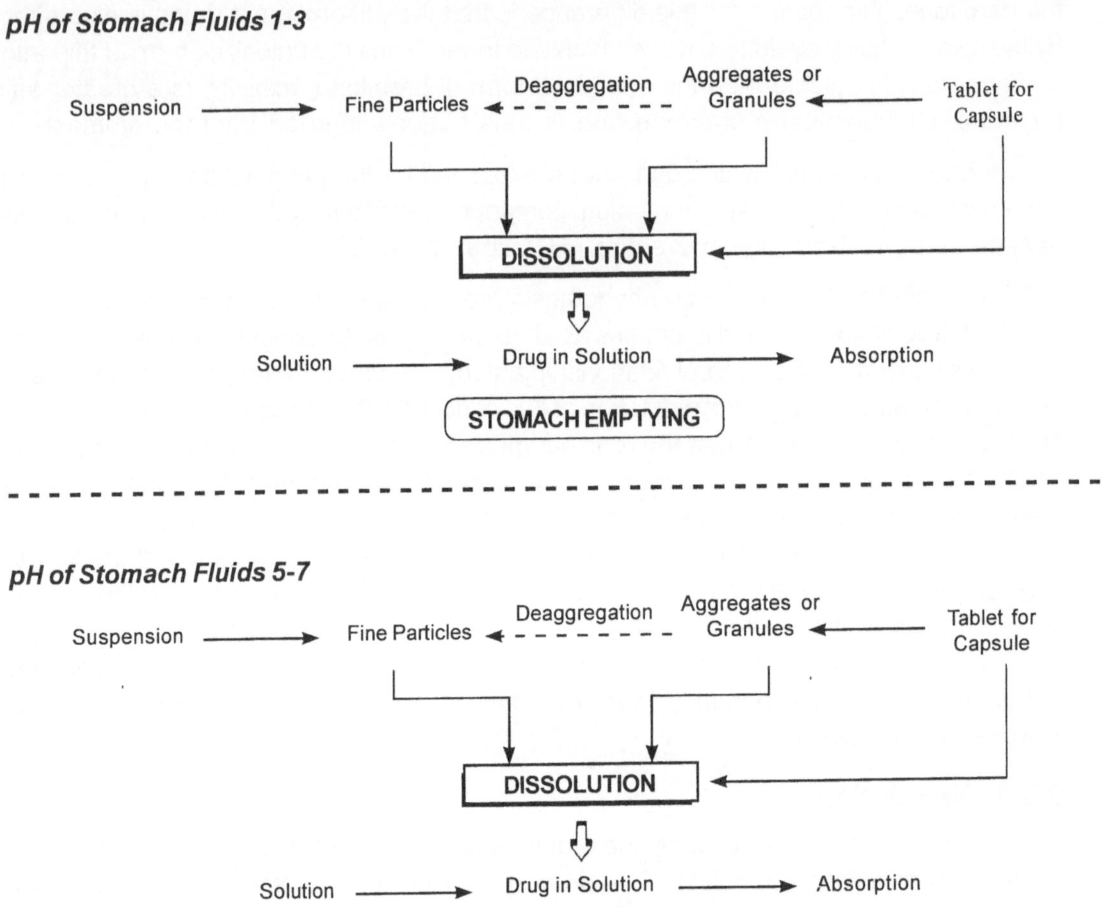

Fig. 2.25 Diagrammatic Representation of the Processes Involved in Drug Absorption From Different Dosage Forms.

Mechanisms of Dissolution

Dissolution is nothing but the rate of solution of a solid in a solvent; that is, it is the transfer of solute molecules from the surface of solid into the bulk of a solvent. In order for the dissolution of a solid to occur, solute molecules must first escape from the surface of the solid and then undergo some form of transport process away from the surface into the bulk of the solvent. Three types of dissolution models are proposed depending on the relative significance of two processes mentioned above and the means by which the transport is effected. These three models which, either alone or in combination, can be used to describe the dissolution rate mechanisms. The three models are:

1. Diffusion Layer Model or Film Theory
2. Interfacial Barrier Model or Limited Solvation Theory and
3. Danckwerts' Model or Surface Renewal Theory

Diffusion Layer Model or Film Theory

The simplest of the three models is the diffusion layer model, in which it is assumed that there is a static liquid film adjacent to the solid surface. The reaction at the solid/liquid film interface is assumed to be rapid, so that the rate of dissolution is governed entirely by the diffusional transport of the solute molecules through the liquid film. Once the solute molecules pass the liquid film/bulk film interface, rapid mixing occurs and the concentration gradient is destroyed. The model is depicted in Fig. 2.26(a).

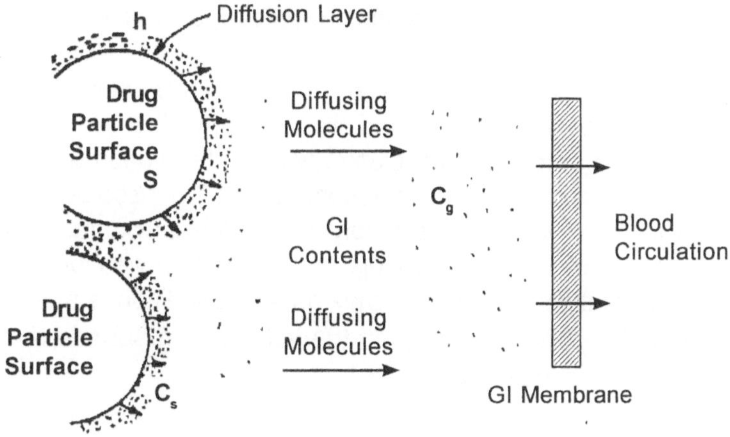

Fig. 2.26(a) Schematic diagram of the dissolution process.

The rate at which the dissolution of a drug takes place from a particle into its surrounding fluid according to this model can be assessed by the Noyes-Whitney equation. The assumptions made in developing the Noyes-Whitney equation are:

1. Drug particles are spherical in shape and equal in size,
2. The dissolution process is controlled by diffusion of molecules or ions,
3. There is no chemical reaction between the drug and the components of the fluid in which the drug is present, and
4. The thickness of the diffusion layer (h) and the saturation solubility of drug in diffusion layer (Cs) are constant irrespective of the particle size.

According to Noyes and Whitney, the rate of dissolution (dm/dt) is given by,

$$\frac{dm}{dt} = \frac{DA\,(Cs - Cg)}{h} \quad .....(2.10a)$$

Where:

dm/dt = rate of the dissolution of the particles

D = diffusion coefficient of the drug in solution in the GI fluids (greater the value, faster the dissolution. But is inversely proportional to viscosity of the medium)

A = effective surface area of the drug particles (greater the surface area, faster the dissolution and can be increased by micronization)

h = the thickness of the diffusion layer (stationary layer of the solvent) around the drug particles (more the thickness, lesser is the diffusion and dissolution, can be reduced by agitation)

Cs = saturation solubility of the drug in the diffusion layer

Cg = concentration of the drug in solution in the bulk of GI fluids

(Cs-cg) = concentration gradient (greater the concentration gradient faster is the dissolution)

Equation 2.10a represents a first order dissolution process, where the driving force is the concentration gradient (Cs-Cg) and dissolution is said to be under non-sink condition which is true in case of in–vitro dissolution (where dissolution is done in limited dissolution medium). During such dissolution, after sometimes, the dissolution slows down because of drug concentration but *in-vivo* dissolution (dissolution in human stomach) is always rapid than in-vitro because of the moment of dissolved drug (from dissolution site to blood) resulting in Cg=0, thus dissolution will be at its max as sink condition is maintained.

Since during sink condition (keeping the volume and surface area constant),

$$dC/Dt = K$$

where K = constant

Fig. 2.26a schematically illustrates the relationship of the terms in equation 2.10a to the dissolution process. It should be emphasized that this crude model does not completely describe the dissolution process. The model has, however, helped to explain many experimental results. Each term in the equation influences the rate of dissolution of a drug in GI fluids. As the dissolution of drug particles take place, the particle size and surface area are also changed. Hixon and Crowell developed an equation to account for these changes during dissolution and is known as *Hixon and Crowell's Cube Root Law of dissolution.*

$$W_o^{1/3} - W_t^{1/3} = k\,t \qquad .....(2.10b)$$

Where, W_o = original mass of the drug

W_t = mass of the drug remained at time t

K = dissolution rate constant

Interfacial Barrier Model or Limited Solvation Theory

In this model, it is assumed that the reaction at the solid surface is not instantaneous, due to a high free energy of activation required for solubility of a solid. Therefore, the rate of solubility of solid in the liquid film becomes rate limiting rather than diffusion of dissolved molecules. The situation is illustrated in Fig. 2.26(b) for the case where the now relatively rapid transport process occurs by diffusion through a static liquid film. Equation for describing the dissolution rate of a solid by this model is,

$$dm/dt = Ki\,(Cs - Cg) \qquad .....(2.10c)$$

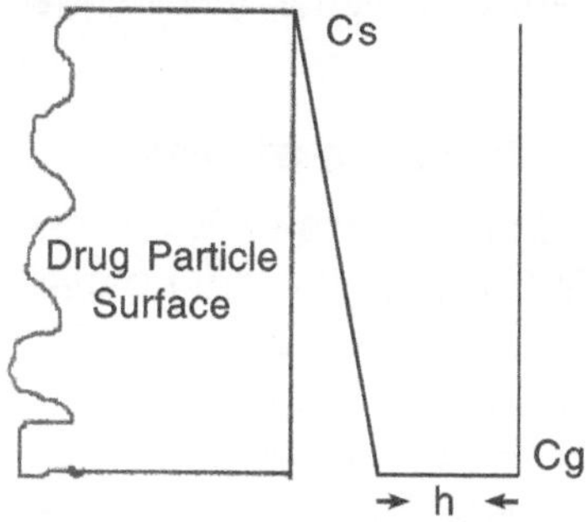

Fig. 2.26(b) Mechanisms of Dissolution-Interfacial Barrier Method.

Where, dm/dt, Cs and Cg are as defined previously and Ki is the effective interfacial transport rate constant.

Danckwerts'Model or Surface Renewal Theory

Dankwerts' never agreed for the existence of a saturated diffusion layer and proposed that the transport of a solute away from the solid surface is achieved by means of macroscopic packets of solvent which attach themselves to the surface, absorb the solute by normal diffusion, and are then replaced by fresh packets of solvent. Since fresh solvent packets attack the new solid surface each time to effect dissolution, the theory is also known as *Surface Renewal Theory* (Fig. 2.26(c)).

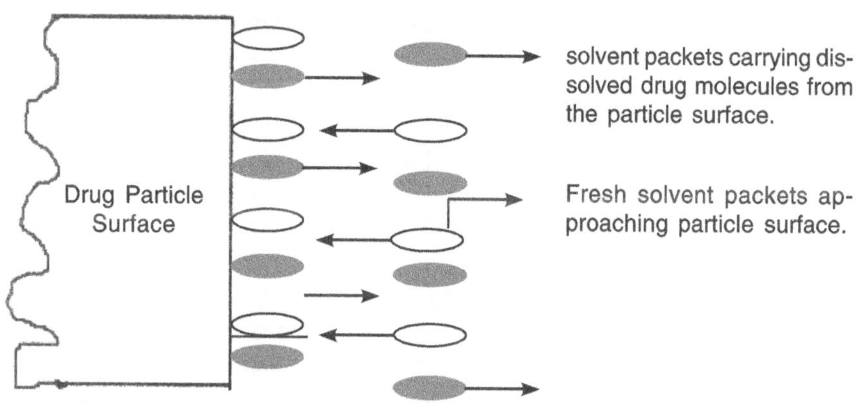

Fig. 2.26(c) Mechanisms of dissolution-Danckwert's model.

The turbulence present in the dissolution medium at the solid/liquid interface is responsible for the rapid movement of solvent packets or macroscopic mass of eddies that reach the solid/liquid interface in random manner. Because of the rapid movement of these solvent packets, the drug concentration in them never reaches Cs. The general expression used for the rate of dissolution of a solid by Danckwerts' model is,

$$dm/dt = S^{1/2} D^{1/2} (Cs - Cg) \quad .....(2.16d)$$

Where, S is the mean rate at which a fresh surface is produced and all other terms are as defined previously.

2.5.3.1 Factors Affecting the Rate of Dissolution

Particle Size and Effective Surface Area : Particle size and surface area of the molecule inversely proportional *i.e.* The smaller the drug particles, the greater the surface area for a given amount of drug. Thus equation 2.10a predicts that dissolution rate will increase as the effective surface area of the drug in contact with the GI fluid increases (i.e. as the particle size decreases). However, for drugs that are freely soluble in the GI fluids, the particle size may not influence the dissolution rate significantly. Drugs having a limited solubility (< 1%) in the fluids of the GIT often exhibit poor or erratic absorption unless the dosage forms are specially tailored for the drug. Therefore, many poorly soluble and slowly dissolving drugs are marketed in micronized or microcrystalline form. Particle size reduction is thus likely to result in an increased bioavailability, provided that absorption of the drug dissolution rate limited.

Particle size reduction improves the bioavailability of certain drugs such as griseofulvin, spiranolactone, digoxin, and benoxaprofen. Micronization of griseofulvin reduces the daily dose required for therapeutic effect from 1 g to 0.5 g, while the micronization of spiranolactone results in the reduction of the therapeutic dose by twenty fold (from 500 mg to 25 mg). Particle size may also be an important factor in the bioavailability of digoxin. Reduction in digoxin particle size by ball milling from a mean diameter of 30 μm to 3.7 μm leads to an increase in the rate and extent of absorption of the drug.

There are instances in which particle size reduction fails to increase the absorption rate of a drug. One possible explanation for this observation is that the dissolution of the drug may not be a rate-limiting step in the absorption process. Micronization some times dramatically increases the tendency of drug particles to aggregate, which may lead to a decrease in effective surface area (i.e. the portion of the surface actually in contact with the dissolving fluids). A decreased dissolution rate of phenacetin, a hydrophobic drug, is observed with a decreased particle size. In fact, the smaller phenacetin particles had more air adsorbed on their surfaces and actually float on the dissolution medium. When a surface active agent is added to the dissolution medium, the smaller particles were more readily wetted. Thus, their absolute surface area becomes their effective surface area and the rate of dissolution is increased significantly. Physiological surface active agents like bile salts and lysolecithin probably facilitate the dissolution and absorption of poorly water-soluble drugs in the small intestine.

A unique approach to presenting a poorly soluble drug in an extremely fine state of subdivision to the GI fluids is the administration of the drug in the form of solid dispersion. Solid dispersions consist of the drug in a physiologically inert, readily water-soluble material called "carrier". Solid dispersions can be formulated as solid eutectic mixtures. For example, sulphathiazole in a matrix of urea. When this system is exposed to the GI fluids, the water-soluble carrier dissolves quickly and exposes the drug in fine state of subdivision, which undergoes rapid dissolution in the GI fluid. The formation of a solid solution of a poorly water-soluble drug in a water-soluble carrier should offer a greater improvement in dissolution rate and the bioavailability of the poorly water-soluble drug than that of its eutectic mixture. This is because of the fact that the poorly water-soluble drug would be dispersed as single molecules throughout the water-soluble carrier. The increased dissolution rates and the bioavailabilities of griseofulvin are observed when solid dispersions of griseofulvin in high molecular weight polyethylene glycol are evaluated. Formation of a solution of griseofulvin in polyehtylene glycols is responsible for the observed improvement in the dissolution rates and bioavailabilities.

In addition to size reduction, other factors also contribute to the improved dissolution rate and bioavailability exhibited by solid dispersions. They are:

1. an increase in aqueous solubility of the drug due to the presence of drug particles in extremely small size,
2. improved solubility of the drug in the diffusion layer by 'carrier',
3. prevention of aggregation and agglomeration of the drug particles exposed to the GI fluids,
4. excellent wettability and dispersibility of the exposed drug particles in the GI fluids, and
5. possible formation of metastable polymorphic forms (which are more soluble and rapidly dissolving in the GI fluids) of the drug during the formation of the solid dispersion system.

Certain drugs such as penicillin G, Omeprazole, Esomeprazole and erythromycin are unstable in gastric fluids. Thus chemical degradation will be minimized if such drugs do not dissolve readily in gastric fluids. Hence, particle size reduction would not only produce an increased rate of dissolution of a drug in the gastric fluids, but also its degradation. This would result in a decrease in the amount of intact drug available for absorption from the small intestine.

It is interesting to note that in the case of nitrofurantoin, the inclusion of small-sized particles of this drug in tablets give an increased incidence of undesirable side effects. The enhanced bioavailability resulted from particle size reduction was believed to be responsible for these undesirable side effects. This is an example where an improved bioavailability results in over medication of patients.

Saturation Solubility of the Drug, Cs

The next term in the equation 2.10a, that can be manipulated, is Cs, the saturation solubility of the drug. The Cs is influenced by both patient and pharmaceutical variables. The patient variables includes the changes in pH as well as the amounts and types of secretions along the GIT. Additionally both the physical and chemical properties of a drug molecule can be modified to increase or decrease its saturation solubility.

The pH Effect

The solubility of a weak acidic drug or weak basic drug is influenced by the pH of the fluid. Therefore, differences are expected in the solubility and hence the dissolution rate of such drugs in different regions of the GIT.

The dissociation of weak acidic drug is given by:

$$\overset{Ka}{[HA] \qquad\qquad [A^-]\ [H^+]} \qquad .....(2.11)$$

The total solubility of a weak acidic drug is given by,

$$Cs = [HA] + [A^-] \qquad .....(2.12)$$

Where Cs = total solubility of drug in the fluid

[HA] = the intrinsic solubility of unionized acid (denoted as Co)

$[A^-]$ = the concentration of its anion

The concentration of the anion can be written as:

$$[A^-] = \frac{[HA]\,Ka}{[H^+]} = \frac{Co\,Ka}{[H^+]} \qquad .....(2.13)$$

The total solubility of a weak acidic drug is thus:

$$Cs = \frac{Co + Co\,Ka}{[H^+]} = \frac{Co\,(1 + Ka)}{[H^+]} \qquad .....(2.14)$$

In a similar manner, the solubility of a weak basic drug is given by,

$$Cs = \frac{Co + Co\,[H^+]}{Ka} = \frac{Co\,(1 + [H^+])}{Ka} \qquad .....(2.15)$$

Equations 2.14 and 2.15 indicate that the dissolution rate of weak acidic drugs increases with increasing pH (i.e. decreasing $[H^+]$), whereas the dissolution rate of weak basic drugs decreases with an increasing pH. Therefore, the dissolution rate of weak acidic drugs is more in the intestine than in the stomach, whereas weak basic drugs show a greater dissolution rate in the stomach than in the intestine. It is, therefore, important for poorly soluble weak basic drugs to dissolve rapidly in the stomach, since the dissolution rate of undissolved drug in the small intestine may be too low to permit complete absorption.

The relationships that have been described between the dissolution rate and hydrogen ion concentrations (equations 2.14 and 2.15) are only approximations, because they do not fully account for the influence of the unstirred diffusion layer. These equations tend to overestimate the dissolution rate of weak acidic drugs in the small intestine and the dissolution rate of weak bases in the stomach. Under these conditions, the hydrogen ion concentration of the bulk, $[H^+]$, is not equal to the hydrogen ion concentration of the diffusion layer, $[H^+]d$. In general, $[H^+]d > [H^+]$ for weak acidic drugs and $[H^+]d < [H^+]$ for weak basic drugs.

It is possible to approximate the hydrogen ion concentration of the diffusion layer around a drug particle by measuring the pH of a buffer solution of a given pH saturated with that drug. A saturated solution of a weak acidic drug, like that found in the diffusion layer, tends to depress the neutral pH of the intestinal fluids, whereas a saturated solution of a weak basic drug tends to elevate the low pH of the gastric fluid. These fine differences seem to be of little importance for the absorption of weak acidic drugs, or weak basic drugs administered as such, but they are important when drugs are given in the form of salts.

Salt Forms

Most of the drugs available are salts of either weak acids or weak bases as salt formation is the easiest way to increase solubility and dissolution rate. The dissolution rate of a particular salt is usually different from that of the parent compound. Sodium or potassium salts of weak acidic drugs dissolve more rapidly than the free acids, regardless of the pH of the dissolution medium. The effect of salt form on the dissolution rate can not be explained in terms of solubility and bulk pH, but requires a consideration of the pH of the diffusion layer. The pH of the diffusion layer surrounding each particle at a given bulk pH is always greater for sodium or potassium salt of a weak acidic drug than for the corresponding free acid. This is because of the neutralizing action of the strong alkali cations (e.g., K^+ or Na^+ ions) present in the diffusion layer. On the other hand, the pH of the diffusion layer of an HCl or other strong acid salt of a weak basic drug is always smaller than the diffusion layer pH of the corresponding free base.

At a given pH, the solubility of a drug (acid/base or salt) is a constant and the influence of salt formation can be on drug solubility/rate of dissolution and absorption can be explained by considering the pH of the diffusion layer (not the bulk of solution).

Considering the case of salt of weak acidic drug, which has a relatively high solubility at the elevated pH in the diffusion layer, dissolution of the drug particles will take place at a faster rate. The dissolved drug diffuses out of the diffusion layer and comes in contact with the bulk of gastric fluids, where the pH is lower than that of diffusion layer, and may lead to the precipitation of drug in a free acid form. This is because of the low solubility of the drug at a lower pH. Thus the free acid form of the drug in solution, which is in excess of its solubility at the bulk pH of the gastric fluid, will precipitate out leaving a saturated or near saturated solution of free acid in the gastric fluid. It is considered that the precipitated free acid will be in the form of very fine wetted drug particles, which exhibit a very large effective surface area in contact with the gastric fluid. This large effective surface area is many times greater than that would have been obtained if the free acid form of the drug had been administered, which facilitates rapid dissolution of the precipitated particles of free acid under suitable conditions. There are conditions which facilitate a further dissolution of the precipitated free acid form. They are:

1. When a dissolved drug is absorbed, concentration of the drug in the gastric fluids is decreased favoring the dissolution of the fine particles of the drug.
2. Additional gastric secretions increase the fluid volume in which a further dissolution of fine particles takes place.
3. Fine precipitated drug particles emptied slowly from the stomach into the intestine give scope for the dissolution of drug particles remained in the stomach.

As a result of this rapid re-dissolution of fine precipitated drug particles, the concentration of free acid in solution will be maintained at or near to saturation solubility of free acid in the gastric fluids at the bulk pH. Thus the oral administration of a solid dosage form containing a strong alkali salt of a weak acidic drug would be expected to give a more rapid rate of drug dissolution and a more rapid drug absorption than if the free acid form of the drug itself had been included in the dosage form. This is true for the drugs that exhibit a dissolution rate-limited absorption.

Many examples exist of the effects of soluble salts on drug absorption. Some studies also report significant effects on clinical response. Marked differences have been observed in the rate and extent of absorption of novobiocin when administered as such or in the form of a salt. The bioavailability of the dug after oral administration of a sodium salt is twice that of a calcium salt and 50 times that of a free acid.

Oral administration of penicillin V and its potassium and calcium salts resulted in peak plasma levels of the drug that are best correlated with their dissolution rates. Potassium salt of penicillin V produces a higher peak plasma level followed by calcium salt and then the free form.

So far the dissolution of strong alkali salts of weak acidic drugs have been considered to explain how the salt form of a drug shows a rapid dissolution rate than that of its parent drug. The higher rate of dissolution of strongly acidic salt forms of a weak basic drug in GI fluids than that of free base, can be explained by considering the pH of the diffusion layer around drug particle. The presence of strong acidic anions (e.g. Cl^- ions) in the diffusion layer formed around each dissolving salt particle of drugs ensures that the pH in that layer is lower than the bulk pH in either gastric or intestinal fluid. This lower pH will increase the solubility of a drug (Cs) in the diffusion layer. The oral administration of a salt form of a weak basic drug in a solid dosage form generally ensures that dissolution of the drug before it passes into the small intestine where the pH conditions are less favorable to the dissolution of weak bases. Hence, the use of strong acidic salt forms of weak basic drugs generally ensures that stomach emptying (and not dissolution rate) is the rate-limiting step for the absorption of such drugs from the small intestine.

It is not always true that a salt form of a drug will have a higher dissolution rate than its parent drug. Certain salts have a lower solubility and dissolution rate than their parent drug, e.g. the aluminum salts of weak acids, and the pamoate salts of weak bases. In these, insoluble films of either aluminum hydroxide or pamoic acid appear to form over the dissolving solids when the salts are exposed to alkaline or acidic environment, respectively. These insoluble films further reduce the rate of dissolution. The experimental data suggest that salt formation is a potential means of obtaining a slow absorption and prolonged effects of certain drugs. The pamoate salt of imipramine has been marked as a slow-release form of the drug.

If $[H^+]_d$= Hydrogen ion concentration at diffusion layer

$[H^+]_b$= hydrogen ion concentration in the bulk of the solution

Then

For salts of weak acid $[H^+]_d < [H^+]_b$

For salt of weak bases $[H^+]_d > [H^+]_d$

An alternative method of increasing the dissolution rate of a weak acidic drug is **in situ salt formation** where physiologically inert basic compounds are included in a solid dosage form containing the free acid form of the drug. The presence of basic ingredients ensures that a relatively alkaline diffusion layer is formed around each dissolving drug particle. The presence of aluminum dihydroxyamino acetate and magnesium carbonate in aspirin tablets is found to increase the dissolution rate of aspirin in the stomach and the bioavailability of this drug following oral administration. Besides it also has other advantages of reduced gastric irritation and ulcerogenic tendency of the drug and it also overcomes from the difficult of solubility of sodium salt of aspirin.

An alternative method of increasing the dissolution rate of a weak acidic drug in the gastric fluid is the inclusion of physiologically inert basic compounds in a solid dosage form containing the free acid form of the drug. The presence of basic ingredients ensures that a relatively alkaline diffusion layer is formed around each dissolving drug particle. The presence of aluminum dihydroxyamino acetate and magnesium carbonate in aspirin tablets is found to increase the dissolution rate of aspirin in the stomach and the bioavailability of this drug following oral administration.

Some times, problems with chemical stability preclude the use of salts of a drug in a dosage form. Aspirin, for example, is much more prone to hydrolysis in the form of sodium acetylsalicylate. Even solid dosage forms of this salt have poor chemical stability.

At other times, undesirable pharmacological responses observed with the rapid dissolution of salt forms of a drug precludes the use of salts in the dosage form. For example, oral administration of sodium salt of talbutamide reduces blood glucose to about 65 to 70% of control levels. The more slowly dissolving free acid form produced a gradual decrease in blood sugar to about 80% of control levels, when administered orally. Pronounced reduction in the blood glucose level achieved by sodium salt of talbutamide may lead to severe hypoglycemia and even diabetic coma. Hence, the free acid form of tolbutamide is a more useful form of the drug for treatment of diabetes.

Crystal Form

Crystal habit and the internal structure of a drug can affect physicochemical properties, which range from chemical stability to bioavailability. Many drugs can exists in more than one crystalline form, a property known as *polymorphism*. Many physico-chemical properties vary with the internal structure of the solid drug, including melting point, density, hardness, crystal shape, solubility and dissolution rate. A drug may exists in more than one crystalline form, but at a given temperature and pressure only one crystalline form is stable and all other forms found under these conditions are called metastable polymorphs. The metastable polymorphs will tend to transform into the most stable form at rates that depend on the energy differences between the metastable and stable forms. The metastable polymorph is a higher energy form of a drug and usually has a lower melting point, greater solubility and greater dissolution rate than the stable crystal form. As a result, one polymorph may be more active therapeutically than another polymorph of the same drug. In other words, the clinical efficacy of a drug depends on the polymorph administered.

The influence of polymorphism on bioavailability of a drug is best illustrated by chloremphenicol palmitate which exists in three crystalline forms designated as A, B and C. Polymorph A is the stable form, B is the metastable form and C is the unstable form under normal conditions of temperature and pressure. Polymorph C is too unstable to be included in the formulation, but polymorph B is sufficiently stable so that it can be formulated as a dosage form. Bioavailability of orally administered suspensions of polymorphs A and B reveals that polymorph B could produce therapeutic levels in the plasma while polymorph A fails to produce biological activity. This is attributed to the more rapid in-vivo dissolution of the metastable polymorph B of chloremphenicol palmitate. Following dissolution, chloremphenicol palmitate is hydrolyzed to give free chloremphenicol in solution, which is then absorbed. The stable polymorph A of chloremphenicol palmitate dissolves so slowly and consequently is hydrolyzed so slowly to chloremphenicol in-vivo that this polymorph is virtually without biological activity.

Crystalline form II of sulfonamide is about twice as soluble as crystalline form III. Studies in normal human subjects show that the rate and extent of absorption of the sulfonamide are about 40% greater after administration of form II than after administration of form III.

Polymorphism can also be a factor in formulation technology. Cortisone acetate is found to exist in at least five different forms, four of which are found to be unstable in the presence of water and which change to a stable form. Since this transformation of soluble metastable forms to stable form involves appreciable caking of the crystals, only stable form of cortisone acetate should be used in preparing a suspension.

In addition to different polymorphic crystalline forms, a drug may exists in an amorphous form. Amorphous forms are typically prepared by rapid precipitation, lyophilization, or rapid cooling of liquid melts. Since amorphous forms are usually of a higher thermodynamic energy than the corresponding crystalline forms, solubilities as well as dissolution rates are generally greater. Therefore, there is a possibility that amorphous form of a drug may show a higher bioavailability than that of the crystalline form.

A classic example of the influence of an amorphous versus crystalline form of a drug on its gastrointestinal bioavailability is provided by novobiocin. The amorphous form of novobiocin is at least 10 times more soluble than the crystalline form. Studies in dogs fail to detect any absorption of novobiocin after oral administration of the crystalline form. The more soluble amorphous form of novobiocin is readily absorbed following oral administration. An important observation made in the case of an aqueous suspension of novobiocin is that thermodynamically unstable amorphous form converts slowly into the stable crystalline form upon storage. This conversion of the amorphous form of novobiocin to the stable crystalline form results in a loss of the therapeutic effectiveness of the dosage form.

Solvate Formation

A Solvate is a molecular complex that has incorporated the crystallizing solvent molecules into specific sites within the crystal lattice. When the incorporated solvent is water, the complex is called a hydrate. A crystal not containing any water within its structure is termed anhydrous.

In general, hydrates show a less aqueous solubility than their corresponding anhydrous forms. Conversion of an anhydrous compound to a hydrate within a dosage form may reduce the dissolution rate and the extent of absorption. In a study, the anhydrous and trihydrate forms of ampicillin were administered orally as a suspension to human subjects. The more soluble anhydrous form produced higher and earlier peaks in the blood serum levels than the less soluble trihydrate form.

Studies in humans indicate that the rate and the extent of absorption of griseofulvin are significantly increased after administration of a chloroform solvate compared to that observed after administration of the non-solvated form of the drug. These findings are consistent with the greater solubility and dissolution rate of the solvates in a simulated intestinal fluid.

Soluble Prodrugs

While salt formation is limited to molecules with ionizable groups, prodrugs may be formed with any organic molecule having a chemically reactive functional group. Prodrugs are synthetic derivatives of drug molecules that may have an intrinsic pharmacological activity but usually must undergo some transformation in-vivo to liberate the active drug molecule. Because of a rapid dissolution rate, soluble prodrugs exhibit an improved rate and extent of absorption from the GIT.

The widely used benzodiazepine, and diazepam, undergoes a biotransformation to form the active metabolite nordiazepam. Clorazepate is a prodrug of nordiazepam and is marketed as dipotassium salt that is freely soluble in water, in contrast to the poorly soluble nordiazepam. Clorezepate is converted into nordiazepam in gastric fluid and hence shows improved absorption.

Water soluble prodrugs can be produced by adding selected amino acids that are substrates for the enzymes located in the intestinal brush border. Assuming that the enzyme cleavage is not a rate-limiting step, and that the liberated drug molecule would remain in the lipophilic membrane, then the transport of the parent drug should be very rapid. Using the lysine ester prodrug of estrone, a potential increase of five orders of magnitude in absorption rate is found in-vivo using perfused rat intestine.

Complexation

Complexation of a drug in gastrointestinal fluids may alter the rate and, in some cases, the extent of absorption. The drug may form complex with the components of a formulation, regular components of the GIT, or the components of the diet. The influence of the complexation of a drug on its rate and the extent of absorption depends on whether the complex formed is soluble or insoluble in the GI fluids. Further, the soluble complex of a drug should dissociate to liberate the parent drug for absorption. Thus, it appears that it is not the magnitude of the association constant of the complex but the rate at which the complex dissociates that determines whether absorption of the drug is rapid and/or as complete as in the absence of complex formation.

Mucin is a viscous mucopolysaccharide that lines the mucosal surfaces of the stomach and intestine. It forms complexes with certain drugs. Streptomycin, dihydrostreptomycin and quaternary ammonium compounds bind strongly to the mucin forming unabsorbable complexes. Thus complexation with the mucin reduces the bioavaiblability of each of these drugs. Bile salts in the small intestine interact with certain drugs, including neomycin, kannamycin and tubocurarine, to form insoluble, non-absorbable complexes.

Tetracyclines provide an example of drugs whose bioavailabilities are reduced by the formation of poorly soluble complexes with dietary components. Tetracyclines form insoluble complexes with calcium ions and other polyvalent metal ions present in milk, certain foods, or other sources such as antacids. Tetracyclines bioavailability is reduced on concomitant administration with ferrous sulfate due to complexation.

Complexation probably occurs often in pharmaceutical dosage forms. Complex formation between drugs and gums, cellulose derivatives, polyols, or surfactants is common. The extent of absorption of tetracycline is reduced if dicalcium phosphate is included as a diluent in a tablet or a hard gelatin capsule. Amphetamine forms a poorly soluble complex with sodium carboxymethylcellulose, which is responsible for the observed reduction in bioavailability of amphetamine from a dosage form containing sodium CMC as an excipient. Phenobarbital forms an insoluble complex with polyethylene glycol 4000. The dissolution and absorption rates of phenobarbital from tablets containing this polyol are markedly reduced. In many cases, the drug-excipient complexes are soluble in the GI fluids and rapidly dissociate to liberate the 'free' drug. In such cases little or no effect of complexation on drug absorption is noted.

Drug complexes usually differ appreciably from the free drug with respect to water solubility, dissolution and lipid partition coefficient. Therefore, complexation of a poorly absorbable drug with certain compounds to form a lipid soluble complex may be used to improve the absorption of a drug. For example, dialklylamides improves the absorption of prednisone by forming lipid soluble complexes with prednisone. The gastrointestinal absorption of ergotamine tartarate is increased by a simultaneous intake of caffiene. Digoxin absorption from GIT is improved when it is administered as hydroquinone-digoxin complex. Hydroquinone forms a water-soluble, rapidly dissolving complex with digoxin. The complex is quickly and completely dissociated when dissolved.

Adsorption

The concurrent administration of drugs and medicinal products containing solid adsorbents (e.g. antidiarrhoeal mixtures) may result in the adsorbents interfering with the absorption of such drugs from the GIT. The adsorption of a drug onto solid adsorbents such as kaolin, attapulgite or charcoal may reduce the rate and/or extent of drug absorption from the GIT. Adsorption of drugs onto solid adsorbents leads to the reduction in the concentration of the 'free' drug in the GI fluids available for absorption. Whether or not an adsorption of drug onto a solid adsorbent affect the rate and/or extent of drug absorption depends on whether or not adsorbed drug is released into the GI fluids. If the drug-adsorbent interaction is readily reversible, drug will be released from the solid adsorbent into the GI fluid to replace the free drug that has been absorbed from GIT.

Promazine adsorbs onto attapulgite and charcoal when administered concurrently. Attapulgite decreased the rate but not the extent of absorption of promazine. Charcoal significantly reduces both the rate and the extent of absorption of promazine. Studies indicate that promazine-attapulgite adsorbate is readily dissociated during absorption of promazine from the GIT, while promazine-charcoal adsorbate has shown little tendency to dissociate. Bioavailability of lincomycine is reduced when administered with kaolin-pectin preparation. Parallel in-vitro studies showed that the mixture strongly binds lincomycin.

Cholestryramine and colestipol are insoluble anionic exchange resins used to lower the serum cholesterol levels in patients with hypercholesterolemia. These agents bind cholesterol metabolites and bile salts in the intestinal lumen and prevent enterohepatic cycling. Cholestryramine is found to reduce the absorption of the anti-coagulants warfarin and phenprocoumon. Colestipol resin decreased the absorption of chlorthiazid by 50%.

The inert excipients used in the formulation must be evaluated for such interactions with drugs before finalizing the formulation. Talc, which is used as an excipient in tablet formulation, is claimed to interfere with the absorption of cyanocobalamin by virtue of its ability to adsorb this vitamin.

Concentration of the Dissolved Drug in Bulk Solution, Cg

It can be seen from equation 2.10a that the saturation solubility of a drug, Cs in the diffusion layer does not of themselves determine dissolution rate. The determinant is, rather, the difference between Cs and Cg, the concentration gradient, (Cs-Cg). It is generally assumed that Cg is much smaller than Cs. It means dissolution of drugs occur under sink conditions. It should be noted that the volume of the bulk fluids is much larger than the volume of the boundary layer. Thus, a large absolute amount of a drug in the bulk fluids may still give a small value of Cg.

If the concentration of a drug in bulk fluids increases then the concentration the gradient decreases leading to a decreased rate of dissolution of the drug. For example, if a drug is absorbed through the GI membrane very slowly, the drug concentration in the GI fluids may build up. This build up would, by decreasing the concentration gradient, decrease the dissolution rate. The drug solubility in the diffusion layer and in the bulk fluids may differ significantly due to difference in pH of these fluids. A drug may be more soluble in the boundary layer and then precipitate in the bulk fluids, especially if the pH differs between these two sites. However, these precipitated particles should be quite small, and thus may rapidly dissolve. On the other hand, the drug may be more soluble in the bulk fluids than in the boundary layer because of a difference in the pH or complexation with other components. In this case, the gradient may decrease and dissolution may slow down or even stop. In most cases, an increase in Cg which affects the dissolution rate, would only occur when another process, such as membrane transport or stomach emptying becomes the rate-limiting step in drug absorption.

Diffusion Coefficient (D) and Thickness of the Stationary Layer (h)

The terms D and h in the Noyes-Whitney equation are considered to be uncontrollable by the pharmaceutical manufacturers. For a spherical, ideal drug molecule in solution, the diffusion coefficient, D, is given by

$$D = \frac{kT}{6\pi\eta r} \quad .....(2.16)$$

Where:

k = Boltzmann's constant

T = absolute temperature

h = viscosity of the solution

r = radius of the molecule in solution

In equation 2.16 k and 6p are constants. The radius r is a property of a drug molecule which can not be manipulated. The viscosity of the GI fluids in which the drug is present and temperature of the GI fluids can vary and may influence the dissolution rate of a drug. Increasing the viscosity of GI fluids will not only decrease the dissolution of a drug but also decreases the gastric emptying rate, thus the delaying delivery of the drug to the absorption site. Increasing the temperature of the GI fluids will increase the diffusion and hence the dissolution of a drug. Patients might be advised to take oral dosage forms with warm liquids. However, extremely hot liquids will delay stomach emptying.

The thickness of the stationary diffusion layer, h, is assumed to be constant and is independent of particle size. In fact, this is not necessarily true. The diffusion layer probably increases as particle size increases. Furthermore, h will be influenced by the degree of agitation experienced by each drug particle in the GIT. Hence, an increase or decrease in the GI motility would be expected to decrease or increase the thickness of the diffusion layer, thus increasing or decreasing the rate of dissolution of drugs. Noyes-Whitney equation was developed on the assumption that all the particles were spherical and of the same size. Furthermore, pharmaceutical systems often contain more than one active ingredients of different particle size distribution. Thus, the pharmaceutical systems are polydisperse and multiparticulate. Another important point to be noted is that as the dissolution proceeds the particles become progressively small, hence, h can vary considerably initially and throughout the dissolution process. In summary, D and h are largely uncontrollable factors, although they may influence bioavailability.

Drug Stability in GIT

Drugs may undergo extensive acid or enzymatic hydrolysis in the GIT which reduces the bioavailability of such drugs. The extent of hydrolysis of drugs in the GI fluids depends on the residence time of the drugs and hydrogen ion concentration or enzyme concentration. The drugs penicillin G and erythromycin are susceptible to acid hydrolysis. The half-life of degradation of penicillin G is less than 1 min. at pH 1 and about 9 min. at pH 2. The degradation rate of penicillin G decreases sharply with an increasing pH; the drug is stable in the small intestine. Bioavailability of drugs that are not stable in the stomach can be improved by minimizing the dissolution of drugs in stomach and maximizing the dissolution of drugs in the intestine. The concept of delaying the dissolution rate of a drug until it reaches the small intestine has been employed to improve the bioavailability exhibited by erythromycin from the GIT. The drug is administered orally as an enteric coated tablet. The enteric coat resists the gastric fluid, but disrupts or dissolves in intestinal fluid at a relatively alkaline pH. Hence, the drug is protected from gastric hydrolysis.

Digoxin undergoes hydrolysis in the gastric fluids to digoxigenin and its mono- and bis-digitoxosides. The rate of hydrolysis of digoxin increased with an increased hydrogen ion concentration i.e. a decreased pH.

Investigations with a series of erythromycin esters, which are unstable in the stomach, have shown than bioavailability is inversely proportional to the dissolution rate in a simulated gastric fluid (pH 1). The propionyl ester of erythromycin exhibits a greater bioavailability which dissolves slowly at the pH 1. The minimal dissolution rate of this ester in the stomach and rapid dissolution in the small intestine is responsible for the improved bioavailability of erythromycin.

Certain prodrugs must undergo degradation in the GIT to liberate their corresponding parent drug. Clorazapate is converted to nordiazepam, the active form, in the stomach. Failure to achieve a complete conversion results in a decreased bioavailability. Similarly, the esters of chloremphenicol must be hydrolyzed completely in the small intestine to liberate chloremphenicol for absorption. Clinical studies in children indicate that about 70% of chloremphenicol palmitate undergo conversion in the intestine.

In the case of erythromycin estolate, which is the lauryl sulfate salt of the ester erythromycin propionate, the improved bioavailability is because of two reasons.

1. The poorly soluble lauryl sulfate salt remains undissolved and is thus not degraded during its passage through the stomach. In the small intestine, the lauryl sulfate salt dissolves quickly and dissociates to give the ester, erythromycin propionate.
2. Erythromycin propionate is highly lipohilic and hence is absorbed quickly from the small intestine than its free base and reaches the blood circulation. In the blood, the ester erythromycin propionate undergoes hydrolysis to give erythromycin, the active form of the antibiotic.

Any failure to effectively convert a prodrug to parent drug in the GI fluids, gut wall or liver during absorption results in the prodrug reaching the systemic circulation. An important problem that may be encountered when prodrugs reach the systemic circulation in considerable amounts is the appearance of toxicity distinct from that observed with the parent drug. For example, hepato-toxicity is associated with the estolate and ethyl succinate forms of erythrtomycin.

2.5.3.2 Measurement of Dissolution Rates

Many experiments proved that the disintegration time of a solid dosage form is unable to predict the bioavailability of drug from the dosage form. From the basic principles one can expect a linear relationship between drug absorption and dissolution rather than disintegration, particularly for poorly water-soluble drugs. Dissolution tests in-vitro measures the rate and extent of dissolution of a drug in an aqueous medium from a dosage form. Extensive research work on in-vitro dissolution and in-vivo availability of drugs revealed the fact that in-vitro dissolution test can be used to predict the in-vivo performance of the dosage form. There are a number of factors that must be considered when performing a dissolution test.

The size and shape of the dissolution vessel may affect the rate and extent of dissolution. For example, the vessel may range in size from several milliliters to several liters. The shape may be flat or round bottomed so that in one case the tablet may lie in a different position in different experiments and in other case it may be in one position in all the experiments. The flow pattern of fluids and the degree of turbulence created may also be influenced by the shape.

The type of stirrer, its size and position in the vessel affects the amount of agitation in the fluid. Agitation increases the dissolution rate by increasing mixing and by decreasing the thickness of diffusion layer. Stirring rates must be controlled, and specifications differ between drug products.

The temperature of the dissolution medium must also be controlled and variations in temperature must be avoided. Most dissolution tests are performed at 37° C, the body temperature.

The nature and the quantity of the dissolution medium will also affect the dissolution test. Various investigators have used dilute gastric juice, 0.1 N HCl, phosphate buffer, acetate buffer, simulated gastric juice, water, and simulated intestinal juice, depending on the nature of the drug product and the location in the GIT where the drug is expected to dissolve. Which medium is best is a matter of considerable controversy. However, the medium selected for the study must be able to show the in-vitro and in-vivo correlation. In selecting the volume of dissolution medium, the solubility as well as the amount of drug in the dosage form must be considered. Usually, a volume of medium larger than the amount of solvent needed to completely dissolve the drug is used in such test.

The design of the dissolution test apparatus must consider all the factors discussed above. To-date there is no single apparatus and test that can be used for all drug products. Each drug product must be evaluated with a dissolution test that best correlates to its in-vivo bioavailability. The United States Pharmacopoeia has played an important role in the development of dissolution standards for many drug products.

The pharmacopoeia specifies the conditions under which a dissolution test should be carried out for a specific drug product. The specifications include the apparatus, volume and nature of dissolution medium, stirring speed, temperature of dissolution medium, and the time periods after which samples have to be collected for analysis.

Usually, the report on a dissolution test will state that a certain percentage of the labeled amount of the drug product must dissolve within a specified period of time. In practice, the absolute amount of a drug in a drug product may vary from tablet to tablet. Therefore, a number of tablets from each lot are usually tested to get a representative dissolution rate for the product.

2.5.3.2.1 Official Methods of Dissolution

This test is provided to determine compliance with the dissolution requirements where stated in the individual monograph for a tablet or capsule dosage form, except where the label states that the tablets are to be chewed. Requirements for dissolution do not apply to liquid-filled soft gelatin capsules. Of the types of apparatus described herein, use the one specified in the individual monograph.

Rotating Basket Method (Apparatus 1)

The assembly consists of the following: a vessel made up of glass, cylindrical in shape with a hemispherical bottom and a nominal capacity of 1000 ml; a cylindrical basket made up of a stainless steel mesh of No.40 and attached to a motor through a shaft. A speed-regulator is used to allow the shaft rotational speed to be selected and maintained at the rate specified in the individual monograph. The basket holds the sample and rotates in the vessel containing the dissolution medium. The entire flask is immersed in a constant temperature water bath set at 37° C.

The rotational speed and the position of the basket must meet specific requirements set forth in the current pharmacopoeia. The position and alignment of the stirrer are specified in the pharmacopoeia. Dissolution calibration standards are available to make sure that these mechanical and operating requirements are met. Individually test 1 tablet of the *USP Dissolution Calibrator, Non-disintegrating type*, according to the operating conditions specified. The apparatus is suitable if the results obtained are within the acceptable range stated in the certificate for that calibrator in the apparatus tested.

Paddle Method (Apparatus 2)

Apparatus 2 is the same as Apparatus 1, except that a paddle formed from a blade and a shaft is used as the stirring element. The metallic blade and shaft comprise a single entity that may be coated with a suitable inert coating. The paddle is vertically attached to a variable-speed motor that rotates at a controlled speed and creates minimum turbulence due to stirring. The tablet or capsule is placed into a round-bottomed dissolution flask. The dissolution flask is immersed in a water-bath maintained at 37° C. The position and alignment of the paddle are specified in the USP. The paddle method is sensitive to tilting than the basket method, therefore, improper alignment may drastically affect the dissolution results with some drug products. Calibration of the apparatus is carried out using official dissolution calibration tablets.

Methods for Testing Enteric-Coated Products

The USP provides two methods for testing enteric-coated products.

Method A

The apparatus type to be used for testing a particular drug product is specified in the drug monograph. The product is first tested in 0.1 N HCl for 2 hours, and then changed to pH 6.8 by adding 0.2 M tribasic sodium phosphate. Final adjustment of the pH of dissolution medium can be made either with 2N NaOH or HCl if necessary. The test is then generally carried for 45 minutes. No significant dissolution should occur in an acidic medium (less than 10% for any specific sample unit), and a specified percent of the drug must be released in the buffer medium. Specifications are set in the individual drug monographs.

Method B

Dissolution is carried out in the apparatus specified in the individual drug monograph (usually apparatus 1 or 2). This method involves testing the drug product in 0.1 N HCl for 2 hours, and then draining the acidic medium and replacing it with a pH 6.8 buffer medium prepared by mixing 0.2 M tribasic sodium phosphate with 0.1N HCl. The temperature of the buffer medium must be at 37° C before replacement. The acceptance criteria are the similar to those for method A.

Interpretation of Results of Dissolution Test

Unless otherwise specified in the individual monograph, the requirements are met if the quantities of an active ingredient dissolved from the units tested conform to the accompanying acceptance table (Table 2.2). Continue testing through the three stages unless the results conform to either S1 or S2. The quantity, Q, is the amount of the dissolved active ingredient specified in the individual monograph, expressed as a percentage of the labeled content; both 5% and 15% values in the acceptance table are percentages of the labeled content so that these values and Q are in the same terms.

Table 2.2 Dissolution Acceptance Table

Stage	Number of Units Tested	Acceptance Criteria
S1	6	Each unit release not less than Q+5%
S2	6	Average of 12 units (S1+S2) is equal to or greater than Q, and no unit is less than Q-15%
S3	12	Average of 24 units (S1 + S2 + S3) is equal to or greater Q, not more than 2 units are less than (Q-15%), and no unit is less than (Q-25%)

For many drug products, the passing of Q is set at about 75% in 45 min. and this standard has been proposed for all drug products. Setting the dissolution specification for a new drug product requires a thorough consideration of the physical and chemical properties of the drug. However, the dissolution test must ensure consistent bioavailability of the product. Further the test must provide for variations in manufacturing and testing variables so that a product may not be improperly rejected.

The USP monograph for aspirin tablets contains a dissolution test requiring the use of Apparatus 1 at 50 rpm with 500 ml of 0.05M acetate buffer (pH 4.5). Not less than about 80% of the aspirin in each tablet must dissolve in 30 minutes. In the case of the digoxin tablets dissolution test, Apparatus 1 is specified. The test has to be carried out at 120 rpm and the dissolution medium is diluted hydrochloric acid. Not less than 65% of the labeled amount of digoxin must dissolve in 60 minuets. Other tablets for which a dissolution requirement is provided include nitrofurantoin, phenylbutazone, hydrochlorthiazide, quinine sulfate and prednisone.

2.5.3.2.2 Unofficial Methods of Dissolution

Beaker Method

Levy and Hayes in 1960 described this method. In their original work, they used a 400 cm^3 beaker containing 250 cm^3 of dissolution medium, which was agitated by means of a three-bladed polyethylene stirrer with a diameter of 50 mm. The stirrer was immersed to a depth of 27 mm into the dissolution medium and rotated at 60 rpm. Tablets were placed in the beaker and the test was carried out by collecting samples of the dissolution medium at different time intervals. The samples were filtered and analyzed for drug content. The major disadvantages of this method are: 1. a tablet can take different positions on the bottom of the beaker, and 2. the formation of 'mounds' of particles in different positions on the flat bottom of the beaker.

Flask-Stirrer Method

This method was developed by Poole in 1969. The apparatus includes a round-bottomed flask and a stirring element similar to that used in the beaker method. The use of round-bottomed flask helps to avoid the problems that may arise from the formation of 'mounds' of particles in different positions on the flat bottom of a beaker.

Rotating Bottle Method

The equipment consists of a rotating rack that holds bottles in which the products are tested for dissolution. The dissolution medium and drug product are placed in the bottles, the bottles are capped tightly and rotated in a water-bath maintained at 37° C. At selected time intervals the samples are removed from the bottles, filtered through a 40-mesh screen, and the samples are assayed for drug content. Equal volumes of a fresh dissolution medium are added into the bottles and the dissolution test is continued. A dissolution test with a pH 1.2 medium for 1 hour, pH 2.5 medium for the next 1 hour, followed by pH 4.5 medium for 1.5 hours, a pH 7.0 medium for 1.5 hours, and pH 7.5 medium for 2 hours are recommended to simulate the condition of the GIT.

This method was suggested in NF-XIII and has become less popular. The rotating bottle method is used mainly for controlled release beads. For this purpose the dissolution media may be changed, such as from gastric juice to artificial intestinal juice. The main disadvantage is that this procedure is manual and tedious.

Flow-Through Dissolution Method

In this method, a tablet or capsule is placed in dissolution chamber and the dissolution medium is pumped through the dissolution chamber. The flow rate is usually maintained between 10 and 100 ml/min. Laminar flow of the medium is maintained by using a pulseless pump. The dissolution medium may be fresh or recirculated. In the case, where fresh dissolution medium is pumped continuously, the dissolution rate at any time point can be obtained, whereas in the official basket or paddle methods cumulative dissolution rates are obtained. When the dissolution medium is recirculated, cumulative dissolution rates are obtained. A major advantage of the flow through method is the easy maintenance of a sink condition for dissolution. A large volume of dissolution medium may also be used, and the mode of operation is easily adopted to automated equipment.

Rotating and Static Disc Methods (Intrinsic Dissolution Method)

In these methods, the drug that is to be assessed for the rate of dissolution is compressed into a non-disintegrating disc without excipients. The disc is mounted in a holder so that only one face of the disc is exposed to the dissolution medium. The holder and the disc are immersed in the dissolution medium and either held in a fixed position in the static disc method or rotated at a given speed in the rotating disc method. Samples of dissolution medium are collected at predetermined times, filtered and analyzed for drug content.

In both the methods discussed above, the surface area through which the dissolution of the drug takes place is assumed to be constant. Therefore, the dissolution rate of the drug obtained from these methods is expressed as mg/cm^2.min.i.e.the amount of the drug dissolved per unit of time and unit of the surface area. This is referred to as intrinsic dissolution rate and is different from the dissolution rates estimated by using other methods in which the surface area for dissolution is not constant.

2.5.3.3 Control of Variables in Dissolution Testing

There are a number of methods and equipment for the assessment of dissolution rate of drug products. There are several equipment and operating variables associated with dissolution testing. Even if the discussion is restricted to the official methods, the problems of variable control in dissolution testing still exist. Variation of about 25% or more occur with the same type of equipment and procedure. The variables may or may not exert a profound effect on the dissolution rate of the drug, depending upon the particular dosage form.

The basket method is more sensitive to clogging due to gummy materials. Fine drug particles and sticky materials can clog up the basket screen and decrease the dissolution rate by creating a local non-sink condition for dissolution. The centering and alignment of the paddle is critical in the paddle method. Turbulence can create an increased agitation, resulting in a higher dissolution rate. Wobbling and tilting due to worn equipment should be avoided. The basket method is relatively insensitive to the tilting effect. Degassing of the dissolution medium is to be carried out before testing, since the dissolved gases may form air bubbles on the surface of the dosage form and can affect dissolution in both the basket and paddle methods.

For many drug products, the dissolution rates are higher with the paddle method than the basket method. Dissolution rates obtained at 50 rpm with the paddle method may be comparable with the dissolution rates obtained at 100 rpm with the basket method. It was observed that the dissolution rates obtained with the paddle method from theophylline tablets of 4.0 kg hardness at 50 rpm were higher than that of basket method. This difference in the dissolution rates was not observed when the tablets of 6.8 kg hardness were tested at 125 rpm by both the methods. However, the dissolution rates were increased with increase in stirring rate. No simple correlation can be made for dissolution results obtained with different methods.

It is generally impossible to make meaningful conclusions about bioavailability from dissolution data alone, unless an in-vitro and in-vivo correlation has been well established. The use of various testing methods makes it even more difficult to interpret dissolution results, because there is no simple correlation among dissolution results obtained with various methods. In the absence of in-vivo data, the selection of the dissolution method is based on the type of drug product to be tested. For example, a gummy preparation may clog up the basket screen, a low-density preparation may be poorly wetted in the basket method, and therefore the paddle method is preferred.

2.5.3.4 In-vitro and In-vivo Correlations

Bioavailability testing is a complicated and expensive way to ensure the proper performance of drug products. Great economies in time, labor, and money would be possible if in-vitro tests could be developed that would predict bioavailability. Such in-vitro tests, if available, could be used as quality control tests and compendial standards and would help to ensure that every drug product performs as expected. It is not that simple to predict the biological performance of a drug product based on in-vitro test results alone. Bioavailability problems have arisen with tetracycline tablets, nitrofurantoin tablets and digoxin tablets in products that meet all compendial tests and have similar in-vitro performance.

Several research publications describe a good correlation between the in-vitro dissolution profile and bioavailability of the dosage form. Quantitative linear correlations between in-vivo data and dissolution data have been found with different brands of prolonged released amphetamine, aspirin tablets, different esters of erythromycin and different salts of penicillin V. An excellent correlation was observed between the dissolution rate of oxazepam tablet and the peak concentration of oxazepam in the blood following oral administration of the tablet. In another study, it was found that the percent of salicylamide in solution and the mean percentage of the dose excreted in urine were linearly correlated.

Percent of Drug Dissolved In-vitro versus Peak Plasma Concentration : One of the ways of checking the in-vitro and in-vivo correlation is to measure the percent of the drug released from different dosage forms and also to estimate the peak plasma concentrations achieved by them and then to check the correlation between them. It is expected that a poorly formulated dosage form releases a less amount of the drug than a well formulated dosage form, and, hence the amount of the drug available for absorption is less for poorly foumulated dosage form than from a well formulated dosage form. Therefore, the peak plasma concentration, which is a function of the amount of the drug available for absorption, will be higher for a well formulated drug product than that of a poorly formulated dosage form. Several products were tested and a linear correlation was observed between the maximum drug concentration in the body and the percent of the drug dissolved in-vitro.

Percent of Drug Dissolved Versus Percent of Drug Absorbed : If the dissolution rate is the limiting step in the absorption of a drug, and is absorbed completely after dissolution, a linear correlation may be obtained by comparing the percent of the drug absorbed to the percent of the drug dissolved. In choosing the dissolution method, one must consider the an appropriate dissolution medium and use a dissolution stirring rate so that in-vivo dissolution is approximated.

The drug aspirin is absorbed rapidly and completely from the GIT. Therefore, a change in the dissolution rate from a dosage form may be reflected in a change in the amount and rate of drug absorption during the period of observation. It should be remembered that differences in the dissolution rates of dosage forms will be reflected in the rate and extent of the drug only if the drug absorption is dissolution rate limited. If the rate limiting step in the bioavailability of a drug is the rate of absorption of the drug, a change in dissolution rate may not be reflected in a change in the rate and extent of drug absorption from the dosage forms.

Dissolution Rate Versus Absorption Rate: Provided that the rate of drug absorption is dependent on the rate at which the drug is presented in solution, a linear correlation may be expected between the dissolution rate and the absorption rate of the drug. Therefore, a faster dissolution rate may result in a faster rate of appearance of the drug in the plasma.

The absorption rate is usually more difficult to determine than the absorption time. Since the absorption rate and absorption time of a drug are inversely correlated, the absorption time may be used in correlating the dissolution data to the absorption data. In the analysis of in-vitro and in-vivo drug correlation, rapid drug absorption may be distinguished from the slower drug absorption by observation of the absorption time for the dosage form. The quicker the absorption of the drug the less is the absorption time required for the absorption of a certain amount of the drug. The time required for the dissolution of a fixed amount of a drug from the dosage form and the time required for the absorption of the same amount of drug from the dosage form are correlated. In one study, the dissolution time for the drug products were linearly correlated to the absorption times for various amounts of aspirin absorbed from three sustainedly released aspirin products. The results from this study demonstrate that aspirin was rapidly absorbed and was very much dependent on the dissolution rate for absorption.

Percent of Drug Dissolved Versus Serum Drug Concentration: For drugs whose absorption from GIT is dissolution rate limited, a linear correlation may be established between the percent of drug dissolved at specified times and the serum drug concentrations at corresponding times. In a study on aspirin absorption the percent of drug dissolved in the dissolution medium was correlated to the serum concentration of aspirin. The dissolution medium was a simulated gastric juice. Because aspirin is rapidly absorbed from the stomach, the dissolution of the drug is a rate-limiting step. Therefore, differences in the serum concentration of aspirin were observed for the formulations with different dissolution rates.

Percent of Drug Dissolved Versus Percent of the Dose Excreted in Urine: It has been observed that the percent of a drug dissolved and the percent of drug absorbed are linearly correlated. There exists a linear correlation between the amount of drug in body and the amount of the drug excreted in the urine. Therefore, a linear relation may be established between the percent of the drug dissolved and the percent of the dose excreted in the urine. In a study, a linear relationship was obtained between the percentage of salicylamide dissolved in either 15 or 20 minutes and the mean percentage of the dose excreted in the urine.

2.5.3.5 Limitations of Dissolution Test

An established in-vitro and in-vivo correlation holds good for a formulation as long as the quality and quantity of ingredients and the manufacturing procedures used in the production of the formulation are unchanged. However, if significant formulation changes are made, further bioavailability testing might be warranted to re-establish the correlation. Further, the changes that occur in a dosage form during storage may severely affect the established correlation. It has been reported that a good correlation that was established between the in-vitro dissolution rate and the in-vivo availability in humans for fresh methaqualone tablets was not holding good for methaqualone tablets subjected for stability testing.

It should be recognized that the active ingredient in any dosage form may interact with the excipient in a given dosage form or some endogenous material in the gastrointestinal tract. Such complexes may not prevent the dissolution of the active ingredient, but could conceivably prevent its absorption in-vivo.

We still lack scientific sophistication to predict the bioavailability characteristics of drug products, taking into account such factors as gastrointestinal function, pre-systemic metabolism, inter- or intra-subject variability and the mechanisms of drug release from the dosage form, from purely physical data such as drug dissolution profiles. However, a precise, sensitive, and reproducible dissolution test is a useful tool in the quality control process, especially where the relationship between differences in the dissolution rate or the extent and differences in bioavailability properties have been established for a particular product. The alterations in processing conditions or the drug or raw material properties can affect the bioavailability of the product.

2.6 Metabolic Factors

A drug must pass sequentially from the gastrointestinal lumen, through the gut wall, and through the liver, before entering the general circulation. This sequence is an anatomic requirement because blood perfusing virtually all gastrointestinal tissues drains into the liver via the hepatic portal vein. Drug loss may occur in the GIT due to the instability of the drug in the GIT and/or due to complexation of drug with the components of the GI fluids, food, formulation excipients or other co-administered drugs. In addition, the drug may undergo distruction within the walls of the GIT and/or liver.

2.6.1 Drug Loss in GIT

Any reaction that competes with the absorption of a drug may reduce the oral bioavailability of a drug. Table.2.3 lists various reactions that can occur within the GIT. Reactions can be both enzymatic and non-enzymatic. Acid hydrolysis is a common non-enzymatic reaction. Enzymes in the intestinal epithelium and within the intestinal microflora, which normally reside in the large bowel, metabolize some drugs. The reaction products are often inactive or less potent than the parent molecule.

The complexities that occur in-vivo preclude accurate prediction of the contribution of a competing reaction to decreased bioavailability.

Table 2.3 Drugs Affected by Reactions that Occur in GIT.

Reaction	Drug	Remarks
Complexation	Tetracycline	Unabsorbed insoluble complexes with polyvalent
Conjugation Glucuronidation Decarboxylation	Sulfoconjugation Salicylamide Levodopa	Isoproterenol Loss of activity Loss of activity Loss of activity
Hydrolysis **Acid**	Penicillin G Erythromycin Digoxin	Loss of activity Loss of activity Product (digitoxides) have variable activity
Enzymatic	Aspirin Pivampicillin Insulin	Aspirin Salicylic acid formed, active anti-inflammatory Active ampicillin formed: pivampicillin (ester) is inactive Loss of activity
Oxidation	Cyclosporine	Loss of activity
Reduction	Sulfasalazine	Intended for local (intestinal) anti-inflammatory action; parent drug may have some activity; product 5 amino salicylic acid is active
Adsorption	Digitoxin	Adsorption of the drug to cholestyramine leads to poor bioavailability

2.6.2 Drug Loss in Liver

All drugs that are absorbed from the stomach, small intestine and colon pass into the hepatic portal system and are presented to the liver before reaching the systemic circulation. The liver is the primary site of drug metabolism. Hence, this first pass of an absorbed drug through the liver may result in extensive metabolism of the drug and a significant proportion of the absorbed dose of intact drug may never reach the systemic circulation. This phenomenon is known as the **first pass effect** and results in a decrease in bioavailability of those drugs which are rapidly metabolized by the liver (Fig. 2.27).

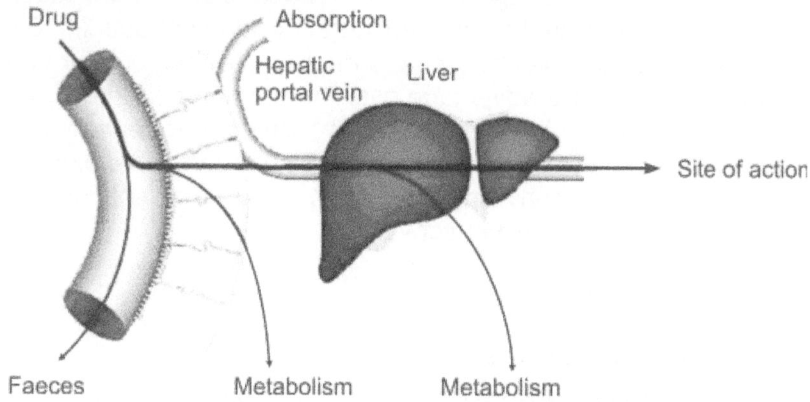

Fig. 2.27 First Pass metabolism.

Drugs that show a substantial first-pass effect due to hepatic elimination are listed in Table 2.4. Apart from this feature, they have little in common. They are of diverse chemical structures, possess different pharmacologic activities, and are metabolized via a number of pathways. When the metabolite(s) formed during the first pass through the liver, they are less potent than the parent drug, and the oral dose required is lager than the I.V. or I.M. dose to achieve the same therapeutic effect. This occurs for many drugs listed in Table 2.4. In the case of isoproterenol, hepatic extraction is so high that it is impossible to achieve the therapeutic level in the blood by the oral route. Pharmaceutical manipulations are insufficient to improve the situation. It is better to administer the drug by the parentral route or to discard the drug in favor of another drug.

Table 2.4 Drugs that Exhibit Low Oral Bioavailability Due to First-Pass Effect

Alprenolol	Hydrolazine	Neostigmine
Amitriptyline	Imipramine	Nicardipine
Chlormethiazole	Isoproterenol	Nicotine
Chlorpromazine	Isosorbide dinitrate	Nifedipine
Cytarabine	Ketamine	Nitroglycerine
Desipramine	Labetolol	Papaverine
Dextropropoxyphene	Lidocaine	Phenacetin
Dihydroergotamine	Lorcainide	Pentazocine
Diltiazem	Mercaptopurine	Pentoxifyline
Doxorubin	Methylphenidate	Propranolol
Encainide	Metoprolol	Scopalamine
Estradiol	Morphine	Testosterone
5-Fluorouracil	Nalbuphine	Verapamil

Avoiding the first pass through the liver probably explains the most of the activity of nitroglycerin administered sublingually for an acute anginal attack. Blood perfusing the buccal cavity bypasses the liver and enters directly into the superior venacava. Similarly, the rectal route has a definite advantage over the oral route for drugs destroyed by gastric acidity or by enzymes in the intestinal wall and microflora. Potentially, the rectal route may also partially reduce the first-pass hepatic loss. Part of the rectal blood supply, particularly the inferior and middle hemorrhoidal veins, bypasses the hepatic portal circulation and dumps directly into the inferior venacava.

2.7 Complicated Factors

2.7.1 Drug-Food Interactions

In general, gastrointestinal absorption is favored by an empty stomach. However, some drugs have to be given with or after a meal in order to avoid gastric irritation or to reduce the side effects. Food will reduce the rate and/or extent of absorption by virtue of reduced gastric emptying rate, which is particularly important for the drugs unstable in gastric fluids and for dosage forms designed to release drug slowly. In addition, food provides a rather viscous environment which will reduce the rate of drug dissolution and drug diffusion to the absorbing membrane. Drugs may also bind to food particles or react with the gastrointestinal fluids secreted in response to the presence of food.

Examples of drug-food interaction include digoxin, acetaminophen, phenobarbital sodium, various sulphonamides and cephalexin, among others. Administration of certain antibiotics after a meal frequently results in a significant decrease in both the rate and the extent of absorption. This has been observed with certain tetracyclines and penicillins, lincomycin and rifampicin.

The absorption of a few drugs is actually promoted when administered after a meal. For example, the absorption of riboflavin is greater when administered after a meal. The absorption of griseofulvin is doubled when administered after a meal containing a high fat content. The bioavailability of chlorthiazide is increased when taken immediately following a meal compared to that found in fasting subjects.

Food may influence drug bioavailability by means of the following mechanisms.

1. **Increased Viscosity of Gastrointestinal Contents:** The presence of food in the gastrointestinal tract will provide a viscous environment which may result in a reduction in the rate of dissolution in the gastrointestinal contents. In addition, the rate of diffusion of a drug in solution from the lumen to the absorbing surface may be reduced by an increase in viscosity. Both of these effects will tend to decrease the bioavailability of the drug.
2. **Alteration in the Rate of Gastric Emptying:** For instance, hot solid meals containing high amounts of fat tend to decrease the gastric emptying rate and thereby delay the on set of drug action.
3. **Stimulation of Gastrointestinal Secretions:** Food stimulates the secretions from the GIT. The gastric secretions (hydrochloric acid and pepsin) and intestinal secretions

(bile salts, bile acids, enzymes etc.,) influence the drug stability and the absorption rate. Degradation of drugs takes place in the GIT due to chemical hydrolysis and enzymatic metabolism and results in a reduced bioavailabilty of such drugs. Bile salts are surface active agents and can increase the absorption of certain drugs by increasing their rate of dissolution in the GI fluids (e.g. griseofulvin). However, bile salts have been shown to form insoluble, non-absorbable complexes with such drugs as neomycin, kanamycin and nystatin.

4. **Competitive Inhibition of Drug Absorption by Food Components:** The specialized absorption mechanisms are developed for the absorption of nutrients. Drugs which show a structural similarity with these nutrients are also absorbed by the same mechanism. Therefore, a competitive inhibition of drug absorption may be observed in the presence of nutrients. One example appears to be levodopa whose absorption may be inhibited by certain amino acids resulting from the break down of the ingested proteins.
5. **Complexation of Drugs With Dietary Components:** Tetracyclines form insoluble and non-absorbable complexes with calcium ions present in the diet. This is the reason for the reduced absorption of tetracyclines when administered along with milk. Foods containing a high iron content also reduce the bioavailability of tetracylines. In general, reduction in bioavailability due to complexation is observed only when drug forms an irreversible or un-absorbable complexes with the dietary components.
6. **Blood Flow to the Liver:** Blood flow to the GIT and liver increases shortly after a meal. This increased blood flow to the liver will increase the rate at which drugs are presented to the liver. The metabolism of some drugs (e.g. propranolol, hydralazine, dextropropoxyphene) is sensitive to their rate of presentation to the liver. The greater the rate of presentation of such drugs to the liver the larger the fraction of the drug that escapes first-pass metabolism. This is because the enzyme systems responsible for their metabolism become saturated at that rate of presentation of drugs to the liver.

2.7.2 Disease States

Gastrointestinal disorders and disease states are likely to influence drug absorption. Gastric fluid pH is elevated in patients with gastric cancer and achlorhydria. Alteration in drug absorption due to changes in the gut pH will most likely to be mediated by its influence on the dissolution rate. Aspirin appeared to be better absorbed in achlorhydric subjects than in normal subjects.

Changes in gastric emptying rate are expected to influence the rate and possibly the extent of absorption, for the reasons discussed previously. Gastric emptying rate is reversibly reduced soon after gastric surgery, as a result of pyloric stenosis and in the presence of various diseases. Riboflavin absorption is increased in hypothyroidism and reduced in hyperthyroidism.

Diarrheal conditions may decrease drug absorption as a result of reduced intestinal residence time. The absorption of several drugs is reduced in response to lactose- and saline-induced diarrhea.

There are various malabsorpiton syndromes known to influence the absorption of certain nutrients. Studies concerned with drug absorption in patients with malabsorption have been limited, and the results of such studies generally have not been remarkable. Reduced absorption of digoxin in patients with sprue, malabsorption, and pancreatic insufficiency has been reported.

As most drugs are best absorbed from the small intestine, any surgical procedure that removes a substantial portion of the small intestine is likely to influence drug absorption. A strong correlation was noted between the length of jejunum remaining in continuity and the area under the digoxin concentration in serum versus time curve.

If there is a reduction in bioavailability of a drug due to any of the pathological conditions or disease states cited earlier, a practical approach to solve this problem is to optimize the absorption of the drug from the GIT. To do this, a practical approach might well be to administer the drug in a form readily available for absorption. In most cases, if possible, administration of a drug in form solution will represent the best way to achieve maximal absorption, as this will eliminate the time needed for drug dissolution of a solid oral dosage form in the gut. When absorption can not be sufficiently improved by use of a drug solution, alternative routes of administration must be considered (e.g., an intra- venous or an intra-muscular route).

2.7.3 Age

The majority of data accumulated in the literature concerned with drug absorption is obtained from studies conducted in young adults. Information about drug absorption in subjects of two extremes of age spectrum (i.e. pediatric and geriatric populations) is very less. For a variety of reasons one would expect the absorption process in the later groups to be different from that in young adults. Unfortunately, at present there is too little information to present valid general statements.

Clinical experiments can not be carried out in the pediatric population (neonates, infants and children) because of ethical considerations. A further complication is the rapid development of organ functions, which is likely to influence results even over a relatively short experimental period (e.g. 2 to 4 weeks), especially in neonates and infants.

Acid secretion in the stomach is related to the development of the gastric mucosa, therefore, gastric fluid is less acidic in the new born than in adults. This condition appears to last for some time, as pH values similar to the adult are not reached until after about 2 years. The higher gastric fluid pH and smaller gut fluid volume may influence the dissolution rate and the stability of acid-unstable drugs.

The gastric emptying rate in neonates appears to be slow at least in first 6 months when compared to adults. Accordingly, the absorption of riboflavin was found to be steady in neonates and fast in infants. Intestinal transit tends to be irregular and may be modified by the type of food ingested and the feeding pattern.

Intestinal surface area and total blood flow to the GIT are smaller pediatrics than in adults and may influence the efficiency of absorption. The drug absorption from suppositories may be incomplete and irregular in young because of irregular bowel movements. It is always better to use drugs in a solution form rather than a solid dosage form for a better absorption in the young.

There is a need to conduct experiments in elderly population to understand drug disposition, because of a number of important and unique characteristics of elderly population (e.g., they consume more drugs per capita, they suffer from more diseases and physical impairments, and their percentage of the population is increasing, etc.,).

There are substantial changes in a variety of physiologic functions in the elderly which may influence drug absorption, including a greater incidence of achlorhydria, altered gastric emptying, reduced gut blood flow, and a smaller intestinal surface area. There are, in addition, other factors that may influence absorption, such as a greater incidence of GI diseases, altered nutritional intake and eating habits, and ingestion of a drug which may affect the absorption of other drugs. Although data are still somewhat limited, the general impression is that the rate of absorption is frequently reduced, while there is little if any change in the extent of absorption.

2.8 Formulation Factors

Physiological factors and physicochemical properties of a drug itself have shown to influence the rate and/or the extent of drug absorption from GIT. Since drugs are administered in a suitable dosage form, the components of the dosage form and production methodologies can also influence the bioavailability of a drug. Drugs are almost never administered alone to a patient but in the form of dosage forms which have been carefully designed to deliver the drug to the biological system so as to achieve desired therapeutic effect. Modern dosage form is a drug delivery system whose selection is as important and critical as the selection of the drug itself for the treatment of a disease. The difference in the rate or extent of absorption of a drug from one formulation to another may range from 2 to 5-fold. A difference of more than 60-fold has been observed in the absorption rate of spiranolactone from the worst formulation to the best formulation.

2.8.1 Influence of Excipients

Excipients are physiologically inert substances that are included in a formulation along with the drug to facilitate the preparation, patient acceptability, drug stability and functioning of the dosage form as a drug delivery system. Although excipients are considered to be inert, they can potentially influence the rate and/or extent of absorption of drugs.

For example,

Drug	Excipient	Effect
Tetracyclines	dicalcium phosphate	Form water-insoluble, unabsorbable complexes
Amphetamine sodium	carboxymethylcellulose	Form water-insoluble, unabsorbable complexes
phenobarbitone	polyethylene glycol 4000	Form water-insoluble, unabsorbable complexes
Ranitidine	Sucrose	Decrease absorption
Tolbutamide	Pregelatinized corn starch	Increased absorption leading to toxic effect
Furosemide	Sodium starch glycolate	increase the bioavailability of furosemide

Diluents

An outbreak of phenytoin intoxication occurred in Australia when the diluent lactose was used in a capsule dosage form of sodium phenytoin instead of calcium sulfate dihydrate. This was due to the fact that calcium sulfate dihydrate formed the calcium-phenytoin complex and reduced the GI absorption. Therefore, when lactose was used as a diluent, the entire dose of sodium phenytoin was available for absorption. This lead to very high levels of phenytoin in plasma that exceeded the maximum safe levels and produced toxic side effects.

In a study evaluating formulations of the non-steroidal anti-inflammatory drug (NSAID) aspirin, the effect of gluconolactone as a direct compression diluents was compared with the established diluent, anhydrous lactose. There was less hydrolysis of aspirin when it was formulated with gluconolactone thus more drug was available for absorption.

Surfactants

Surfactants are often employed as wetting agents, suspension stabilizers, emulsifying agents or solubilizing agents in dosage forms. Surfactants are found to be capable of either increasing, decreasing or exerting no effect on the absorption of drugs across the biological membrane. Furthermore, they might also be able to produce significant changes in the biological activity of drugs by perhaps exerting an influence on drug metabolizing enzymes or on the binding of drugs to the receptor proteins.

It is interesting to note that surfactant increases the absorption of a poorly water soluble drug at lower concentration, but decrease at higher concentrations. At lower concentrations they may improve the dissolution rate of the drug and also disrupt the integrity and function of a membrane. These membrane-disrupting effects of surfactants increase the membrane penetration of the drug. Inhibition of absorption of poorly water soluble drugs by surfactants at higher concentrations is due to the micellar solubulization of drugs. Micellar solubulization of drugs causes a reduction in 'free' drug concentration in the GI fluids leading to a decreased rate and/or extent of drug absorption.

Polysorbate 80 enhances the absorption of Phenacetin from a suspension dosage form by preventing aggregation and thus increasing the effective surface area and the dissolution rate of the drug particles in the GI fluids.

Besides, therapeutic use of Tween 20Tween 80, Myrj 52, and Brij 30 were also found to inhibit intestinal P-gp, MRPs, and other pump proteins and thus may be used to improve the oral bioavailability of epirubicin or other anticancer molecules that are candidate for PGP efflux. MDR-reversing agents in drug formulations, pharmaceutical excipients may exhibit lower systemic side-effects and improve oral absorption of drugs in MDR spectrum. The combined use of anticancer drugs with these excipients may have significant implications in circumventing multidrug resistance in cancer chemotherapy. It provides a potential strategy for improving bioavailability in the optimization of formulations for drugs performing Pluronic P85 increases permeability of a broad spectrum of intestinal absorption and secretion.

Surfactants could influence drug absorption from the GIT by altering the gastric residence time of a drug by exerting a physiological action. Therefore, surfactants can influence the absorption of a drug by variety of mechanisms of which some may enhance drug absorption while others may reduce it. The observed effect on drug absorption will depend on which of the different actions is the over-riding one. The ability of a surfactant to influence drug absorption will also depend on the physicochemical characteristics and concentration of the surfactant, the nature of the drug and the type of biological membrane involved.

Vscosity - Enhancers

Viscosity-enhancing agents are often employed in the formulation of liquid orals to control such properties as palatability, ease of pouring and in the case of suspensions, the rate of sedimentation of the dispersed particles.

Viscosity-enhancers can influence drug absorption from the GIT by several mechanisms. Any Complex formation between a drug and a hydrophilic polymer could reduce the concentration of drug in the solution which is available for drug absorption. The oral administration of viscous solutions or suspensions may produce an increase in viscosity of the GI fluids. Such an increase in viscosity could lead to the following general effects:

1. A decrease in the gastric emptying rate, i.e. an increase in gastric residence time,
2. A decrease in intestinal motility, i.e. an increase in the intestinal transit time,
3. A decrease in dissolution rate of the drug, and
4. A decrease in the rate of movement of drug molecules to the absorbing membrane.

Effects 1 and 2 may contribute to increased absorption of a drug. An extended gastric residence time, or a slower intestinal transit time produced by an increase in viscosity, would allow a longer period in which drug dissolution could occur in the GIT and this could lead to an increase in the extent of absorption of a drug from a solid dosage form. The net effect of the increased viscosity on the absorption of a particular drug from the GIT will thus depend on whether or not the absorption-enhancing effects outweigh the absorption-reducing effects of increased viscosity. Normally, effect 3 would not be applicable to solution dosage forms unless the dilution of the administered solution in the GI fluids causes a precipitation of the drug. In general, effects 1,2 and 4 influence the absorption of drugs from viscous solutions.

In the case of suspensions containing drugs whose bioavailabilities are dissolution-rate limited, an increase in viscosity could also lead to a decrease in the rate of dissolution of the drug in GI fluids. The reduction in bioavailability of nitrofurantoin from aqueous suspensions containing methylcellulose is a net result of the effect 1,2,3 and 4. In addition nitrofurantoin forms complex with methylcellulose leading to a further reduction in the absorption of nitrofurantoin.

2.8.2 Role of the Dosage Form

In addition to the amount and physicochemical properties of each excipient included in a formulation, the type of dosage form and its method of preparation or manufacture can influence bioavailability. In general, the bioavailability of a drug tends to decrease in the following order: solution> hard gelatin capsule> uncoated tablet> coated tablet. Although this ranking of the types of oral dosage forms is not universal, it does provide a useful guidance.

Solutions

With rare exceptions, drugs are absorbed more rapidly when given as a solution than in any other oral dosage form. Formulation of a drug as a solution normally eliminates the in-vivo dissolution step and presents the drug in the most readily available form for absorption. The rate-limiting step in the absorption of a drug from a solution dosage form is likely to be gastric emptying, particularly when the drug is given after a meal.

Dilution of an aqueous solution of a poorly soluble drug in the gastric fluids can result in precipitation of the drug because of various reasons. This is particularly true when the aqueous solubility of the drug has been increased by means of formulation techniques or by using the soluble salt form of the drug.

When an acidic drug is given in solution in the form of a salt, there is the possibility of precipitation in the gastric fluid. However, in most cases, the extremely fine nature of the precipitate permits a more rapid rate of dissolution. However, with highly water-insoluble drugs, like phenytoin or warfarin, this may not be the case; one may find that the absorption rate or the extent of absorption from a well formulated suspension of the free acid is greater than from a solution of the sodium salt.

Most of the times, solutions of poorly water-soluble drugs are prepared by adding co-solvents, like alcohol or propylene glycol, complexing agents that form water-soluble complexes with the drug, or surfactants in a sufficient quantity to exceed the critical micelle concentration and to effect solubulization. After administration, dilution of co-solvents, dissociation of soluble complexes or break down of micelles in gastrointestinal fluids may result in the precipitation of the drug. Experimental evidence suggests that in most cases re-dissolution of precipitate takes place rapidly.

As discussed earlier, the viscosity of a solution dosage form, particularly if a viscosity-enhancing agent has been included, influences the bioavailability of the drug.

Suspensions

Suspension is a useful dosage form for administering an insoluble or poorly water-soluble drug. A well formulated suspension is regarded as being an efficient oral drug delivery system, second in efficiency only to the solution dosage form. Usually, the absorption of a drug from a suspension is dissolution-rate limited. Drug dissolution from a suspension is rapid because of a large effective surface area, presented to the GI fluids at the site of absorption. In contrast to hard gelatin capsule and tablet dosage forms, dissolution of all drug particles commences immediately on dilution of the dose of suspension in the GI fluids. A drug contained in a tablet or a hard gelatin capsule may ultimately achieve the same state of dispersion in the GI fluids, but only after a time lag.

Several studies have demonstrated the superior bioavailability characteristics of suspensions compared to those of solid dosage forms. The rates of absorption of trimethoprim and sulfamethoxazole were found to be higher from suspension than those obtained form the capsule or tablet dosage forms of these drug combinations. However, there were no significant differences between preparations in the extent of absorption of the either drug. Similar observations have been reported with penicillin V and phenobarbitol.

Factors associated with the formulation of aqueous suspension dosage forms which can influence the bioavailability of drugs from the GIT include:

1. The particle size and effective surface area of the dispersed drug,
2. The crystal form of the drug,
3. Formation of a non-absorbable complex between the drug and its excipient,
4. The inclusion of a surface active agent in the formulation, and
5. The viscosity of the suspension.

Information concerning the potential influence of the above factors on the rate and extent of absorption of a drug is presented in earlier sections of this chapter.

Capsules

The capsule dosage form has the potential to be an efficient drug delivery system. Two types of gelatin capsules are used for the encapsulation of drugs with suitable excipients.

Soft Gelatin Capsules

The soft elastic capsule has a gelatin shell somewhat thicker than that of hard gelatin capsules, but the shell is plasticized by the addition of glycerin, sorbitol or a similar polyol. Unlike the hard gelatin capsules, the soft gelatin capsule may be used to contain aqueous solutions of a drug, or drugs that are liquids (e.g. the anti-tussives drug, benzonatate) or semi-solids (e.g. certain vitamins). Drugs encapsulated in soft gelatin capsules are dissolved or dispersed in a non-toxic, non-aqueous vehicle which may be water miscible or water immiscible. Generally, vegetable oils represent the water-immiscible class, whilst polyethylene glycols and certain non-ionic surfactants (e.g. polysorbate 80) represent water miscible class.

After oral administration, the soft gelatin shell dissolves and splits in the GI fluids and the contents of the capsule come in contact with the GI fluids. If the vehicle used in the formulation is water-miscible vehicle, it dissolves and/or disperses in GI fluids and liberates the drug. The liberated drug may exist in the GI fluids as a solution or as fine particles depending upon the solubility of the drug in the GI fluids. The drug is thus liberated in a form which is conducive to rapid absorption. Many poorly water-soluble drugs exhibited greater bioavailabilities when administered in water-miscible vehicles in a soft gelatin capsule than in hard gelatin capsules or tablets.

In the case of soft gelatin capsule containing drugs in solution or suspension in water-immiscible vehicles, release of the contents will almost certainly be followed by dispersion in the GI fluids. Emulsifiers are included in the formulation to aid the dispersion process. Bile secreted into the intestine also helps the dispersion process. If the drug is in a solution form in a digestible oil, the drug may be absorbed along with the oil by fat absorption process. If the drug is less oil soluble or is dissolved in non-digestible oil, partitioning of the drug from the oil phase into the GI fluids will be the rate-limiting step in drug absorption. Inclusion of emulsifying agents probably increases the rate of partitioning of the drug from the oil into GI fluids by increasing the surface area of contact between oil and GI fluids.

If a drug is suspended in an oily vehicle, drug release into the GI fluids involves dissolution of the drug in oily vehicle and its partition across the oil/water interface. Another possibility by which drug release could take place from such systems is that the solid drug particles may travel across the oil/aqueous interface, enter the GI fluids and undergo dissolution.

Factors that can influence the bioavailability of drugs from a soft gelatin capsule formulation include:

1. Type of vehicle used i.e. water-miscible or water-immiscible and whether the vehicle is a digestible oil or a non-digestible oil.
2. Form of the drug in the vehicle i.e. whether the drug is in solution or in suspension.
3. Particle size of the drug in case the drug is suspended in the vehicle.
4. Inclusion of a surface active agent either as a wetting agent, as an emulsifying agent or as a solubulizing agent.
5. Inclusion of a suspending agent which can increase the viscosity of the formulation.
6. Inclusion of other additives which may form non-absorbable complexes with the drug.

Hard Gelatin Capsules

Hard gelatin capsules contain drugs in powder form or as a compressed powder mass with appropriate excipients. In general, one can expect that a well formulated hard gelatin capsule dosage form will exhibit bioavailability better than or at least comparable to the bioavailability of the same drug from a compressed tablet. Drug particles in a capsule are not subjected to high compression forces that tend to compact the powder and to reduce the effective surface area. Therefore, a well formulated gelatin capsule is one which provides a rapidly dissolving gelatin shell and a quickly dispersing capsulated mass so that fine drug particles come in contact with the GI fluids for dissolution. However, the formulation of a drug in a finely divided form surrounded by a water-soluble shell does not guarantee a better bioavailability. The net dissolution rate of a drug observed from capsule results from the rates of different processes such as:

1. The dissolution rate of the hard gelatin shell in GI fluids,
2. The rate of penetration of GI fluids into the encapsulated mass,
3. The rate at which the encapsulated mass disperses in the GI fluids, and
4. The rate of dissolution of the dispersed drug particles in the GI fluids.

Diluents are necessary in a capsule dosage form, particularly when the drug is hydrophobic. The diluent serves to facilitate the rate of penetration of GI fluids into an encapsulated mass, disperse the drug particles, minimizes aggregation and the maximize effective surface area and the dissolution rate. However, the diluent should not exhibit a tendency to adsorb or complex with the drug since either can impair absorption from the GIT. For example, when dicalcium phosphate is used as a diluent in the formulation of a tetracycline capsule it forms, an insoluble and unabsorbable complex and reduces the bioavailability of tetracycline.

The incorporation of a wetting agent in the formulation may improve the dissolution rate of a poorly water-soluble drug by increasing the area of contact between the drug particles and the GI fluids. Another way of improving the wetting characteristics of poorly water-soluble drugs includes treating the drug with a solution of a hydrophilic polymer such as methylcellulose. Capsules containing phenytoin treated with methylcellulose show a greater dissolution rate and absorption rate than the capsules containing an untreated drug.

Excipients used in the formulation may influence the dissolution rate of drug from capsules. Magnesium stearate is used as a lubricant for the capsule filling operation. Because of its hydrophobic nature, magnesium sterate often retards the penetration of the GI fluids into the encapsulated mass after the dissolution of the gelatin shell. However, this problem can be solved by the inclusion of a surfactant as a wetting agent and a hydrophilic diluent in the formulation.

Both the formulation and the type and conditions of the capsule filling process can affect the packing density and liquid permeability of the encapsulated mass. If the encapsulated mass packing density is high (i.e. decrease in porosity), the liquid penetration into the encapsulated mass and the effective surface area for dissolution of drug particles decreases significantly if the drug is hydrophobic in nature.

Formulation factors which can influence the bioavailabilities of drugs from any hard gelatin capsule include:

1. Crystal form of the drug,
2. Particle size of the drug and the effective surface area available for dissolution,
3. Use of salt form of a drug in place of a parent drug (weak acid or weak base),
4. The types and quantities of various excipients,
5. Drug-excipient interactions (e.g. adsorption, complexation),
6. Chemical stability of the drug in the dosage form and in the GIT,
7. The type and conditions of the filling process,
8. The properties of the capsule shell and its interaction with the formulation,
9. The packing density of encapsulated mass, and
10. Packaging and storage conditions.

Tablets

In tablet manufacture, the drug and the excipients are mixed, granulated and punched into a tablet or the powder mix containing directly compressible vehicle is punched directly into a tablet. In either case the effective surface area of the drug particles reduces significantly due to the granulation and compression processes. After oral administration, a tablet undergoes disintegration and deaggregation in the GI fluids to regenerate well dispersed primary drug particles. Most of the bioavailability problems encountered with a tablet dosage form are due to the difficulty in regenerating well-dispersed drug particles in the GI fluids and/or slow dissolution rate of the drug from the tablet dosage form.

Formulation ingredients and the manufacturing procedures followed in the production of tablets influence the bioavailability of a drug. For example, inclusion of a suitable disintegrant before and after the granulation improves the disintegration, where as use of higher amounts of a binder leads to the production of hard granules that are difficult to disintegrate. Use of high compressional forces during the compaction of the granules or the powder mix produces tablets with greater hardness and prevents easy breakdown of the tablet leading to a decreased bioavailability.

Coated tablets, tablets developed for special purposes such as sustained release or timed-release may show a different absorption pattern depending upon the formulation. For example, enteric coated, tablets specifically release the drug in the small intestine.

Factors that influence the biological performance of the uncoated tablet dosage form includes:

1. The physicochemical properties of the drug,
2. The tablet excipients used in the formulation,
3. The method of manufacture used,
4. The type of tablet press used and the compressional force applied, and
5. The packaging and storage conditions.

Absorption of Drugs from Extravascular Sites Other Than Per Oral

Even though a majority of drugs are administered by the oral route, several drugs are administered by other non-invasive routes such as buccal, rectal, intramuscular etc., for one or more of the following reasons.

1. To prevent drug degradation in the GIT due to unfavorable pH and/or enzymes.
2. To prevent gut metabolism of drugs.
3. To prevent presystemic hepatic metabolism of drugs.
4. To improve the rate and extent of drug absorption (i.e. Biovailability).
5. To deliver the drugs those are not absorbed through GI mucosa (e.g. proteins).
6. To achieve a sustained action (e.g. intramuscular injection of penicillin).

It is important to note that the barriers involved in drug absorption from the site of these routes are similar in nature to that found in GI membrane. Therefore, a passive diffusion of the drug across these barriers is the basic absorption mechanism involved forms these sites.

Sublingual/Buccal Administration: Generally, tablets are administered by the sublingual and buccal route

Sublingual Route: The dosage form is placed beneath the tongue. 'Sublingual', literally 'under the tongue', from Latin, refers to a pharmacological route of administration in which certain drugs are entered directly into the bloodstream via absorption under the tongue. Many pharmaceuticals are prepared for sublingual administration. These commonly include cardiovascular drugs, steroids, barbiturates, some enzymes and increasingly frequently, certain vitamins and minerals.

Buccal route: The dosage form is placed between the cheek and teeth or in the cheek pouch.

Drugs administered by this route are supposed to produce systemic drug effects, and consequently, they must have good absorption from the oral mucosa. The oral mucosal regions are highly vascularized therefore a rapid on set of action is observed from these routes. For example, the anti-anginal drug nitroglycerin is administered by the sublingual route for a rapid set of action. The blood that perfuses oral regions drains directly into the general circulation. Thus, drug absorption from the oral cavity avoids the first-pass metabolism. Drugs destroyed in GIT, metabolized in gut wall and/or liver can be administered by these routes. Further, peptides and proteins and other high molecular weight drugs that are not absorbed easily from the GIT may be administered by these routes. Examples of drugs administered by these routes include antihypertensives like nefidipine, steroids like progesterone and methyltestosterone, peptides like oxytocin, and analgesics like morphine.

The important points to be considered in developing dosage forms for sublingual and buccal routes of administration are:

1. The drugs with palatable organoleptic properties such as taste and odor should be used.
2. The therapeutic dose of the drug should be low.
3. The drug selected should dissolve rapidly in saliva and should have a high saturation solubility in the saliva.
4. The drug must have good absorption properties through the oral mucosa.
5. The drug and excipient used in the formulation should not stimulate salivation. This reduces the fraction of the drug that is swallowed rather than being absorbed through the oral mucosa.

The absorption of drugs from the oral cavity is generally by passive diffusion. The physiological factors such as salivation, salivary pH, temperature and pathological conditions in the mouth influence the drug absorption.

Summary of the different Buccal dosage forms described in the literature

Dosage Forms	Structure	Release	Effect	Active Ingredients
Matrix tablets	Monolithic matrix	Sustained/bidirectional	Local/systematic	Local administration: metronidazole. Systemic administration: propamolol, timolol, metoclopramide, morphine sulphate, nitroglycerin, odein, insulin, calcitonin, glucagone-like pepcide
	Coating matrix (coated on the outer side or on all but one faces)	Monodirectional	Systemic	
	Two-layer matrix	Bidirectional	Local (mainly)	
	Two-layer matrix coated with impermeable layer	Monodirectional	Systemic	
Patches	Laminated film with coating layer	Monodirectional	Local/systemic	Local administration: diclofenac, tannic acid, boric acid. Systematic administration: tyrocropin-releasing hormone, octrrotide, oxygen, buserelin, calcitonin, leuenkephalin
Lipophilic gles	Cubic and lamellar liquid crystalline phases of glyceryl monooleare	-	Systemic	Systemic administration: (D-Ala2, D-Leu5)enkephalin
Transfersomes	Phospholipid deformable vesicles	-	Systemic	Systemic administration: insulin

Rectal Administration

The psychological feelings of patients made this route unpopular. However, this route of administration is useful for children, old people and unconscious patients. Drugs may be administered by this route for either local or systemic effects. A wide variety of drugs are administered by this route for systemic actions, e.g., analgesics, anti-spasmodics, sedatives, tranquilizers, and anti-bacterial agents.

Factors Affecting Drug Absorption from Rectal Route

Physiological Factors

1. **Blood Circulation to Rectum :** Three veins collect the blood from lower part of the colon and rectum. They are the upper, middle, and lower hemorrhoidal the veins. The lower hemorrhoidal veins surrounding the rectum enter into the inferior vana cava and thus bypass the liver. The upper hemerrhoidal vein does connect with the portal veins leading to the liver. More than half (50- 70%) of rectally administered drugs were reported to be absorbed directly into the general circulation. The lymphatic circulation also helps in absorbing a rectally administered drug in diverting the absorbed drug from the liver.
2. **pH and Lack of Buffering Capacity of the Rectal Fluids :** The pH of the rectal mucosa plays a significant rate-controlling role in drug absorption. Since rectal fluids are essentially neutral in pH (pH = 7) and have no effective buffer capacity, the dissolving drugs determine the pH existing in the anorectal area. Hence, the pH of the rectal fluids is altered by dissolving the drug and/or the excipients used in the formulation. Studies on rectal absorption of drugs reveal that the rectal mucosa is preferentially permeable for unionized drugs.
3. **Rectal Contents :** One of the rate-limiting steps in drug absorption is the diffusion of the drug to the site on the rectal mucosa at which absorption occurs. This diffusivity is influenced not only by the nature of dosage form but also by the physiological state of the colon, that is, the amount and chemical nature of the fluids and solids (fecal matter) present.
4. **Diluents' Volume:** Diluents' volume is also an important determinant of rectal drug uptake, as demonstrated with methohexital administered rectally for pre-procedure sedation. Equivalent deep sedation was achieved with 25 mg/kg of a 10% solution (0.25 mL/kg) and with 15 mg/kg of a 2% solution (0.75 mL/kg). Peak blood levels of the drug, however, were significantly higher for a longer time in the children treated with the 2% solution.

Despite the limitations associated with drug absorption in the rectum, many drugs usually administered by the intravenous and oro-gastric routes have also been administered rectally. Sedatives commonly administered by this route include midazolam, diazepam, and ketamine. In children, the rectal route is convenient for the administration of benzodiazepines to treat status epilepticus because an intravenous line is not required. The rectal dose generally must be higher than the dose administered intravenously or orally. The extent of the increase depends on the factors that affect absorption.

The most important concern with this route of administration are

1. Irregular uptake; clinically important patient-to-patient variability exists. The absorption of the drug may be delayed or prolonged, or uptake may be almost as rapid as if an intravenous bolus were administered, which may cause adverse cardiovascular or central nervous system effects.
2. the slow onset of effect (minutes) and the prolonged duration of effect (hours). The peak blood levels vary considerably from patient to patient. The potential for rapid and almost complete absorption has serious implications when drugs with cardiac or pulmonary depressant effects are administered.

The state of the anorectal membrane also plays a role in drug absorption. This membrane wall is covered with a relatively continuous mucous blanket, which can act as a mechanical barrier for a free passage of the drug through the pore space where absorption occurs.

Physicochemical Characteristics of the Drug

1. **Lipid-Water Partition Coefficient:** Drugs having high lipid-water partition coefficients exhibit higher rates of absorption through rectal mucosa which acts as a lipoidal membrane. Therefore, unionized forms of drugs are better absorbed than their corresponding ionized forms.
2. **Particle Size:** In general, the smaller the particle sizes of a drug, the more readily the dissolution of the drug particle and the greater the chance for rapid absorption.

Intravaginal Administration

The vagina is a muscular tube extending between the uterus and the external genitalia with an average length of 7.5 to 9 cm. The vagina normally contains resident bacteria supported by the nutrients found in the cervical mucus. As a result of their metabolic activities, the normal pH of the vagina ranges between 3.5 and 4.5, and this acid environment restricts the growth of many pathogenic organisms.

The vaginal walls contain a network of blood vessels and layers of smooth muscle, and the lining is moistened by the secretions of the cervical glands and by the movement of water across the permeable epithelium.

Drugs administered via vaginal route are generally absorbed by

(i) transcellularly via concentration dependent diffusionthrough the cells

(ii) paracellularly mediated by tight junctions

(iii) vesicularly or receptor mediated transport.

Absorption of drug from vaginal delivery systems occurs in two main steps: drug dissolution in vaginal lumen and membrane penetration. Any biological or formulation factor that affects drug dissolution and membrane transport could potentially affect the absorption profile from vaginal drug delivery systems. Overall, vast and multifarious factors and processes are involved in drug absorption from the vaginal route

Formulation systems experimented for vaginal drug delivery

Therapeutic drug	Intended use	Dosage form	Animal model	Comments
Nonoxynol-9	Spemicide/topica l contraceptive	Gel, foam, cream	Rabbit	Detergent type spermicide, irritation and increased risk of infections
Miconazole nitrate	Anti-fungal	Cream, suppository, swelling controlled release system	*In vitro*	-
Prostaglandin E_2	Cervical ripening	Crosslinked PEG hydrogel, suppository	*In vitro*	Onset of labor not always predictable
Lactobacilli strains	Urogenital tract infections	Bi-layered tablet	*In vitro*	Restoration of normal vaginal flora, good bacterial viability in tablets
Progestin, levonorgestrel, norethindrone acetate	Contraceptives	Vaginal ring	Human	Uterine bleeding, hormonal side effects, expulsions
Estradiol	Hormone replacement therapy	Vaginal ring	Human	Risk of endometrial proliferation
Relaxin	Cervical ripening	Gel	Human	Decreased incidence of cesarean deliveries, reduced matemal-fetal morbidity
LHRH	Hormone-dependent mammary tumors, fertility control	Suppository	Rat	Chronic administrations suppress secretion of ovarian steroids
Leuprolide	Ovulation inducing activity	Solution, suppository, jelly	Rat	Activity increased by 5 times with addition of absorption enhancers
Insulin	Diabetes mellitus	Solution, gel	Rat, rabbit	Low bioavailability

Intravaginal route was originally used for the administration of drugs to act locally in the treatment of bacterial or fungal infections or prevent contraception. Now, this route is also used for the systemic delivery of many drugs including contraceptives and steroids. Factors that influence the absorption of drugs from the vagina include the pH of the vaginal fluids, micro-organisms that normally reside in the vagina and vaginal secretions.

Intraoccular Administration

Drugs are commonly applied to the eye for a localized effect of the medication on the surface of the eye or on its interior. Most frequently sterile aqueous solutions are employed; however, non-aqueous solutions, suspensions, and ophthalmic ointments are also commonly used. Recently, ophthalmic inserts impregnated with a drug, have been developed to provide for a continuous release of drugs.

The formulations are administered in the conjunctival sac. The capacity of this sac is small, hence, small volumes in concentrated form are administered for an effective therapy. For a local action on the surface of the eye, the drug should dissolve in the lacrimal fluid. The lacrimal fluid drains continuously from the top of the eye lid to the bottom and is collected into the lacrimalduct and then passes into the nasal cavity. The pH of the lacrimal secretions influences the absorption of weak electrolytes. However, the pH of formulation also plays a role in drug absorption. In general a low pH promotes lacrimal secretion, increases lacrimal fluid drainage into the nasal cavity, and causes drug loss. High pH of the formulation decreases the flow of the lacrimal fluid and increases the drug absorption because of an increased contact time of the drug and lack of dilution of the formulation by tears. The barrier for drug penetration into the interior of the eye is the cornea that has both lipophilic and hydrophilic character with respect to drug penetration. Hence, drugs with optimum lipohilicity and hydrophilicity exhibit rapid and better absorption.

The effective "dose" of medication administered ophthalmically may be varied by the strength of medication administered, the volume administered, the pH of the dosage form, the viscosity enhancers present in dosage form, the retention time of the medication in contact with the surface of the eye and the frequency of administration.

Intranasal Administration

Generally drugs are administered by the intranasal route for the treatment of local conditions such as perennial rhinitis, allergic rhinitis, nasal decongestion etc., Recent studies on absorption of drugs through nasal mucosa revealed that the absorption of lipophilic drugs takes place mainly by passive diffusion and the absorption of polar drugs by pore transport. The rate of absorption of lipophilic drugs is found to be dependent on their molecular weight. Drugs with a molecular weight less than 400 daltons exhibit a higher rate of absorption while drugs with a molecular weight of around 1000 daltons show a moderate to satisfactory rate of absorption. The type of formulation used, the pH of the nasal secretions (generally ranges 5.5 to 6.5), and pathophysiology of the nasal mucosa influence the rate of drug transport.

Advantages

- Large nasal mucosal surface area for dose absorption
- Rapid drug absorption via highly-vascularized mucosa
- Rapid onset of action
- Ease of administration, non-invasive
- Avoidance of the gastrointestinal tract and first-pass metabolism
- Improved bioavailability
- Lower dose/reduced side effects
- Minimal aftertaste
- Improved convenience and compliance
- Self-administration

Presently, the nasal route is becoming popular for the systemic delivery of some peptide and protein drugs. This is because of the high permeability of the nasal mucosa, rich vasculature and the ease of administration. The use of intranasal drugs is not without limitations as it may cause temporary nasal irritation which may lead to discomfort.

Until recently, the modes of administering intransal preparations have been limited to nasal drops, non-pressurized nasal sprays (mists), inhalants, and intranasal gels (jellies), creams and ointments. A new alternative to these traditional intranasal preparations is the pressurized metered nasal aerosol. Intranasal aerosol offers numerous advantages, including the delivery of a measured dose of a drug, excellent depth of penetration into the nasal passageway with a minimal inadvertent penetration into the lungs, reduced droplet or particle size, lower dosage than that of the comparable systemic preparations, maintenance of sterility from dose to dose, greater patient compliance, decreased mucosal irritability, and greater flexibility in product formulation.

Pulmonary Administration

The drugs may be administered for their local action of the bronchial tree or for their systemic effects through absorption from the lungs. Inhalations, sprays and aerosols are used to deliver the drugs to the lungs. The large surface area of the alveoli, high permeability of the alveolar epithelium for drug penetration, and a rich vasculature are responsible for rapid absorption of drugs by this route. However, this route is not commonly used for systemic effects of drugs. A majority of drugs administered by this route are meant for acting on pulmonary system, for example, bronchodilators (isoproterenol sulfate, salbutamol), anti-allergics (cromolyn sodium) and anti-inflammatory (betamethasone, dexamethasone).

When drugs are administered as aerosols containing fine particles, particle size, the pH of the bronchial fluids and pathophysiological condition of the alveolar epithelium are the determinants of the drug absorption. In general particles greater than 10 mm are retained in the throat and upper airways, whereas fine particles reach the pulmonary epithelium. Metered aerosols are used to avoid variation in administered doses observed with conventional aerosols and inhalations.

Topical Administration

The skin is the outer surface of the animal body that comes in contact with the environment. It protects the interior of the body. It consists of three distinct layers called epidermis, dermis and the subcutaneous fat tissue. The epidermis consists of, from outer to the inner stratum corneum, stratum lucidum, stratum granulosum, stratum spinosum and stratum germinativum. The dermis is a highly vascularized region filled with a connective tissue, hair follicles, base of the sebaceous glands and nerve endings. Once drugs reach this region, they will be transported into the systemic circulation continuously, because of sink conditions prevailing in this region.

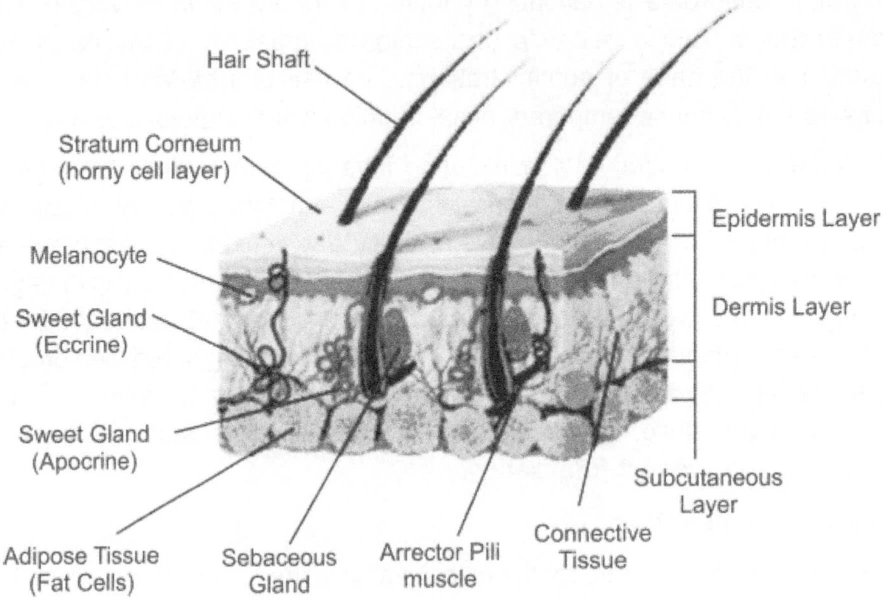

Fig. 2.28 Skin anatomy

Whether a topically applied drug is meant for local action or for a systemic effect, it has to reach the vascular region of the skin, dermis. The principle barrier for drug penetration is the "stratum corneum" of epidermis. Stratum corneum is composed of dehydrated, keratinized, dead horny epithelial cells and is about 20-40 mm thick.

The absorption of drugs through the skin is known as percutaneous absorption. Drugs can penetrate the intact skin through the walls of the hair-follicles, through the sweat glands or the sebaceous glands, between the cells of the horny layer and through the stratum corneum cells. However, the main route for the penetration of drugs is generally through the epidermal layer, rather than through the hair follicles or the gland ducts, since the surface area of the latter is rather minute compared to the area of the skin containing neither of these anatomical elements. Therefore, it can be concluded that percutaneous absorption of a drug mainly depends on the ability of the drug to penetrate the stratum corneum. In other words, the stratum corneum is the rate-limiting barrier in passive percutaneous absorption of drugs.

Factors Influencing Percutaneous Absorption of Drugs

1. **Drug Release From Dosage Form:** The first step in percutaneous absorption is that the drug present in the dosage form should reach the skin surface at an adequate rate and in sufficient concentration.
2. **Drug Concentration in the Formulation:** In general, the more the concentration of a drug in the formulation, the greater will be the rate of drug absorption through the skin.

3. **Drug Oil/Water Partition Coefficient:** In general, the greater the solubility of a drug in oil, the greater its percutaneous absorption. However, the aqueous solubility of a drug determines the concentration presented to the absorption site.
4. **Drug Affinity to the Skin Tissue:** In order to have a better absorption, a drug should have preferential partition towards the membranes of the skin than the vehicle in which it is presented. On the other hand, the drug must not have such a great affinity for the tissue that it remains tightly bound and fails to penetrate as deeply as is required of. For instance, a local anesthetic must penetrate to the level of nerve fibers to be effective.
5. **Surface Area:** More drug is absorbed through percutaneous absorption when the drug substance is applied to a larger surface area.
6. **Site of Application:** Percutaneous absorption appears to be greater when the drug is applied to the skin with a thin horny layer than with one that is thick. Thus, the site of application may have a bearing on the degree of drug absorption. The absorption from such sites as the palms of the hands and the soles of the feet is poor due to thick stratum corners.
7. **Hydration of the Skin:** The hydration of the skin is one of the most important factors in percutaneous absorption. The hydration of stratum corneum appears to increase the rate of passage of all substances that penetrate the skin. Increased absorption is probably due to the softening of the tissue and the consequent "sponging" effect with an increase in the size of the pores, allowing a greater flow of substances, large and small, through them.
8. **Nature of the Vehicle Used:** Drug absorption appears to be best from vehicles that easily cover the skin surface, mix readily with the sebum and bring the drug in contact with the tissue cells for absorption. Vehicles used greatly influence the absorption of readily "absorbable" drugs. The absorption of drugs is better from animal and vegetable oils than from mineral oils because the former types penetrate the skin readily. Similarly, organic solvents can enhance the absorption of a drug dissolved in them through their penetrability.

   In general, vehicles that cause hydration of the skin improve the percutaneous absorption of drugs. Oleaginous vehicles effectively increase the skin hydration and thereby increase the drug penetration through skin. Water-in-oil emulsion type vehicles are probably next in effectiveness to oleaginous vehicles in enhancing the hydration of the skin. Vehicle containing humactants like glycerin, reduce the moisture content of the skin by drawing the moisture from the skin, when conditions of a low humidity prevail.
9. **Rubbing or Inunction:** In general, the amount of rubbing in or inunction of the topical application will have a bearing on the amount of drug absorbed; the longer the period of inunction, the greater the absorption.
10. **Contact Period:** The longer the time of contact of a dosage form with the skin, the greater will be the absorption of the drug.

11. **Permeation Enhancers:** Certain chemicals like DMSO, propylene glycol, azone etc., are found to enhance the percutaneous absorption of drugs by disrupting the network of the horny layer. Hence, these chemicals are used in transdermal drug delivery systems and also in other topical preparations to increase the drug absorption.
12. **Other Factors:** Absorption of drugs is rapid from regions where numerous hair follicles exists than from the region with less hair follicles (e.g. scalp). Absorption of drugs is rapid from a damaged skin due to the lack of stratum corneum, the barrier for percutaneous absorption. Therefore, injuries, mild burns, rashes and inflammation promote drug absorption.

Intramuscular Administration

Absorption of drugs from muscle tissue is rapid and the absorption rate is perfusion rate-limited. The higher the blood flow rate to the tissue, the greater will be the absorption rate of a drug. This dependence of absorption on perfusion may be explained by the nature of the barrier (the capillary wall) between the site of injection (interstitial fluid) and the blood. This capillary wall, a much more loosely knit structure than the epithelial lining of the gastrointestinal tract, offers little impedance to the movement of drugs into blood, even for polar ionized drugs. For example, gentamicin, a water-soluble, ionized polar base has greater difficulty penetrating the gastrointestinal mucosa but is rapidly and completely absorbed from an intramuscular site. This low impedance by the capillary wall in the muscle applies to drugs, independent of pKa, degree of ionization and molecular size up to approximately 5000g/mole.

In contrast to small molecules, size, polarity and charge pose a particular problem for administration of proteins, and large polypeptide drugs; their transport across many membranes is hindered. Drugs injected into the muscle reach the systemic circulation by two mechanisms: diffusion through the interstitial fluids and fenestrations in the lining of the vascular capillaries and by convective flow of the interstitial fluids through lymphatic channels. Molecular size is of primary importance for passage across the capillary endothelium. Polypeptides of less than approximately 5000 g/mole primarily pass through the capillary pathway. Those of greater than about 20,000 g/mole are less able to traverse the capillary wall; they primarily enter the blood via the lymphatic pathway. Lymph flow is slow and causes absorption from nonvascular parental sites to continue for many hours. The nonvascular parental routes offer the advantage of providing a prolonged input for short half-life proteins. However, absorption kinetics from both intramuscular and subcutaneous administration has been shown to be highly dependent on the site of injection, temperature, and degree of rubbing at the injection site.

Now, there is a need for the development of novel delivery systems for protein drugs because of their short half-lives and decomposition in the gastrointestinal tract. Smaller polypeptides have been shown to be absorbed across the nasal membranes. High molecular weight polypeptides and proteins may require more creative methods to ensure consistent and more complete bioavailability or may require the development of more specific methods for delivering these drugs to the site of action.

Subcutaneous Administration

All the points discussed under intramuscular administration are also applicable to subcutaneous administration except that the rate of absorption of drugs from subcutaneous tissue is less than that observed from the muscle due to a less blood flow rate to this region. This can be considered as an advantage when slow on set and sustained action are desired (e.g. insulin). Blood flow to the subcutaneous tissue can be increased by massage, application of heat, co-administration of vasodilators locally and thereby drug absorption from this site can be improved. Decrease in drug absorption can be achieved by immobilization of limb, cooling at the site of injection, co-administration of vasoconstrictors. In general, low volumes of injection are used for the subcutaneous route. Inclusion of enzyme hyaluronidase enables the administration of large volumes and also improves the rate of drug absorption by increasing the area of contact between the drug and the tissue.

Likely Questions Issues

1. What is the rate-limiting step in bioavailability?
2. With the help of a neat sketch, explain the common anatomical features of the stomach?
3. What are the primary functions of the stomach?
4. How is the surface area available for absorption in the intestine increased tremondously?
5. What is the nature of a cell membrane?
6. What are the different pathways of drug absorption?
7. What are the different mechanisms of drug absorption? Write about the passive diffusion.
8. How sink conditions are maintained at the absorption site in the GIT?
9. What is an active transport?
10. Write about the specific characters of active transport process?
11. Compare and contrast passive diffusion and a carrier mediated transport.
12. What is the difference between an active transport and a facilitated diffusion?
13. Most of the drugs are absorbed by passive diffusion while a majority of nutrients are abosorbed by an active transport. Explain the reason for this general observation.
14. How are ionizable drugs absorbed?
15. With the help of a neat sketch, explain the barriers for drug absorption from the GIT.
16. How do the components of GI fluids affect the drug absorption?
17. For which drugs a rapid gastric emptying is desirable and for which drugs it should be slow?
18. List the factors that influence the gastric emptying rate.
19. What is the influence of the intestinal transit time on the abosrption of a drug whose site of absorption is the small intestine?

20. For which type of drugs the blood flow rate to the GIT influences the absorption.
21. In general, there exist a linear relationship between the drug oil/water partition coefficient and the rate of drug absorption from the GIT. Write about the exceptions to this general rule with reasons.
22. What are the assumptions made in developing the pH-partition hypothesis?
23. What are the limitations of pH-partition theory?
24. Explain the absorption of weak acidic drugs based on the pH-partition theory.
25. Reduction of particle size of phenacetin fail to increase the dissolution rate. Why?
26. Increase in the effective surface area by micronization is not advisable for certain drugs. What are they?
27. How do you improve the saturation solubility of drugs?
28. Why the salts of drugs show a higher solubility?
29. How the amorphous, metastable polymorphs, anhydrates and solvates show rapid dissolution than their counterparts?
30. Explain the terms in the Noyes-Whitney equation.
31. What do you understand by the terms "diffusion coefficient" and "thickness of the stationary layer"?
32. Write a note on drug stability in the GIT.
33. List the official and unofficial methods of dissolution testing.
34. What are the various factors to be considered in designing a dissolution test apparatus?
35. Discuss the similarities and differences between the Rotating Basket Method and Paddle method.
36. Give the table used to interpret the results of the dissolution test.
37. Write the procedure to be followed for testing the dissolution of enteric coated tablets.
38. What do you mean by intrinsic dissolution rate? How is it determined?
39. How do you control the variables in dissolution testing?
40. Write a note on in-vitro and in-vivo correlations.
41. What are the limitaions of a dissolution test?
42. What are the metabolic factors that affect drug absorption from the GIT?
43. Write a note on the role of drug-food interactions in drug absorption.
44. Pediatrics and geriatrics differ significantly with respect to drug absorption from adults. Justify the statement.
45. Surfactants can increase or decrease the drug absorption. Explain how?
46. Explain the absorption of drug from soft gelatin capsule.
47. What are the reasons for administering the drugs by extravacular routes other than per oral?

48. What are the advantages of sublingual/buccal route of administration?
49. What are the important points to be considered in developing sublingual/buccal dosage forms?
50. What are the physiological factors affecting drug absorption from the rectum?
51. Write a note on intravaginal administration of drugs.
52. What are the factors that influence the "effective dose" of an intraoccularly administered dosage form?
53. Write a note on pulmonary drug administration.
54. What are the various formulations administered intranasally?
55. Which is the principle barrier for percutaneous absorption?
56. What are the factors influencing percutaneous absorption of drugs?
57. Explain the absorption of drugs from the muscular tissue.
58. Write a note on subcuatneous administration of drugs.
59. Ibuprofen, a weak acid has a pKa of 4.4 and diazepam is a weak base with a pKa of 3.7. Assuming that the pH of stomach, small intestine, blood equal to 3.0, 5.8, 7.4 respectively, comment on their site (s) of absorption.
60. What are the different mechanisms of dissolution?
61. Explain Danckwert's dissolution model.
62. Give Hixon-Crowell equation or what is cube root law?

Further Readings

1. Buccal drug delivery: A challenge already won? (2005) Silvia Rossi, Giuseppina Sandri and Carla M. Caramella, Drug Discovery Today: Technologies Volume 2, Issue 1, Pages 59-65.
2. C.J. Kenyon, G. Hooper, D. Tierney, Butler J. Devane J, I.R. Wilding; (1995), The effect of food on the gastrointestinal transit and systemic absorption of naproxen from a novel sustained release formulation; Journal of Controlled Release, 34, 31-36
3. Davis SS; (2005), Formulation strategies for absorption windows, Drug Discovery Today.; 10(4):249-57.
4. Emma L. McConnell, Hala M. Fadda, AbdulW. Basit; (2008), Gut instincts: Explorations in intestinal physiology and drug delivery; International Journal of Pharmaceutics; 364, 213–226.
5. Jantratid, E., Janssen, N., Reppas, C., Dressman, J.B., 2008. Dissolution media simulating conditions in the proximal human gastrointestinal tract: an update. Pharm. Res. 25, 1663–1676.
6. John, V.A., Shotton, P.A., Moppert, J., Theobald, W., 1985. Gastrointestinal transit of Oros drug delivery systems in healthy volunteers: a short report. Br. J. Clin. Pharmacol. 19 (Suppl. 2), 203S–206S.

7. Kellow, J.E., Borody, T.J., Phillips, S.F., Tucker, R.L., Haddad, A.C., 1986. Human interdigestive motility: variations in patterns from esophagus to colon. Gastroenterology 91, 386–395.
8. Kerlin, P., Phillips, S., 1982. Variability ofmotility of the ileum and jejunum in healthy humans. Gastroenterology 82, 694–700.
9. Kerlin, P., Zinsmeister,A., Phillips, S., 1982.Relationship of motility to flow of contents in the human small intestine. Gastroenterology 82, 701–706.
10. Lawrence X. Yu, Gordon L. Amidon (1998), Characterization of small intestinal transit time distribution in humans; International Journal of Pharmaceutics, 171; 157–163.
11. Measurement of gastrointestinal pH in normal ambulant human subjects; (1988); D.F. Evans, G. Pye, R. Bramley, A.G. Clark, T.J. Dyson and J.D. Hardcastle. *Gut, 29:* 1035 1041.
12. Streubel A, Siepmann J, Bodmeier R, (2006); Drug delivery to the upper small intestine window using gastroretentive technologies, Curr Opin Pharmacol.6(5):501-8.
13. The vagina as a route for systemic drug delivery; (2005); Alamdar Hussain, Fakhrul Ahsan; Journal of Controlled Release 103; 301 – 313.
14. Yoshie Masaoka, Yusuke Tanaka, Makoto Kataoka, Shinji Sakuma and Shinji Yamashita; (2006); Site of drug absorption after oral administration: Assessment of membrane permeability and luminal concentration of drugs in each segment of gastrointestinal tract: European Journal of Pharmaceutical Sciences; 29, 240-250.
15. Yoshie Masaoka, Yusuke Tanaka, Makoto Kataoka, Shinji Sakuma, Shinji Yamashita; (2006), Site of drug absorption after oral administration: Assessment of membrane permeability and luminal concentration of drugs in each segment of gastrointestinal tract; European journal of pharmaceutical sciences; 29,240–250.

3

Drug Distribution

Drug distribution refers to the reversible transfer of drug from one location to another within the body. Definitive information on the distribution of a drug requires its measurement in various tissues. Such data has been obtained in animals, but is essentially lacking in humans. Much useful information on the rate and extent of distribution in humans can be derived from blood or plasma data.

Pharmacokinetic variability means that the same dose of a drug results in different blood levels in different individuals. Pharmacokinetic variability is the result of inter-individual differences in the absorption and disposition of drugs. The term disposition refers to the fate of a drug after absorption. On reaching the blood stream, drugs are simultaneously distributed throughout the body and eliminated. Elimination includes biotransformation (metabolism) and excretion of drugs. Distribution usually occurs much more rapidly than elimination. Drug molecules are distributed throughout the body by means of the circulation of the blood. The entire blood volume is pumped through the heart each minute. Therefore, a drug is diluted into the total blood volume within minutes of its entry into the blood.

The drug molecules are distributed throughout the body by the systemic circulation consisting of a series of blood vessels, including the arteries which carry the blood to the tissues; and veins, which return the blood back to the heart. An average adult (70-kg) has about 5 liters of blood (3 liters of plasma and 2 liters of blood cells). About 50% of the blood is in the large veins or venous sinuses. An average cardiac out put is about 5.5 liters/min. in subjects at rest and it may be 5 to 6 times higher during exercise.

Even though a drug is circulated via the blood to all the tissues, its distribution in all the tissues is not uniform. Several factors influence drug distribution to various tissues of the body. They are listed below.

1. Physicochemical properties of the drug
    - Molecular size
    - Oil/water partition coefficient (Ko/w)
    - Degree of ionization that depends on pKa
2. Physiological factors
    - Organ/Tissue size
    - Blood flow rate
    - Physiological barriers to the diffusion of drugs
        - Blood capillary membrane
        - Cell membrane
        - Specialized barriers
        - Blood-brain barrier
        - Blood-cerebrospinal fluid barrier
        - Placental barrier
        - Blood-testis barrier
3. Drug binding in the blood
4. Drug binding to the tissue and other macromolecules

3.1 Physicochemical Properties of the Drug

Molecular size, oil/water partition coefficient and degree of ionization are the important physicochemical properties of the drugs that influence their distribution in the body. Most of the drug molecules easily cross the capillaries and reach the interstitial fluid (extra-cellular fluid, ECF) bathing the cell. Drugs with molecular weights upto 500 to 600 daltons quickly diffuse out of the vascular system and reach the ECF.

However, the capillary membranes vary in their permeability characteristics depending upon the tissue. For example, the capillary membranes in the liver and kidneys are more permeable to drug movement than capillaries in the brain. The sinusoidal capillaries of the liver are very permeable and allow the passage of large-molecular-weight molecules.

Once the drug is present in the ECF, it is transported into the cell mainly by passive diffusion. The factors that influence the penetration of drugs into the cells are the same as those observed in gastrointestinal absorption of drugs. Small, water-soluble molecules and ions diffuse through aqueous channels or pores in the cell membrane. Water-soluble molecules and ions with a molecular weight of more than 50 daltons can not enter the cell easily, except by special transport mechanisms. Lipid-soluble molecules are dissolved in the cell membranes and diffuse into the cell due to the concentration gradient. The relative amounts of unionized and ionized forms of weak acidic or basic drugs in ECF depends on the pH of the blood and the ECF. Hence, the pKa of the drugs play critical role in drug distribution of polar drugs by influencing the degree of ionization. Therefore, the penetration of weak acidic or basic drugs into tissues depend on the pH of the ECF and blood. However, the pH of the blood and the ECF is maintained remarkably uniform at 7.4.

The partition coefficient of a drug between the organ and the blood is a measure of the ability of a drug to concentrate in the tissue. The volume of thyroid gland tissue is about 20 ml. If the partition coefficient of the drug between the thyroid and the blood is 1, the drug in the tissue would rapidly come into equilibrium with the blood, but relatively little drug would be found in the thyroid. However, for certain drugs containing iodine moieties, partition coefficient is enormous and a significant amount of the drug will distribute into this small gland relatively rapidly. Therefore, the higher the partition coefficient value of a drug, the more it will concentrate in the organ.

The oil/water coefficient (Ko/w) is a measure of lipophilicity of a drug. The higher the lipophilicity of a drug the easier it will be for the drug molecule to penetrate the lipid cell membrane. Therefore, lipophilic drugs show high distribution rates than polar drugs. However, the unionized form of a drug is lipophilic than ionized form, hence, the pKa of the drug determines the relative amounts of ionized and unionized forms of the drug in addition to the pH of the blood and the ECF. The overall permeability of a drug through the lipoidal membranes depends on both the pKa and Ko/w. The *effective partition coefficient* of a drug is defined as the product of the fraction unionized at pH 7.4 and Ko/w of unionized drug. Two drugs may have similar Ko/w values, but the difference in pKa values leads to a change in their effective partition coefficients and hence different distribution patterns.

An interesting experiment was conducted in dogs for demonstrating the pH dependent cellular distribution of phenobarbital, a weak acid. When the plasma pH is lowered by carbon dioxide inhalation, there is a decrease in the plasma concentration of phenobarbital. Under these conditions, a greater fraction of the drug is in the unionized form (acidic pH increases the fraction of unionized form) and a larger amount of the drug moves into the cells. Sodium bicarbonate ingestion causes alkalosis and produces an elevation of phenobarbital levels in the plasma. This is because of the movement of the drug from the cells to the ECF. Therefore, acidosis deepens phenobarbital anesthesia, whereas alkalosis lightens it. This is the reason for using sodium bicarbonate in the treatment of barbiturate intoxication. This treatment also produces urinary alkalosis which promotes the urinary excretion of weakly acidic drugs.

3.2 Organ/Tissue Size

A particular organ in the body may acts as a site of distribution or as a site of both distribution and elimination. The relative importance of the various organs as storage and/or elimination sites depends on how fast the drug gets to each organ and how much space or volume is available to hold the drug. The greater the size of a tissue, the higher the drug accumulation in that tissue.

3.3 Blood Flow to the Organ

Another important factor that governs the rate of accumulation of a drug in an organ is the rate of the blood flow to that organ. The rate of uptake of a drug by an organ is called **organ clearance**. It is obvious that an organ can not clear the drug from the blood any faster than the drug delivered to the organ via the blood flow (for details see Chapter 4).

Distribution, like absorption can be rate-limited by either perfusion or permeability. A *perfusion-rate limitation* prevails when the tissue membranes present essentially no barrier to distribution. This condition is observed with small lipophilic drugs diffusing across the most membranes of the body and, by almost all drugs, except macromolecules diffusing across loosely knit membranes, such as capillary walls of the muscle and subcutaneous tissue. Perfusion is generally expressed in units of milliliters of the blood per minute per volume of the tissue (ml/min/ml of tissue). When all the factors remain constant, well-perfused tissues take up a drug much more rapidly than do poorly perfused tissues. There is a direct correlation between the tissue perfusion rate and the time required to distribute a drug to a tissue.

Therefore, a rapid equilibrium is observed with lipid-soluble drugs between the blood and the kidney, liver, heart, and brain, all of which are highly perfused with blood. Skeletal muscle and adipose tissue are perfused with the blood at a slower rate and hence, equilibrium between the drug in these tissues and the blood is attained slowly.

Lipid-soluble drugs rapidly penetrate the tissues highly perfused with the blood and show a quick on-set of action. However, redistribution of these lipid-soluble drugs into less well perfused tissues, rather than metabolism or excretion, may limit the duration of action of such drugs. For example, lipid-soluble drug, thiopental produces anesthesia within seconds after I.V. administration because of rapid equilibration between the blood and brain. However, the thiopental levels in brain decline rapidly even though the drug is metabolized slowly in the brain and as a result the duration of action is short. The rapid decline in the levels of thiopental in the brain is due to the re-distribution of the drug to the other tissues, particularly the skeletal muscle and fat.

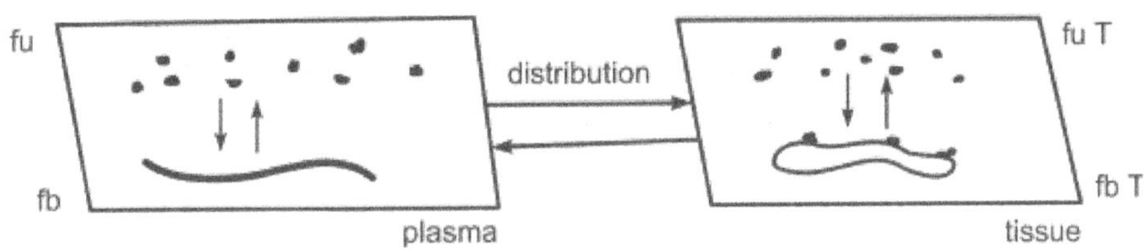

Fig. 3.1 Equilibrium between bound/unbound drug in plasma/tissue.

fb is the fraction bound where

$$fb = \frac{[\text{bound}]}{[\text{total}]} = 1 - fu$$

A *permeability-rate limitation* is observed for polar drugs diffusing across the tightly knit lipoidal membranes. Differences in the ease of entry are a function of both oil/water partition coefficient and the degree of ionization. For example, salicylic acid and phenobarbital show differences in time required to reach an equilibrium between the blood and the CSF, even though their partition coefficients are not much different. This is because of the fact that the weaker acid, phenobarbital, exists mainly in unionized form in the plasma at pH 7.4 than salicylic acid. This difference can be predicted by considering their effective partition coefficient at pH 7.4 (Table 3.1).

Table 3.1 Influence of Ko/w and pKa of Drugs on Distribution of Drugs into the CSF.

Drug	pKa	Fraction Unionized at pH 7.4 form	Partition coefficient of unionized at pH 7.4	Effective partition coefficient (min.)	Time to reach 50% equilibrium
Phenobarbital	8.1	80	0.05	0.040	4
Salicylic acid	3.0	0.004	0.12	0.0005	115
Thiopental	7.6	0.6	3.3	2.0	1.4
Barbital	7.5	0.6	0.002	0.0012	27

3.4 Physiological Barriers to the Diffusion of Drugs

The distribution of various compounds that enter the blood to different tissues is restricted because of the presence of the specialized barriers. This is developed in the body to protect the sensitive tissues from the effect of a variety of chemicals that enter the blood by several routes.

3.4.1 Blood Capillary Membrane

The processes by which drugs transverse the capillary membrane include **passive diffusion** and hydrostatic pressure. Passive diffusion is the process by which drug molecules move from a region of high concentration to a region of low concentration and is described by *Fick's Law of diffusion.*

$$\text{Rate of diffusion} = \frac{dQ}{dt} = \frac{-D\,K\,A\,(Cp - Ct)}{h}$$

Where:

Cp = drug concentration in the plasma

Ct = drug concentration in the tissue

A = surface area of the membrane

h = thickness of the membrane

K = the lipid/water partition coefficient

D = diffusion coefficient of the drug in the membrane

The negative sign indicates that the transfer of the drug takes place from inside the blood capillary into the tissue.

The average hydrostatic pressure of the blood capillary is +18mm Hg and the mean pressure in the tissue is -6 mm Hg, resulting in a net total pressure of 24mm Hg higher in the capillary over the tissue. This pressure is nullified by the osmotic pressure of the blood, which contributes a suction pressure of 24mm Hg, putting the plasma fluid back into the capillary. Thus, the net result is that the pressure in the tissue and most parts of the capillary are equal, with no net flow of water. However, at the arterial end of the capillary, the pressure of the blood is about 8 mm Hg higher than that of the tissue. The higher pressure at the end of the arterial capillary is called **hydrostatic** or **filtration pressure**. This pressure difference causes the filtration of the fluid from the capillary end into the tissue. This filtered fluid is later returned to the venous capillary due to a lower pressure of about the same magnitude in the venous blood. The lower pressure of the venous blood compared to the tissue fluid is termed **absorptive pressure**. Therefore, hydrostatic pressure represents a pressure gradient between the arterial end of the capillaries entering the tissue and venous capillaries leaving the tissue. Hydrostatic pressure is responsible for penetration of water-soluble drugs into spaces between endothelial cells and possibly kidneys, in which a high arterial pressure and a high blood flow allow for small drug molecules to be filtered in the glomerulus of the renal nephron.

Certain body fluids may be relatively inaccessible to drugs in the blood stream; These include cerebrospinal fluid (CSF), bronchial secretion, pericardial fluid, and the middle ear fluid. The degree of access of antibiotics to these fluids may be a limiting factor in treating infections. Inflammation, often secondary to infection, increases drug penetration.

Drug concentration in the body fluids also depend on the degree of drug binding in the fluid. Drug concentration in the CSF and saliva, which are usually protein free, often is low, equivalent to free (unbound) drug concentration in the plasma. Drug concentration in the extra-cellular fluid may be less than that in the plasma, because the ECF has a lower albumin concentration than the plasma. Drug concentration in the synovial fluid varies with the degree of inflammation, because albumin concentration in this fluid fluctuates with the severity of the disease process.

3.4.2 Cell Membrane

Once the drug is present in ECF, it is generally transported by passive diffusion into the cell. The factors that influence the penetration of drugs into cells are same as those observed in the gastrointestinal absorption of drugs. The cell membrane acts like a lipid barrier for the transport of drugs. Permeability of drugs through this membrane limits the entry into the cell.

3.4.3 Blood-Brain Barrier (BBB)

The capillaries in the brain and spinal cord are different in their permeability characters from those found in the rest of the body. The capillary endothelial cells are surrounded by a layer of *glial cells*, which have tight intercellular junctions. This added layer of cells around the capillary membranes acts as a thicker lipid barrier and slows the diffusion and penetration of water-soluble and polar drugs into the brain and spinal cord. This lipid barrier is called the **blood-brain-barrier** (BBB) and is depicted in Fig. 3.2.

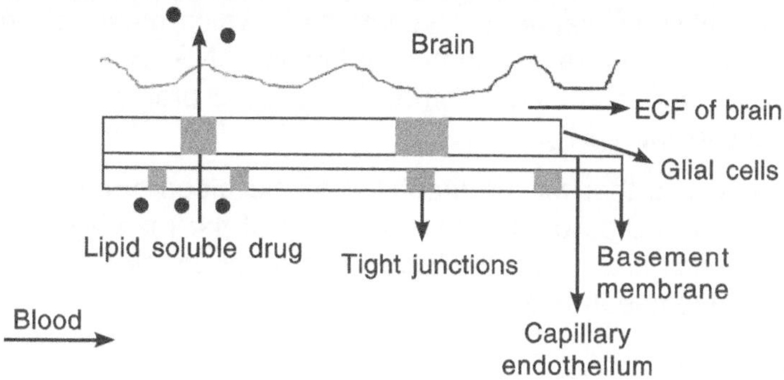

Fig. 3.2 Schematic representation of transport of lipid soluble drug across blood brain barrier.

The BBB represents an important boundary between the peripheral and central nervous system in the form of a permeability barrier to the passive diffusion of substances from the blood stream into various regions of the CNS. Evidence of the barrier is provided by the greatly diminished rate of access of chemicals from the plasma to the brain. In general, only lipid soluble drugs can diffuse into the interstitial fluid of the brain and spinal cord. Water soluble compounds can not cross the endothelial lining without the assistance of carriers. Many different transport mechanisms are involved. For example, there are separate transport systems for glucose, large amino acids, and glycine (the smallest of the amino acids).

The transport process is both selective and directional. Large amino acids and glucose are transported out of the blood, whereas glycine is transported into the blood. There are functional reasons for directional transport. The neurons have a constant need for glucose that must be met regardless of the relative concentrations in the blood and interstitial fluid. However, glycine is a neurotransmitter, and its concentration in neural tissue must be kept relatively low, much lower than that in the circulating blood. Nevertheless, most of the transport mechanisms of the blood-brain barrier involve facilitated diffusion and so occur down the concentration gradient. The blood-brain barrier remains intact throughout the CNS, but less prominent in the portion of the hypothalamus and in the membranous root of the diencephalon and medulla.

The penetration rate of a drug into the brain depends on its degree of ionization in the plasma and its lipid solubility. Highly lipid-soluble drugs such as thiopental reach the brain immediately from the plasma, whereas polar drugs, like barbital, penetrate the CNS at a lower rate. Penicillin G, is a weak organic acid with pKa 2.6 which exists in a completely ionized form in the plasma. The rate of penetration of penicillin into the brain is slow due to their poor lipid solubility. The blood-brain-barrier may severely limit treatment with antibiotics, cancer chemotherapeutic agents, and other polar drugs. Pro-drug approach is useful in enhancing drug delivery to the CNS. Parkinsonism is associated with a depletion of dopamine in the brain. The inability of dopamine to cross blood-brain-barrier restricts its use in the treatment of Parkinsonism. 0Therefore, a precursor of dopamine, levodopa, which can penetrate the barrier is used in the treatment of this disease. Levodopa is metabolized in the brain to dopamine.

Drugs such as anticonvulsants or psychotropics, which must act on the brain should have good lipid-solubility for a rapid penetration into the CNS. Because of the lipid-solubility of these drugs, they can distribute to other tissues and precipitate side effects, if these drugs do not crossed the BBB quickly.

It has been observed that the permeability of the blood-brain-barrier is increased in meningeal infections because of an abnormal state of the membranes. Increased levels of drugs such as penicillin G, ampicillin have been found in the CSF of patients with viral, bacterial or other meningeal inflammatory states.

3.4.4 Blood-Cerebrospinal Fluid Barrier

The *chroid plexus* is the site of cerebrospinal fluid production. In the lower brain stem, a region of the choroid plexus in the roof of the fourth ventricle projects between the cerebellum and pons. In the anterior brain stem, two extensive folds of the choroid plexus originate in the roof of the diencephalon and extend through the interventricular foramina. These folds cover the floors of the lateral ventricles.

Large epyndymal cells cover the capillaries of the choroid plexus and contact the cerebrospinal fluid of the ventricles. Through a combination of active and passive transport these cells secrete cerebrospinal fluid at a rate of about 1200 ml/day. The composition of the CSF is closely regulated.

The junctions between the endothelial cells of the blood capillaries are open and easily permeable to drugs. Therefore, drugs reach the extracellular fluid (ECF) easily from the blood at the blood-CSF barrier. However, the choroid plexus cells have tight junctions between them and do not allow the penetration of polar drugs. Hence, lipid soluble drugs can only penetrate the lipoidal barrier (Fig. 3.3). Since the CSF is almost free from proteins, the CSF concentration of lipid-soluble drugs usually reflect a free drug concentration in plasma. Drug levels are usually higher in the brain tissue than in the CSF. Phenytoin concentrations in epileptic patients are 6 times higher in the temporal lobe than in the CSF.

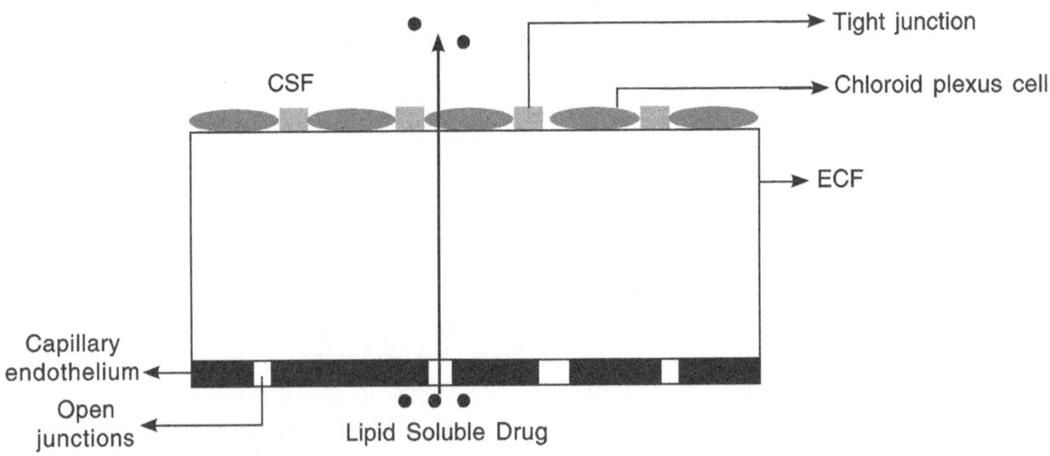

Fig. 3.3 Diagram showing the transport of lipid soluble drug across blood cerebrospinal fluid barrier.

3.4.5 Placental Barrier

Blood flows to the placenta through the paired umblical arteries and returns in a single umblical vein. It has been estimated that the chorionic villi provide around 90 square meters of surface area for active and passive exchange between the fetal and maternal blood streams. The maternal and the fetal blood vessels are separated by the placental barrier that consists of a fetal trophoblast basement membrane and the endothelium. Studies on the placental transfer of a several compounds revealed that the barrier is not as effective as BBB in restricting the entry of polar compounds. Many drugs having a molecular weight less than 1000 daltons and considerable lipid solubility can easily cross the barrier by passive diffusion. Since some degree of fetal exposure is likely to occur with virtually all drugs, and since the consequences of such exposure is usually unknown, it is necessary to restrict the administration of drugs to a pregnant woman, especially during the first trimester of pregnancy. Chronic medication presents the greatest concerns. The higher the blood level of drug in a pregnant patient on chronic medication, the greater is the risk to the fetus. Examples of drugs that cross the placental barrier include narcotic analgesics, sulfonamides, anticonvulsants, barbiturates, antibiotics, steroids etc.

The shortest time possible for a drug to equilibrate between maternal blood and the fetal tissue has been estimated to be about 40 minutes. Polar drugs whose passage across the placenta is impeded by a low lipid solubility, large molecular size, ionization, and a high protein binding, probably require hours for equilibration. Fetal exposure to drugs that are rapidly eliminated by the mother is also likely to be small.

3.4.6 Blood-Testis Barrier

The seminiferous tubules are isolated from the general circulation by a *blood-testis barrier* comparable to the blood-brain barrier. Extensions of sustentacular cells (*sertoli cells*) form a layer that surrounds the seminiferous tubule beneath the spermatogonia. Tight junctions between the adjacent sustentacular cells prevent free diffusion from the interstitial fluid to the seminiferous tubule. Transport across the sustentacular cells is tightly regulated so that the conditions inside the tubule remain very stable.

3.5 Drug Binding in Blood

Within the blood, drug can bind to many components including blood cells and plasma proteins. The drug can also bind with tissue proteins or other macromolecules such as melanin and DNA to form a drug-macromolecule complex. The formation of a drug-protein complex is termed as *drug-protein binding*. The drug-protein binding process is generally a reversible process. However, certain drugs may bind to proteins irreversibly. For example, the reactive intermediate metabolites of acetaminophen at higher doses, bind irreversibly with liver proteins and cause hepatotoxicity.

Most drugs bind or interact with proteins by a reversible process. Reversible drug-protein binding means the drug binds to the protein with weaker chemical bonds such as ionic, Van der Waals, hydrogen, and/or hydrophobic bonds. The amino acids that constitute the protein chain contain hydroxyl, carboxyl, or other sites available for reversible drug-protein interactions.

Albumin, α_1-acid glycoprotein, lipoproteins, immunoglobulins (Ig G), and erythrocytes within the blood are the most important macromolecules that bind the drugs. The most important contribution to drug binding in the plasma is made by *albumin* which constitutes about one half of the total plasma proteins. Albumin is synthesized by the liver. Its molecular weight ranges between 65,000 and 69,000 daltons. Albumin is present in the plasma and in extra-cellular fluid of various tissues. Total plasma albumin for a 70-Kg man is about 120g. Total interstitial albumin is approximately 156g. Thus almost 60% of the total albumin in the body is found out side the plasma. Albumin concentration in the plasma is maintained at a relatively constant level of 3.5 to 4.5% w/v. Lower levels are found during pregnancy and in certain diseases. Albumin is responsible for maintaining osmotic pressure of the blood and for the transportation of endogenous and exogenous substances. As a transport protein for endogenous substances, albumin complexes with free fatty acids (FFA), bilirubin, various hormones (such as cortisone, aldosterone, and thyroxine), tryptophan, and other compounds. Most of weak acidic drugs and neutral drugs bind to albumin.

α_1-acid glycoprotein (orosomucoid) is a low molecular weight (approximately 40,000 daltons) protein and is a globulin. The average plasma concentration of α_1-acid glycoprotein ranges between 40mg/100 ml and 100mg/100ml. Its concentration in the plasma increases in malignant diseases, inflammation and stress, and decreases in hepatic diseases and the nephrotic syndrome. α_1-acid glycoprotein binds primarily basic drugs such as lidocaine, propranolol, imipramine and quinidine.

Globulins (α, β, γ globulins) may be responsible for the transport of endogenous substances, but play a limited role in drug binding. A globular protein known as corticosteroid-binding-globulin (CBG) or transcortin is highly specific to certain steroids such as prednisolone. Transcortin also binds thyroxine and vitamin B_{12}. Gamma globulins are important in immunological reactions, but have negligible role in drug binding.

Lipoproteins are macromolecular complexes of lipids and proteins. Lipoproteins are classified based on their density. They are responsible for the transport of plasma lipids. They may be participated in drug binding interactions, if the binding sites on albumin become saturated.

Erythrocytes or red blood cells (RBCs) may bind both endogenous and exogenous compounds. Erythrocytes constitute about 45% of the volume of the blood. Drug uptake by erythrocytes is a function of plasma protein binding. A linear correlation has been observed between the blood or RBC/plasma concentration ratio and free drug concentration of propranolol, phenytoin, haloperidol and quinidine in plasma.

Penetration of a drug into the RBC is dependent on the free concentration of the drug in the plasma. Increased levels of a free drug concentration in the plasma linearly increased the drug levels of phenytoin and acetazolamide in the erythrocytes.

For drugs that bind to RBCs strongly, the haematocrit will influence the total amount of drug in the blood. For these drugs, the whole blood drug concentration should be measured. Measurable amounts of the drug may be present in RBCs for a long time if the binding of the drug to the RBCs is an irreversible process.

Total plasma concentration is usually measured in plasma. The total drug concentration in blood can be estimated by equation

$$C_B = C_{RBC} \cdot HCT + C_P (1\text{-}HCT)$$

HCT = hematocrit

C_{RBC} = the drug concentration in RBC.

3.5.1 Plasma Protein Binding and Drug Distribution

The drug bound to the plasma protein is not available for distribution, hepatic metabolism, renal elimination and pharmacological action. The high molecular weight of drug-protein complex restricts the passage across the blood capillaries and its low lipid-solubility prevents the passage across cell membranes. Only an un-bound drug or a free drug circulating in blood can cross the blood capillaries and cell membranes and hence, is available for distribution, glomerular filtration and hepatic metabolism.

Drug-protein binding interaction is a reversible process. As the free drug concentration in blood decreases, the drug-protein complex dissociates to liberate the free drug and maintain equilibrium. Therefore, a drug bound to protein is considered to be in temporary storage. Because of reversible binding of a drug to the proteins, free drug levels of a drug are maintained for a longer time in the blood. Accordingly, the biological half-life of highly protein bound drug is longer than that of a drug having a negligible or no protein binding.

Although drug binding to plasma proteins is usually rapidly reversible, some studies reported irreversible binding to albumin, for e.g., the acyl glucuronide metabolite of zomepirac and tolmetin.

3.5.2 Plasma Protein Binding and Drug Effects

Free drug concentration in the plasma is responsible for the observed pharmacological effect or therapeutic response. Plasma drug concentrations are generally reported as the total drug concentration in the plasma, including both a protein-bound drug and an unbound (free) drug concentrations. The minimum therapeutic levels for most drugs listed in literature refer to the total drug concentrations in plasma or serum. In the past, because of difficulties in the measurement of free drug concentrations in plasma, the total plasma concentrations were used in the development of an appropriate drug dosage regimen for the patient. Presently, ultrafiltration of the plasma or serum enables an easy estimation of a free drug concentration in the plasma or serum.

The total drug concentration of a drug that undergoes protein binding in the plasma is usually higher than in the ECF, cerebrospinal fluid, synovial fluid, lymph and other body fluids, since the protein concentration in these fluids is less than in the plasma. The concentrations of albumin in the plasma is about 4%. ECF and synovial fluids have about 1g/100 ml. Normal CSF contains so little protein that it is often viewed as an ultrafiltrate of the plasma. The free drug in the plasma is in equilibrium with the drug in the CSF and hence, free drug levels of a lipid-soluble drug in plasma reflect the drug concentrations in the CSF. Elevation of albumin levels in the synovial fluid from patient with arthritis or other degenerative joint diseases has been observed. The total drug concentration in synovial fluid is a function of total albumin content. In a study it was observed that the ratio of total ibuprofen in the synovial fluid to that in serum correlated with the albumin concentration ratio. However, free drug concentration in synovial fluid was similar to the free serum levels. This indicates that an unbound drug can easily penetrate into the synovial fluid.

Experimental results in rats suggest that the anticoagulant effect of warfarin is more nearly a function of its free rather than of its total concentration in the plasma. Similar results were observed for the anticonvulsant action of phenytoin.

3.5.3 Protein Binding and Drug Elimination

A free or unbound drug in the plasma is available for distribution, metabolism and urinary excretion. The relationship of reversible drug-protein biding in the plasma, drug distribution and elimination is depicted in Fig. 3.4. The driving force for drug excretion in urine is the free drug concentration in the plasma. The glomerular capillaries permit the passage of most of drug molecules but restrict the passage of plasma proteins and the drug-protein complex. Therefore, only free or unbound drug is filtered. The elimination half-lives of drugs which are excreted mainly by glomerular filtration, are generally increased when the percent of a drug bound to the plasma proteins is increased. If a drug is neither secreted nor reabsorbed by the tubules and is not protein bound, its renal clearance is a measure of the golmerular filtration rate (GFR). If a drug is protein bound, the renal clearance of the total drug in the plasma is less than GFR but the renal clearance of a free drug in the plasma is equal to GFR.

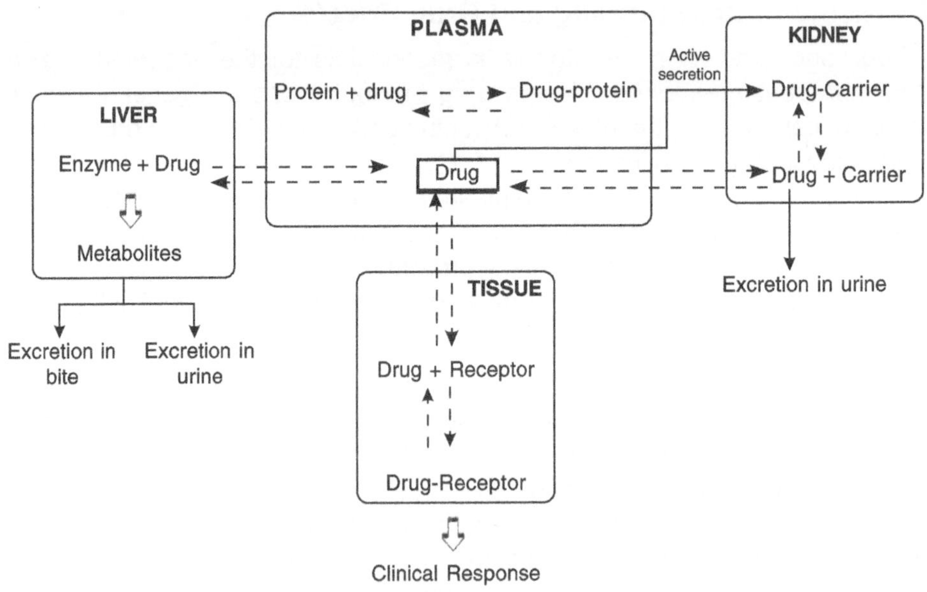

Fig. 3.4 Effect of Reversible Drug-Protein Binding Interaction on Drug Distribution, Metabolism, Urinary Excretion and Pharmacological or Therapeutic Effect.

A protein bound drug is unable to enter the hepatocytes resulting in a reduced drug metabolism by the liver. In addition, the bound drug is not available as a substrate for liver enzymes or other enzymes thereby further reducing the rate of metabolism. In general drugs that are highly bound to plasma protein have reduced overall drug clearance.

Blood vs plasma clearance

Pharmacokinetic parameters should preferably be determined from blood but usually drug concentration is measured in plasma or serum.

The free fraction is different in tissues vs plasma, but the unbound concentration is the same at equilibrium.

$$f_p . C_P = f_B . C_B$$

The determination of the blood/plasma ratio helps to estimate the importance of the drug distribution in the erythrocytes.

A linear correlation between the blood/plasma ratio and the degree of plasma protein binding (f_U) is reported for propranolol, phenytoin, quinidine, and haloperidol.

Drug binding to erythrocytes is usually rapidly reversible. Drugs that bind strongly to red blood cells may exhibit concentration dependent uptake from plasma. Drugs reported to bind strongly to the erythrocytes (B/P ratio>1) include promazine, chlorpromazine, propronalol, salicylates, Phenobarbital, and phenytoin.

The pharmacokinetic parameters are usually calculated from plasma rather than from whole blood. When drug binding is similar in plasma and RBC, C_B H" C_P since f_B H" f_P

However, if the binding in plasma is greater than in RBC, $C_B < C_P$, then $AUC_B < AUC_P$ and plasma clearance provides an underestimate of the blood clearance. Maximum errors are of the order of 40%.

At B/P ratio >1, clearance determined from plasma concentration would significantly overestimate of blood clearance and could exceed hepatic blood flow.

3.5.4 Clinical Significance of Drug-Protein Binding

The fraction of a drug bound to the plasma protein can change with the dose of the drug administered and the patient's plasma protein concentration. The plasma protein concentration is controlled by a number of variables. They are,

- Protein synthesis
- Protein catabolism
- Distribution of albumin between intravascular and extravascular space
- Excessive elimination of plasma protein, particularly albumin
- A number of diseases, age, trauma, and related circumstances

When a highly protein-bound drug is displaced from its binding site by a second drug or agent, a sharp increase in the free drug in the plasma may occur, leading to toxicity. With drugs that are not highly bound to the plasma proteins, a small displacement from the protein causes a transient increase in the free drug concentration, which may cause a transient increase in pharmacological action. Drug displacement from the protein by a second drug can occur by the competition of the second drug for similar binding sites.

For example salicylates, for instance, decrease the binding capacity of thyroxin, the thyroid harmone, to proteins. Through this action the, the displaced drug becomes less protein bound and their activity (abd toxicity) may be increased. The intensity of the pharmacological response is related to the ratio of the bound drug to free active drug and to the therapeutic index of the drug. Warfarin, an anticoagulant, is 97% bound to plasma protein leaving 3% in free form to exert its effect. If a second drug, such as naproxen, which is strongly bound to plasma proteins, is administered and results in only 90% of the warfarin being bound, 10% of warfarin will be in free form. Thus, the blood level of free warfarin (3 to 10%) will triple and possibly result in serious toxicity.

Alteration of the protein structure by the drugs may also change the capacity of the protein to bind drugs. For example, acetylation of the lysine residue of albumin by aspirin changes the binding capacity of albumin for phenylbutazone. The displacement of endogenous substances from plasma proteins by drugs is usually of little consequence. However, in infants the displacement of bilirubin by drugs (e.g. NSAIDs) can cause mental retardation and even death due to the difficulty of bilirubin elimination in the new born. The nature of drug-drug and drug-metabolite interactions is also important in drug-protein binding.

Practice Problem

It was observed in patients that a new drug under investigation caused 5% displacement of oxazepam (95% bound) and phenobarbital (55% bound) from their respective binding sites. What are the consequences of these interactions ?

Using the data in the given problem, the following table can constructed.

Drug	Before displacement	After displacement	Percent increase in free drug
Oxazepam			
Percent bound	95	90	
Percent unbound	5	10	+100
Phenobarbital			
Percent bound	55	50	
Percent unbound	45	50	+10

For a highly bound drug, oxazepam, an increase of 5% in a free drug is actually a 100% increase in the free drug level in comparison with the initial drug level. For a weakly bound drug, phenobarbital, an increase of 5% free drug concentration is only a 10% increase in the free drug level when compared to initial free drug level. For a patient treated with phenobarbital, a 10% increase in the free drug level would probably not effect the therapeutic outcome. However, for a patient medicated with oxazepam, a 100% increase in the free drug level may precipitate toxic effects of the drug.

3.5.5 Kinetics of Protein Binding

The kinetics of a reversible drug-protein binding can be described by the law of mass action.

$$\text{Drug} + \text{Protein} \rightleftharpoons \text{Drug-Protein-Complex}$$

or

$$D_F + P_F \underset{K_2}{\overset{K_1}{\rightleftharpoons}} PD \quad .....(3.1)$$

At a dynamic equilibrium, the rates of forward reaction and backward reaction are equal. The D_F is the free drug or unbound drug concentration and P_F is the concentration of free protein. If the number of binding sites on the protein is one, then the molar concentrations of the bound drug and protein are equal (i.e., $[PD] = [P_B] = [D_B]$). K_1 and K_2 are the rate constants for association and dissociation, respectively.

According to law of mass action, the equilibrium association constant, Kas, can be expressed as the ratio of the molar concentration of the products and the molar concentration of the reactants.

$$Kas = \frac{K_1}{K_2} = \frac{[PD]}{[P_F][D_F]} = \frac{[D_B]}{[P_F][D_F]} \quad .....(3.2)$$

The magnitude of the Kas yields information on the degree of drug protein binding. Very large Kas indicates that the drug binds strongly to the protein and, hence, free drug concentration of such a drug is low. Therefore, a very large dose of the drug is required to achieve a reasonable therapeutic concentration of a free drug.

The total drug concentration in the plasma, D_t, is the sum of both bound and unbound drug concentrations.

$$D_t = D_F + D_B \quad .....(3.3)$$

Similarly,

$$P_t = P_F + P_B \quad .....(3.4)$$

$$P_F = P_t - P_B \quad .....(3.5)$$

Substituting the value of P_F in equation 3.2, we get

$$Kas = \frac{[D_B]}{[D_F]([P_t]-[P_B])} \quad .....(3.6)$$

or

$$Kas = \frac{[D_B]}{[D_F]([P_t]-[P_B])} \quad .....(3.7)$$

Since, $[P_B] = [D_B]$

However, if the protein contains 'n' number of binding sites, then,

$$\text{Kas} = \frac{[D_B]}{[D_F](n[P_t]-[D_B])} \quad .....(3.8)$$

The degree of binding is frequently expressed as the bound-to-total concentration ratio. This ratio has limiting values of 0 and 1.0. Drugs with values greater than 0.9 are said to be highly bound. As stated previously, an unbound drug, rather than a bound drug, concentration is frequently important in therapeutics. Therefore, the fraction of the drug in the plasma unbound, fu, is of greater utility than the fraction of the bound.

$$\text{fu} = \frac{[D_u]}{[D_t]} = \frac{[D_F]}{[D_F]+[D_B]} \quad .....(3.9)$$

For most of drugs, for a given amount of drug in the body, the greater the binding of the drug to the plasma proteins, the larger the total drug concentration in the plasma. One of the reasons in pharmacokinetic variability of a drug is due to variations in the extent of plasma protein binding.

The fraction of the unbound in the plasma, fu, depends on the total drug concentration, the protein concentration and the magnitude of Kas. In principle, the number of binding sites on a protein molecule is limited. Therefore, as the drug concentration in the plasma increases, the number of free sites on the protein decreases progressively and the fraction of free drug increases. Drugs with a high association constant and drugs that are given in large doses may exhibit concentration-dependent changes in the fraction of free drug in the plasma. In practice, however, the fraction of unbound drug in the plasma for most drugs administered in therapeutic doses is essentially constant over the entire drug concentration range.

3.5.6 Determination of Binding Sites and Binding Constants

In order to study the protein binding nature of the drugs, a determinable quantity 'r' is defined, as follows:

$$r = \frac{\text{moles of drug bound}}{\text{total moles of protein}} \quad .....(3.10)$$

Moles of a bound drug is equal to [PD] = $[D_B]$ and the total moles of protein $[P_t] = [P_F] + [PD]$, the Equation 3.10 becomes,

$$r = \frac{[PD]}{[PD]+[P_F]} \quad .....(3.11)$$

But, according to Equation 3.2, [PD] = Kas $[P_F]$ $[D_F]$. Substituting the value of [PD] in Equation 3.11, the following expression is obtained.

$$r = \frac{\text{Kas}\,[P_F][D_F]}{\text{Kas}\,[P_F][D_F]+[P_F]} \quad .....(3.12)$$

or

$$r = \frac{\text{Kas}\,[D_F]}{1+\text{Kas}\,[D_F]} \quad .....(3.13)$$

Equation 3.13 describes the simplest situation, in which a drug and a protein interact at 1:1 ratio. Further, it is assumed that only one independent binding site for each mole of the drug is present on the protein molecule. If there are "n" identical independent binding sites are present per protein molecule, then the following equation is used.

$$r = \frac{n\,Kas\,[D_F]}{1+Kas\,[D_F]} \qquad .....(3.14)$$

Protein molecules may contain more than one type of binding sites on which the drug molecules can bind with different association constants. For example four different sites on human albumin have been identified for drug-binding, namely, *warfarin and azapropazone binding site* (Site 1), *diazepam binding site* (Site 2), *digitoxin binding site* (Site 3) and *tamoxifen binding site* (Site 4). Dicoumarol binds primarily at Site 1 and secondarily at Site 2. In such cases, Equation 3.14 expands to the following:

$$r = \frac{n_1\,K_1\,[D_F]}{1+K_1\,[D_F]} + \frac{n_2\,K_2\,[D_F]}{1+K_2\,[D_F]} \qquad .....(3.15)$$

Where, the numerical subscripts represent different types of binding sites and their respective number and association constants.

- The assumptions made in developing these equation are:
- Drug molecules bind to the protein at independent binding sites.
- The affinity of a drug for one binding site does not influence binding to other sites.
- The number and association constants are different for different types of binding sites.

In reality, drug-protein biding sometimes exhibits a phenomenon of *cooperativity* i.e. the binding of the first drug molecule at one site on the protein molecule influences the successive binding of other drug molecules. The binding of oxygen to hemoglobin is an example of cooperativity.

In vitro Methods

In general, purified albumin is used in the kinetic study of protein binding since most of the drugs bind to albumin. It is possible to determine experimentally both the free drug, $[D_F]$ and the bound drug, $[D_B]$ or [PD], as well as the total protein concentration ($[P_F]$ + [PD]).

1. **Direct Plot Method:** Equation 3.14 shows that as a free drug concentration increases, the number of moles of the drug per mole of the protein become saturated and reach a plateau. Therefore, a direct plot of the r verus $[D_F]$ can be used to find out the number of binding sites on protein 'n' (plateau value). Association constant, Kas, is obtained by finding the drug concentration required to saturate the half of the total binding sites available (i.e. n/2). See Fig. 3.5.

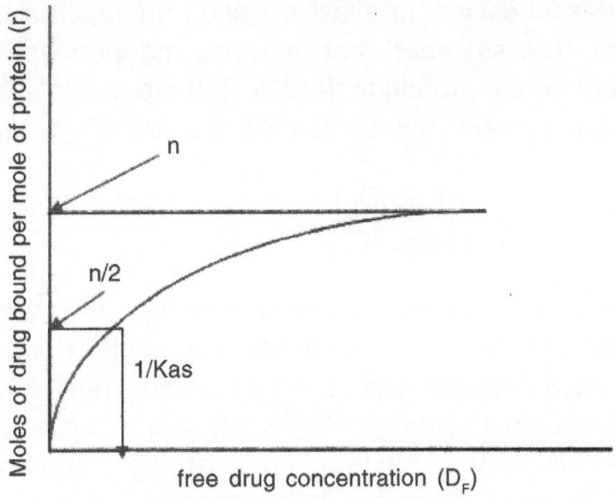

Fig. 3.5 Direct plot of r versus (D_F).

2. **Double Reciprocal Plot:** Equation 3.14 can be linearized by rearrangement and the resultant linear equations are useful for determining the number of binding sites and association constants by graphical method. The reciprocal of Equation 3.14 gives the following equation.

$$r = \frac{1+Kas\,[D_F]}{n\,Kas\,[D_F]} \quad .....(3.16)$$

or

$$\frac{1}{r} = \frac{1}{n\,Kas\,[D_F]} + \frac{1}{n} \quad .....(3.17)$$

A plot of 1/r versus 1/[D_F] is called a *double reciprocal plot* (Fig. 3.6). Equation 3.17 is like a straight line equation with an intercept (i.e. y = mx + c). Therefore, a number of biding sites may be determined from y intercept, and the association constant may be obtained from the slope. Failure to obtain a straight-line by a double reciprocal plot indicates the complex nature of drug-protein binding.

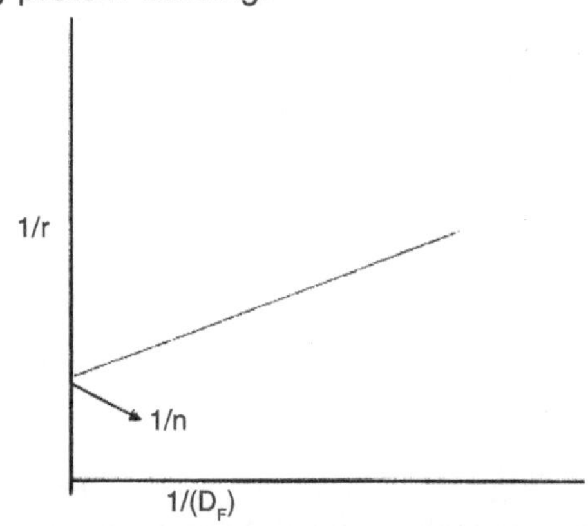

Fig. 3.6 Double reciprocal plot for the determination of number of binding sites and associated constant.

3. **Scatchard Plot:** Scatchard plot is a rearrangement of Equation 3.14 and it spreads the data to give a better line for the estimation of the binding sites and binding constants. Rearrangement of Equation 3.14 yields,

$$r = \frac{n\,Kas\,[D_F]}{1+Kas\,[D_F]}$$

$$r + r\ Kas\ [D_F] = n\ Kas\ [D_F]$$

$$r = n\ Kas\ [D_F] - r\ Kas\ [D_F]$$

$$\frac{r}{[D_F]} = n\ Kas - r\ Kas \qquad .....(3.18)$$

A graph obtained by plotting $r/[D_F]$ versus r gives a straight line with x and y intercepts equal to n and n Kas, respectively, and the slope is equal to Kas (Fig. 3.7).

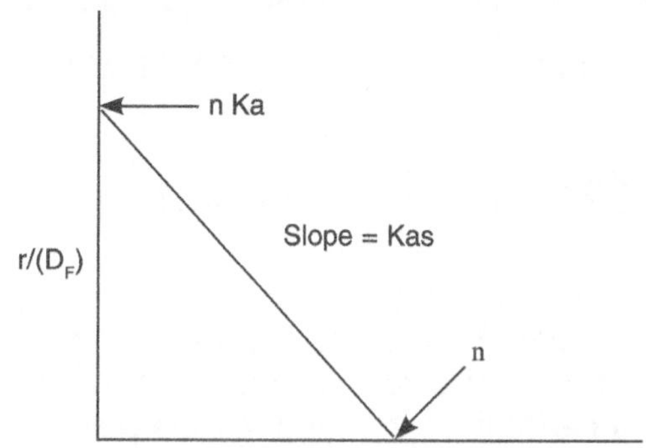

Fig. 3.7 Scatchard plot for the determination of number of binding sites on protein (n) and association constant (ka) of drug-protein binding.

Curvilinear scatchard plot indicates that the drug-protein binding is not equimolar and more than one binding site is present for the drug on the protein. The binding of salicylic acid and dicoumarol are examples where more than one binding site is involved (Fig. 3.8). In these cases, there are at least two different, independent binding sites (n_1 and n_2), each with its own independent association constant (K_1 and K_2). Equation 3.15 best describes this type of drug-protein interaction.

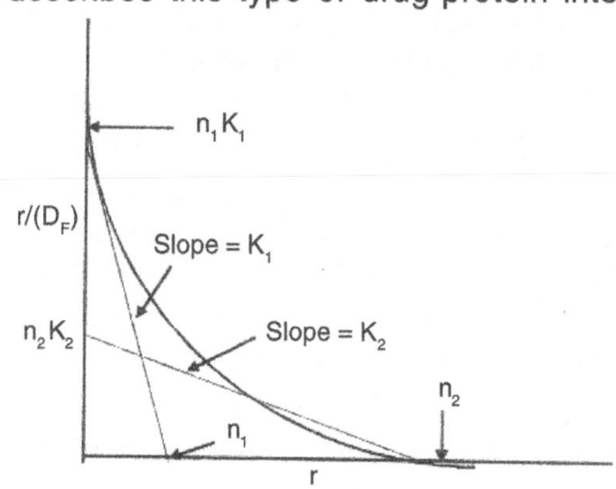

Fig. 3.8 Curvilinear scatchard plot showing more than one type of binding site.

In vivo Methods

A double reciprocal plot and scatchard plots can be used for the estimation of binding sites and association constants even when the exact nature and amount of protein is not known. The fraction of the drug bound, fb, can be determined experimentally and is equal to the ratio of the concentration of the bound drug, $[D_B]$ and the total drug concentration, $[D_t]$, in the plasma.

$$fb = \frac{[D_B]}{[D_t]} \qquad .....(3.19)$$

Now, the value of r can be calculated using the following equation.

$$r = \frac{[D_B]}{[P_t]} = \frac{n\,Kas\,[D_F]}{1+Kas\,[D_F]} \qquad .....(3.20)$$

Rearrangement of this equation gives the following expression, which is analogous to the scatchard equation.

$$\frac{[D_B]}{[D_F]} = n\ Kas\ P_t - Kas\ [D_B] \qquad .....(3.21)$$

It is possible to determine the free and bound drug concentrations in the plasma experimentally. A plot of $[D_B]/[D_F]$ versus $[D_B]$ gives a straight line whose slope is equal to the association constant, Kas. The values obtained for n and Kas give a general estimate of the affinity and binding capacity of the drug, as the plasma contains a complex mixture of proteins. In addition, estimation of the total protein content of the plasma may be used for understanding the nature of the drug-protein binding.

3.6 Drug Binding to Tissue and Other Macromolecules

Certain drugs may bind to specific tissue proteins in addition to plasma proteins. They may also bind to other macromolecules such as melanin or DNA. The higher the binding of a drug to the tissue or other macromaolecules, the lower will be the plasma concentration of the drug. This results in an increased apparent volume of distribution.

Drug binding to tissue is poorly understood because of difficulties in performing such studies. Unlike plasma protein binding, tissue binding of a drug can not be measured directly. The tissue must be disrupted, resulting in the loss of its integrity. However, tissue binding studies are important in understanding the distribution of drugs.

Few studies have been carried out using animal tissue. Tissue binding has no significant effect on drug clearance, but increases the residence time of drug in the body. A decrease in tissue binding decreases the half-life of a drug. The role of tissue binding in the pharmacological effects of drugs is yet to be known.

3.7 Apparent Volume of Distribution

The apparent volume of distribution, Vd, is frequently used to estimate the extent of drug distribution in the body. The apparent volume of distribution has no physiological meaning. There is usually a considerable difference between the apparent volume of distribution of a drug and the actual volume in which it distributes. The apparent volume of distribution is simply the ratio between the amount of drug in the body and the drug concentration in the blood. Therefore, depending on the ability of drug to distribute to various tissue, the degree of protein binding and tissue binding of the drug, the volume of distribution of the drug may range from 3 liters/70 kg body weight to 40,000 liters/70 Kg body weight or more, a value far in the excess of the total body size.

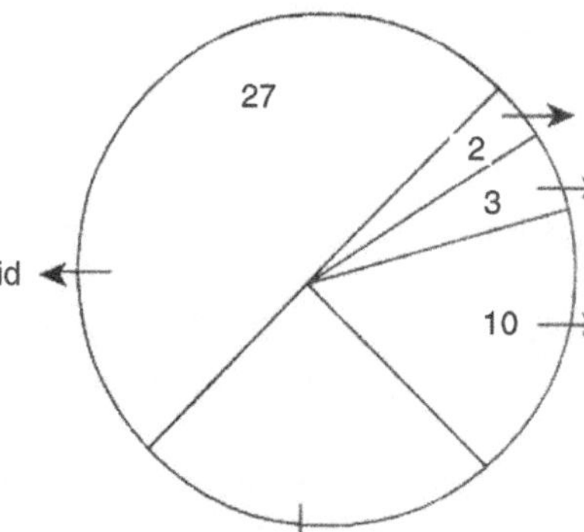

Fig. 3.9 Various body fluids volume in liters in a healthy adult weighing 70kg

Fig. 3.9 shows the volumes of different body fluids. Total body water (TBW) may be divided into 3 compartments; blood, extra-cellular fluid and intracellular fluid. Total body water is about 60% of total body weight. TBW in a normal adult weighing 70 Kg is about 42 liters, in which plasma water, ECF and intracellular water constitute 7%, 36% and 57%, respectively.

The volume of plasma water, ECF and intracellular fluid can be determined experimentally using tracer compounds which show negligible protein and tissue binding and distribute in specific fluids. Certain dyes, such as Evans blue, are essentially confined to the circulating plasma and can be used to determine the plasma volume and also blood volume, if the haematocrit value is known. Certain substances distribute rapidly throughout the ECF, but do not cross cell membranes (e.g., chloride and bromide ions). Therefore, they may be used to estimate the extra-cellular water volume. Certain lipid-soluble compounds without binding or with negligible binding such as antipyrine, or duteriated water (D_2O) can be used to estimate the total body water. The important points to be considered in the estimation of volumes of the body water are:

1. the protein binding and tissue binding nature of the tracer used (i.e., the extent of binding of the tracer to a particular macromolecule), and
2. the distribution pattern of the tracer in the specific body compartment or compartments.

The concentration of a drug in the blood or plasma is used to estimate the apparent volume of distribution. Hence, the apparent volume of distribution of a drug depends on the ability of the drug to cross biological membranes, protein binding and tissue binding of the drug. If a drug is preferentially bound to plasma proteins, the apparent volume of distribution is smaller than the real volume of distribution. On the other hand, preferential binding of drugs at extra-vascular sites results in an apparent volume of distribution larger than the true volume of distribution. Therefore, the volume of distribution is a function of four major factors:

1. the size of the organ into which the drug distributes.
2. the partition coefficient of the drug between the organ and circulating blood.
3. the blood flow to the distributing organs and
4. the extent of binding of the drug both in blood and in various tissues.

Apparent volume of distribution, Vd is calculated using the following equation.

$$Vd = \frac{\text{Amount of drug in the body at equilibrium}}{\text{Plasma drug concentration}} = \frac{X}{Cp} \quad .....(3.22)$$

If plasma volume, Vp and apparent volume of distribution of the drug, Vd are known, the fraction of the drug in plasma and outside the plasma (extracellular and intracellular fluids) can be estimated. Note that the amount of drug in plasma is Vp Cp and the amount of the drug in the body is Vd Cp. Therefore,

$$\text{Fraction of drug in plasma} = \frac{Vp}{Vd} \quad .....(3.23)$$

Similarly,

Fraction of the drug in the body outside the plasma including blood cells is given by,

$$\text{Fraction of drug in body outside plasma} = \frac{(Vd - Vp)}{Vd} \quad .....(3.24)$$

The above equations are developed without considering the binding of the drug in the blood. Within the blood, the drug can bind to many components including blood cells and plasma proteins. Therefore, drug molecules in blood can exist in a bound form (drug bound to blood cells and plasma proteins) and in unbound form (as soluble form in plasma water). As a consequence of binding, the concentration of the drug in whole blood (Cb), in plasma (Cp) and in plasma water as a free drug (Cf) can differ significantly. Remember that Cb>Cp>Cf. Now, it is possible to define different volumes of distribution of a drug. The unbound or free drug volume of distribution, Vf, is given by,

$$Vf = \frac{X}{Cf} \quad .....(3.25)$$

Similarly, whole drug in blood volume of distribution, Vb can be written as,

$$Vb = \frac{X}{Cb} \quad .....(3.26)$$

and the volume of distribution of the drug based on its plasma concentration is Vd.

$$Vd = \frac{X}{Cp} \qquad .....(3.27)$$

As the amount of a drug in the body is independent of the site of measurement, it follows from equations 3.25, 3.26 and 3.27 that

$$Vd\ Cp = Vb\ Cb = Vf\ Cf \qquad .....(3.28)$$

The values of these volume terms can differ markedly for a given drug. *The term most often quoted in the literature is based on the measurement of a drug in the plasma (i.e. Vd).*

Free drug concentration, rather than bound or total drug concentration is frequently more important in therapeutics. Therefore, the fraction of drug in plasma unbound, f_{up},

$$f_{up} = \frac{Cf}{Cp} \qquad .....(3.29)$$

The fraction of a drug in the body located in the plasma depends on its binding to both the plasma and tissue components, as shown schematically in Fig. 3.10. A drug may have a great affinity for plasma proteins, but may still be located in the tissue if the tissue has an affinity even greater than that of plasma protein binding.

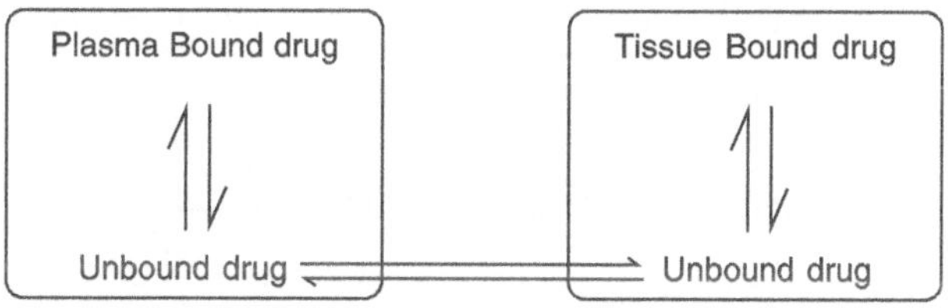

Fig. 3.10 Equilibrium between the unbound drug in plasma and in tissue compartments.

Tissue binding may be inferred from measurement of drug binding in plasma. Consider the following mass-balance equation.

Amount in body = Amount in plasma + Amount in outside plasma

$$Vd \cdot Cp = Vp.Cp + Vt\ .Ct \qquad .....(3.30)$$

Where, Ct is the total drug concentration in the tissue and Vt is the aqueous volume outside of the plasma. Dividing the Equation 3.30 by Cp,

$$Vd = Vp + Vt\ \frac{Ct}{Cp} \qquad .....(3.31)$$

The fraction of the unbound or free drug in the tissue, f_{ut} is given by,

$$f_{ut} = \frac{C_{ft}}{Ct} \qquad .....(3.32)$$

Where, C_{ft} = free drug concentration in the tissue.

It can be seen from the Fig. 3.9 that at equilibrium the unbound drug concentration in both plasma and the tissue are equal (i.e. Cf = C_{ft}). Therefore,

$$\frac{f_{up}}{f_{ut}} = \frac{Ct}{Cp} \quad .....(3.33)$$

Substituting f_{up}/f_{ut} in the place of Ct/Cp in Equation 3.31,

$$Vd = Vp + Vt\,\frac{f_{up}}{f_{ut}} \quad .....(3.34)$$

It is possible to develop appropriate equations for the calculation of various parameters for a normal adult weighing 70 kg and having normal physiological fluid volumes (Table 3.2).

Table 3.2 Approximate Equations for the estimation of Various Parameters Related to Drug Distribution in a 70-kg Healthy Adult.

Fraction of Drug in Body	Approximate Equation
In plasma	3/Vd
Outside plasma	(Vd – 3)/Vd
Unbound in body water	$\frac{42\,f_{up}}{Vd}$
Unbound in extracellular fluids	$\frac{15\,f_{up}}{Vd}$
In extracellular fluids	$\frac{7.5\,(1+f_{up})}{Vd}$
Out side extracellular fluids	$\frac{Vd-7.5\,(1+f_{up})}{Vd}$
Bound to proteins in plasma	$\frac{3\,(1-f_{up})}{Vd}$
Bound to extracellular proteins	$\frac{7.5\,(1-f_{up})}{Vd}$
Bound outside the extracellular fluids (in tissues)	$\frac{(Vd-35)\,(f_{up}-7.5)}{Vd}$

Practice Problem

An in-vitro protein binding study was conducted for a new anticancer drug and the following data were obtained. Determine the number of biding sites (n) and the association constant (Kas) from the given data using the Scatchard equation.

r	$[D_F] \times 10^4$ M
0.40	0.33
0.80	0.89
1.20	2.00
1.60	5.33

Answer:

Step 1: The Scatchard equation is given by,

$$\frac{r}{[D_F]} = n\ Kas - r\ Kas$$

Therefore, calculate the values for $r/[D_F]$

r	$[D_F] \times 10^4$ M	$r/[D_F]$
0.40	0.33	1.21
0.80	0.89	0.90
1.20	2.00	0.60
1.60	5.33	0.30

Step 2: Plot a graph of $r/[D_F]$ versus r on rectangular coordinates. Join the points to get a straight line and extend the line to get the x and y intercepts. The X and Y intercepts yield n and n Kas respectively. The slope of the line is equal to Kas.

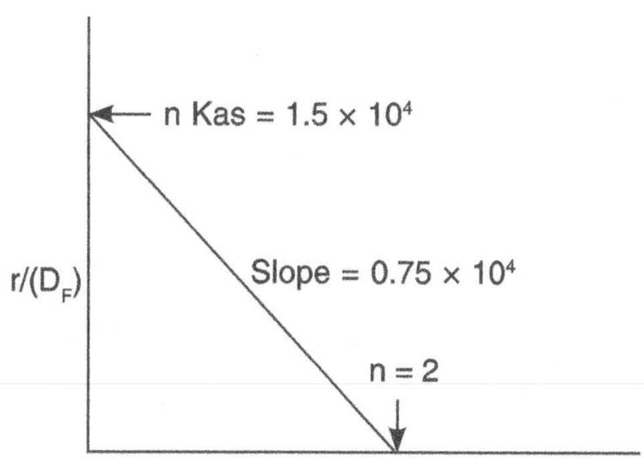

Kas can also be calculated from y intercept. They intercept = n Kas = 1.5×10^4 and n = 2

Therefore, Kas = $1.5 \times 10^4/2 = 0.75 \times 10^4$

Likely Questions

1. What are the important physicochemical properties of the drugs that limit their distribution?
2. How plasma pH influences the duration of action of phenobarbital?
3. List the physiological factors that affect the drug distribution.
4. Explain the permeability rate-limited and perfusion rate-limited drug distribution.
5. Drug distribution depends both on pKa and Ko/w. Explain.
6. Why intravenous administration of thiopental causes a quick on set of action and a rapid termination of action?
7. The Ko/w of thiopental and barbital are 3.3 and 0.002, respectively. The unionized fraction of both the drugs is 0.6 at pH 7.4. Comment on their distribution pattern.
8. Explain the Fick's law of diffusion.
9. What do you mean by hydrostatic pressure and absorptive pressure in drug distribution?
10. Drug concentration in the CSF is a measure of free drug concentration in plasma. What is your comment on this statement?
11. With the help of a diagram, explain a drug transport across the blood-brain barrier.
12. What are the reasons for directional transport across the blood-brain barrier?
13. Why levodopa, a prodrug of dopamine, is used in the treatment of Parkinsonism?
14. Explain the blood-cerebrospinal fluid barrier.
15. Write a note on (a) Placental barrier (b) Blood-testis barrier.
16. Why chronic administration of drugs to pregnant women is not advisable?
17. Why a protein bound drug is both pharmacokinetically and pharmacodynamically inactive?
18. List the various components of blood to which drugs normally bind.
19. Why is plasma albumin considered an important protein for drug binding?
20. What is the influence of protein binding on drug distribution?
21. Write the effect of protein binding on drug action.
22. Draw a diagram that shows the influence of protein binding on drug distribution, pharmacological action, biotransformation and excretion.
23. What is the influence of plasma protein binding on apparent volume of distribution of drugs?
24. How is the plasma protein concentration controlled?

25. Why the displacement of a highly protein bound drug from its binding sites by a second drug precipitate toxic effects?
26. Derive an equation for the fraction of the unbound drug in the plasma, f_{up}?
27. Give an equation that accounts for more than one type binding site on the protein?
28. What is a double reciprocal plot?
29. How is the Scatchard plot useful in determining the number of binding sites and association constants?
30. If the Scatchard plot is curvilinear, what it suggests?
31. How will you determine the different types of binding sites and association constants?
32. Write a note on in-vivo method for the estimation of n and Ka.
33. How will you determine volumes of different body fluids?
34. What are the factors that influence the apparent volume of distribution of drugs?
35. Which of the drugs listed below might be predicted to cause an adverse response due to the concurrent administration of a drug that causes 85% displacement of them from their respective binding sites? Why?

Drug	Percent Bound
Chloramphenicol	53
Phenytoin	93
Erythromycin	75
Morphine	35

36. Explain why the plasma concentration of *free* naproxen *increases* in a patient with a chronic alcoholic liver disease and probably other forms of cirrhosis; whereas, the *total* plasma drug concentration *decreases.* Percent of naproxen bound to plasma proteins is greater than 99.
37. The volume of distribution of drugs A, B and C are 10, 40 and 300 liters, respectively. Determine the percent unbound drug present outside plasma.

References

1. Ansel's Pharmaceutical Dosage Forms and Drug Delivery Systems, eighth edition, by Loyd V. Allen, Jr., Nicholas G. Popovich, Howard C. Ansel.
2. Encyclopedia of Pharmaceutical Technology, volume 13, editors- James Swarbrick, James C. Boylan, page no 162-163
3. Faed, E.M., Protein binding of drugs in plasma, interstitial fluid and tissues: effect on pharmacokinetics. Eur J Clin Pharmacol. 1981;21(1):77-81.

4. Gibaldi M, Koup JR. Pharmacokinetic concepts - drug binding, apparent volume of distribution and clearance. Eur J Clin Pharmacol. 1981;20(4):299-305.
5. Gibaldi, M., Mc namara, P.J., Apparaent volume of distribution and drug binding to plasma proteins and tissues. Eur. J. Clin. Pharmacol. 13; 373 (1978)
6. *Oie, S. Drug distribution and binding. J Clin Pharmacol. 1986 Nov-Dec;26(8):583-6.*
7. Pharmacokinetics ,second edition, edited by Milo Gibaldi, Donald Perrier, page no : 319-352. Informa Health Care U.S. 2007.
8. Remington, The Science and Practice of Pharmacy, 21st edition, volume 1 pages 1166-1167

4

Drug Elimination

Drug elimination means irreversible removal of the drug from the body by all possible routes of elimination. Elimination occurs by excretion and metabolism. **Drug excretion** refers to the removal of unchanged drug (intact drug). For most drugs, excretion occurs predominantly via kidneys. Some drugs, like gentamycin or cephalexin, are eliminated from the body almost entirely by renal excretion. Gaseous anesthetics, or volatile substances are excreted via lungs into expired air. Other minor pathways for drug excretion may include the excretion of the drug into the bile, sweat, saliva, milk or other body fluids.

Drug metabolism or **biotransformation** is the major mechanism for elimination of drugs from the body. Metabolism is the process by which the drug is chemically modified in the body and the end product of this modification is called **metabolite**. Generally, the liver is the major and some times only, site of drug metabolism. However, a drug may be metabolized extensively in one or more other tissues, such as kidneys, lungs, blood, skin and gastrointestinal wall. Biotransformation is usually enzymatic, but some drugs may be metabolized by non-enzymatic processes. Enzymes responsible for the metabolism of drugs are mainly located in the liver.

4.1 Renal Excretion

The basic anatomic unit of renal function is the *nephron*. There are 1 to 1.5 million nephrons in each kidney and are collectively responsible for the removal of metabolic waste and the maintenance of water and electrolyte balance. The basic components of a nephron are the glomerulus, proximal tubule, loop of Henle, distal tubule, and collecting tubule (see Fig. 4.2). All collecting tubules are connected and finally comes out as ureters form each kidney and are opened into the urinary bladder.

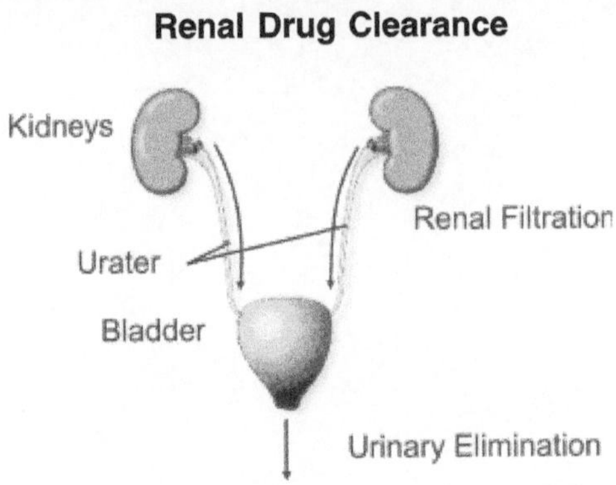

Fig. 4.1 Renal clearance of the drug.

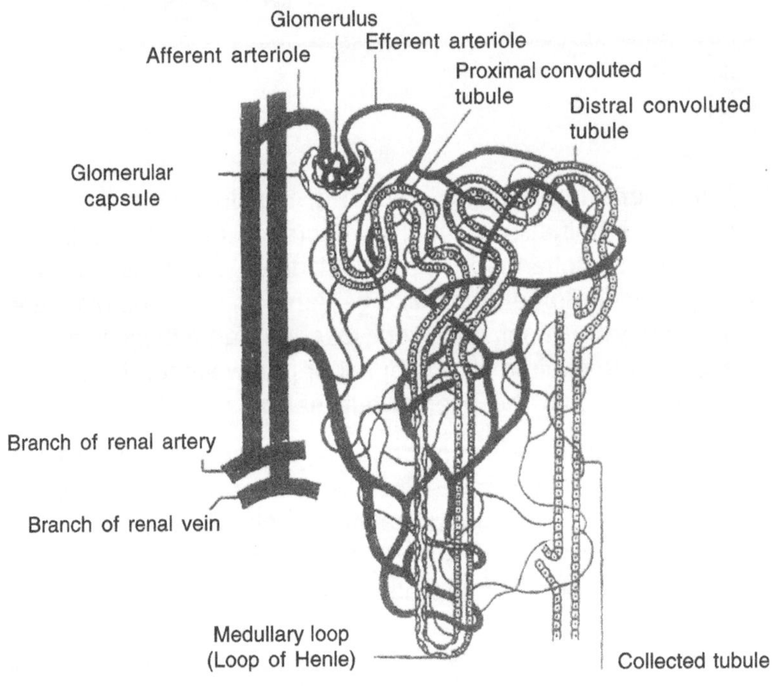

Fig. 4.2 Diagram of a nephron including the arrangement of the blood vessels.

Approximately, 20 to 25% of the cardiac out put or 1.2 liters to 1.5 liters of blood per minute go to the kidneys. About 10% of this volume is filtered at the glomeruli. Therefore, about 120 ml of plasma water is filtered each minute. The rate at which plasma water is filtered, 120ml/min in a 70-Kg 20-year-old man, is conventionally called the glomerular filtration rate, GFR.

The pores of glomerular capillaries are sufficiently large to permit the passage of compounds with molecular weights less than 20000 g/mole. Therefore, most of the drugs and even small proteins such as insulin and myoglobin can pass through the capillaries easily. Compound having molecular weight greater than 20,000 g/mole find difficulty in passing through the capillaries. Indeed, virtually no albumin (molecular weight 69,000 g/mole) is normally found in the ultrafiltrate. Accordingly, only an unbound or free drug in plasma water is filtered but not a protein bound drug.

Taking normal GFR as 120 ml/min into consideration, about 180 liters of fluid is filtered through the kidneys per day. However, 1 to 1.5 L is excreted as urine and the remainder is absorbed in the renal tubules. Renal tubules reabsorb not only the water but also various electrolytes and essential nutrients. Reabsorption of water results in high urinary concentrations of certain solutes, including drugs that are not reabsorbed in the renal tubules. As a result, high amounts of metabolic wastes such as urea, phosphate, sulfate, etc., and drugs and their metabolites are excreted through urine.

The essential nutrients and water are reabsorbed at various sites including the proximal tubule, loop of Henle, and distal tubules. Both active reabsorption and secretion mechanisms are involved. In the case of drugs, an unionized, lipid soluble drugs are reabsorbed rapidly and extensively, whereas polar drugs and ions are not reabsorbed.

Some drugs such as penicillin G are excreted into the renal tubule by active tubular secretion. Therefore, the renal excretion of a drug is a complex phenomenon involving one or more of the following processes: glomerular filtration, active tubular secretion, and passive reabsorption.

4.2 Renal Blood Flow

The renal blood flow (RBF) is the volume of blood flowing through the renal vasculature per unit time. The renal blood flow can be determined by estimating the renal clearance of paraaminohippuric acid (PAH). PAH is poorly lipid soluble, it does not penetrate erythrocytes, it is not reabsorbed from the tubules, and more importantly it is completely filtered in the glomerulus in a single pass through the kidneys. Therefore, the renal clearance of PAH is a measure of the renal plasma flow rate (RPF). Another compound used for this purpose is iodopyracet (Diodrast). The renal plasma flow rate (RPF) and renal blood flow rate are related as given below,

$$RPF = RBF - (RBF \times Hct) \quad .....(4.1)$$

Where, Hct is the hematocrit. Hematocrit is the fraction of blood cells in the blood and is about 0.45. Normally, blood cells constitute 45% of the total blood volume.

$$RBF = RPF\ (1 - Hct) \quad .....(4.2)$$

Normal RPF can be calculated based on the normal values of RBF (1.2 L/min.) and hematocrit (0.45). According to equation 4.1,

$$RPF = 1.2 - (1.2 \times 0.45) = 0.66 \text{ L/min. or } 660 \text{ ml/min.}$$

Accordingly, the renal clearance of PAH is a measure of renal plasma flow rate (600-700 ml/min.).

4.3 Renal Clearance

Drug present in the body is subjected to elimination by all possible pathways of elimination. Drug elimination can be expressed as the amount eliminated per unit time. Consider that 100 mg of a drug is administered as I.V.bolus. Suppose that the volume of distribution of the drug is 10 L. The blood concentration will be 10 ug/ml at zero time. The blood concentration after 1 hour is found to be 8 ug/ml. It means, 20 mg of drug [(10 ug/ml x 10 L) - (8 ug/ml x 10 L)] is eliminated per hour. The rate of elimination of the drug is expressed in terms of the volume of fluid cleared of the drug per hour i.e., 20 mg of drug is equivalent to 2 L of volume of the fluid in which the drug is initially distributed. Therefore, **drug clearance** is equal to 2 L/hour.

Drug clearance is defined as the volume of the fluid cleared of the drug per unit time. Similarly, renal clearance is defined as the volume of plasma that is completely cleared of drug per unit time by kidneys. This concept may be applied to any organ that eliminates the drug (e.g. hepatic clearance, biliary clearance). Renal clearance, (Cl_R), often constitutes a significant fraction of the total drug clearance (Cl_T).

For drugs that are eliminated solely by the renal route, the $Cl_R = Cl_T$

The rate of urinary excretion of a drug by filtration is proportional to its plasma free drug concentration.

$$\frac{dx_u}{dt} \propto C \qquad .....(4.3)$$

$$\frac{dx_u}{dt} = Cl_R\, C \qquad .....(4.4)$$

$$Cl_R = \frac{dx_u / dt}{C} \qquad .....(4.5)$$

Where:

dx_u/dt = instantaneous rate of urinary excretion of the drug

C = plasma concentration of unbound the drug

Cl_R = renal clearance of unbound drug

It is difficult to practically obtain an instantaneous rate of excretion of the drug, dx_u / dt. Therefore, an average rate of excretion of the drug during a time period (DXu/Dt) and plasma concentration of the drug at the mid point of urine collection (C') are used to calculate renal clearance of the drug.

$$Cl_R = \frac{(\Delta Xu / \Delta t)}{C'}$$

Differences in the renal clearance of enantiomers

Renal clearance, like hepatic clearance, can be stereoselective. Examples are disopyramide and terbutaline where clearance of the two enantiomers differs by approximately 2-fold. Equally, however, there are other examples, tocainide being one where there is no difference in the renal clearance of enantiomers. This difference is likely due to differences in the affinity of the enantiomers for the transporters involved in tubular seceretion. Thus for the majority of compounds that are filtered in the glomerulus and are not actively secreted, there will be no difference in the elimination of the enantiomers.

4.3.1 Determination of GFR

Glomerular filteration rate (GFR) is the volume of fluid filtered from the renal glomerular capillaries into the Bowman's capsule per unit time.

GFR is typically recorded in units of volume per time[2].

$$\text{GFR} = \frac{\text{urine concentration} \times \text{urine flow}}{\text{Plasma concentration}}$$

Determination of clearance of endogenous creatinine using its plasma and urinary concentration (standard clearance) or Cockroft and Gault equation (estimated clearance) is commonly performed for assessment of glomerular filtration rate.

In order to determine glomerular filtration rate (GFR) of an individual, a compound having following characters is required.

1. It should not bound to plasma proteins or to any other macromolecules.
2. It should not be either secreted or reabsorbed across the renal tubules.

Creatinine, the endogenous end product of creatine metabolism and inulin, polysaccharide, meet the above requirements. Therefore, the renal clearance of inulin or creatinine is a measure of the glomerular filtration rate (GFR). Under normal conditions, GFR is relatively stable and insensitive to changes in the renal blood flow.

A number of equations have been derived to estimate the creatinine clearance from the plasma creatinine value. One such (Crockcroft and Gault, 1976) is:

$$\text{Clearance (mL/min)} = \frac{(140 - \text{age in years}) \times \text{Wt (kg)}}{814 \times \text{plasma [creatinine] (mmol/L)}}$$

This gives a reasonably good correlation with measured values provided that the plasma creatinine value is not within the normal range, the renal failure is not so severe, and there is no inhibition of tubular secretion of creatinine by medications.

4.3.2 Renal Clearance of Drug and GFR

The renal clearance of a drug relative to GFR provides information on the mechanisms of renal excretion. Renal clearance of a drug just by glomerular filtration may be estimated from the fraction of free drug in the plasma. The product of GFR (120 ml/min.) and the fraction of free drug or unbound drug in the plasma is the renal clearance of the drug by filtration. Renal clearance values, calculated as above, exceeding 120 ml/min are indicative of tubular secretion. Expected renal clearance of penicillin G, taking the fraction of free drug in the plasma (0.4) into consideration, is 48 ml/min. But the renal clearance of penicillin G (500 ml/min.) exceeds the expected value (48 ml/min.). This is because of tubular secretion of penicillin G.

Renal clearance values that are below 120 ml/min., even when the degree of plasma protein binding is taken into consideration, are indicative of tubular reabsorption. The drug, phenytoin, undergoes protein binding. The renal clearance of phenytoin (5 ml/min.) is less than the expected (50 ml/min.), indicating tubular reabsorption.

The other way of comparing drug renal clearance and GFR is the calculation of clearance ratio. Clearance ratio is the ratio of drug renal clearance to the renal clearance of inulin (i.e., GFR). A clearance ratio less than 1 indicates that the drug probably undergoes tubular reabsorption. A clearance ratio greater than 1 indicates the existence of tubular secretion, and the renal clearance ratio is equal to 1 means the drug is excreted by filtration only (not always true, see below).

Although renal clearance of drugs give some insight into the mechanisms of renal excretion, conclusions can not be drawn just based on these values. The renal clearance of a drug is a net result of the possible processes involved in the excretion of that drug. Secretion and reabsorption have opposite effects on renal clearance. For example, sulfisoxazole undergoes tubular secretion and reabsorption in a man but to the similar extent. Therefore, the renal clearance of sulfisoxazole will be equal to the expected value, and leads to the wrong conclusion that the drug is excreted only by filtration. Therefore, relative magnitudes of each process influence the renal clearance of a drug. From a physiological point of view, renal clearance may be considered as the ratio of the sum of the glomerular filtration and active secretion rates less the reabsorption rate divided by the plasma drug concentration.

$$Cl_R = \frac{\text{filtration rate} + \text{secretion rate} - \text{reabsorption}}{\text{plasma drug concentration}}$$

Tubular Secretion

Tubular secretion is an active transport process by which drugs diffuse against concentration gradient from the blood to the renal tubule and requires an energy input for the process to occur. The process exhibits some degree of structural specificity and hence, drugs with similar structures may compete for the same carrier system. Carrier systems exist for secreting weak acids (anions) such as thiazide diuretics bile salts, penicillin G, prostaglandins, salicylates and bases (cations) such as triamterene, acetylcholine, atropine, dopamine, epinephrine, morphine, quinine including quaternary ammonium compounds from the plasma into the tubular lumen. The secretory processes are located predominantly in the proximal tubule. The carrier system is capacity limited and may be saturated.

Protein binding influences the elimination of a half-life of the drug that is excreted solely by glomerular filtration. In contrast, protein binding has very little effect on elimination of a half-life of a drug excreted mostly by active secretion, because there is a rapid transport of the unbound drug (free drug) and rapid dissociation of the drug-protein complex. For example, dicloxacillin, although extensively bound to the plasma protein and not subject to hepatic metabolism, is rapidly eliminated by active secretion.

Competitive inhibition of secretion of one drug by another is observed with an active transport process and this character has been used to prolong the half-life of drugs like penicillin that are eliminated to a considerable extent by tubular secretion. Probenecid, a weak organic acid, competitively inhibits the tubular secretion of penicillin G and other penicillins. Probenecid has been used clinically to increase the duration of action of penicillins. Another example of competitive inhibition of excretion is cimetidine and procainamide, probenecid and gemifloxacin.

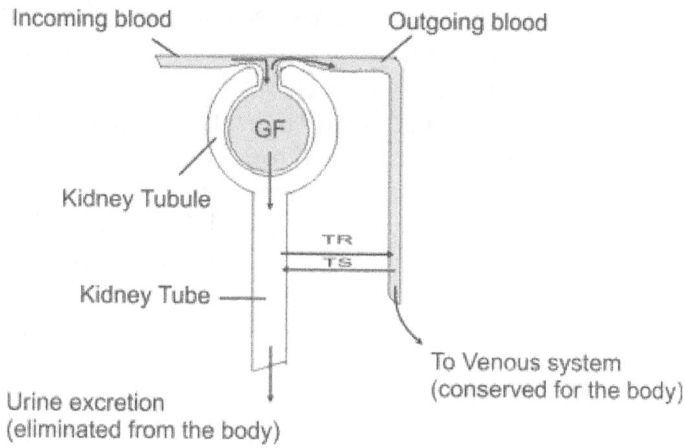

Fig. 4.3 Tubular secretion (TS) and tubular reabsorption (TR) of the drug.

Tubular Reabsorption

Drugs reach the renal tubule either by glomerular filtration or by both glomerular filtration and active secretion. Most drugs are subject to tubular reabsorption. The tubular reabsorption of drugs is usually a passive process, while the essential nutrients such as glucose are reabsorbed by active process. Depending on the extent of reabsorption, drugs may have renal clearance values of zero (for drugs that are completely absorbed), less than the GFR if the drug enters the tubules only by filtration, or more than the GFR if the extent of reabsorption is less than tubular secretion plus the GFR. The renal tubule membranes favor the transport of lipid-soluble drugs. Drugs that are poorly lipid-soluble or ionized are poorly reabsorbed.

The reabsorption of weak acidic or weak basic drugs is influenced by the pKa of a drug and the pH of the fluid in the renal tubule (i.e., urine pH). Both these factors together determine the proportions of both ionized and unionized forms of the drug. In general, the unionized form of a drug is more lipid soluble than the ionized form and penetrates the lipoid membranes easily. Therefore, the relative proportion of the unionized form of a drug decides the rate and extent of reabsorption of the drug from the renal tubules back into the body. Tubular reabsorption of drugs is usually a passive process.

The pH of the blood is maintained at 7.4, the pKa of a drug is constant but the normal urine pH may vary from 4.5 to 8.0. Urine pH is affected by diet, pathophysiology of the kidneys and drug intake. Diets rich in carbohydrate will result in a higher pH, whereas diets rich in protein content will result in a lower urinary pH. Respiratory or metabolic acidosis produces acidic urine while respiratory or metabolic alkalosis produces alkaline urine. Drugs such as ascorbic acid and antacids such as sodium bicarbonate produce acidic urine and alkaline urine respectively, when administered in large quantities. Diurnal variation in the pH of the urine is observed, i.e., urine pH is relatively low during sleep, but increases after awakening.

Even though reabsorption of filtered solutes takes place from both proximal and distal tubules, reabsorption of drugs takes place mainly from distal tubules. Therefore, urine pH is assumed to be equal to the pH of the site of reabsorption in renal tubules. Since the weak acidic drugs mainly exist in a unionized form in acidic pH, the reabsorption of weak acidic drugs is expected to be higher in acidic pH. Consequently, the renal clearance of weak acidic drugs is low in acidic pH and high in alkaline pH. Similarly, weak basic drugs are reabsorbed in alkaline urine pH and eliminated in acidic urine pH. Urinary pH is important only when the drug in question is a weak acid or base of which a significant fraction is excreted. The plasma levels will change inversely to the excretory rate. For example, it has been shown clinically with quinidine that alkalinization of the urine not only decreases the urine concentration but also increases the plasma concentration and toxicity.

The pKa of the drug is also one of the determinants of renal clearance. Relatively strong acids and bases exist completely in ionized form over the entire pH range of the urine and hence show little tubular reabsorption. Weak acidic drugs and weak basic drugs exhibit pH-dependent tubular reabsorption in the critical range of pKa values. The critical range of pKa values for weak acidic drugs is 3.0 to 7.5 and for weak basic drugs is 7.5 to 10.5.

Active Tubular Reabsorption

As stated earlier in this chapter, most of the drugs are reabsorbed from the renal tubules by passive processes, but there are some exceptions to this general statement. Uric acid is thought to be reabsorbed by an active transport system since its reabsorption is found to be inhibited by uricosuric drugs (probenecid, Sulfinpyrazone). Capacity-limited renal elimination of riboflavin suggests that this vitamin undergoes reabsorption by an active process. Lithium and fluoride appear to undergo active tubular reabsorption.

A complicated observation is that a drug may primarily inhibit active reabsorption at one dose and active secretion at another, frequently lower, dose. For example, small amounts of salicylates will decrease total urate excretion, while high doses have a uricosuric effect. This is offered as an explanation for the apparently paradoxical effects of low doses and high doses of drugs on the total excretory pattern of compounds that are handled by renal active transport.

4.4 Hepatic Elimination of Drugs

4.4.1 Anatomy and Physiology of the Liver

The liver is located in the right side of the abdominal cavity. It consists of large right and left lobes that merge in the middle. The liver is perfused by the blood from both the hepatic artery and large hepatic portal vein. The hepatic artery carries oxygen to the liver and accounts for about 25% of the blood supply. The hepatic portal vein that collects blood from various segments of the GI tract carries nutrients and accounts for about 75% of the liver blood flow (Fig. 4.4).

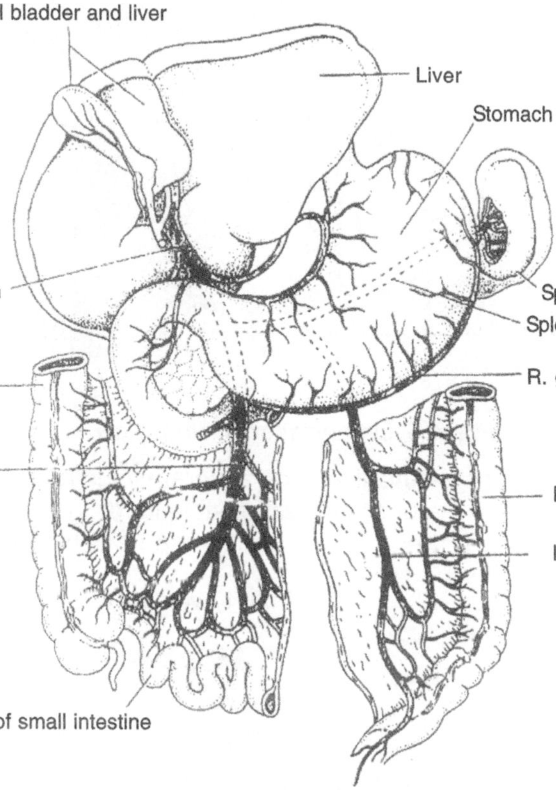

Fig. 4.4 Blood flow to the liver. Blood collected from GIT to liver.

The liver is organized in lobules, within which blood flows past hepatic cells via sinusoids from branches of the portal vein and also the hepatic artery to the central vein of each lobule (Fig.4.5). The endothelium of the senusoids has large fenestrations, and the plasma is in close contact with liver cells (Fig. 4.6). There is usually only one layer of hepatocytes between senusoids, so the total area of contact between liver cells and plasma is very large. The central veins coalesce to form the hepatic vein. Blood leaves the liver via the hepatic vein, which empties into the inferior vena cava. The average transit time for blood across the liver lobule from portal venule to the central vein is about 8.4 seconds. Numerous macrophases called **Kupffer cells** are anchored to the endothelium of the senusoids and project into the lumen. Kupffer cells are phagocytic tissue macrophases that are part of the reticuloendothelial system; they engulf wornout red blood cells and foreign material.

Each liver cell is also apposed to several bile canaliculi. The canaliculi drain into intralobular bile ducts, and there coalesce via interlobular bile ducts to form the right and left hepatic ducts. These ducts join outside the liver to form the common bile duct. The cystic duct drains the contents of the gallbladder. The hepatic duct unites with the cystic duct to form the common bile duct. The common bile duct enters the duodenum at the duodenal papilla. Its orifice is surrounded by the sphincter of Oddi and it usually unites with the main pancreatic duct just before entering the duodenum.

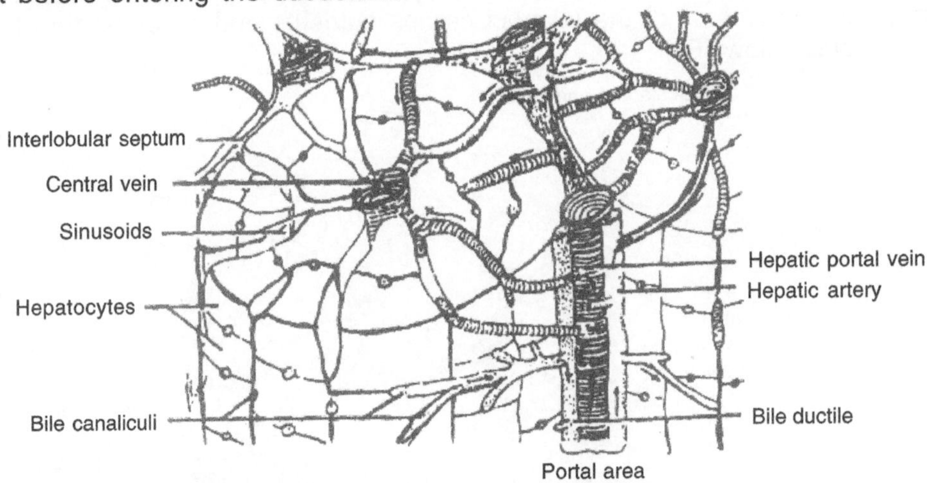

Fig. 4.5 Organization of blood flow in the liver.

The principle functions of the liver are several including detoxification of many drugs and toxins. The liver is the major organ responsible for drug metabolism. However, intestinal tissues, kidneys, lungs and the skin also contain appreciable amounts of biotransformation enzymes.

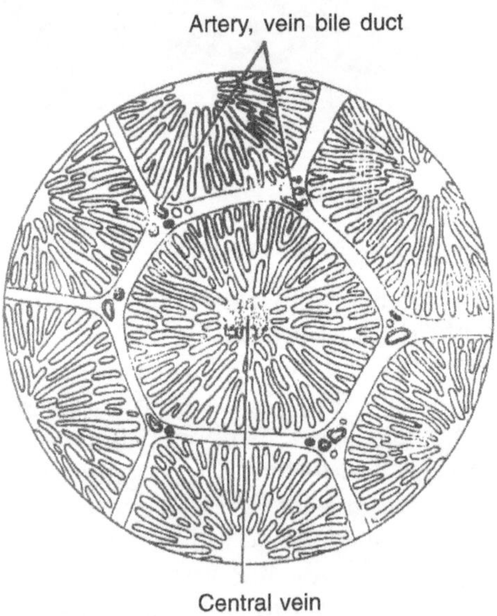

Fig. 4.6 A magnified transverse section of liver lobules.

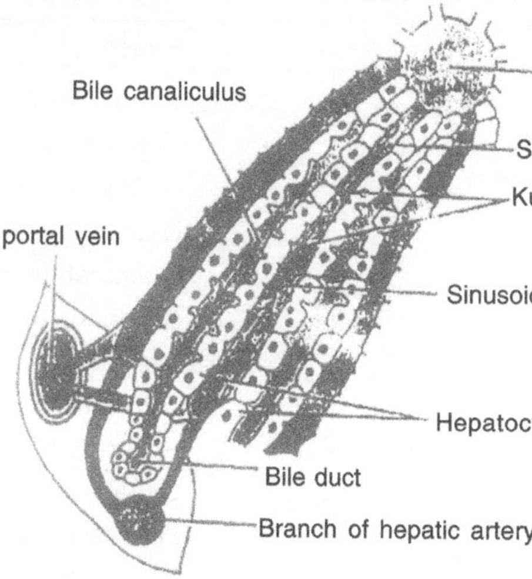

4.5 Drug Metabolism

Drug metabolism or biotransformation refers to the biochemical (enzymatic) conversion of a drug to another chemical form. Biotransformation is usually enzymatic, but some of the drugs may be chemically changed by a non-enzymatic process, as in the case of ester hydrolysis. Several of the transformations occur in the endoplasmic reticulum of the liver and of certain other tissues. On homogenizing these tissues, the endoplasmic reticulum is disrupted with the formation of small vesicles called **microsomes**. For this reason, metabolizing enzymes of the endoplasmic reticulum are called **microsomal enzymes**. Drug metabolism, therefore, may be classified as microsomal and non-microsomal.

Drug latentiation: When a delayed or prolonged response to a drug is desired or an unpleasant taste or local reaction is to be avoided, it is a common pharmaceutical practice to prepare an inactive or non offending precursor, such that the active form may be generated in the body. This practice has been termed drug latentiation. Chloramphenicol palmitate, dichloralphenazone and the estolates of various steroid harmones are examples of deliberately latentiated drugs.

Because inactive metabolites do not always result from biotranformation, the term detoxification should not be used as a synonym for biotransformation*.

The pathways of metabolism may be divided into two major groups of reactions, **Phase I** and **Phase II** reactions. Phase I or synthetic or functionalization reactions occur first and introduce or expose a functional group on the drug molecule. Phase II or synthetic or conjugative reactions involve conjugation of endogenous substances with the drug molecule via functional groups. A list of major reactions is presented in Table 4.1.

Table 4.1 Reactions Classed as Phase I or Phase II Metabolism.

Phase I	**Phase II**
Oxidation (microsomal) Aromatic Hydroxylation Aliphatic Hydroxylation Epoxidation N-Dealkylation O-Dealkylation S-Dealkylation Oxidative deamination N-oxidation S-oxidation Phosphothionate oxidation Dehalogenation	Conjugation with Sugars (a) Glucuronidation O-Glucuronides N-Glucuronides (b) Conjugation with other sugars Sulfation Methylation Acetylation Amino Acid conjugation Glutathione conjugation Fatty acid conjugation Condensation reactions
Oxidation (non-microsomal) Alcohol Dehydrogenase Aldehyde Oxidation Xanthine Oxidase Amine Oxidases Alkylhydrazine Oxidase Aromatases	
Reduction Azo reduction Nitro reduction Reductive dehalogenation	
Hydrolysis Ester hydrolysis Amide hydrolysis Hydrazine and Carbamate Hydrolysis	
Hydration Other minor reactions	

Although important exceptions exist, most biotransformations result in metabolites that are polar and considerably less active than the parent compounds. A lipid-soluble drug crosses cell membranes and is easily reabsorbed by the renal tubular cells, exhibiting a tendency to remain in the body. The conversion of a lipid-soluble drug to a more polar metabolite enables the drug to be eliminated more quickly than if the drug remains a lipid-soluble. The apparent volume of distribution of a metabolite is usually less than that of a parent drug. Metabolites are excreted in the urine more readily than their precursors because often they are not subject to tubular reabsorption. The primary objective of drug metabolism is to eliminate the drug from the body.

4.5.1 Phase I Reactions

The basic objective of the phase I reactions is to introduce or expose a functional group on the drug molecule. The molecule is now available for Phase II reactions. Phase I reactions occur first and the metabolite generally contains hydroxyl, amine or carboxyl group. Phase I metabolism includes oxidation (by microsomal and non-microsomal enzymes), reduction, hydrolysis, hydration and other rare miscellaneous reactions (Table 4.1). Examples of the more important Phase I drug metabolism pathways in a man are given in Table 4.2.

Table 4.2 Metabolic pathways for Drugs in Man.

Type of Reaction	Example
I. Oxidation 1. Microsomal (a) Aromatic hydroxylation 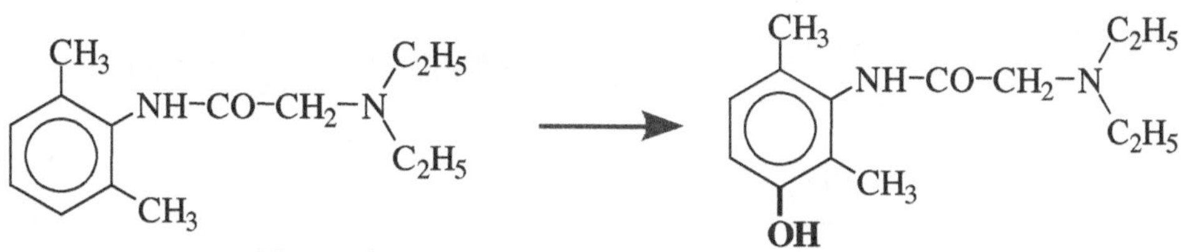 Lignocaine	
(b) Aliphatic hydroxylation 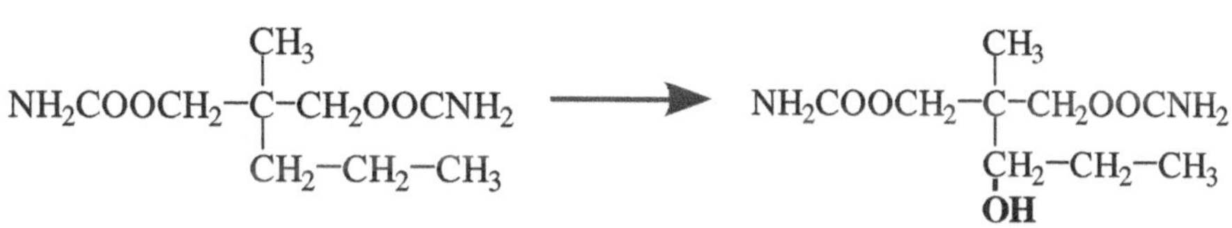 Meprobamate	
(c) Epoxidation 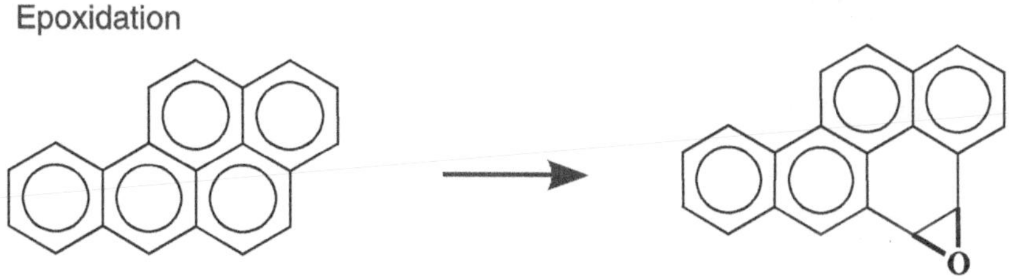 Benzo[a]pyrene	

Type of Reaction	Example
(d) N-dealkylation	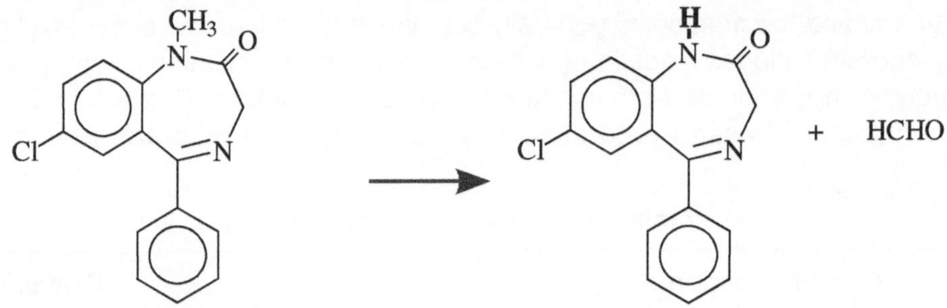 Diazepam
(e) O-dealkylation	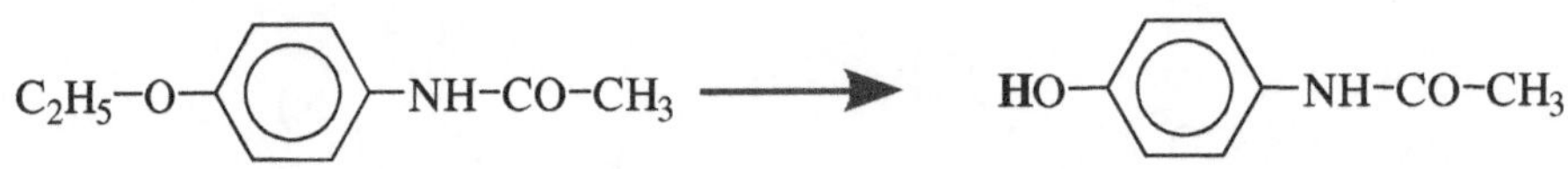 Phenacetin
(f) S-dealkylation	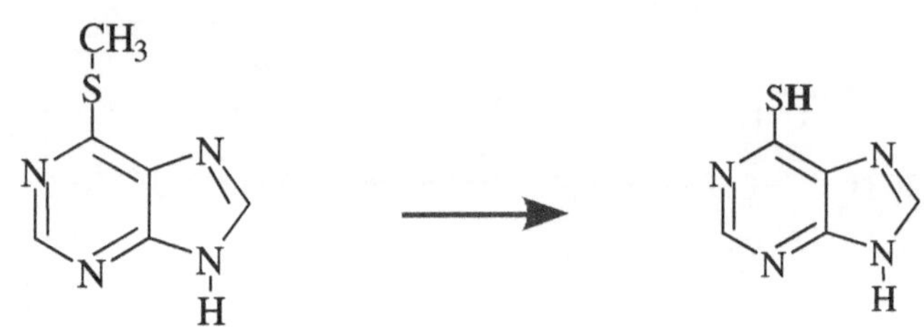 S-methylthiopurine
(g) Oxidative deamination	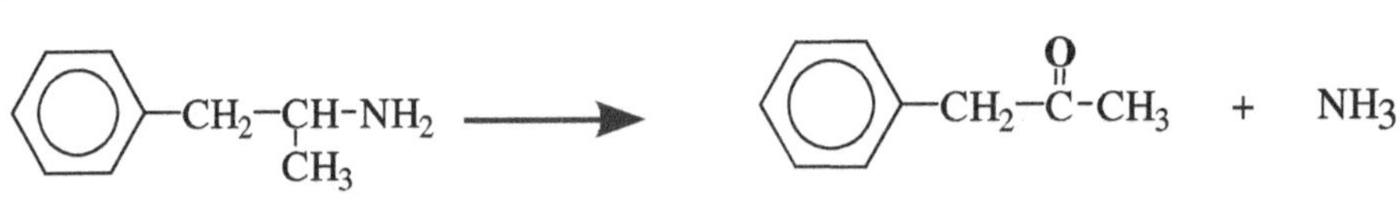 Amphetamine

Table 4.2 ***Contd...***

Type of Reaction	Example

(h) N-Oxidation

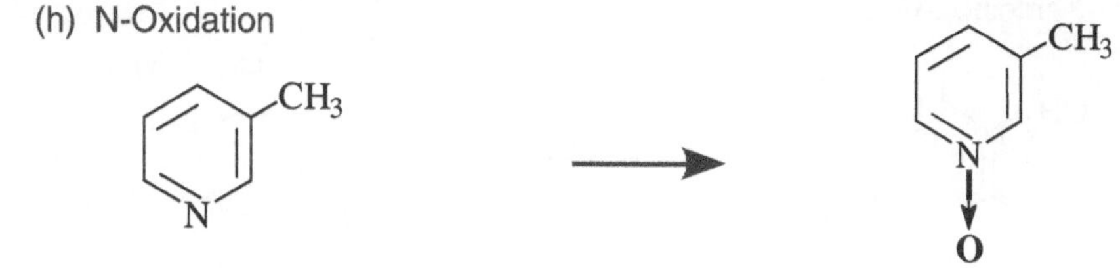

(i) S-Oxidation

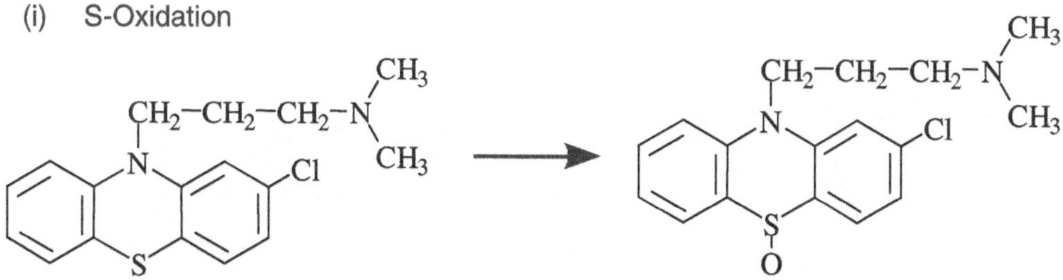

Chlorpromazine

(j) Phosphothionate oxidation

Parathion

(k) Dehalogenation

$$CF_3-CHBrCl \longrightarrow CF_3-CH_2-\mathbf{OH} \longrightarrow CF_3-COOH$$

Halothane

2. Non - microsomal

(a) Alcohol dehydrogenase

$$CH_3-CH_2-OH \longrightarrow CH_3-CHO$$

Ethanol

(b) Aldehyde oxidation

$$CH_3-CHO \longrightarrow CH_3-\mathbf{COOH}$$

Acetaldehyde

Table 4.2 ***Contd...***

Type of Reaction	Example
(c) Xanthine oxidase	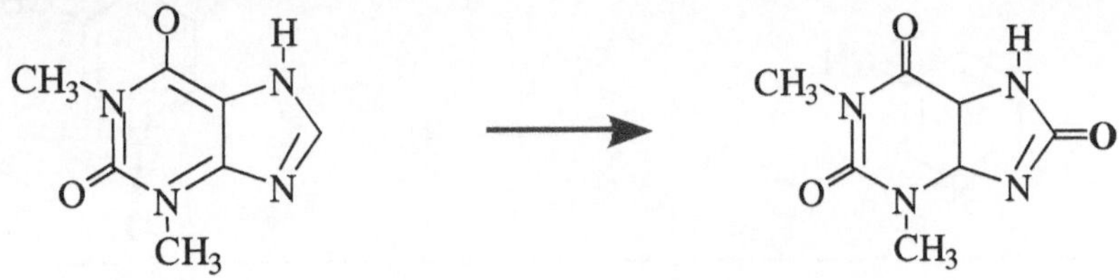 Theophylline
(d) Amine oxidase	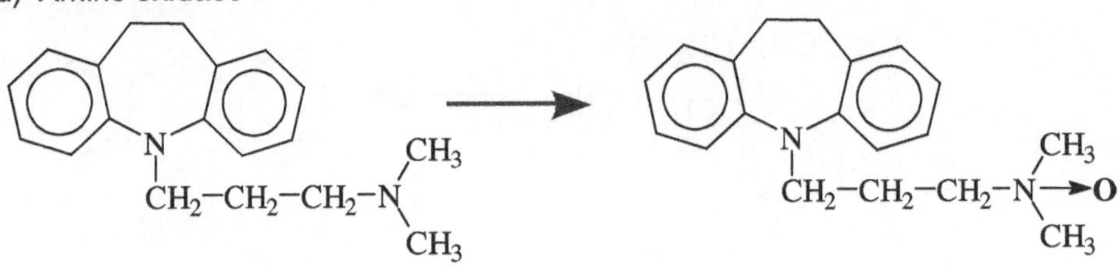 Imipranine
(e) Alkylhydrazine oxidase	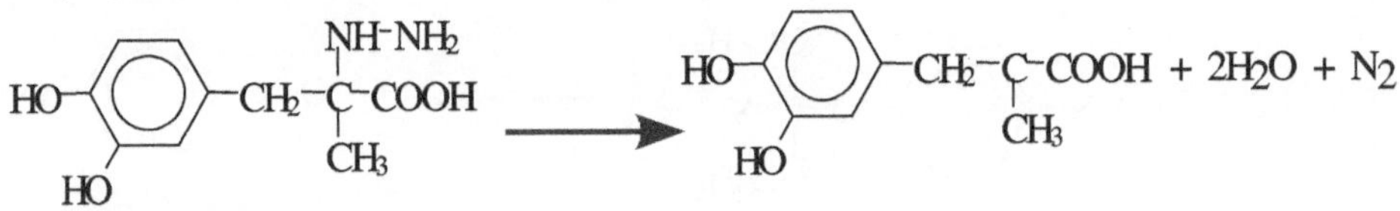 Carbidopa
(f) Aromatases	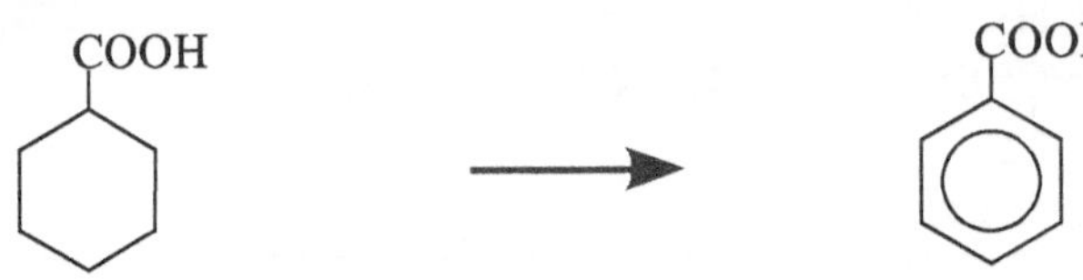 Drug containing cyclohexane carboxylic acid
II. Reduction	
(a) Azo reduction	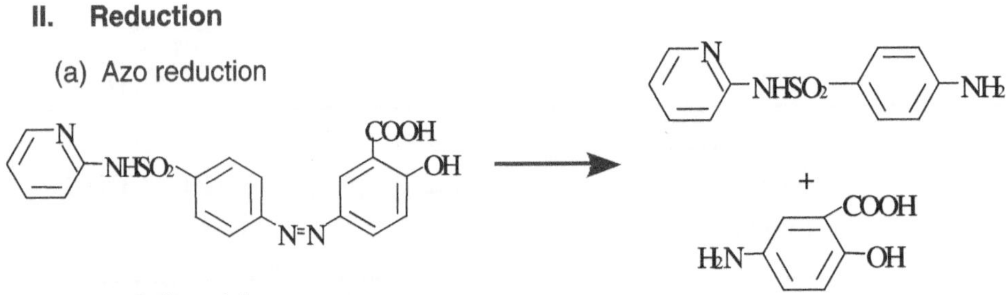 Sulfasalzine

Table 4.2 *Contd...*

Type of Reaction	Example
(b) Nitro reduction 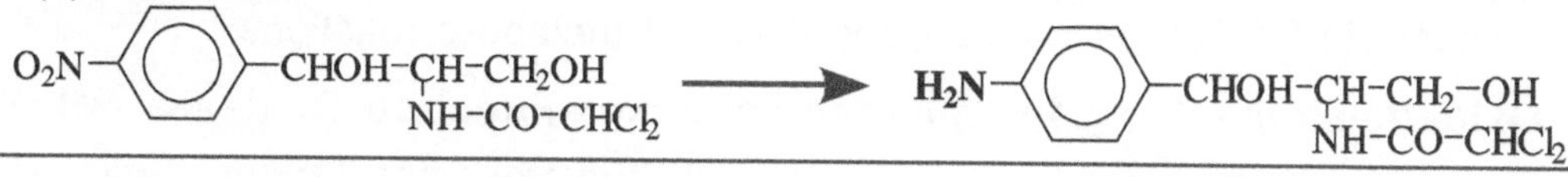	
(c) Reductive dehalogenation 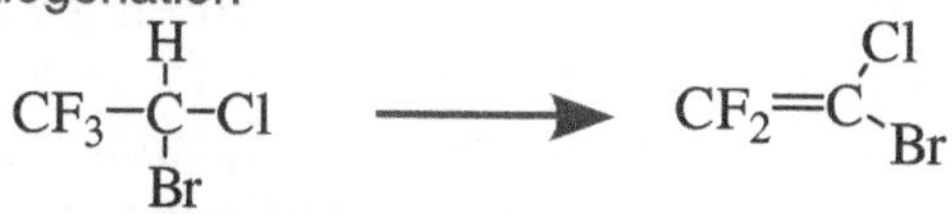 Halothane	
III. Hydrolysis (a) Ester hydrolysis 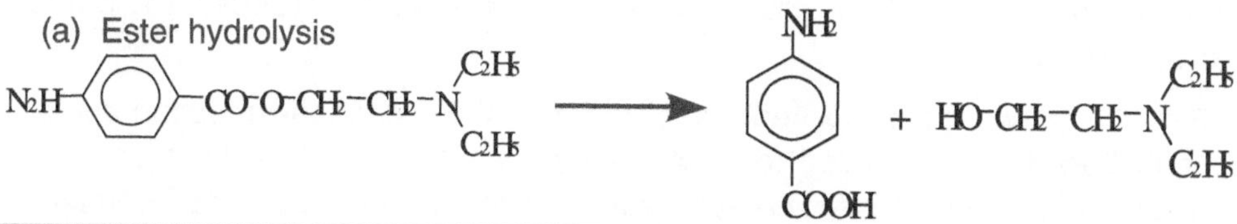	
(b) Amide hydrolysis 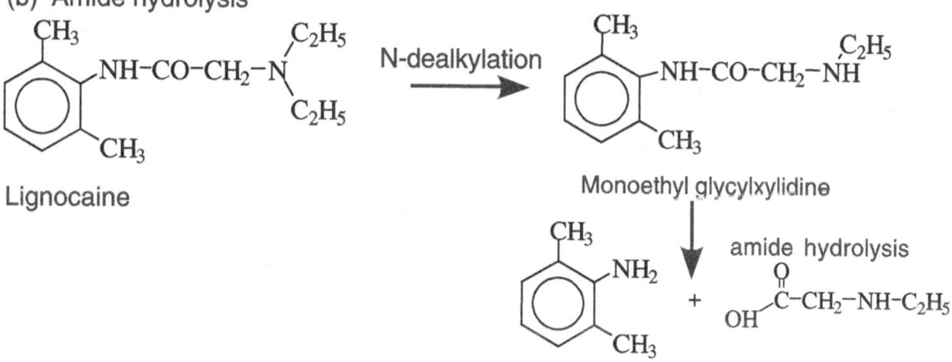	
(c) Hydrazine and carbamate hydrolysis 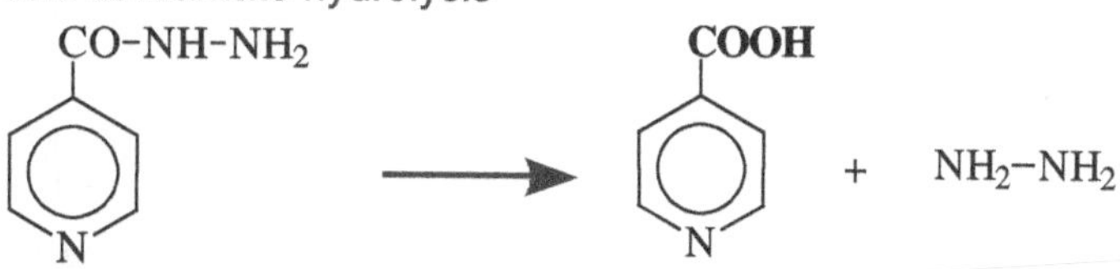 Isoniazid	
IV. Hydration 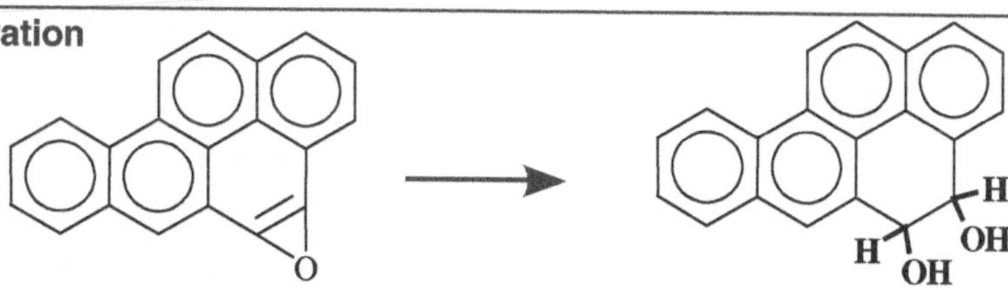 Benzo[a]pyrene 4,5 -epoxide	

4.5.1.1 Enzymes Involved in the Biotransformation of Drugs

Microsomal and non-microsomal enzymes present in the liver and other tissues are responsible for various Phase I and Phase II metabolic reactions.

Oxidation's Involving the Microsomal Mixed-Function Oxidases (MFO's)

The mixed-function-oxidase system found in microsomes (endoplasmic reticulum) of many cells (notably those of liver, kidney, lung and intestine) performs many different functionalization reactions. The mixed-functions-oxidase enzymes are structural enzymes that constitute an electron transport system that requires reduced NADPH, molecular oxygen, cytochrome P-450, NADPH-cytochrome P-450 reductase, and phospholipid. Cytochrome P-450 is a heme protein containing iron. Cytochrome P-450 is a group of enzymes that are responsible for many of the oxidations and also reduction reactions. Many drugs, as well as steroid hormones, are oxidized by this microsomal system.

Fig. 4.7 shows the simplified cytochrome P-450 oxidation-reduction cycle. Binding of the substrate to the oxidized form of the cytochrome P-450 is the first step involved in the oxidation of xenobiotics. The substrate-oxidized cytochrome P-450 complex is reduced by the NADPH-cytochrome c reductase by transfering one electron to the complex. This is the rate-limiting step in the oxidation of xenobiotics. The reduced substrate-cytochrome P-450 complex combines with a molecule of oxygen and the substrate is oxidized, releasing the oxidized cytochrome P-450.

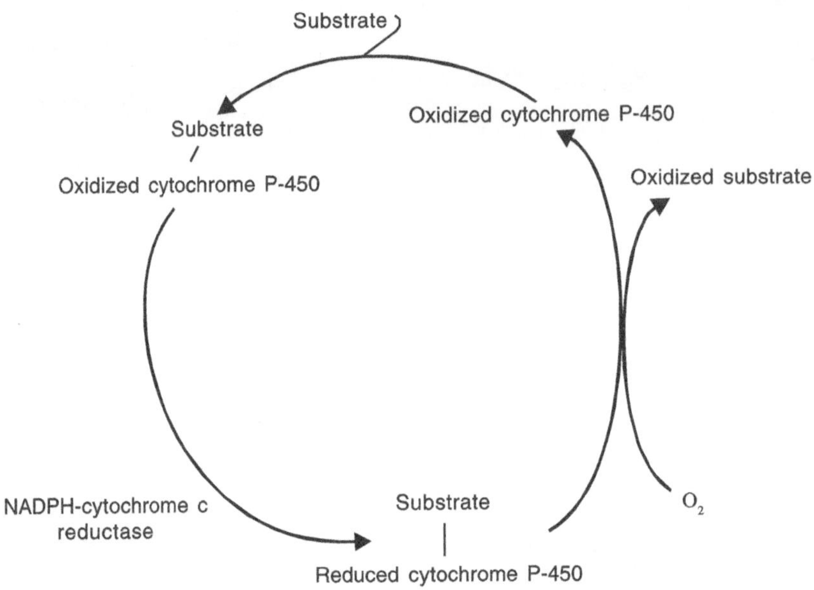

Fig. 4.7 A magnified transverse section of liver lobules.

Oxidation Involving Enzymes Other than MFO's

Oxidation of certain drugs, such as alcohols and xanthines, may be catalyzed by non-microsomal enzymes. Enzymes in the body not related to MFO's include alcohol dehydrogenase, aldehyde dehydrogenase, xanthine oxidase, amine oxidases, aromatases and alkylhydrazine oxidase. Drugs such as mercaptopurine and azothioprine are metabolized by non-microsomal enzymes.

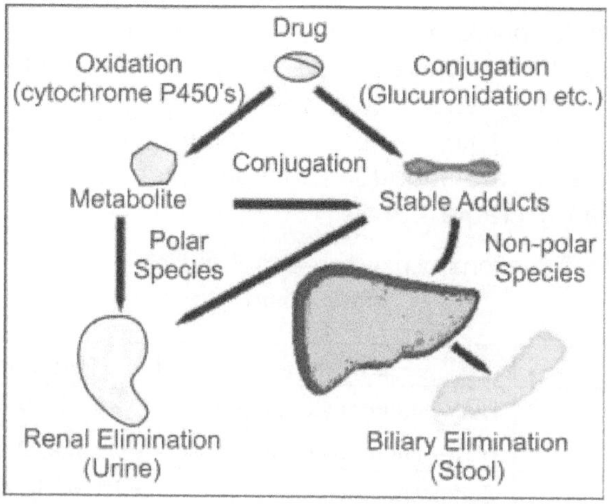

Fig. 4.8 drug metabolism pathways.

Reduction

Reduction is a relatively uncommon pathway of drug metabolism. Hepatic microsomes catalyze various reductive reactions and require NADPH for this purpose. Azo and nitro-reduction is catalyzed by cytochrome P-450 (but can also be catalyzed by NADPH-cytochrome c-reductase). Chloral hydrate is reduced to its active metabolite, trichloroethanol by alcohol dehydrogenase. Reduction of prednisone and cortisone results in the formation of their active metabolites prednisolone and hydrocortisone. Azo dyes, used as coloring agents in pharmaceutical products and food, are reduced to form amines, both in the liver and by the intestinal flora.

Hydrolysis

Hydrolysis of esters, amides, hydrazides and carbamates is a common pathway of drug metabolism. Liver microsomes and microsomes of other tissues contain non-specific esterases that catalyze these hydrolytic reactions. The plasma also contains non-specific acetylcholine esterases, pseudocholinesterase and other esterases.

Hydration

Hydration can be regarded as a specialized form of hydrolysis, where water is added to the compound without causing the compound to dissociate into a number of components. Epoxides are converted into dihydrodiols by the enzyme, epoxide hydratase (also known as epoxide hydrase or hydrolase). The precarcinogenic polycyclic hydrocarbon epoxides in particular undergo this reaction (e.g. benzo[a]pyrene 4,5 epoxide).

4.5.2 Phase II Reactions

As mentioned previously, Phase I reactions introduce or expose a functional group on the drug molecule. Once a polar constituent is revealed or placed into the molecule, then a Phase II or conjugation reaction may occur. If a drug molecule contains a functional group, conjugation reactions may occur without phase I metabolism of the drug (e.g. salicylic acid). However, the drug may also undergo Phase I reactions, and then Phase II reactions. Conjugation reactions use conjugating reagents, that are derived from biochemical compounds involved in carbohydrate, fat, and protein metabolism. Phase II biotransformation reactions involve a diverse group of enzymes acting on diverse types of compounds, generally leading to a water-soluble product which can be excreted in the urine or bile. Table.4.3 lists the types of conjugation, enzymes involved and functional groups required for conjugation reaction. Examples of the phase II pathways of metabolism are given in Table 4.4.

Table 4.3 Conjugation Reactions, Enzymes and Functional Group Involved in Phase II Metabolism.

Reaction	Enzyme	Functional Group
Glucuronidation	UDP-Glucuronyltransferase	-OH, -COOH, $-NH_2$,-SH
Glycosidation	UDP-Glucuronyltransferase	-OH, -COOH, -SH
Sulfation	Sulfotransferase	-OH, $-NH_2$,$-SO_2NH_2$
Methylation	Methyltransferase	-OH, $-NH_2$,
Acetylation	Methyltransferase	-OH, $-NH_2$,$-SO_2NH_2$, -COOH
Aminoacid conjugation	---------	-COOH
Glutathione conjugation	Glutathione-S-transferase	epoxide, organic halide
Fatty Acid	---------	-OH
Condensation	---------	various

Table 4.4 Example of phase II metabolic pathways.

Types of Reaction	Examples
1. Conjugation with sugars (a) Glucuronidation (i) O-Glucuronides	

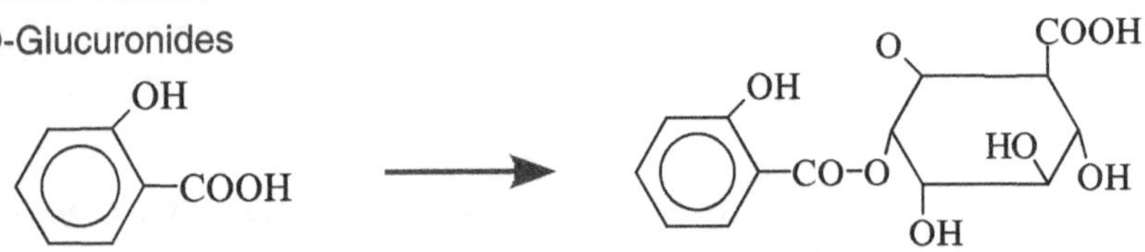

Salicylic acid

Table 4.4 *Contd...*

Types of Reaction	Examples
(ii) N-Glucuronides	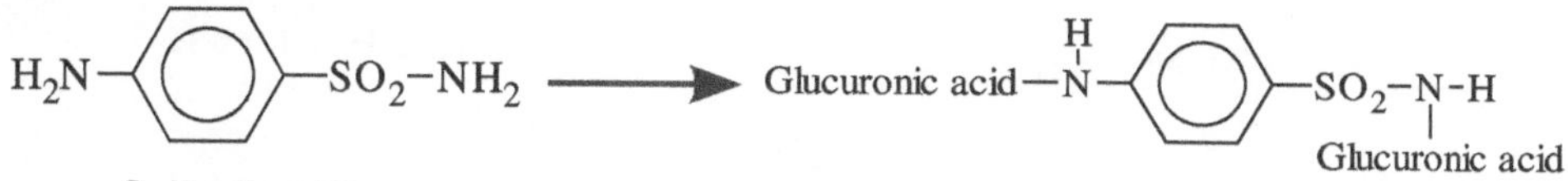 Sulfanilamide
(iii) S-Glucuronides	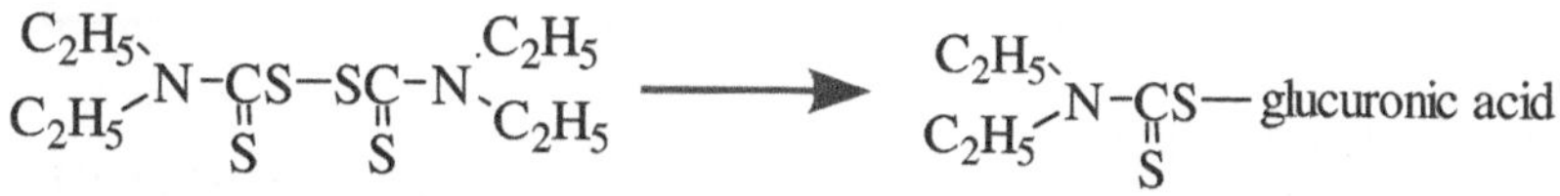 Antabuse
(b) Other sugars	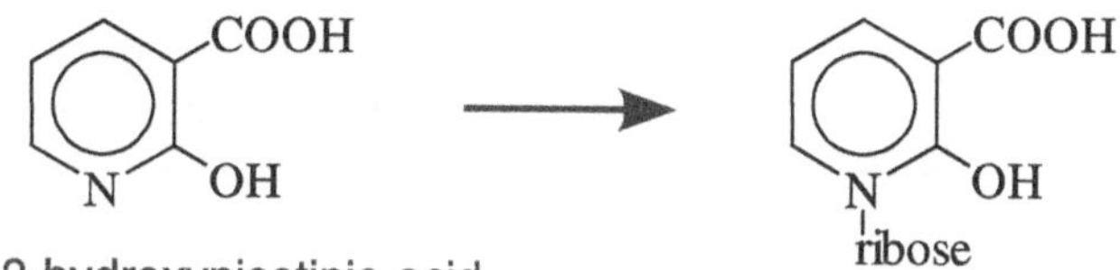 2-hydroxynicotinic acid
2. Sulfation	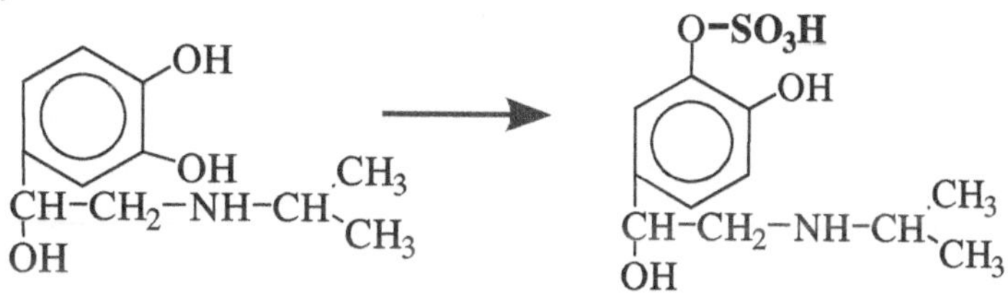 Isopreoterenol
3. Methylation	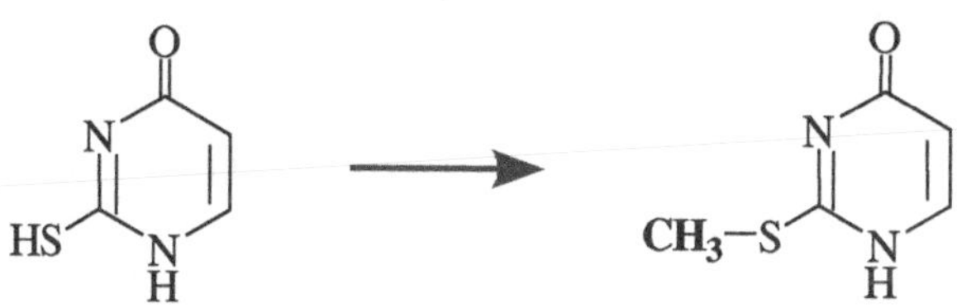 Thiouracil

Table 4.4 ***Contd...***

Types of Reaction	Examples
4. Acetylation 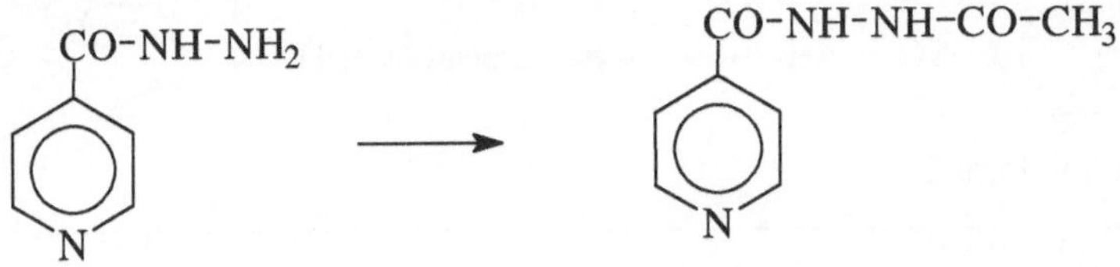 Isoniazid	
5. Amino acid conjugation 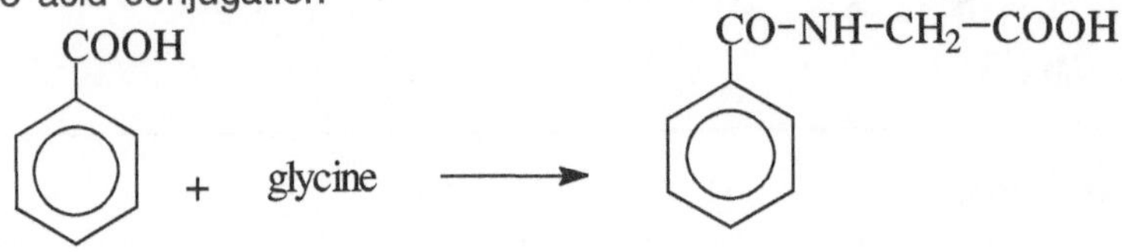 Benzoic acid	Hippuric acid
6. Glutathione conjugation 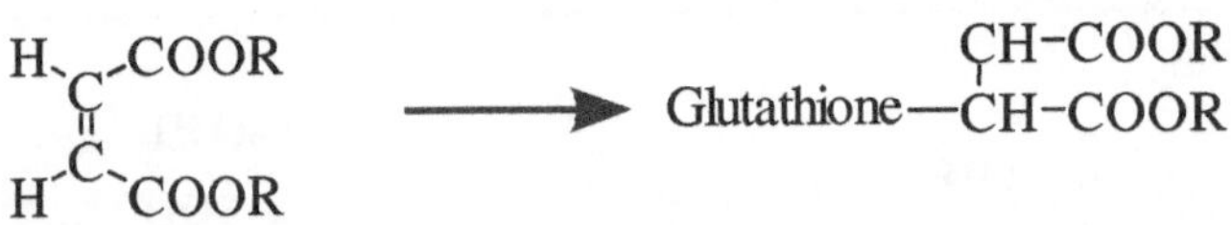 Esters of maleic acid	
7. Fatty acid conjugation 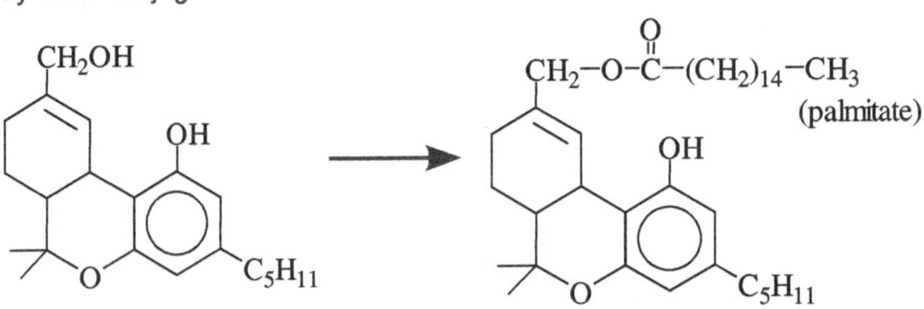 11-hydroxy - Δ^9 - tetrahydro - cannabinol	

Table 4.4 ***Contd...***

Types of Reaction	Examples
8. Condensation reactions	

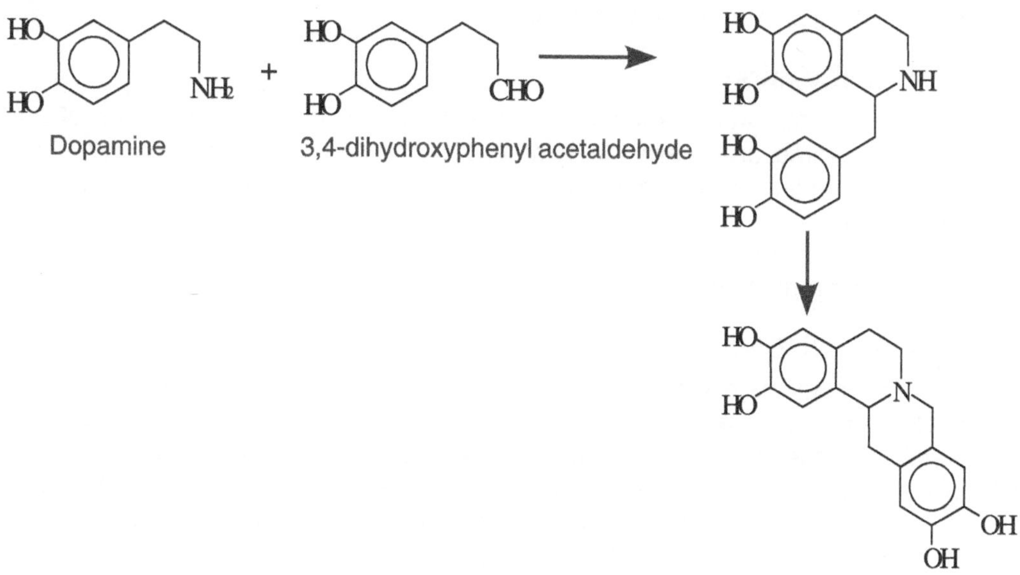

Dopamine 3,4-dihydroxyphenyl acetaldehyde

4.5.2.1 Glucuronidation

The major route of sugar conjugation is glucuronidation (conjugation with a-D-glucuronic acid), although conjugation with glucose, xylose and arabinose are also possible. Glucuronide formation is quantitatively the most important form of conjugation for drugs and endogenous compounds. Glucuronidaton involves the reaction between the high-energy form of the conjugating agent, uridine diphosphate glucuronic acid (UDPGA) and drugs containing hydroxyl, carboxyl, amine or thiol groups. The reaction is mediated by the microsomal enzyme glucuronyltransferase. It is interesting to note that inversion takes place during the reaction with the a-glucuronic acid forming a b-glucuronide. The formed O-glucuronides are often excreted in the bile and thus released into the gut where they can be broken down to the parent compound by b-glucuronidase and possibly reabsorbed. This is the basis of enterohepatic circulation of drugs. Glucuronides are water-soluble acids that are easily excreted in the urine. Some ester glucuronides are labile and can be hydrolysed in the urine or plasma to the parent drug. Accumulation and hydrolysis of the glucuronide conjugate of clofibrate in patients with renal disease result in high blood levels of clofibrate.

4.5.2.2 Sulfation

Conjugation with sulfate is a common pathway of metabolism of phenols, but also occur for alcohols, amines, to a lesser extent, thiols. The sulfate donor is 3'-phosphosdenosine-5'-phosphosulfate (PAPS), which is produced by a two stage reaction from ATP and sulfate.

The phenol, alcohol and arylamine transferases are fairly non-specific and metabolize a wide range of drugs and xenobiotics but the steroid sulfotransferases are specific for a single steroid or a number of steroids of a particular type. Sulfate conjugates are water-soluble and have a high renal clearance.

4.5.2.3 Methylation

Even though methylation reactions are mainly meant for the metabolism of endogenous substances, some drugs are methylated by non-specific methyl transferases. The high energy intermediate, S-adenosylmethionine (SAM), is required to form methyl conjugates. SAM is produced from L-methionine and ATP under the influence of the enzyme, L-methionine adenosyltransferase. In general, unlike other conjugation reactions, methylation leads to a less polar product and thus the metabolite is not easily excreted from the body.

4.5.2.4 Acetylation

Acetylation reactions are common for aromatic amines and sulfonamides and require the co-factor, acetyl-CoA. Acetyl-CoA is obtained either from the glycolysis pathway or via direct interaction of acetate and coenzyme A. Acetylation takes place mainly in the liver and it is interesting to note that these reactions occur in Kupffer cells and not in hepatocytes where most of the biotransformation reactions occur. Acetylation can also take place in reticuloendothelial cells of the spleen, lung and gut, and the enzyme is referred to as N-acetyltransferase.

The acetylated product is usually less polar than the parent drug. The renal toxicity of the earlier sulfonamides is attributed to the precipitation of less polar acetylatedsulphonamides. In addition, a less polar metabolite will be reabsorbed in the renal tubule and has a longer elimination half-life. For example, the active metabolite of procainamide, N-acetylprocainamide has a longer half-life than that of procainamide. The N-acetyltransferase enzyme responsible for metabolism of isoniazid and other drugs has been found to exhibit genetic polymorphism. Two distinct sub-populations have been observed to inactivate isoniazid, called "slow inactivators' and 'rapid inactivators".

4.5.2.5 Amino acid Conjugation

Aromatic acids are activated by combining with ATP to form coenzyme A derivatives before conjugation with amino acids. Amino acid conjugation is, thus, a special form of N-acylation. The usual amino acids involved are glycine, glutamine, ornithine, arginine and taurine. It has been observed that ureotelic animals (those excreting uric acid) use predominantly ornithine in the amino acid conjugation reactions. The enzymes involved are not well understood. Bile acids also undergo amino acid conjugation reaction. The conversion of benzoic acid to hippuric acid and salicylic acid to salicyluric acid are examples of this metabolic pathway.

4.5.2.6 Glutathione Conjugation

Glutathione (GSH) is a tripeptide of glutamyl-cysteine-glycine that is recognized as a protective device within the cell for the removal of potentially toxic electrophilic compounds. GSH reacts non-enzymatically and enzymatically via glutathion-S-transferase, through the nucleophilic sulfhydral group with reactive electrophilic oxygen intermediates of certain drugs formed during oxidative biotransformation reactions. These reactive electrophilic intermediates may react with nucleophilic macromolecules such as proteins in the cell, leading to a cell injury and cellular necrosis. The list of compounds conjugated to glutathione include epoxides, haloalkanes, nitroalkanes, alkenes and aromatic halo- and nitro- compounds.

The enzymes catalyzing these reactions are the glutathione-S-transferases which are located in the cytosol of the liver, kidney, gut and other tissues. The general steps involved in glutathione conjugation are given below.

1. Conjugation of glutathione (Gln-Cys-Gly) with the drug molecule through the sulfhydral group of cysteine in the presence of glutathione-S-transferase.

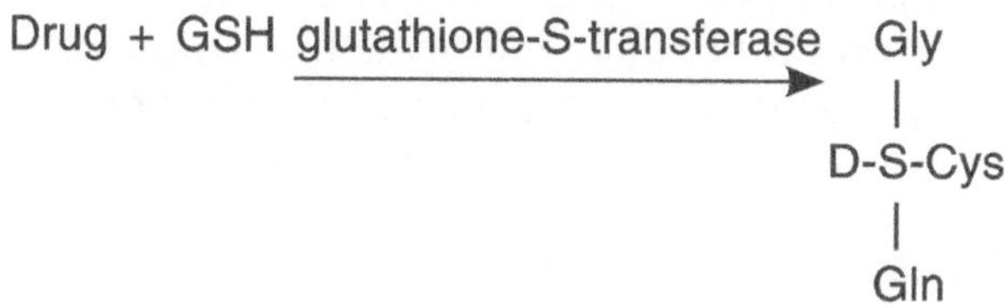

2. Removal of glutamyl by glutamyl transpeptidase

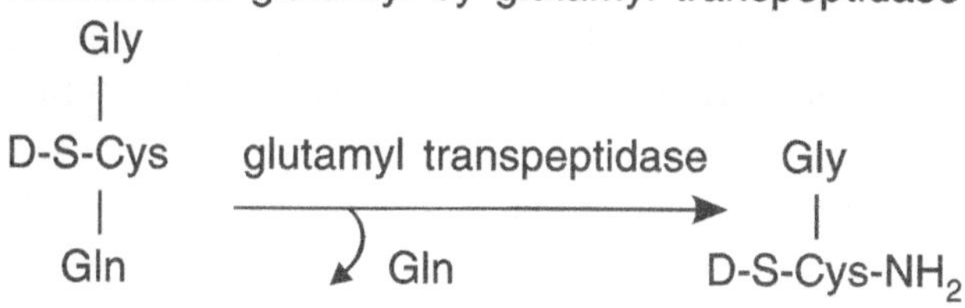

3. Removal of glycine by peptidase

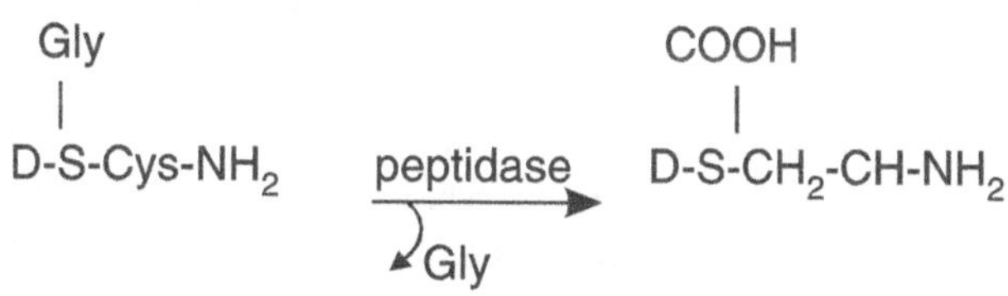

4. N-acetylation of the cysteine conjugate to form N-cetylated cysteine (mercapturic acid).

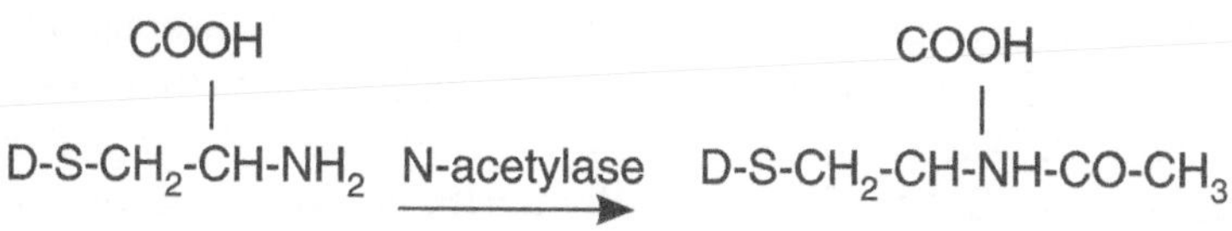

It has been observed that glutathione conjugates undergo a biliary secretion. In the gut, the conjugates undergo breakdown by a C-S lyase produced by instestinal microflora resulting in transfer of the -SH group from the glutathione to the drug molecules. Methylation on -SH group also takes place in the instestine and the S-methylated drug molecule is reabsorbed, reaches the liver and oxidized to a methylthio-derivative and then excreted. This type of metabolism is observed with certain sulfur containing compounds or compounds that form sulfur containing conjugates, such as caffeine, propachlor and 2-acetamido-4-chloromethylthiazole.

The enzymatic formation of GSH conjugates shows saturation kinetics. Therefore, high doses of drugs such as acetaminophen may form high amounts of electrophilic intermediates. These intermediates covalently bind to hepatic cellular macromolecules, resulting in cellular necrosis. N-acetylcysteine, which contains the sulfhydryl group, is used as an antidote for acetaminophen intoxication.

4.5.2.7 Fatty Acid Conjugation

The fatty acids involved in the conjugation reactions are stearic and palmitic acids. Liver microsomal enzymes catalyze these reactions. Little information is available about the mechanism involved and compounds that undergo this type of conjugation. Fatty acids conjugation has been shown to occur for 11-hydroxy-D^9-tetrahydrocannabinol.

4.5.2.8 Condensation Reactions

These recently discovered reactions may not be enzymatic but purely chemical and have been found for amines and aldehydes. Tetrahydropapaveroline, which is a potent dopamine antagonist, is a condensation product of dopamine and its metabolite, 3,4-dihydroxyphenylacetaldehyde. Tetrahydropapaveroline is a naturally occurring alkaloid.

4.5.3 Metabolism of Enantiomers

About 40% of drugs contain one or more asymmetric (chiral) centers in the molecule. For each chiral center, there are two possible mirror images of enantiomers, the R- and S-forms, which often differ in their pharmacokinetic and pharmacodynamic properties. Because of difficulty and cost of separation, a majority of synthetic chiral drugs are marketed as racemic mixtures.

Each isomeric form may have different pharmacological actions and different side effects. For example, the natural thyroid hormone L-thyroxin stimulates the basal metabolic rate, while the synthetic D-thyroxin does not influence the basal metabolic rate but lowers the cholesterol level in the blood.

Since enzymes, as well as drug receptors exhibit stereo-selectivity, isomers of drugs may show differences not only in pharmacological activity but also biotransformation and pharmacokinetics. For example, S(-) warfarin is more potent anticoagulant than R(+) warfarin. The half-life of S(-) warfarin is less than R(+) warfarin. Carprofen, a nonsteroidal anti-inflammatory drug, exists in both S and R configuration. The S-form of carprofen is more potent and its clearance is faster than that of the R-form. The (+)-isomer of amphetamine is eliminated more rapidly than the (-)-isomer. The extent of protein binding is often different for each stereoisomer. For example, the S-form of dispyramide is more highly protein bound in man than R-form. A list of some common drugs which exist as enatiomers is given in Table.4.5.

Table 4.5 Common Drugs that Exist as Enantiomers

Amphetamine	Flecainide	Terbutaline
Atropine	Hexobarbitol	Thyroxine
Brompheniramine	Ibuprofen	Tocainide
Cocaine	Motoprolol	Verapamil
Carprofen	Morphine	Warfarin
Dispyramide	Nadolol	
Doxylamine	Propoxyphene	
Ephedrine	Propranolol	

4.5.4 Regioselectivity

Regioselectivity refers to the metabolism of the drug molecule at a specific region. It means the enzymes will catalyze a reaction that is specific for a particular region in the drug molecule. For example, isoproterenol undergoes methylation at meta position preferentially to form a 3-O-methylated metabolite. O-methylation at para position is very little. Therefore, certain enzymes are not only sterioselective but also regioselective.

Table 4.6 Sources of Variation in Intrinsic Clearance

- Genetic factors
- Genetic differences within population
- Racial differences among different populations
- Environmental factors and drug interactions
  - Enzyme induction
  - Enzyme inhibition
- Physiological conditions
  - Age
  - Gender
  - Diet/Nutrition
  - Pathophysiology
- Drug dosage regimen
- Route of drug administration
- Dose dependent (non-linear) pharmacokinetics

4.5.5 Variation of Biotransformation Enzymes in Humans

A number of biological and environmental variables are responsible for variation in metabolism in humans. Table.4.6. lists various biological and environmental variable that influence the intrinsic clearance of compounds form the body. **Pharmacogenetics** is the subject that deals with genetic differences in drug elimination. Whole population can be grouped as slow acetylators and fast acetylators based on their ability to metabolize isoniazid. The difference is referred to as genetic polymorphism. Slow acetylators are often prone to isoniazid-induced neurotoxicity. Procainamide and hydralazine are other two drugs that are acetylated and demonstrate genetic polymorphism. A well documented example of genetic polymorphism occurred with phehytoin. Two phenotypes, efficient metabolizer (EM) and poor metbaolizer (PM) were identified in the population. The PM frequency in the Caucasians was about 4%, and among the Japanese about 16%. Another example of genetic differences in drug metabolism is the glucose-6-phosphate-dehydrogenase deficiency, which is observed in approximately 10% black Americans. The incidence of side effects with mephobarbital was higher in the Japanese possibly due to a slower oxidative metabolism.

Environmental factors and exposure to chemicals may alter the basal level of enzymatic activity. The aromatic hydrocarbons, such as 3-methylcholanthrene and benzpyrene released during cigarette smoking stimulate the enzymes involved in theophylline metabolism. Therefore, the biological half-life of theophylline is shorter in smokers. Phenobarbitol stimulates the liver microsomal enzymes responsible for various metabolic pathways, including oxidation, reduction and hydrolysis. Phenobarbital enhances the metabolism of meperidine to normeperidine.

Inhibition of hepatic enzyme activity is observed by a variety of agents including carbon monoxide, heavy metals, and certain drugs such as cemitidine. Enzyme inhibition by cemitidine may lead to higher plasma levels and longer elimination of co-administered phenytoin or theophylline.

The physiological conditions of the host-including age, gender, nutrition, diet and pathophysiology- also affects the level of hepatic enzyme activities. In addition to the physiological condition, route of administration, time of administration and dose administered may also alter the pharmacokinetics and pharmacodynamics of a drug.

4.5.6 Species Differences in Drug Metabolism

Drug metabolism studies in laboratory animals are carried out during the early preclinical phase of drug development to identify the major metabolic pathways of a new drug. These studies are often useful in suggesting the most likely drug metabolites to be found in man. For most drugs, different animal species may have different metabolic pathways. Drug metabolism studies in laboratory animals and man were carried out with different compounds to find out the species that closely resembles the man with respect to drug metabolism. The studies concluded that the rhesus monkey resembles man closely in terms of the urinary metabolite patterns. The urinary metabolite patterns in the dog and rat were less useful in predicting results in humans.

Species differences in the activity of microsomal enzyme systems are usually so great as to render the results of studies in laboratory animals meaningless. For example, amphetamine is mainly hydroxylated in the rat, whereas in humans and dogs it is largely deaminated. Sulfadimethoxine is mainly acetylated in rats, but in humans the major urinary metabolite is a glucuronide. Even though the biotransformation pathways are the same in different animal species, the rates of metabolism may differ significantly. Many drugs are metabolized much more rapidly in rats and dogs than in man. As a result, a certain dose of a drug may have little pharmacological activity in a test animal, but elicit an adequate response in humans. These differences have to be taken into consideration during the development of a new drug. These considerations are also important for the toxicological evaluation of drugs in laboratory animals.

4.6 Induction and Inhibition of Drug Metabolizing Enzymes

Humans are being exposed to many chemicals, either in the environment, for medical reasons or as a result of the life styles. The chemical substances are derived from a variety of sources and include pharmaceutical products, cosmetics, food additives and industrial chemicals. Microsomal drug metabolism can be stimulated or inhibited by a large number of drugs and chemicals.

4.6.1 Enzyme Induction

Microsomal enzyme induction is a complex process associated with an increase in liver weight, proliferation of the endoplasmic reticulum, and increase in microsomal protein and cytochrome P-450. In general, enzyme induction caused by drugs and chemicals can be grouped into two, exemplified by phenobarbital and aromatic hydrocarbons such as 3-methylcholathrene and benzpyrene. Phenobarbital-type inducers stimulate the liver microsomal enzymes that are responsible for a wide variety of metabolic pathways, including oxidation, reduction, and glucuronide formation. On the other hand, polycyclic hydrocarbons stimulate a limited group of metabolic reactions. Pretreatment with phenobarbital enhances the metabolism of pethidine while pretreatment with polycyclic aromtic hydrocarbons does not. Enzyme induction caused by cigarette smoke (due to benzo[a]pyrene and 3-methylcholanthrene in smoke) increases the metabolism of theophylline, but phenobarbital does not. However, pretreatment of experimental animals with either phenobarbitone or polycyclic aromatic hydrocarbon, benzo[a]pyrene, results in a substantial increase in zoxazolamine (muscle relaxant) metabolism. Table.4.7. provides a partial list of drugs that are proved to cause enzyme induction.

Table 4.7 List of Some Drugs that Cause Enzyme Induction.

Classification	Examples
Analgesics	Nikethamide
Antipyretic and Analgesic	Antipyrine
Anti-inflammatory	Phenylbutazone
Antibiotics	Rifampicin
Anticonvulsants	Carbamazepine
Antifungal drugs	Griseofulvin
Antimalarials	Quinine
Sedatives and hypnotics	Phenobarbitone
Diuretics	Spiranolactone

Some drugs induce microsomal enzymes that are involved in their own metabolism; this phenomenon has been called self-induction or auto-induction. For example, the anticonvulsant drug carbamazepine stimulates the production of enzymes responsible for its own metabolism and hence, its metabolic clearance increases on continuous administration until the microsomal enzymes are maximally induced.

4.6.2 Enzyme Inhibition

Inhibition of a drug metabolism by other drugs or xenobiotics is a well recognized phenomenon. This inhibition of drug metabolism by drugs or xenobiotics can take place in several ways including the destruction of pre-existing enzymes, inhibition of enzyme synthesis by complexing and thus inactivating the drug-metabolizing enzyme, by complexing a co-factor such as $NADPH_2$ needed for enzyme activity or by interacting with the drug itself. In addition, the product of the enzyme reaction, the metabolite, competes with the substrate leading to the inhibition of the parent drug metabolism. This type of inhibition is called **product inhibition.**

Table 4.8. shows the list of some drugs and xenobiotics known to produce enzyme inhibition. Certain drugs including monoamine oxidase (MAO) inhibitors and xanthine oxidase inhibitors are used clinically to inhibit specific enzyme systems. Unfortunately most of these drugs lack specificity and may inhibit more than one enzyme system. The anti-ulcer drug cimetidine has become one of the most potent and comprehensive inhibitor of microsomal drug metabolism used in clinical medicine.

Table 4.8 Some of the Drugs and Xenobioticcs Known to Produce Enzyme Inhibition.

Drugs	Xenobiotics
Allobarbital	Ethylene
Secobarbital	Acetylene
Amphetamine	Piperonal
Cemetidine	Safrole
Isoniazid	Peperonylbutoxide
Dapsone	Carbontetrachloride
Fenfluramine	Parathion
Sulfanilamide	7, 8-benzoflavone
Chloremphenicol	
Amantadine	
Indomethacin	
MAOinhibitors(Isocarboxazid, Phenelzine)	
Xanthine oxidase inhibitors (Allopurinol)	

Enzyme inhibition may be reversible or irreversible. The type of inhibition is usually classified by enzyme kinetic studies and by observing the changes in Km (Michaelis-Menton Constant) and Vmax (maximum velocity of an enzymatic reaction). Enzyme kinetic studies use the Michaelis-Menton equation. Accordingly, enzyme inhibition may be classified as competitive inhibition, non-competitive inhibition and other types.

In the case of **competitive inhibition**, the inhibitor and drug compete for the same active site on the enzyme. An increase in the drug concentration may displace the inhibitor from the enzyme and partially or fully reverse the inhibition. Therefore, competitive inhibition is also known as **reversible inhibition**.

In the case of **non-competitive inhibition**, the inhibitor may inhibit the enzyme by combining at a site on the enzyme that is different from the active site (i.e., allosteric site). Non-competitive inhibition can not be reversed by increasing the drug concentration (i.e., **irreversible inhibition**).

Other types of enzyme inhibitions, such as mixed enzyme inhibition and uncompetitive enzyme inhibition, can be identified by observing changes in Km and Vmax (Table.4.9.).

Table 4.9 Identification of Types of Enzyme Inhibition.

Type	Km	V_{max}
Competitive	Changes	No change
Non-competitive	No change	Changes
Other (mixed enzyme inhibition and uncompetitive enzyme inhibition	Changes	Changes
Doxylamine		
Ephedrine		

4.6.3 Enzyme Kinetics of Drug Metabolism

Conversion of a drug into metabolites by biotransformation reactions requires enzymes. Enzyme concentration and drug concentration at the site of metabolism are important determinants of the metabolic rate of a drug in addition to drug affinity towards the enzyme. In the body, the biotransformation enzyme concentration is constant at a given site and the drug concentration varies with the dose and time. The drug affinity towards a particular enzyme is an inherent property of the drug molecule.

When the drug concentration is low relative to enzyme concentration at the site of metabolism, there are abundant enzyme molecules to catalyze the reaction. The rate of metabolism depends mainly on the drug concentration and it follows the first-order kinetics. When the drug concentration is higher than that of enzyme at the site of metabolism, all the available enzyme molecules will be complexed with the drug molecules and the rate of metabolism may change to zero-order process. This is because of the **saturation of enzyme system**. In other words, the system is working at its full capacity. The drug concentration at which enzyme saturation occurs depends on the drug and its affinity to the enzyme.

Let us consider metabolism of a drug which interacts with the enzyme on an equimolar basis (i.e., one mole of drug interacts with one mole of the enzyme) to form an enzyme-drug intermediate, which further reacts to yield a metabolite of the drug as shown below.

$$[E] + [D] \underset{K2}{\overset{K1}{\rightleftharpoons}} [ED] \xrightarrow{K3} \text{metabolite} + E$$

Where [E] = Enzyme concentration; [D] = drug concentration; [ED] = Enzyme-drug complex concentration and K1, K2, K3 = First-order rate constants.

Michaelis and Menton developed an equation that describes the rate of metabolism of a drug by an enzyme. In developing the equation, they assumed that the rate of an enzymatic reaction is dependent upon the concentrations of both the enzyme and the drug, and that an enzyme-drug intermediate is initially formed, followed by the formation of the metabolite and regeneration of the enzyme. Since K1, K2 and K3 are first-order rate constants, the following rate equations may be written.

Rate of formation of enzyme-drug complex

$$= K1\,[E]\,[D] \qquad .....(4.7)$$

Rate of dissociation of enzyme-drug complex or

rate of regeneration of the enzyme

$$= K2\,[ED] + K3\,[ED] \qquad .....(4.8)$$

Therefore, the rate of change in the concentration of enzyme-drug complex (d(ED)/dt) is given by,

$$d(ED)/dt = K1\,[E]\,[D] - (K2\,[ED] + K3\,[ED]) \qquad .....(4.9)$$

According to mass balance, total enzyme concentration, [Et], is equal to the sum of the concentrations of a free enzyme [E] and enzyme complexed with the drug [ED].

$$[Et] = [E] + [ED] \qquad .....(4.10)$$

or

$$[E] = [Et] - [ED] \qquad .....(4.11)$$

Therefore, we can write equation 4.9 as,

$$d(ED)/dt = K1\,([Et] - [ED])\,[D] - [ED]\,(K2 + K3) \qquad .....(4.12)$$

At a steady state, the rate of formation of enzyme-drug complex is equal to the rate of dissociation of enzyme-drug complex. Hence, at a steady state, the rate of change in the concentration of enzyme-drug complex, d(ED)/dt is equal to zero. (i.e., d(ED)/dt = 0)

Therefore,

$$0 = K1\,([Et] - [ED])\,[D] - [ED]\,(K2 + K3) \qquad .....(4.13)$$

$$K1\,([Et] - [ED])\,[D] = [ED]\,(K2 + K3) \qquad .....(4.14)$$

$$K1\,[Et]\,[D] = K1\,[ED]\,[D] + [ED](K2 + K3) \qquad .....(4.15)$$

$$[Et]\,[D] = [ED]\,[D] + [ED]\,\frac{(K2+K3)}{K1} \qquad .....(4.16)$$

$$[Et]\,[D] = [ED]\,\frac{([D]+K2+K3)}{K1} \qquad .....(4.17)$$

Let $$Km = \frac{(K2+K3)}{K1} \quad .....(4.18)$$

$$[Et]\ [D] = [ED]\ ([D] + Km) \quad .....(4.19)$$

Solving the equation 4.19 for [ED], we get

$$[ED] = \frac{[Et]\ [D]}{([D]+Km)} \quad .....(4.20)$$

Multiplying both the sides by K3,

$$K3\ [ED] = \frac{K3\,[Et]\,[D]}{([D]+Km)} \quad .....(4.21)$$

K3 [ED] is nothing but the rate of formation of a metabolite or the rate of velocity of decomposition of the ED into a metabolite and an enzyme. Hence, K3 [ED] is the velocity or rate of enzymatic reaction, v. When the drug concentration is high relative to enzyme, then the reaction proceeds at a maximum velocity or rate called Vmax. It means, the reaction proceeds at a constant velocity and the enzyme system is saturated. A product of K3 and [Et] is Vmax.

$$Vmax = K3\ [Et] \quad .....(4.22)$$

Similarly, $$v = K3\ [ED] \quad .....(4.23)$$

The velocity of metabolism is given by the equation.

$$v = \frac{Vmax\,[D]}{([D]+Km)} \quad .....(4.24)$$

Equation 4.24 is known as Michaelis-Menton equation and describes the rate of metabolite formation. Km is known as **Michaelis constant** and is defined as the concentration of a substrate (drug) when the velocity (v) of the reaction is equal to one-half maximal velocity, or 0.5 Vmax (see Fig..4.6). 1/Km reflects the affinity between substrate (drug) and enzyme. The constant Vmax is a function of the total amount of the metabolizing enzyme.

Equation 4.24 is developed taking the equimolar interaction between the drug and enzyme into consideration and assuming that the enzyme is metabolizing only the drug under consideration. If the same enzyme is also metabolizing any other substrate simultaneously, this equation is not valid. Further, a drug may be metabolized by several enzymes simultaneously to form many metabolites.

Experience suggests that the usual dose of most drugs results in plasma concentrations that are much smaller than the Km values associated with their metabolism. Since [D] << Km (Km >> [D]), the term [D] can be neglected in the denominator of equation 4.24, to get:

$$v = \frac{Vmax\,[D]}{Km} = K\ [D] \quad .....(4.25)$$

Where, K is the apparent first-order metabolic rate constant. Accordingly, the elimination of most drugs that are eliminated totally or in part by biotransformation can be described by the first-order kinetics.

However, some drugs, including phenytoin, ethotoin, salicylate and ethanol have one or more Km values that are comparable to or less than their usual concentrations in the plasma following therapeutic doses. Therefore, the elimination of these drugs can not be described by the first-order kinetics. At higher drug concentrations, [D]>>Km and the equation 4.24 can be written as,

$$v = \frac{Vmax}{Km} = \text{constant} \qquad .....(4.26)$$

It means, when [D]>>Km, the reaction proceeds at a constant rate or follows a zero-order kinetics. The enzymatic system is said to be saturated and capacity-limited metabolism is observed.

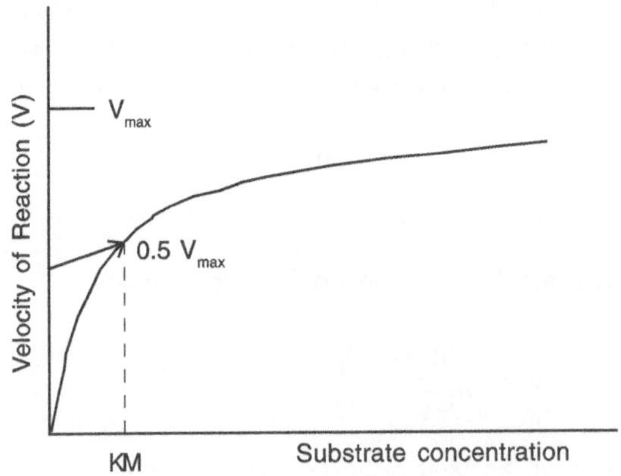

Fig. 4.9 Michaelis-menten enzyme kinetics. The nonlinear relation between enzyme reaction velocity and the drug concentration, resulting in hyperbolic curve. The Km is the drug (substrate) concentration when the velocity of reaction is at 0.5 V_{max}.

A plot of drug concentration versus metabolic rate gives a hyperbolic curve (Fig.4.9) indicating non-linear relationship. Reciprocal of the Michaelis-Menton equation is used to obtain a linear relationship.

$$\frac{1}{v} = \frac{Km}{V_{max}} \frac{1}{[D]} + \frac{1}{V_{max}} \qquad .....(4.27)$$

Equation 4.27 is used to estimate the parameters Vmax and Km and is known as the **Lineweaver-burk** equation. A plot of 1/v versus 1/[D] is used to estimate Vmax and Km (Figure 4.10). Lineweaver-Burk plots are also used to study the enzyme inhibition kinetics (Figure 4.11.a, b and c). The Michaelis-Menton equation of competitive inhibition is given by,

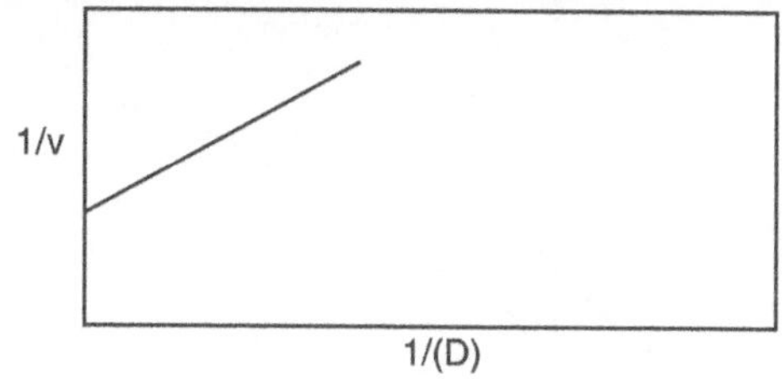

Fig. 4.10 Lineweaver burkplot of 1/v versus 1/(D) for determining Km and V_{max}. Intercept = $1/V_{max}$ and slope = Km/V_{max}.

$$v = \frac{Vmax\ [D]}{[D]+Km(1+I/Ki)} \qquad .....(4.28)$$

Where, I is the inhibitory concentration and Ki is the inhibition constant. For a non-competitive inhibition,

$$v = \frac{Vmax\ [D](1+I/Ki)}{[D]+Km} \qquad .....(4.29)$$

Michaelis-Menton equation can be rearranged in different ways to yield a linear relationship between v and [D].

$$\frac{[D]}{v} = \frac{1[D]}{Vmax} + \frac{Km}{Vmax} \qquad .....(4.30)$$

$$v = \frac{-Km\,v}{[D]} + V_{max} \qquad .....(4.31)$$

The equations 4.30 and 4.31 are useful for the estimation of Vmax and Km (see Fig. 4.10).

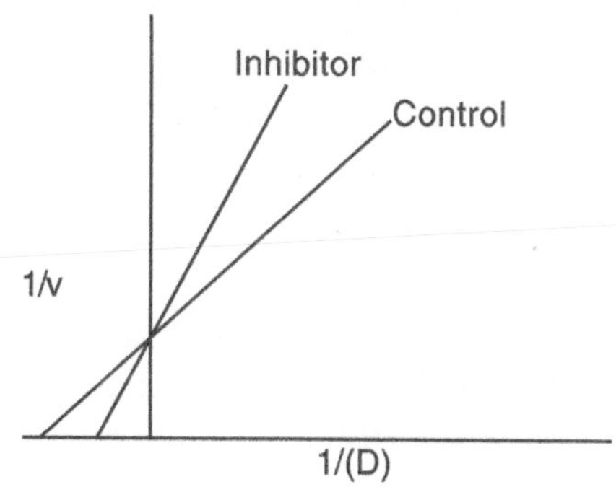

Fig. 4.11 (a) Lineweaver-burk plot used to identify the competitive enzyme inhibition.

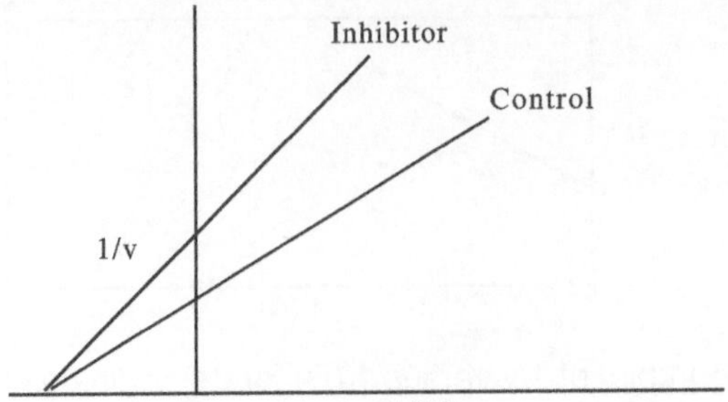

Fig. 4.11 (b) Lineweaver-burk plot used to identify the non competitive enzyme inhibition.

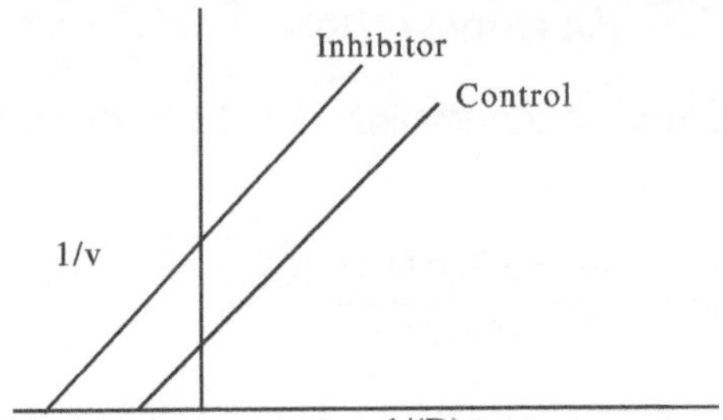

Fig. 4.11 (c) Lineweaver-burk plot used to identify the uncompetitive enzyme inhibition.

4.7 Hepatic Clearance (Clh)

The clearance is a general concept that may be applied to any organ and is used as a measure of elimination of a drug by the organ. Renal clearance was explained earlier in this chapter. **Hepatic clearance** may be defined as the volume of blood that perfuse the liver that is cleared of drug per unit time.

Organ clearance of the drug is given by:

$$CLorgan = Qo\ Eo \qquad .....(4.32)$$

Where, Qo is the blood flow to the organ and Eo is the extraction ratio of the organ. The **Extraction ratio**, Eo, can be estimated by the equation,

$$Eo = \frac{Cin - Cout}{Cin} \qquad .....(4.33)$$

Where, Cin is the drug concentration in the arterial blood (that is going into the organ) and Cout is drug concentration in the venous blood (that is coming out of the organ). Extraction ratio of an organ can also be calculated form the equation given below.

$$Eo = \frac{Cl_{int}}{Qo + Cl_{int}} \qquad .....(4.34)$$

Where, Cl_{int} is the **intrinsic clearance** of the organ, that is, the maximum ability of the organ to remove the drug from the blood when there are no flow limitations.

Hepatic clearance, Clh, is related to both the liver blood flow and the extraction ratio of the liver.

$$Clh = Qh\ Eh \qquad .....(4.35)$$

Where, Qh is the blood flow to the liver and Eh is the extraction ratio of the liver.

For some drugs, the extraction ratio is high (greater than 0.7) and the drug is removed by the liver almost rapidly as the organ is perfused by the blood containing the drug. Drugs with very high hepatic extraction ratios exhibit a hepatic blood flow dependent metabolic rate. For example, propranolol, a b-adrenergic blocking agent, decreases the hepatic blood flow by decreasing the cardiac output, and thereby decreases its own hepatic clearance. Drugs that have high hepatic extraction ratios generally, undergo first-pass metabolism.

For drugs with low extraction ratios (e.g., phenylbutazone, procainamide, theophylline), the hepatic clearance is less affected by the hepatic blood flow. Since, Eh = $Cl_{int}/(Qo + Cl_{int})$, the hepatic clearance, may also be calculated from the equation, 4.36.

$$Clh = \frac{Qh\,[Cl_{int}]}{Qh + Cl_{int}} \qquad .....(4.36)$$

Intrinsic clearance (Cl_{int}) is a measure of inherent activities of the mixed-function oxidases and biliary secretion. Hence, changes or alterations in mixed-function oxidase activity or biliary secretion affect the rate of drug removal by the liver. Intrinsic clearance of a drug is affected by several factors, including enzyme induction, enzyme inhibition, age of the individual, nutritional and pathological factors. Drugs that show low extraction ratios and are eliminated mainly by metabolism demonstrate a marked variation in the overall elimination half-lives within a given population chiefly due to genetic differences in intrinsic hepatic enzyme activity.

Hepatic clearance may also be expressed as the rate of drug removal divided by the plasma drug concentration in artery.

$$Clh = \frac{\text{Rate of drug removal by the liver}}{\text{Plasma concentration of drug (Cin)}}$$

Rate of drug removal by the liver = Clh x Cin

It should be noted that only a free drug in the blood can cross the cell membranes and reach the interior of the cell but not a protein bound drug. An increase in the free drug concentration in the blood will make more drug available for hepatic extraction and subsequent metabolism or biliary secretion. Therefore, protein binding of drugs has to be considered in calculating the hepatic clearance of drugs.

4.7.1 Influence of Protein Binding on Hepatic Clearance

In equation 4.36, the hepatic clearance is related to the blood flow to the liver and the hepatic intrinsic clearance. Equation 4.36 is derived assuming no protein binding, while in fact Cl_{int} should be defined in terms of the maximum ability of the liver to remove the free drug (unbound), resulting in the following:

$$Clh = \frac{Qh\,[f\,(Cl_{int})]}{Qh + f(Cl_{int})} \qquad .....(4.37)$$

Where, f is the fraction of free drug in the blood. When the intrinsic clearance of the liver is very high compared to the blood flow, such that $f(Cl_{int}) >> Qh$, the extraction ratio approaches 1 and Clh @ Qh.

$$Clh = \frac{Qh\,f\,(Cl_{int})}{f(Cl_{int})} \cong Qh \qquad .....(4.38)$$

Thus, if a drug is cleared exclusively in the liver with an extraction ratio approaching unity, hepatic clearance will be very sensitive to changes in the liver blood flow and essentially independent of protein binding, because the drug is removed from the plasma binding sites during circulation through the liver. Similarly, for drugs eliminated in the kidneys by an active transport process, the elimination appears to be independent of the extent of protein binding. However, for most drugs, the blood flow is significantly greater than the intrinsic organ clearance ($Qh >> Cl_{int}$) and then equation 4.37 is reduced to

$$Clh = \frac{Qh\,f\,(Cl_{int})}{Qh} = f\,(Cl_{int}) \qquad .....(4.39)$$

It means that the hepatic clearance is directly related to the degree of protein binding. This is certainly true for the renal clearance of drugs that are eliminated by passive filtration mechanisms in the kidney. In these cases, if no drug is reabsorbed through the kidney tubule, Cl_{int} may be approximated to the glomerular filtration rate (GFR) depending on the extent of the drug protein binding.

4.8 Pharmacological Activity of Metabolites

For most drugs, biotransformation results in the formation of a more polar metabolite that is pharmacologically inactive and is eliminated rapidly than the parent drug. For some drugs the metabolite may be pahrmacologically active or produce toxic effects (Table 4.10).

Table 4.10 Pharmacological Activities of Metabolites.

Drug		Metabolite
Active drug to Inactive metabolite		
Amphetamine	→	Phenylacetone
Phenobarbitol	→	Hydroxyphenobarbitol
Active drug to active metabolite		
Phenacetin	→	Acetaminophen
Amitryptyline	→	Nortryptyline
Imipramine	→	Desimpramine
Active drug to active metabolite with different pharmacological activity		
Mepiridine (analgesic)	→	Normeperidine (CNS stimulant)
Prodrug to Active Metabolite		
Chlorazepate	→	Nordiazepam
Hetacillin	→	Ampicillin
Active drug to Reactive metabolite		
Acetaminophen	→	Reactive metabolite (hepatotoxicity)
Methoxyflurane	→	Reactive metabolite (renal toxicity)

It can be seen from the Table 4.10 that metabolites differ significantly from their parent compounds with respect to pharmacological activity and polarity. **Prodrugs** are inactive and must be biotransformed in the body to metabolites that have pharmacological activity. More recently prodrugs have been designed to improve stability and absorption or to prolong duration of action. Prodrug levodopa used in the treatment of parkinsonism, is more lipid soluble, crosses the blood-brain-barrier easily and converted into active L-dopamine by the decarboxylase enzyme in the brain. The neurotransmitter L-dopamine does not easily penetrate the blood-brain-barrier and, therefore, can not be used as a therapeutic agent.

4.9 Disposition of Metabolites

Since the prime objective of biotransformation reactions is to convert a drug into more polar and pharmacologically inactive metabolites, most biotransformations result in metabolites that are more polar and inactive. However, certain important exceptions do exists as discussed earlier in this chapter. The apparent volume of distribution of polar metabolites such as glucuronides, sulfates etc., is less than that of the parent drug. Metabolites are excreted in urine more readily than their parent drugs because of the lack of tubular reabsorption of polar metabolites. Renal excretion plays an important role in the elimination of metabolites. Renal impairment may lead to the accumulation of drug metabolites in the body. If a metabolite is pharmacologically active, accumulation of the metabolite may result precipitation of toxic effects.

4.10 First Pass Effect

Drugs given orally are absorbed from the stomach or small intestine and transported via the mesenteric vessels to the hepatic portal vein and then to the liver prior to the systemic circulation. Some drugs are metabolized extensively in the intestinal mucosal cells during absorption or in the liver cells during their first transit and therefore exhibit a poor systemic availability when administered orally. This rapid metabolism of an orally administered drug prior to reaching the general circulation is termed **first-pass effect** or **presystemic elimination**.

Many drugs show a low oral bioavailability due to first-pass effect in the liver. Drugs that undergo the first-pass hepatic metabolism includes desipramine, diltiazem, isoproterenol, lidocaine, nitroglycerine and propranolol. Blood perfusing buccal cavity bypasses the liver and enters directly into the superior vena cava. Nitroglycerin, an antianginal drug, is administered sublingually to avoid the first-pass effect. Part of the rectal blood supply, particularly in the inferior and middle hemerrhoidal veins, bypasses the hepatic portal circulation and dumps directly into the inferior vena cava. Therefore, certain drugs are administered as suppositories to avoid the first-pass effect.

4.11 Biliary Excretion

As explained earlier in this chapter, the bile is secreted by the hepatocytes, stored in the gall bladder and emptied into the duodenum in response to food intake. Bile primarily consists of water, bile salts, bile pigments, electrolytes, and to lesser extent cholesterol and fatty acids. Some drugs may be secreted by the liver cells into the bile. Production of bile as well as excretion of drugs into bile appear to be an active transport process. Separate active biliary secretion processes have been reported for organic anions, organic cations, and polar, uncharged molecules. Biliary secretion of methotrexate is inhibited competitively by probenecid.

In men, the bile flow rate ranges from 0.5 to 0.8 ml/min. The drug concentration in bile may be as high as 1000 times the plasma drug concentration. Therefore, some drugs may have biliary clearances of 500 ml/min. or higher. The most important factor influencing the excretion of a drug in bile is the molecular weight of the compound. Drugs that are mainly excreted in the bile have molecular weights in excess of 500g/moles. Drugs with molecular weights between 300 and 500 are excreted both in urine and in bile. Drugs with molecular weights of less than 300 are almost exclusively excreted via the kidneys into urine. A direct relationship between the molecular weight and the biliary excretion of 18 cephalosporins in rats has been observed.

Another factor that influences the biliary excretion of drugs is the presence of a strong polar group. Most of the times metabolites of drugs, especially glucuronides are excreted into the bile. In general, metabolites are more polar than the parent drug, and glucuronides of drugs are more polar as well as have high molecular weight than their parent drugs which favor their secretion into bile.

Compounds that enhance bile production may increase the biliary excretion of drugs. Phenobarbital is found to increase the biliary excretion of drugs by two mechanisms. First, by increasing the formation of glucuronides via enzyme induction and second, by enhancing the bile flow. In contrast, compounds that decrease bile flow or pathophysiological conditions that cause cholestasis will decrease the biliary drug excretion. The extent of the biliary excretion of a drug depends upon the route of administration. For example, drugs given orally may be extracted by the liver into the bile to a greater extent than if the drugs are given intravenously.

Biliary elimination may play a role in the inter-individual differences in drug response observed in healthy subjects and in patients with certain diseases. Cholestatic disease states, in which normal bile flow is reduced, will influence drug elimination by this route resulting in increased risk of drug toxicity .

Relationship between hepatic and biliary clearances

Hepatic clearance (Cl_h) of a drug is the sum of its hepatic metabolic clearance (Cl_{hm}) and its biliary clearance (Cl_{bl})

$$Cl_h = Cl_{hm} + Cl_{bl}$$

Cl_{bl} of a drug can be experimentally determined by measuring the amount of unchanged drug excreted in bile over an extended period of time:

$$Cl_{bl} = \frac{\text{amount of unchanged drug excreted in the bile from time 0-t}}{AUC_{0\text{-}t,iv}}$$

$AUC_{0\text{-}t,\ iv}$ is the AUC in blood from time 0-t and t is usually more than 24 hr for sufficient bile collection after intravenous administration of drug.

4.12 Enterohepatic Circulation

A drug or its metabolite(s) secreted into bile is stored in the gallbladder and eventually emptied into the duodenum. The drug or its metabolite(s) present in the small intestine may be excreted into the feces or reabsorbed back into the systemic circulation. The cycle in which a drug is absorbed, excreted into the bile, and reabsorbed is known as **enterohepatic circulation** (Fig.4.12). This cycle may be repeated many times, until biotransformation, renal excretion, and fecal excretion ultimately eliminate the drug from the body. In this way, enterohepatic cycling may increase the persistence of drugs in the body. Some drugs excreted as glucuronide conjugates are hydrolyzed in the small intestine back to the parent drug by the action of a b-glucuronidase enzyme released by the intestinal bacteria. The liberated parent drug is reabsorbed back into the systemic circulation. Examples of the drugs that are enterohepatically circulated are morphine and the penicillins.

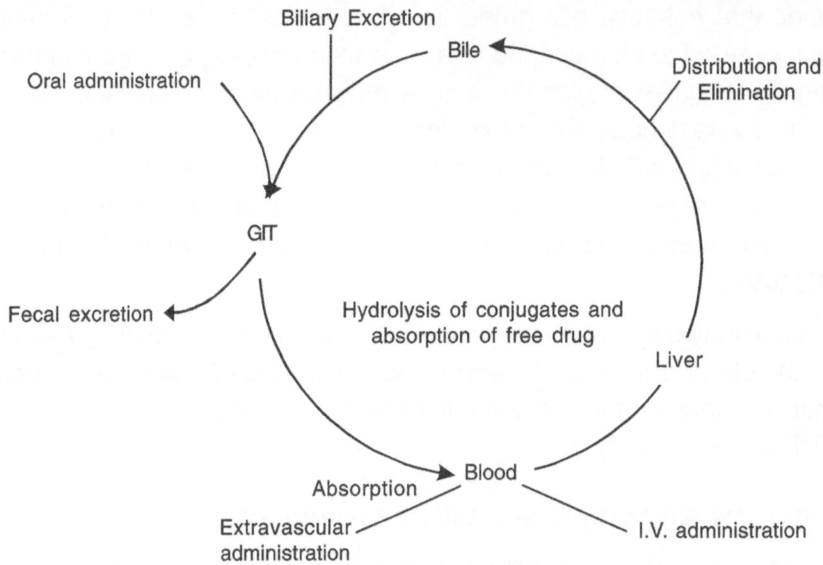

Fig. 4.12 Schematic Representation of Entero-Heptatic Cycling of Drugs.

Biliary excretion and thereby enterohepatic cycling of a drug can be expected if it appears in the feces following its intravenous administration. Enterohepatic circulation after a single dose of a drug is not as important as after multiple doses or a very high dose of a drug. Drugs that undergo enterohepatic circulation some times exhibit a small secondary peak in the plasma drug concentration-time curve following oral administration. The first peak occurs as the drug in the GIT is depleted; a secondary peak then emerges as biliary excreted drug is reabsorbed.

Recent studies have been directed towards finding enterohepatic cycling in men by interrupting the cycle in the intestine. Oral administration of cholestyramine, a non-absorbable ion-exchange resin that strongly binds acidic and neutral drugs, decrease the half-lives of digitoxin and warfarin. These drugs undergo enterohepatic cycling and cholestyramine interrupts the cycle and promotes their fecal excretion. Oral administration of charcoal, a non-specific adsorbent decrease the half-lives of dapsone, phenobarbital, carbamazepine and phenylbutazone.

4.13 Extrahepatic Metabolism

The liver is the main organ involved in drug metabolism. However, other sites of metabolism include the skin, lung, gastrointestinal mucosal cells, microbial flora in the distal portion of the ileum and the large intestine. The kidney may also be involved in certain drug metabolism reactions. Many tissues mentioned above contain microsomal and soluble drug metabolizing enzymes, whose role in drug disposition is poorly understood.

Drug metabolism in the skin could decrease the therapeutic efficacy and duration of action of topically applied drugs, intended to act locally, or produce the first-pass effect for drugs intended for systemic effects.

Drug metabolism in the gastrointestinal tract following oral administration is the most important contributor of extrahepatic drug metabolism. The consequence of this presystemic metabolism is incomplete bioavailability. Isoproterenol is 1000 times less active after oral administration than after of I.V. administration. This difference is due to intestinal metabolism of isoproterenol following oral administration. Similar observations have been made with terbutaline and morphine. It has been observed that the major metabolite formed following oral administration of a drug is different from that formed after I.V. administration. b-glucuronidases present in the intestine hydrolyze the glucuronide conjugates secreted in bile and liberate the parent drugs leading to enterohepatic cycling. Esterases in the intestine hydrolyze the drugs containing the ester group and thereby influence their bioavailability.

The intestinal flora present in the distal small intestine and colon are involved in the metabolism of certain drugs or drugs that are subject to biliary excretion. The drug sulfasalazine is metabolized by the intestinal bacteria to form sulfapyridine and 5-aminosalicylate. The cleavage is believed to be important for the therapeutic effects of the drug to liberate 5-aminosalicylate.

4.14 Minor Pathways of Excretion

Urinary excretion and biotransformation of the drugs are the major pathways of drug elimination. However, there are other minor pathways for the elimination of the drug from the body. Some times these pathways may contribute a significant fraction to drug elimination. For example, pulmonary excretion of general anesthetics.

Salivary Excretion of Drugs

Salivary excretion of drugs is of little quantitiative importance in drug elimination. Lipid solubility, pKa, plasma protein binding of drug and the pH of saliva influence the salivary excretion of a drug. The pH of the saliva ranges between 6.2 to 8.0 and the average pH of saliva is about 6.5 which is lower than the pH of the plasma (7.4). Because of a lower pH of saliva, the saliva/plasma free drug concentration ratios are less than unity for weak acids, and more than one for weak bases. Drugs are transferred into saliva mainly by passive diffusion. The lipid soluble unionized form of the drug diffuses into the saliva from the plasma. Since the saliva is free from proteins, drug levels in saliva reflect the free drug levels in the plasma. Some drugs are actively secreted into the saliva from the plasma. For example, lithium and metoprolol concentrations in the saliva are several times higher than in the plasma.

The saliva/plasma drug concentration ratio (Cs/Cp) is found to be fairly constant for certain drugs. For example, a good to excellent correlations between drug concentrations in saliva and plasma or serum have been reported for antipyrine, diazepam, theophylline, quinidine, acetaminophen, tolbutamide, carbamazepine and digoxin. Therefore, salivary concentration of a drug is used as an indicator of free or total drug concentration in plasma. Further, salivary excretion of drugs is used for the estimation of pharmacokinetic parameters of drugs. However, large differences in Cs/Cp ratio do exist among patients and within individual patients due to variability in saliva pH, which ranged from 6.2 to 8.0. This variability lead to little popularity of salivary kinetic studies.

An equation that shows the relationship between the lipid solubility, pKa, plasma protein binding of drug, saliva pH and Cs/Cp ratio is given below:

For weak acid

$$\frac{Cs}{Cp} = \frac{1+10^{(pHs-pKa)}}{1+10^{(pHp-pKa)}} \times \frac{f_{up}}{f_{us}}$$

For weak bases

$$\frac{Cs}{Cp} = \frac{1+10^{(pKa-pHs)}}{1+10^{(pKa-pHp)}} \times \frac{f_{up}}{f_{us}}$$

Cs = Drug concentration in saliva

Cp = Drug concentration in plasma

pHs = Saliva pH

pHp = Plasma pH

f_{up} = Fraction of unbound drug in plasma

f_{us} = Fraction of unbound drug in saliva

As mentioned previously, saliva is free from proteins and hence the value of f_{us} is equal to unity.

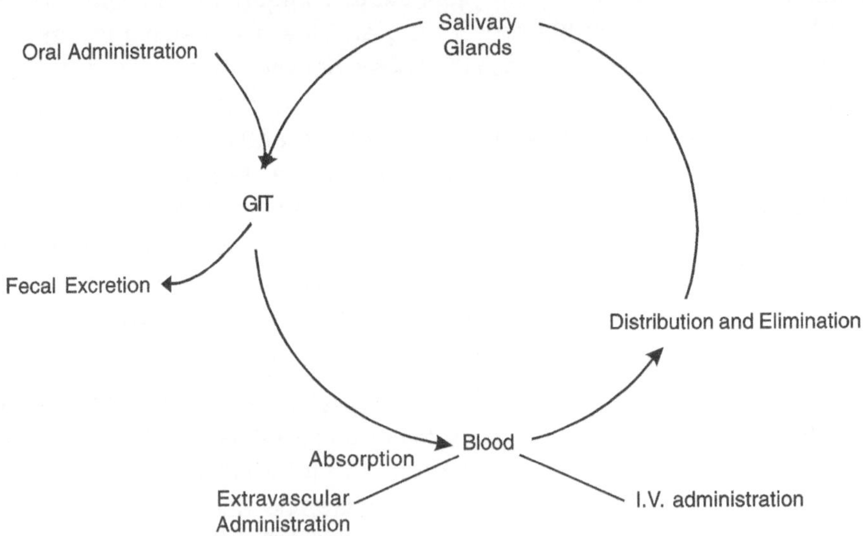

Fig. 4.13 Salivary-GIT cycling of drug given by various routes of administration.

At rest roughly 70 percent of the saliva entering the mouth originates within the submandibular glands, 25 percent arrives from the parotid glands, and 5 percent comes from the sublingual glands. The composition of saliva varies depending on the stimulus provided, and its production may reach 7 ml/min. at meal times. Therefore, considerable amounts of drugs reach the oral cavity and then pass into the GIT from which it can be reabsorbed leading to the cycling of drugs e.g. antibiotics and clonidine (Fig. 4.10). Salivary excretion of antibiotics is considered to be responsible for lingua nigra or black hairy tongue in patients receiving these drugs. Gingival hyperplasia in epileptic patients is related to the salivary excretion of phenytoin. The bitter taste after administration of drugs is also due to the salivary excretion of drugs.

Pulmonary Excretion

General anesthetics like ether, halothane, volatile substances administered in the form of inhalation are absorbed into the blood through the lungs by passive diffusion. The simple principles of gaseous exchange operate in their excretion by diffusion into the expired air. Factors such as the solubility of drug in blood, its volatility and concentration in blood, blood flow rate to lungs and body temperature govern their pulmonary excretion. Liquids like ethanol and benzene are also excreted through the lungs because of their volatility and low solubility in blood.

Secretion of Drugs into Milk

The epithelium of the mammary gland separates milk from the plasma and acts as a lipoid membrane for the transport of various substances. The pH of milk ranges between 6.4 and 7.6 with an average of 6.6. The passive diffusion of a drug from blood to milk depends on the drug concentration in maternal blood, the lipid solubility and the degree of ionization of the drug, the degree of protein binding and the pH of the milk. Because of the lower pH of the milk, weakly basic drugs concentrate more in milk and have a milk/plasma ratio greater than unity whereas the weakly acidic drugs have a milk/plasma drug concentration ratio less than unity, and exhibit low levels in milk.

In general, the daily production of milk is about 850 ml and greatly varies depending upon the general health of the mother and the frequency of breast feeding. Excretion of drugs into milk is not more than 1% of the administered dose and hence does not affect the new born. It has been observed that the amount of a drug that reach the new born via milk is far less than the amount required to elicit therapeutic or toxic effects. However, certain drugs may cause side effects depending upon the dose and frequency of administration. For example, potent drugs like morphine and ergotamine, antibiotics like tetracyclines, sulfonamides and even nicotine present in tobacco are found to reach the new born via milk in considerable quantities and precipitated toxic/side effects.

Gastrointestinal Excretion

Drugs administered by the oral route are absorbed and reach the systemic circulation. The unabsorbed drug is excreted in feces. If the conditions are favorable, drugs can be excreted into the GIT by passive diffusion and may be eliminated. This is reversal of absorption. The metabolites and the conjugates excreted into the GIT via bile are also eliminated through the GIT. Some conjugates may be hydrolyzed by the intestinal microbial flora and are absorbed again into the systemic circulation leading to entero-hepatic circulation. Nicotine and quinine are found to be excreted into the stomach.

Genital Excretion

The genital secretions may contain drugs since the epithelium separating the blood and these special structures is also lipid in nature and passive diffusion of drugs is possible. However, very little information is available on the genital excretion of drugs. Some drugs have been detected in semen.

Excretion Through Sweat

One of the ways of controlling the body temperature is by controlling the rate of sweating. Sweat contains water, elelctrolytes, sebum etc. The diffusion of drugs into the sweat also follows a simple passive diffusion and all the factors involved in passive diffusion are also apply here. It has been reported that excretion of drugs and their metabolites through the skin are also responsible for urticaria and dermatitis and other related hypersensitivity reactions. Several drugs like antipyrine, salicylic acid and heavy metals like lead and arsenic are excreted in sweat.

Likely Questions

1. Define renal clearance.
2. What are the principle processes involved in the urinary excretion of drugs ?
3. How will you determine the GFR?
4. Explain why the plasma protein binding will prolong the renal clearance of a drug that is excreted by glomerualr filtration, but does not affect the renal clearance of a drug excreted by both glomerular filtration and active tubular secretion.
5. How the renal clearance of drugs is useful in assessing the mechanism of urinary excretion? What are the limitations for this?
6. Discuss the factors influencing the passive reabsorption of drugs from the renal tubules.
7. Mention the characters of a substance used for the determination of : (a) GFR and (b) The renal blood flow.
8. Explain the effect of alkalization and acidification of the urine on the renal clearance of a drug with a pKa of 9.4.
9. Define the term biotransformation.
10. What is the basic function of Phase I reactions?
11. Why Phase II reactions are called as *true detoxification* (synthetic) reactions?
12. Why is the liver considered as the major organ involved in detoxification?
13. What are the various sites of drug metabolism in the body?

14. Write a note on metabolism of enantiomers.
15. What is regioselectivity ?
16. List the various factors that are responsible for variation in enzymes in humans.
17. What is enzyme induction? How many types of enzyme inducers are there?
18. What is auto-induction?
19. How will you differentiate the competitive and noncompetitive inhibition?
20. Give Michaelis-Menton equation and explain the terms in it?
21. Show that the order of an enzymatic reaction is dependant on drug concentration.
22. What is Lineweaver-burk equation? What is its use in enzyme kinetics?
23. How will you calculate the hepatic clearance of drugs?
24. Give an equation that shows the relation between hepatic clearance, hepatic blood flow rate and intrinsic clearance of a drug.
25. What is the influence of protein binding on hepatic clearance?
26. What is the first-pass effect?
27. What is the influence of molecular weight of a compound on its biliary excretion?
28. Draw a diagram showing the enterohepatic cycling of drugs.
29. Write a note on extrahepatic metabolism.
30. Give an equation for saliva/plasma drug concentration ratio.
31. What are the factors that influence the salivary excretion of drugs?
32. List the minor pathways of drug elimination.
33. How drug enters the milk from the blood? The pKa of tolbutamide is 5.4. If the pH of saliva is 6.5, the pH of plasma is 7.4, the fraction unbound drug in plasma and saliva are 0.09 and 1.0 respectively, calculate.

References

1. A premier of chemical pathology, by Evelyn SC Koay, Noel Walmsley. Page no: 76.
2. Biliary excretion of drugs in man, Rollins DE, Klaassen CD, Clin Pharmacokinetics 1979 Sep-Oct;4(5):368-79.
3. Biliary excretion, Handbook of Essential Pharmacokinetics, Pharmacodynamics and Drug Metabolism for Industrial Scientists, page 169, http://www.springerlink.com/content/j1h411263070kwq7/.
4. Cimetidine-procainamide pharmacokinetic interaction in man: Evidence of competition for tubular secretion of basic drugs, by A. Somogyi· A. McLean and B. Heinzow, volume 25, number 3/ may , 1983.

5. Clinical Pharmacokinetics- Concepts and Applications, second edition, edited by Malcolm Rowland, Thomas N. Tozer, page no : 148-176.
6. Competitive Inhibition of Renal Tubular Secretion of Gemifloxacin by Probenecid, Cornelia B. Landersdorfer, Carl M. J. Kirkpatrick, Martina Kinzig, Jürgen B. Bulitta, Ulrike Holzgrabe,[3] George L. Drusano, and Fritz Sörgel , Antimicrob Agents Chemother.September 2009, p. 3902-3907, Vol. 53, No. 9.
7. Handbook of bio-analysis and drug metabolism, edited by Gary Evans., page no 26-27.
8. Methods of GFR determination—creatinine clearance after cimetidine administration in clinical practice.

   Author/s: Kabat-Koperska, Joanna (J); Motyl, Waldemar (W); Domanski, Leszek (L); Safranow, Krzysztof (K); Golembiewska, Edyta (E); Kedzierska, Karolina (K); Ciechanowski, Kazimierz (K);

   Journal: Acta medica Austriaca (Acta Med Austriaca), 29 Apr 2004.
9. Modern pharmacology with clinical applications, by Charles R. Craig, Robert E. Sitzel, Page no 41-42.
10. Modern pharmacology with clinical applications, by Charles R. Craig, Robert E. Sitzel, Page no 42-43.
11. Pharmacokinetics, second edition, edited by Milo Gibaldi, Donald Perrier, page no: 319-352. Informa Health Care U.S. 2007.
12. Remington- The Science and Practice of Phrmacy, 21st edition, volume 1, page no: 1163.
13. Remington, The Science and Practice of Pharmacy, 21st editon, volume 1 pages 1166-1167.
14. Renal function, Wikipedia, the free encyclopedia. http://en.wikipedia.org/wiki/Renal_function.

5

Pharmacokinetics: Basic Concepts

Introduction

Pharmacokinetics is the subject that deals with the rates (kinetics) of movement of a drug and/or its metabolite(s) in the body and forces acting on the process. Absorption, Distribution, Metabolism and Excretion of drugs, collectively known as 'ADME', are the processes in which a drug moves in the body at various rates (Table 5.1). Relative rates of these "ADME processes" determine the time course of the drug in the body, the most important of the receptor sites which are responsible for the pharmacological action of drugs. Pharmacokinetics explains the rates of the movement of drugs in the body with the help of a suitable mathematical model. The application of these Pharmacokinetic principles in the safe and effective management of individual patient is called **clinical pharmacokinetics**.

In pharmacokinetics, the concentration of a drug in plasma or any physiological fluid such as urine, saliva, milk etc., is determined with respect to time following its administration. The concentration of a drug in a physiological fluid versus time data is used to study the dynamics of the drug in the body with the help of mathematical equations, derived on the basis of a model and set of assumptions.

5.1 Drug Levels in Blood

After extravascular administration, the drug reaches the blood circulation by a process known as absorption. A plot of blood concentration of the drug versus time is utilized in understanding various important parameters of therapeutics. Fig. 5.1 shows the blood level profile of a drug following a oral route of administration.

Table 5.1: Definition of Absorption, Distribution, Metabolism and Excretion processes.

Process	Definition
Absorption	Absorption is defined as the net transfer of drug from the site of absorption into the circulating fluids of the body. For oral absorption, two steps are required: (1) crossing the epithelium of the gastrointestinal membrane either by transcellular or paracellular pathways and entering the bloodstream via capillaries, and (2) passing through the hepatoportal system intact into systemic circulation. If the drug is metabolized prior to reaching systemic circulation, it is said to have undergone presystemic or first-pass metabolism.
Distribution	Distribution is defined as the net transfer of drug from the circulating fluids of the body to various tissues and organs.
Metabolism	Metabolism is the bioconversion of drug to another chemical form or metabolite, mostly by endogenous enzyme systems involving Phase 1 reactions, such as oxidation (often by the cytochrome P-450 system), reduction, hydrolysis, or dealkylation, or by Phase 2 reactions, such as acetylation, sulfation, or glucuronidation.
Excretion	Excretion is the removal of drug from the body primarily via urine and occasionally via feces, bile, sweat, or exhaled air.

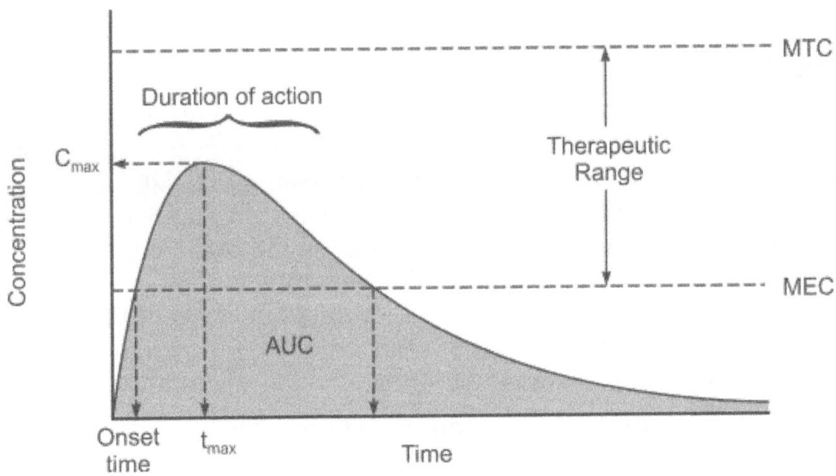

Fig. 5.1 Blood concentration – time profile of a drug following oral administration.

Various terms used in the illustration are described as under:

Minimum Effective Concentration (MEC): Also termed as Minimum Therapeutic Level, is defined as the minimum concentration of a drug in the blood required to elicit a desired therapeutic effect.

Maximum Therapeutic Concentration (MTC): Also known as **Maximum Safe Level,** is defined as the blood level of a drug beyond which side effects or untoward effects will result.

Therapeutic range or window: is the range of drug concentration in blood from the minimum therapeutic level (minimum effective level) to the maximum safe level (minimum toxic level).

As long as the drug levels are maintained within the therapeutic window, therapeutic effect is observed without side effects or toxic effects.

Onset time or Onset of Action: may be defined as the time period required to achieve the minimum effective concentration following the administration of the dosage form.

The onset of the action depends on (1) the administered dose, (2) the release of the drug from the dosage form, (3) the rate of absorption, and (4) the rate of elimination of the drug from the body.

Termination of Action: may be defined as the time period after which the drug levels in blood fall below the minimum therapeutic level and no therapeutic effect is observed.

Duration of Action: The duration of action may be defined as the length of time for which the blood level remains above the maximum therapeutic level and below the maximum safe level or more specifically within the therapeutic window.

Maximum Concentration (C_{max}): is the maximum concentration of the drug in the blood that can be observed following administration of the dosage form. This is an important pharmacokinetic parameter, where rate of absorption equals the rate of elimination. Prior to C_{max}, rate of absorption is greater than the rate of elimination. Post C_{max}, the elimination phase (i.e., metabolism and excretion) dominates over the absorption phase.

Peak Time (t_{max} or t_p): may be defined as the time period at which a maximum concentration of the drug is observed in the blood following administration of the dosage form.The T_{max} value is an important indicator of rate of absorption.

Area under the curve: is defined as the total integrated area under the plasma level-time curve and expresses the total amount of drug that comes into the systemic circulation. This is also another vital pharmacokinetic parameter, which indicates the extent of drug absorption.

Fraction of the Dose Absorbed (F): is the ratio of the amount of drug ultimately reaching the systemic circulation to the total dose administered.

The value of F will be unity if the total administered dose reaches the blood circulation. Many dosage forms often show F values less than unity because of the under mentioned factors:

1. Slow release of the drug from the dosage form and loss of the unabsorbed drug through feces.
2. Degradation of the drug in the GIT due to chemical or enzymatic processes.
3. The drug undergoes the first pass effect. A drug may be stable in the GIT, and absorbed from the GIT completely, but if the drug undergoes extensive metabolism in the liver during its first passage, then the amount of drug reaching the blood stream will be less than the administered dose.

So, a simple blood concentration vs time plot following the administration of a dosage form gives a lot of information about the biological performance of the drug. However, there are so many other pharmacokinetic parameters also, which are useful in designing, developing and evaluating the dosage form.

Desired Characters of an Ideal Drug

In order to achieve the best therapeutic effect, one expects a drug should have the below features,

1. should be absorbed quickly from the absorption site.
2. should arrive at the site of action rapidly and in sufficient quantity.
3. should remain there for a sufficient duration of time.
4. be removed from the site of action eventually.
5. not get distributed to any other tissue.
6. should have a large therapeutic index.

It is generally difficult to obtain all these characters in a drug. Most of the times, the site of action is unknown or not understood. Even if the site is known, it is generally difficult, if not impossible, to determine the drug concentration at the active site in human beings. Whole animal studies involving sacrifice and tissue analysis are possible in animals. They may suffer from some disadvantages also. In addition to the cost factor encountered in the sacrifice of animals as a function of time, there is also the problem of variation between animals. A pharmacokinetic study will attempt to overcome this disadvantage by using each volunteer as his own reference and studying the time course of the drug in the human physiological fluids such as blood/serum/plasma or urine or milk, or saliva.

The basic assumption made in these studies is that there exists a linear relationship between the drug concentration in the blood and the tissue (site of action) and any change in drug concentration in the blood quantitatively reflect the changes at the tissue level. This assumption is justified in most of the cases since every tissue is perfused with blood continuously.

In brief, pharmacokinetics is concerned with quantitatively accounting for the where abouts of a drug after it has been introduced into the body. By analyzing the content of accessible fluids, one uses kinetics to make deductions regarding the amount of the drug in non-accessible regions-perhaps even the site of action. Various pharmacokinetic parameters are calculated based on a mathematical model that are useful in many fields of pharmaceutical sciences.

5.2 Mathematical Model

Mathematical models are a collection of mathematical quantities, operations and relations together with their definitions. A mathematical model used must be realistic and practical, since mathematics are applied to a highly inconsistent biological system. The set of assumptions made in deriving a mathematical equation must be logical and practical.

Qualities of a mathematical model are:

1. **Validity:** It should have practical applicability and should be valuable in describing the events chosen accurately with high precision.
2. **Generality:** Once developed, a mathematical model should have a general application to all the drugs that behave similarly under a given set of conditions or assumptions. This is one of the best qualities of a mathematical model.
3. **Prediction Ability:** It should allow the calculation of new parameters which are not in actual data and should predict the qualitative and quantitative changes in these parameters under a given condition. The parameters like the rate constants, half-lives of drug, etc., can be calculated.
4. **Computability:** The application of a model to biological science in general and pharmacokinetics in particular is dependent on the degree of computability. The assessment of the data should be easy and must not involve lengthy mathematical equations and quantities, making calculation of parameters with a simple calculator practically impossible.
5. **Consistency of Results:** Reproducibility certainly is an important quality of a mathematical model. Unless the results are reproducible, the model is of little use.

Why the Data Should be Fit in a Mathematical Model

The data obtained in a pharmacokinetic study is analyzed by fitting it into a mathematical model. There are many reasons for this and the important ones are :

1. **To Summarize the Data Observed:** It is difficult to understand the data observed as it is and hence the data are summarized in the form of parameters. For example, a drug was given intravenously and the blood concentration versus time data were obtained. By fitting this raw data into a suitable mathematical model, the elimination rate constant, K, can be calculated. Now, the data is summarized in the form of K. If the dose injected and K are known, the data can be regenerated and also an entirely new data at particular time points can be obtained, which was not present originally in the data.
2. **Flexibility:** The data can be analyzed by fitting the data in a suitable mathematical model. The same data can be analyzed by another model. For example, a urine data obtained by a study can be analyzed either by the Sigma-minus method or by excretion rate method.
3. **To calculate the unknown Parameters:** By using the available data, various quantities and pharmacokinetic parameters can be calculated which are valuable and not present in actual data. For example, biological half-life, absorption half-life of a drug, etc.
4. **To Predict Valuable Information:** The pharmacokinetic parameters estimated from the data by fitting it in a suitable mathematical model are useful in predicting valuable information regarding the dosage form performance. For example, blood concentration

vs time data obtained following a single dose can be utilized in predicting the blood concentration time profile following multiple dosing.

5. **To compare Different Formulations of a Drug:** Various formulations developed after extensive research and development are to be evaluated with respect to their biological performance and the best formulation has to be introduced into the market. The task is achieved by conducting experiments on human volunteers and calculating various pharmacokinetic parameters such as peak time (t_p), maximum concentration (C_{max}), area under the curve (AUC) from the data.
6. **To Compare the Drugs with Similar Pharmacological Action:** Assuming that therapeutic efficacy is directly proportional to the drug concentration in the blood, fitting the blood concentration *vs* time data of two different drugs with a similar pharmacological activity, the intrinsic activities of drugs and their pharmacodynamics can be compared.
7. **To Define Therapeutic Window:** With the help of pharmacokinetic values obtained from blood concentration time data, toxicologist can make a correlation between the concentration of a drug in the body and toxic effects. The minimum and maximum therapeutic levels of a drug in the body can be predicted within reasonable limits.
8. **To Get Answer to Various Questions Pertinent to Drug:** Further, there are so many fundamental questions with respect to a drug, which are answered only by pharmacokinetics; they are:
    1. Is the drug absorbed and to what extent ?
    2. Do other things such as food, other drugs, interfere with the absorption of the drug ?
    3. What is the nature of the dose-response plot ?
    4. How the drug behaves at different doses ?
    5. What are optimum dosage regimens for the drug ?
    6. Has the drug undergone gut metabolism, and/or the first pass effect ?
    7. What is the distribution pattern of the drug in the body ?
    8. How is the drug eliminated and the rate of elimination ?
    9. What are the factors that affect the rate of elimination of the drug ?
    10. Is the pharmacological action observed is due to the parent drug or a metabolite?
    11. Is there a correlation between the pharmacological response and pharmacokinetic data ?
    12. Does the situation change with multiple dosing ?

5.3 Pharmacokinetic Models

Pharmacokinetics is the study of the time course of drug absortion, distribution, metabolism and excretion, which move at different rate in the body. Therefore, various mathematical models can be devised to simulate the rate processes of drug ADME. These mathematical models are useful in the development of relationship to describe drug concentrations in the body as a function of time. Because drug concentrations are dependent on time, the two variables drug concentration and time, are termed as **dependent** and **independent** variables, respectively. In practice, pharmacokinetic parameters are not measured directly but are determined experimentally from a set of dependent and independent variables collectively known as **data**. From these data, a pharmacokinetic model is estimated/ postulated and tested for validity and the pharmacokinetic parameters are obtained.

The model chosen for the analysis of the data is based on a hypothesis and set of assumptions that describe biological events in the mathematical form. Care has to be taken when to rely totally on pharmacokinetic model to predict the drug action. In general, the data are analyzed with the simplest pharmacokinetic model and statistical methods are used to find the 'model fit' to the data. If the model does not fit accurately the experimental observations, a new and more complex model (hypothesis) is usually proposed and subsequently tested. However, in clinical setup, it is important to realize that the pharmacokinetic data should not replace clinical observations in the patient and sound judgment by the clinician in decision making. Pharmacokinetic analysis can be broadly classified into following approaches :

1. Compartment models
2. Physiologic pharmacokinetic model (flow model)
3. Non-compartmental pharmacokinetics
4. Non-linear pharmacokinetics

5.3.1 Compartment Model

In a pharmacokinetic analysis of the data, the living system (human body) is assumed to consist of a number of interconnected compartments. A *compartment* is defined as a group of tissues which behaves uniformly with respect to the drug movement. Each tissue may have a different concentration of drug but they all are in an equilibrium in such a way that a change in drug concentration in these tissue is linear or similar. These compartments are virtual and not a real physiologic one, which only provide reflection of the biosystem.

The human body is divided into kinetically homogeneous hypothetical compartments based on the vascularity and the distribution pattern of the drug. Each compartment behaves differently regarding the drug concentration time course data.

1. **Highly Perfused**: Also known as central compartment. Highly perfused lean tissue group, consisting of blood cells, heart, lungs, hepatoportal system, kidneys, glands and also certain tissues protected by specialized lipid membranes such as the brain and the spinal cord. Drug elimination is assumed to take place from this compartment.
2. **Moderately/Poorly perfused**: are termed as Peripheral compartments. Examples include, a poorly perfused lean tissue group, consisting of the muscle and skin; fat group, consisting of adipose tissue including bone marrow.
3. A negligible perfused tissue group, consisting of bones, teeth, ligaments, tendons, cartilages and hair.

A graphical analysis of the plasma concentration time data following an I.V. injection can be used to estimate the number of compartments. The log concentration versus time graph shows lines with different shapes corresponding to different compartments. A statistical analysis of the plasma concentration time data is another method used to find out the number of compartments. Computer programmes are available for this purpose. In general, the kinetics of most drugs can be described by a hypothetical model consisiting of one, two or at the most three functional compartments. It is usually assumed that the rate of drug movement between compartments follow first-order kinetics.

In one compartment model, drug is both added and eliminated from a central compartment. When an intravenous dose of drug is given, the drug enters directly into the central compartment. Elimination of drug occurs from the central compartment because the organs involved in drug elimination, primarily kidney and liver, are well perfused tissues.

In a two-or multi-compartment model(s), drug can move between the central or plasma compartment to and from the tissue compartments. In these models, the total amount of drug in the body is simply the sum of the drug present in the central compartment plus the drug present in the the tissue compartment(s). Knowing the parameters of either the one- or two-compartment model, one can estimate the amount of drug left in the body and the amount of drug eliminated from the body at any time. The compartmental models are particularly useful when the little information is known about the tissues. Table 5.2 enlists the various properties of a compartment.

Table 5.2 Characteristics of a "Compartment".

	Highlights of a compartment
1.	A compartment contains tissues and organs that are "kinetically homogenous"
2.	Within each compartment, distribution to tissues is immediate and rapidly reversible
3.	Although kinetically homogenous, tissues within a compartment have different drug concentrations
4.	Drug with in a compartment is assumed to be "well stirred".
5.	Between compartments, barriers are considered diffusion rate limiting.
6.	Compartments are connected through First-order rate processes
7.	Distribution to any tissue in any compartment depends upon blood flow, blood volume, partitioning, tissue binding, and plasma protein binding

The compartments can be arranged either parallel to each other (**mamillary model**) or in series to each other (**caternary model**).

Mammillary Model

The mammillary model is the most common compartment model used in pharmacokinetics. The model consists of one or more peripheral compartments connected to a central compartment. The central compartment consists of plasma and highly perfused tissues in which the drug distributes rapidly. The drug introduced into a compartment reaches central compartment and from there it distributes to all other compartments which are connected to central compartment. Elimination of the drug is assumed to occur from the central compartment since the major organs involved in drug elimination, primarily kidney and liver, are present in the central compartment.

Fig. 5.2 shows several types of compartment models. Compartment 1 represents the plasma or central compartment, and compartments 2, 3 and 4 represent tissue compartments or peripheral compartments. The pharmacokinetic rate constants are represented by the letter K and the number represent the direction of the drug movement between the compartments. For example, K_{12} means the rate constant with respect to drug movement from compartment 1 to compartment 2. The models are ***open systems*** because drug can be eliminated from the system.

The drawing of models gives a visual representation of the rate processes involved, shows how many pharmacokinetic rate constants are necessary to describe the process adequately, and enables the pharmacokineticist to develop differential equations to describe drug concentration changes in each compartment.

Model 1. One-compartment open model I.V injection

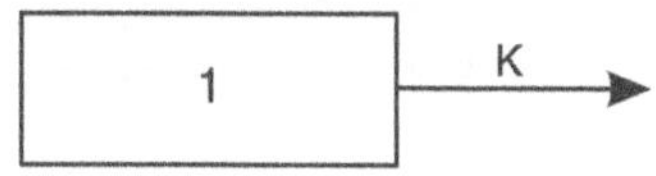

Model 2. One-compartment open model with the first-order absorption

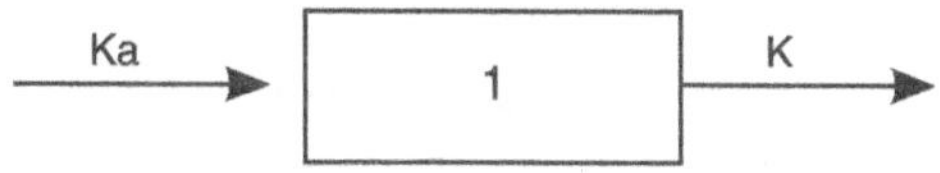

Model 3. Two-compartment open model, I.V. injection

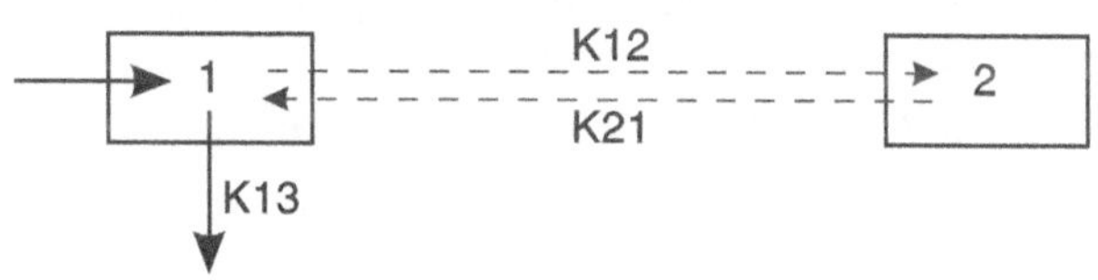

Model 4. Two-compartment open model with the first order absorption

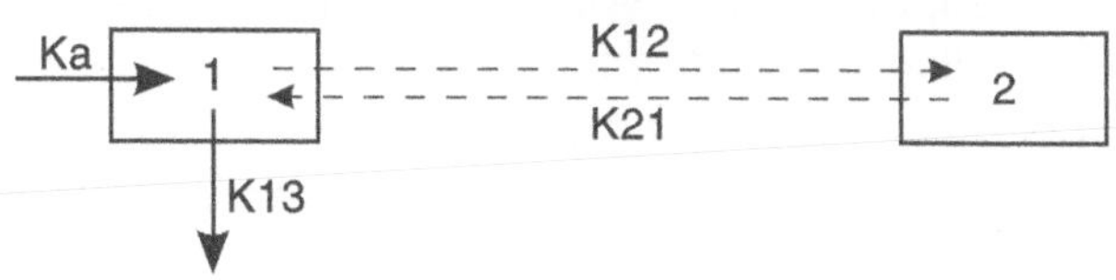

Fig. 5.2 Various compartment models.

Two parameters are needed to describe Model 1 (Fig. 5.2). The volume of the compartment and the elimination rate constant, K. However, in case of Model 4, the pharmacokinetic parameters consist of the volume of Compartment 1 and 2 along with the rate constants – Ka, K13, K12 and K21 – a total of six parameters.

In studying these models, it is important to know whether drug concentration data may be obtained directly from each compartment. For models 3, and 4 (Fig. 5.2) data concerning compartment 2, can not be obtained easily because the tissues are not easily sampled and may not contain homogenous concentrations of the drug. If the amount of the drug absorbed and eliminated per unit time is obtained by sampling compartment 1, then the amount of the drug contained in the tissue compartments can be estimated mathematically. For this purpose, appropriate mathematical equations for describing these models and evaluating the various pharmacokinetic parameters are to be used.

Caternary Models

Another type of compartment model called caternary model, consists of compartments joined to one another in a row or series like the compartments of a train (Fig. 5.3). In contrast, the mammillary model consists of one or more compartments around a central compartment like satellites. Since most of the functional organs of the body are directly connected to the plasma, caternary model is not used as often used as the mammillary model.

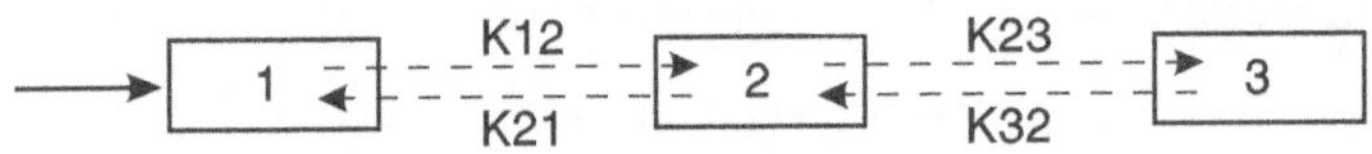

Fig. 5.3 Example of caternary model.

Salient features of compartmental modeling

1. Helps in predicting the drug concentration-time profile in both normal and diseased state
2. Helps in ascertaining a good dosage regimen
3. Helps in meaningful interpretation of a biological response to a dose
4. Provides visual interpretation of various rate processes involved in drug ADME
5. Provides information about how about many pharmacokinetic parameters are required to describe the process adequately.
6. Delineates the entire ADME process into quantitative relationships
7. Helpful in determining drug concentrations especially when little is known about individual tissues.

However, this approach suffers from **various pitfalls** like

1. The compartments are only hypothetical and donot bear any relationship between physiologic function or anatomic structure.
2. Involves lot of mathematical computations
3. Prediction accuracy primarily depends upon the correctness of the curve fitting
4. Compartment models for one drug differ with route of administration.
5. Results from animal species cannot be extrapolated to human.

5.3.2 Physiologic Pharmacokinetic Model (Flow model)

Physiologic pharmacokinetic models, also known as blood flow or perfusion models, are pharmacokinetic models based on known anatomic and physiologic data. The models kinetically describe the data with the consideration that the blood flow is responsible for distributing a drug to various parts of the body. Uptake of a drug into organs is determined by binding of the drug in these tissues. In contrast to the tissue volume of distribution, the actual tissue volume is used. Because there are many tissue organs in the body, each tissue volume must be estimated and its drug concentration described. The model would potentially predict realistic tissue drug concentration, which the compartment model fails to do. Unfortunately, much of the information that is required for adequately describing a physiologic pharmacokinetic model is experimentally difficult to obtain. In spite of the limitation, a physiologic pharmacokinetic model does provide a much better insight of how physiologic factors may change drug distribution from one animal species to another. Other major differences are as follows:

First, no data fitting is required in the perfusion model. Drug concentrations in the various tissues are predicted by the organ tissue size, blood flow, and experimentally determined drug-tissue-blood ratios (i.e., partition of the drug between the tissue and the blood).

Second, blood flow, tissue size, and the drug tissue - blood ratio may vary due to certain pathophysiologic conditions. Thus the effect of these variations on drug distribution must be taken into account in physiologic pharmacokinetics models.

Third, and most important of all, physiologically based pharmacokinetic models can be applied to several species, and with some drugs human data may be extrapolated. Extrapolation is not possible with compartment models, because the volume of distribution in such models is a mathematical concept that does not relate simply to the blood volume and blood flow. To date, numerous drugs (including digoxin, lidocaine, methotrexate, and thiopental) have been described with perfusion models. Tissue levels of some of these drugs can not be predicted successfully with compartment models, although they generally, describe blood levels well. An example of a perfusion model is shown in Fig. 5.4.

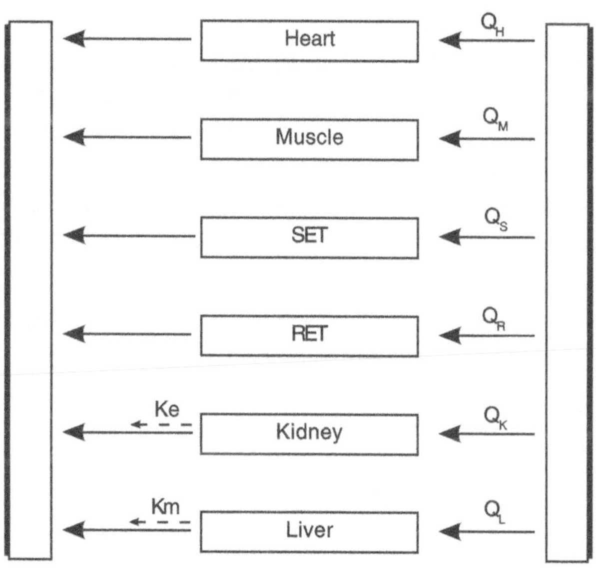

Fig. 5.4 Pharmacokinetic model of drug perfusion.

The number of tissue compartments in a perfusion model varies with the drug-to-drug. Typically, the tissues or organs that have no drug penetration are excluded from consideration. Thus, such organs as the brain, the bones, and other parts of the central nervous system are often excluded, as most drugs have little penetration into these organs. To describe each organ separately with a differential equation would make the model very complex and mathematically difficult. A simpler but equally good approach is to group all the tissues with similar blood perfusion properties into a single compartment. A perfusion model has been successfully used to describe the distribution of lidocaine in blood and various organs. In this case, organs such as lung, liver, brain and muscle were individually described by differential equations, whereas other tissues were grouped as RET (rapidly equilibrating tissue) and SET (slowly equilibrating tissue).

The differential equations that describe drug distribution are usually solved by numerical integration with the model as a base, and the entire time course of drug levels in various tissue organs can be simulated.

The real significance of a physiologically based model is the potential application of this model in the prediction of human pharmacokinetics from animal data. The mass of various body organs or tissues, extent of protein binding, drug metabolism capacity, and blood flow in humans and other species are often known or can be determined. Thus, physiologic and anatomic parameters can be used to predict the effects of drugs on a humans and their effects on animals in cases where human experimentation is difficult or restricted.

5.3.3 Noncompartmental pharmacokinetics

A pharmacokinetic analysis of blood concentration of a drug versus time data using compartment models involves application of mathematical equations developed based on a set of assumptions. Noncompartmental methods, also known as **model independent** methods, do not need such assumptions. In fact, these methods can be applied to virtually any compartmental model, provided that it follows the linear pharmacokinetics. These methods are hardly new and provide a simpler and a general approach for pharmacokinetic analysis. Noncompartmental methods for calculating absorption, distribution, and elimination parameters are based on the theory of statistical moments.

Statistical moment theory: Statistical moment theory provides a unique way to study time-related changes in drug concentration in the plasma and/or tissues. The time course of drug concentration in plasma can usually be regarded as a statistical distribution curve. With in this, the zero moment of a drug concentration in the plasma versus time curve is the total area under the curve from time zero to infinity ($AUC_{0\infty}$). The zero moment of a drug concentration in a plasma-time profile is the total area under the curve resulting from a plot of drug concentration versus time. The first moment of a plasma concentration-time profile is the total area under the curve, resulting from a plot of the product of drug concentration and time versus time ($AUMC_{0\infty}$).

In calculating various pharmacokinetic parameters, the plasma concentration versus time data is plotted (Fig. 5.5) and the AUC from t=0 to the last sampling time, t*, is calculated by means of the trapezoidal rule (See Appendix I). Table 5.3 shows concentration data obtained during and after 1 hour constant rate of intravenous infusion. Also listed are the values of (C)x(t) (concentration multiplied by time). These values are plotted against time in Fig. 5.5. The area under the (C)x(t) versus t plot from t=0 to the last sampling time, t*, is called the first moment of drug concentration with respect to time (AUMC). The area under the curve from t* to ∝ for both the curves may be estimated using appropriate equations to obtain $AUC_{t^*}^{\infty}$ and $AUMC_{t^*}^{\infty}$. Addition of these areas to $AUC_0^{t^*}$ and $AUMC_0^{t^*}$ result in total areas under zero moment and first moment curves, AUC_0^{∞} and $AUMC_0^{\infty}$, respectively. Various pharmacokinetic parameters are calculated using the above values.

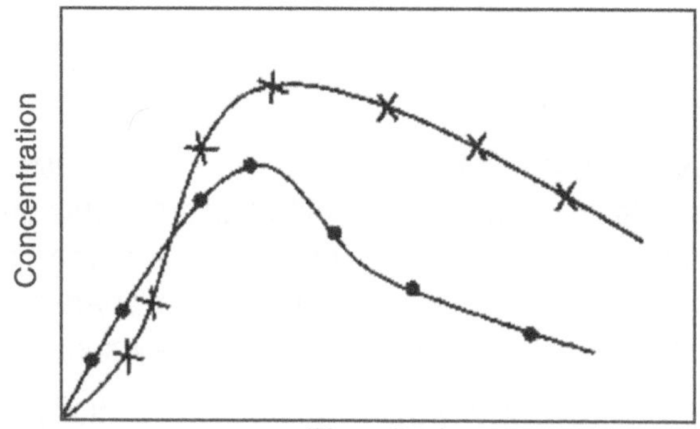

Fig. 5.5 Plots of drug concentration (μg/ml) (•) and drug concentration-time (μg-hr/ml) (X) versus time, during and after 1 hour constant rate intravenous infusion. The area under the drug conc. versus time plot to infinity is $AUCo^{\alpha}$, the area under the drug conc. time versus time plot to infinity is $AUMCo^{\infty}$.

Table 5.3 Drug Concentration and the Product of Drug Concentration and Time at Different Sampling Times.

Time (t) (hr)	Concentration (c) (mg/ml)	Concentration –time (c.t) (mg/ml) (hr)
0.5	3.2	1.6
1.0	5.9	5.9
2.0	4.2	8.4
3.0	3.0	9.0
4.0	2.1	8.4
5.0	1.5	7.5
6.0	1.1	6.6
8.0	0.5	4.0

5.3.4 Non-Linear Pharmacokinetics

The estimation of various pharmacokinetic parameters such as absorption rate constant, elimination rate constant, plasma clearance etc., is based on the assumption that these parameters does not change upon the administration of a drug in different doses or when multiple doses of a drug are given. With some drugs, increased doses or chronic medication can cause deviations from the linear pharmacokinetic profile observed with single low doses of the same drug. This nonlinear pharmacokinetic behavior is also termed **dose-dependent pharmacokinetics**. The time of administration of a drug may influence the pharmacokinetic parameters of the drug, which are termed as **time-dependent pharmacokinetics**. In addition, nonlinear pharmacokinetics may be observed due to a pathologic alternation in drug absorption, distribution, and elimination. Hence, this topic is discussed in detail later in this book.

5.4 Pharmacokinetic Study

At a fundamental level, pharmacokinetics is a tool to optimize the design of biological experiments with drugs and chemicals. Biopharmaceutic and pharmacokinetic studies of drugs and drug products are useful in understanding the relationship between the physicochemical properties of a drug product and the pharamacologic or clinical effect. Fig. 5.6 is a general scheme describing this dynamic relationship.

Biopharmaceutics considers the inter-relationship of the physicochemical properties of drug, the dosage form in which drug is given, and the route of administration and the rate and extent of systemic drug absorption. Thus, biopharmaceutics includes factors that influence the release of drug from a drug product, the rate of dissolution of the drug, and the eventual bioavailability of the drug. **Pharmacokinetics** involves the kinetics of drug absorption, distribution, excretion, and metabolism. Elimination of a drug means both excretion and metabolism. The description of drug distribution and elimination is often termed **drug disposition**.

In order to estimate pharmacokinetics of a drug or drug product, drug concentration in a biological sample versus time data are required. Actually the concentration of the drug at the receptor site versus time data are required to make a meaningful interpretation of a biological response to a dose. Practically it is not possible to obtain the biological sample from a human being at which drug acts and hence few biological fluids, such as blood/plasma/serum, urine, milk, saliva etc., are utilized in any pharmacokinetic study. In most of the pharmacokinetic studies plasma concentration of drug-time data are used to estimate various pharmackinetic parameters and to assess the biological effects. The assumption in using the plasma drug concentration-time data to assess biological response is that there exists a dynamic equilibrium between the plasma and tissue (receptor site) drug levels, and a change in drug levels in the plasma qantitatively reflects a change in the tissue drug levels.

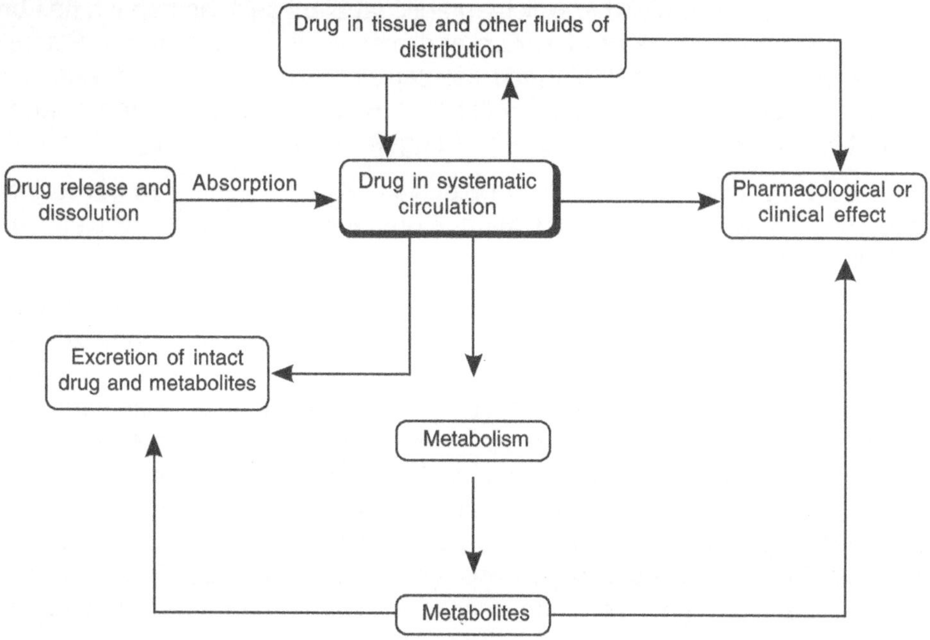

Fig. 5.6 Scheme demonstrating the dynamic relationship between the drug and pharmacological effect.

A drug or a drug product is administered to human volunteers by a selected route of administration. The number of subjects, the period of study, biological sample, number of samples to be collected, time intervals at which samples have to be collected should be decided prior to the study. The biological fluid collected at different time intervals is analyzed for drug content. The drug concentration in a biological fluid versus time data is utilized for pharmacokinetic analysis.

5.4.1 Sampling of Biological specimens

Only a few biologic specimens may be obtained safely from the patient to gain information regarding the drug concentration in the body. *Invasive* methods include sampling blood, spinal fluid, synovial fluids, tissue biopsy, or any biologic material that requires parentral or surgical intervention in the patient. In contrast *non-invasive* methods include sampling of urine, saliva, feces, expired air, or any biological material that can be obtained without parentral or surgical intervention. The measurement of drug concentration in each of these biologic materials yields different information.

Measurement of drug concentration in the blood, serum, or plasma is the most direct approach employed to assess the pharmacokinetics of the drug in the body. The whole blood contains cellular elements including red blood cells, white blood cells, platelets and various other proteins such as albumin and globulins. In general, serum or plasma is used for drug measurement. To obtain serum, the whole blood is allowed to clot and the serum is collected from the supernatant after centrifugation. Plasma is obtained from the supernatant of the whole blood to which an anticoagulant such as heparin has been added. Therefore, the protein content of serum and plasma is not the same. Plasma perfuses all the tissues of the body including the cellular elements in the blood. Assuming that the drug in the plasma is in dynamic equilibrium with the tissues, then changes in drug concentration in the plasma will reflect changes in the tissue drug concentration.

Spinal fluid, synovial fluid and tissue biopsies are occasionally removed for diagnostic purposes. They may be used to ascertain the presence of a drug in sufficient concentration in the biological specimen.

Measurement of a drug in urine is an indirect method to ascertain its bioavailability. The rate and extent of drug excreted in the urine reflect the rate and extent of systemic drug absorption. The use of urinary drug excretion measurements to establish various pharmacokinetic parameters is discussed elsewhere in this text. Measurement of the drug in feces may reflect the drug that has not been absorbed after an oral dose or may reflect that has been biliary secreted after systemic absorption. In mass balance studies estimation of a drug content in feces is carried to account for the entire dose given to the patient. For any mass balance study, both urine and feces are collected and their drug content is measured. For specialized dosage forms, which release the drug by a process of leaching without disintegration and dissolution, fecal collection is performed to obtain the dosage form. The dosage form is assayed to account for the unreleased drug.

Measurement of drug concentration in saliva has been carried for several drugs for therapeutic drug monitoring. If the ratio of drug concentration in saliva to drug concentration in plasma is constant, therapeutic drug monitoring can be carried out with salivary drug concentration. This concept is based on the fact that the drug in saliva is in an equilibrium with the drug in plasma so that a change in drug concentration in saliva reflects a change in plasma drug concentration

5.4.2 Significance of Measuring Plasma Drug Levels

The drug concentration in the tissue, which contains a receptor, is often related to the observed intensity of the pharmacologic or toxic effect of a drug. Because most of the tissue cells are richly perfused with tissue fluids or plasma, estimation of the plasma drug level is an appropriate method of monitoring the course of therapy.

Monitoring the concentration of drugs in blood or plasma ascertains that the calculated dose actually delivers the plasma level required for the therapeutic effect. Clinically, individual variations in the pharmacokinetics of drugs are quite common. Moreover, the patients physiologic functions may be affected by disease, nutrition, environment, concurrent drug therapy, and other factors. The relationship between plasma drug concentrations and pharmacological response is best explained by pharmacokinetic models. For example, measurement of drug concentration in a single blood sample for a patient will not give any useful information. In order to apply this information properly, it is important to know when the blood sample was drawn? what dose of the drug was given? What was the route of administration? If a proper information is available, the use of pharmacokinetic equations and models may describe the blood level time curve accurately.

Monitoring of drug plasma concentrations allows for the adjustment of the drug dosage in order to individualize and optimize therapeutic drug regimens. In the presence of alteration in physiologic functions due to a disease, monitoring plasma drug concentrations may provide a guide to the progress of the diseased state and enable the investigator to modify the drug dosage accordingly. Clinically, a sound medical judgment and observation are most important. Therapeutic judgments should not be based solely on the plasma drug concentrations.

In many cases, the pharmacodynamic response to the drug may be more important to measure than just plasma drug concentration. For example, the electrophysiology of the heart including an electrocardiogram (ECG) is important to assess patients medicated with cardiotonic drugs such as digoxin. For an anticoagulant drug such as dicumarol, prothrombin clotting time might indicate whether a proper dose was achieved. Most diabetics taking insulin will monitor their blood or urine glucose levels.

For drugs that act irreversibly at the receptor site, plasma drug concentrations do not accurately predict pharmacodynamic response. Drugs used in cancer chemotherapy often interface with nucleic acid or protein biosynthesis to destroy tumor cells. For those drugs, the plasma drug concentration does not relate directly to the pharmacodynamic response. In this case, other pathophysiologic parameters are monitored in the patients to prevent adverse toxicity.

5.4.3 Data Required for Pharmacokinetic Analysis

The following data are required for any pharmacokinetic analysis and interpretation of results.

- Drug or Drug product
- Sensitive Analytical Method for measurement of the drug in the biological specimen
- Route of Administration
- Dose Administered
- Sampling interval
- Biological specimen (generally plasma or urine)

The plasma samples collected at different time intervals following a specified dose of drug product administered by a selected route of administration will be analyzed by a sensitive analytical method to get the drug concentration in the plasma versus time profile. These data are subjected to a pharmacokinetic analysis to obtain various pharmacokinetic parameters.

Likely Questions

1. What are the qualities of a mathematical model?
2. Why the plasma drug concentration-time data should be fit in a mathematical model?
3. Define (a) Therapeutic window, (b) Duration of action (c) Maximum concentration (C_{max}) and peak time at which C_{max} occurs (t_p) following an oral administration.

4. What are the desired characters of an ideal drug for the best therapeutic effect?
5. How the human body is divided into compartments? What are they?
6. Why a mammillary model is generally used rather than caternary model in compartmental pharmacokinetics?
7. What are the advantages of a physiological pharmacokinetic model over other models?
8. Write about sampling of biological specimens.
9. Write a note on Statistical Moment Theory.
10. What is the siginificance of measuring the plasma drug level ?

Suggested Readings

1. Jambhekar, S. S., Breen, P. J. Basic Pharmacokinetics. Pharmaceutical Press Inc., UK.
2. Schoewald, R. D. Pharmacokinetic Principles of Dosing Adjustments: Understanding the Basics. CRC Press Pharmacy Education Series. 2001, CRC Press LLC, USA.
3. Shargel, L., Wu-Pong, S., Yu, A. B. C. Applied Biopharmaceutics & Pharmacokinetics. Fifth Ed. McGraw-Hill Publishers, USA. 2005

6

One Compartment Open Model

One Compartment Open Model

When a drug is given extravascularly, the drug moves in the human body through the process of absorption, distribution, metabolism and elimination (ADME). However, the drug is eliminated from the body completely after some time. The body is said to be 'open' with respect to the drug movement. The movement of the drug in the body can be described mathematically by various equations, most of which incorporate exponential terms (i.e. e^x or e^{-x}). This suggests that ADME processes are "*first order*" in nature at therapeutic doses and, therefore, drug transfer in the body is possibly mediated by"passive diffusion." Therefore, there is a directly proportional relationship between the observed plasma concentration and/or the amount of drug eliminated in the urine and the administered dose of the drug. This direct proportionality between the observed plasma concentration and the amount of drug eliminated and the dose administered yields the term "***linear pharmacokinetics***". Because of the complexity of ADME processes, an adequate description of the observations is sometimes possible only by assuming a simplified model; the most useful model in pharmacokinetics is the compartment model.

One compartment open model, the simplest of the models, depicts the body as a single homogenous unit. This model is particularly useful for drugs that rapidly distribute between plasma and other body fluids and tissues upon entry into the systemic circulation. However, this model does not assume that drug concentration in each tissue is the same at any given point of time. The one compartment open model assumes that any changes that occur in the plasma levels of the drug reflect proportional changes in the tissue drug levels.

Pharmacokinetic models are developed based on certain assumptions. It should be remembered that application of mathematics to physiological system means we are trying to correlate mathematics and physiological events, so the assumptions made should be realistic and practical. Other experimental conditions for the validity of assumptions should be studied and noted. The following assumptions are made in deriving mathematical equations for one compartment open model:

1. The process of drug absorption from the absorption site may be explained by the first-order kinetics.

   Explanation : *Most drugs are absorbed by a passive diffusion mechanism that is governed by the first order process i.e., the rate of drug absorption is proportional to the drug concentration at the site of absorption. For drugs which are absorbed solely by active transport, facilitated diffusion etc., this assumption is not valid.*

2. Once a drug enters the systemic circulation, it rapidly distributes to other body fluids and tissue, and a dynamic equilibrium is achieved instantaneously between the drug in the blood and the drug in other tissues.

   Explanation : *The drug which distributes to highly perfused tissues like the heart, lungs, liver, kidney, etc., can distribute quickly and attain an equilibrium between the drug levels in the plasma and other body fluids and tissues.*

   If the drug is distributed to poorly perfused tissues, the time required for its distribution and equilibrium may be considerable. Hence, this simple model is not useful for pharmacokinetic analysis of the data obtained with such drugs.

3. Any changes that occur in the plasma levels of a drug reflect proportional changes in the tissue drug levels.

   Explanation : *since there exists a dynamic equilibrium between drug concentration in the plasma and drug concentration in the tissues, a change in the drug level of the plasma certainly brings a proportional change in the levels of the tissue.*

4. Elimination of the drug from the body follows an apparent first order kinetics and its rate constant, K, is known as an apparent first order rate constant.

   Explanation : *Drug elimination can occur from the body by many processes, including renal, biliary, biotransformation, excretion in the expired air, etc.*

Glomerular filtration in the kidney and passive diffusion into bile are simple first-order filtration process, where as tubular secretion, biotransformation (metabolism), and biliary secretions frequently involve active processes. Enzymes are involved in metabolism processes and hence, at higher concentration of a drug these processes may become saturated. The kinetics of such a saturated process cannot be described by simple first order kinetics. However, the drug concentrations achieved in plasma with therapeutic doses of the drug may not saturate the processes. Hence, the active processes involved in drug elimination may be approximated with first order equations. Further, the sum of the rate constants of all the processes involved in elimination of the drug gives an overall apparent first order rate constant, K.

$$K = Ke + K_{f1} + K_{f2} + Kb + \ldots\ldots \qquad \ldots\ldots(6.1)$$

where Ke and Kb are the first order rate constants of renal and biliary excretion respectively and K_{f1} and K_{f2} are apparent first order rate constants for metabolism. The constants are usually referred to as apparent first order rate constants to convey that the kinetics may be approximated by the first order kinetics.

In order to develop mathematical equations that describe drug concentration in the body fluids versus time profile, the following points should be available.

1. The dose of a drug administered, X0
2. The route of administration of drug. In general, in pharmacokinetics, vascular and extravascular routes of administration are considered. Extravascular route contains an additional drug movement process, known as absorption. Under the route of administration, three types of cases are generally considered. They are 1. intravenous bolus 2. intravenous infusion and 3. extravascular (oral, intramuscular etc.).
3. Biological fluid collected following the administration of the drug. In general blood/plasma/serum and urine are collected for any pharmacokinetic study.
4. The form of the drug measured in the biological fluid. Unchanged drug or metabolite levels in the biological fluid versus time data can be used for a pharmacokinetic analysis.
5. Whether the kinetic study is for a single dose or for multiple doses.
6. The mathematical equations for sustained action dosage forms, timed release dosage forms, etc., should be developed separately.

Table 6.1 shows the various schemes for developing mathematical models and equations.

Table 6.1 Scheme of study of pharmacokinetic equations in one compartment open model.

Scheme Symbol	Route of administration	Biological fluid	Drug/analyte form
6.1	**I.V. Bolus**		
6.1.1	I.V. Bolus	Blood/plasma/serum	Unchanged drug
6.1.2	I.V. Bolus	Urine	Unchanged drug
6.1.3	I.V. Bolus	Blood/plasma/serum	Metabolite(s)
6.1.4	I.V. Bolus	Urine	Metabolite(s)
6.2	**I.V. Infusion**		
6.2.1		Blood/plasma/serum	Unchanged drug
6.2.2		Urine	Unchanged drug
6.2.3		Blood/plasma/serum	Metabolite(s)
6.2.4		Urine	Metabolite(s)
6.3	**Extravascular Administration**		
6.3.1	Oral Administration	Blood/plasma/serum	Unchanged drug
6.3.2	Oral Administration	Urine	Unchanged drug

6.1 Intravenous Injection (Bolus)

When a drug is given in the form of a rapid intravenous injection (I.V. bolus), the entire dose of the drug enters the body immediately. In most cases the drug distributes via the circulatory system to all the tissues in the body and equilibrates rapidly in the body. The biological fluid selected for study and drug form measured in it are to be considered for developing suitable equations.

Scheme 6.1.1 I.V. Bolus - Unchanged Drug in Blood/Plasma

The schematic representation of drug movement in the body in this case is shown below:

$$\xrightarrow[X0]{\text{I.V. bolus}} \boxed{X = Vd.C} \xrightarrow{K}$$

Where:

X0 = Dose of drug injected

X = Amount of drug present in body at any time 't'.

Vd = Apparent volume of distribution of drug.

C = Concentration of drug in central compartment (plasma) at any time 't'

K = Apparent overall first order elimination rate constant.

Following I.V. bolus, the entire dose is in the body and is eliminated from the body by an apparent first-order process. The rate of decrease of the amount of the drug in the body is only dependent upon the amount of the drug present in the body at any given time following I.V. bolus. Thus we can write as follows,

$$\frac{dX}{dt} \alpha X \qquad .....(6.2)$$

dX/dt is the rate of change of the drug amount in the body with respect to time.

$$\frac{dX}{dt} = -KX \qquad .....(6.3)$$

where 'K' is a *first-order rate constant* and the negative sign indicates that the drug is being lost from the body.

To describe the time course of the amount of the drug in the body after injection, equation 6.3 must be integrated after separating the variables.

$$\int_0^t dx/dt = \int_0^t -Kdt$$

$$|\ln X|_o^t = -K|t|_o^t$$

$$\ln X - \ln X0 = -K(t - o)$$

$$\ln X = \ln X0 - Kt \qquad .....(6.4)$$

By applying logarithms,

$$\log X = \log X0 - Kt/2.303 \qquad .....(6.5)$$

The equations 6.4 and 6.5 can be written in exponential form,

$$X = X0.e^{-Kt} \quad .....(6.6)$$

Where, 'e' represents the base of natural logarithm.

Equations 6.4 to 6.6 are useful in describing the amount of the drug in the body - time data, but we need equations that describe the plasma drug concentration-time profile. The amount of the drug in the body and concentration of the drug in plasma can be related by introducing a term, Vd, i.e., the ***apparent volume of distribution***.

$$X = Vd.\ C \quad .....(6.7)$$

The proportionality constant (Vd) in this equation happens to have units of volume and is known as the apparent volume of distribution of the drug.

Substituting the values of 'X' in equation 6.5, we get

$$\text{Log } C = \log C_0 - Kt/2.303 \quad .....(6.8)$$

Where :

C = Concentration of drug in plasma at any time 't'

C_0 = Concentration of drug in plasma at time, t = 0

A semilogarithmic plot of C versus time gives a straight line with a slope of -K/2.303 (Fig. 6.1) and intercept as C_0.

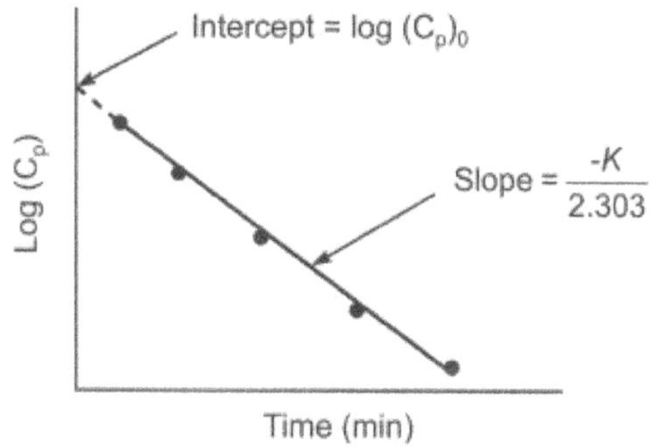

Fig 6.1 Semi-Logarithmic plot of plasma drug concentration-time data following I.V. bolus.

Apparent Volume of Distribution

The hypothetical volume within which a drug is distributed is known as the apparent volume of distribution, Vd. It does not refer to any physiological fluid volume. It is calculated simply by dividing the I.V. dose by drug concentration in plasma, at t = 0, C_0, that implies that the drug concentration in all the fluids and tissues is assumed to be same as in plasma, which is not true. Hence, the value of Vd only represents a theoretical volume in which the drug is assumed to be uniformly distributed. Using X0 and C_0 values, the apparent volume of distribution can be obtained.

$$Vd = \frac{X0}{C_0} = \frac{\text{I.V. dose}}{C_0} \quad .....(6.9)$$

The sole purpose of this parameter is to relate the amount and the concentration of drug in the body at a given time. Therefore, it is important to recognize that the knowledge of this parameter is essential in determining the dose of a drug required to attain the desired initial plasma concentration.

Since values of Vd tend to vary with body weight, therefore, it needs to be normalized w.r.t body weight that allows comparisons among different individuals Such a normalized Vd is the **distribution coefficient**, Ä', calculated by the equation,

$$\Delta' = \frac{Vd}{BW} \qquad .....(6.10)$$

Where BW is body weight. Units are usually ml/g or L/Kg, and care must be taken to employ appropriate units of weight, concentration and volume in Equations. 6.9 and 6.10. Usually, in pharmacokinetic literature, distribution coefficient values are provided as values of "volume of distribution".

Factors that are responsible for any non-homogenous distribution of a drug in its volume of distribution are:

1. binding to plasma proteins
2. dissolution into body lipids
3. pH partition
4. active transport
5. tissue binding, etc.

Consequently, the Vd or Δ' are not useful in finding out the drug distribuiton pattern. However, they may indicate the general ability of a drug to penetrate the membranes, dissolve in fat or bind extensively to extravascular tissues. The more the drug molecules penetrate into tissues and organs following the administration of the dose of a drug, the smaller will be the plasma and/or serum drug concentration and, therefore the higher is the hypothetical volume into which the drug is distributed. The hydrophilic/lipophilic nature of the drug determines the extent to which the drug molecules penetrate into the tissues or the extent of drug distribution. The chemical structure of a compound, in turn, determines the lipophilicity of a drug. In theory, although each drug will have its own volume of distribution and it will be constant for that drug, it is possible for two different drugs to exhibit identical apparent volumes of distribution.

The magnitude of the apparent volume of distribution usually does not correspond to plasma volume, extracellular or total body volume space but may vary from a few liters (7 to 10 L) to several hundred liters (200 L and higher) in a 70 kg subject.

Many acidic drugs, including salicylates, sulfonamides, penicillins and anticoagulants, are either highly bound to plasma proteins or too water soluble to enter into cellular fluid and to penetrate into tissues to a significant degree. These drugs, therefore, have low volumes of distribution and low tissue to plasma concentration ratios. A given dose of these drugs will yield a relatively high plasma concentration. Basic drugs, including tricyclic antidepressants and antihistamines, are extensively bound to extracellular tissues and are also taken up by adipose tissues. The apparent volumes of distribution of these drugs are large, often larger than the total body space; for example, the apparent volume of distribution of amphetamine is approximately 200 L (3 L Kg^{-1}). Figure 6.2 provides the values of the apparent volume of distribution, reported in the literature, for selected drugs.

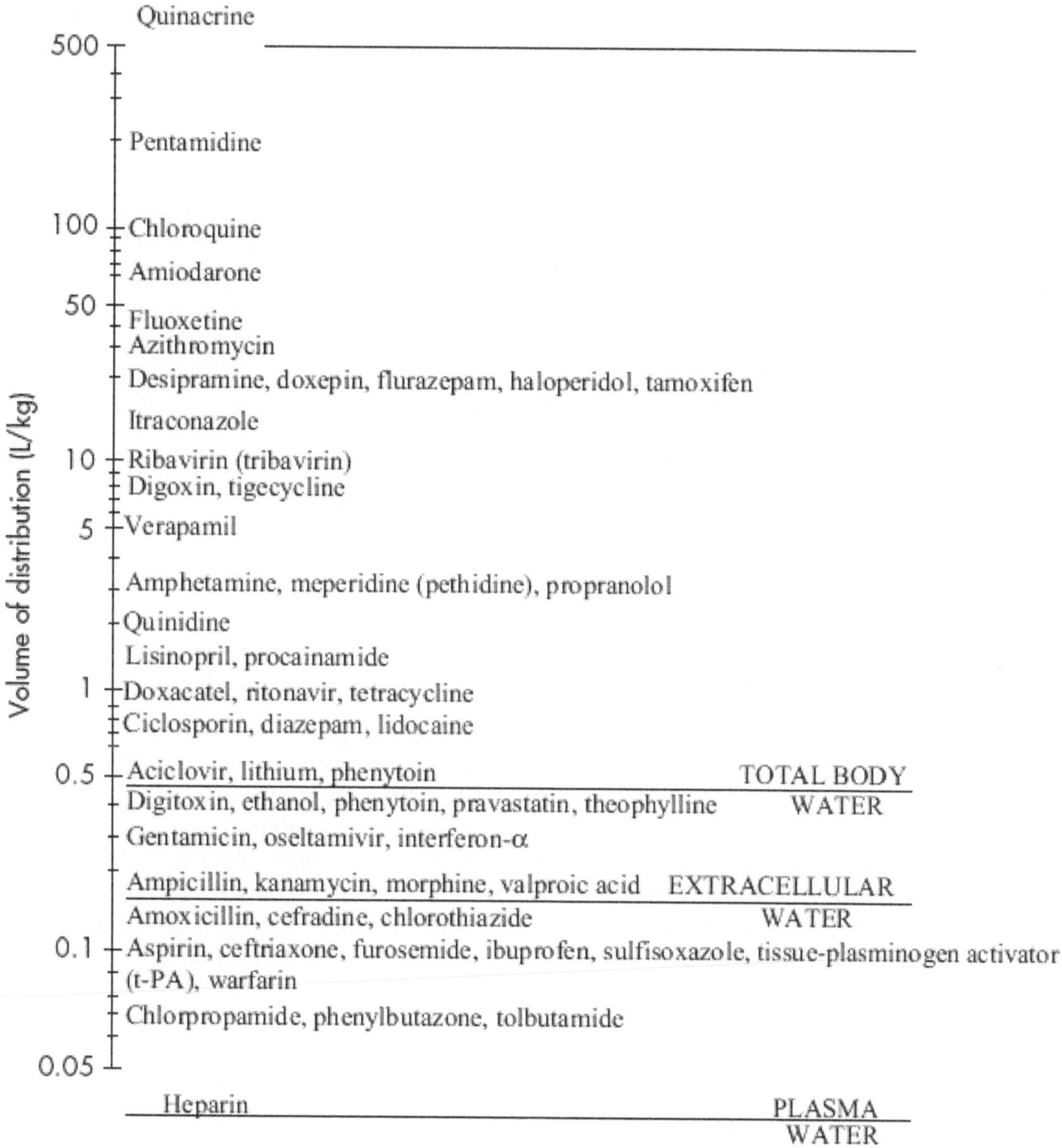

Fig. 6.2 Apparent volume of distribution for select drugs. (Reproduced from Jambhekar and Breen, 2009)

Lipid soluble drugs that are bound negligibly to plasma proteins have a large Vd, and are more concentrated extravascularly. Highly polar, poorly penetrant drugs that are highly bound to plasma proteins will have a smaller Vd. Drugs which bond to tissues will have a large Vd, because of low C_0 values. However, many drugs combine penetrance, lipid solubility and protein binding in such proportions that make it difficult to interpret the meaning of Vd without ancillary information.

Though the apparent volume of distribution is constant for a drug and remains uninfluenced by the dose administered, certain disease states or pathological conditions may bring about changes in the apparent volume of distribution. For example, in edematous conditions the total body water and total extracelllular water increase; this is reflected in a larger apparent Vd value of a drug that is highly water soluble. Similarly, changes in the total body weight and lean body mass may also affect the apparent Vd. Furthermore, since the apparent volume of distribution reflects the extent to which a drug will penetrate into tissues, alteration in the permeability characteristics of tissues will alter the apparent volume of distribution of a drug. It is also important to note that the apparent volume of distribution of a drug may vary with age groups: infants, adults and the geriatric population.

Elimination Rate Constant

$$\text{Log } C = \log C_0 - Kt/2.303$$

Rearranging Equation 6.8 gives following

$$Kt/2.303 = \log C_0/C = \log C_0 - \log C$$

Equation 6.8 is in the form of a straight line equation y = mx + b

Therefore, if log C is plotted against t, as shown in Fig. 6.1, the plot will be a straight line with an intercept (b) of log C_0, and the slope of the line (m) will be -K/2.303. Such plots are commonly used to determine the order of a reaction; that is, if a plot of log C versus time is a straight line, the reaction is assumed to be a first-order process or pseudo first order process. The value of K can be obtained from the slope, which is called ***"apparent over all elimination rate constant"***. The rate constant K has the dimensions of the reciprocal of time, since log C is dimensionless. The slope of the line and the corresponding value of K for a plot such as that shown in Fig. 6.1 may be calculated using the following equation.

$$\text{Slope (m)} = \frac{-K}{2.303} = \frac{\log C_2 - \log C_1}{t_2 - t_1} \quad .....(6.11)$$

where C_1 and C_2 are the plasma concentrations of the drug at time t_1 and t_2, respectively.

The slope of the line can also be calculated more accurately, using the following equation.

$$\text{Slope (m)} = \frac{n\,\Sigma(xy) - \Sigma x\,\Sigma y}{n\,\Sigma(x^2) - (\Sigma x)^2} \quad .....(6.12)$$

where x represents the values of time and y represents the corresponding log C values of drug. $\bar{x}$ and $\bar{y}$ are the arithmetic means of the values of time and log C, respectively. The elimination rate constant represents overall drug elimination from the body, which includes renal excretion of unchanged drug (u) and/or the formation of metabolites (m). Hence,

$$K = K_u + K_m$$

Biological Half-life

Biological half-life of a drug, $t_{1/2}$, is defined as the time required for the concentration to reduce to a half of its initial value. For example, the concentration of the drug in plasma is 10 mg/ml, therefore the time required for the drug concentration in plasma to reduce to 5 mg/ml is termed as biological half life, $t_{1/2}$. The half-life for a first order process or pseudo first order process is a constant . Thus, a first order process never reaches completion, since even the lowest concentration would only fall to a half of its value in one half-life. It means the drug concentration in plasma never reaches zero.

For most practical purposes, a first-order process may be deemed "complete" if it is 95% or more complete. Table 6.2 shows that five half-lives must elapse to reach this point. Thus the elimination of a drug from the body may be considered to be complete after five half-lives have elapsed (i.e., 97% completion). The half-life of a drug determines the residence time of the drug in the body and is useful to find out the time at which the drug levels fall below the therapeutic levels. The half-life of a drug is used to calculate the dosage regimen.

Table 6.2 Relation between number of half-lives elapsed and completeness of process.

Number of Half-lives Elapsed	Initial Concentration Remaining (%)	"Completeness" of Process (%)
0	100.0	0.0
1	50.0	50.0
2	25.0	75.0
3	12.5	87.5
4	6.25	93.75
5	3.13	96.88
6	1.56	98.44
7	0.78	99.22

A simple relationship between the elimination rate constant, K and biological half-life, $t_{1/2}$ may be derived as follows:

$$\text{Log } C = \log C_0 - Kt / 2.303$$

rearranging the above equation,

$$\log \frac{C_0}{C} = \frac{Kt_{1/2}}{2.303} \quad \text{when } \frac{C_0}{C} = 2, \text{ then } t = t_{1/2},$$

thus $$\log 2 = \frac{K\,t_{1/2}}{2.303} = 0.3$$

$$K\,t_{1/2} = 0.3 \times 2.303 = 0.693$$

∴ $$K = \frac{0.693}{t_{1/2}} \qquad .....(6.13)$$

and $$t_{1/2} = \frac{0.693}{K} \qquad .....(6.14)$$

Area Under the Curve (AUC)

Area Under the Curve (AUC) is an important pharmacokinetic parameter often estimated by several methods. It is the area under a plasma drug concentration-time curve. AUC can be measured by various sophisticated mathematical techniques. The most common method for estimating the area is the use of Trapezoidal rule (for detail see Appendix-I). The curve is divided into trapeziums based on data and the sum of areas of all trapeziums gives Area Under the Curve up to the last sampling (AUC_0^t). The remaining area under the curve from the last time point to t = ∝ is calculated by integration method (for details see Appendix - II). Figure 6.3 shows pictorially the application of trapezoidal rule for computation of AUC.

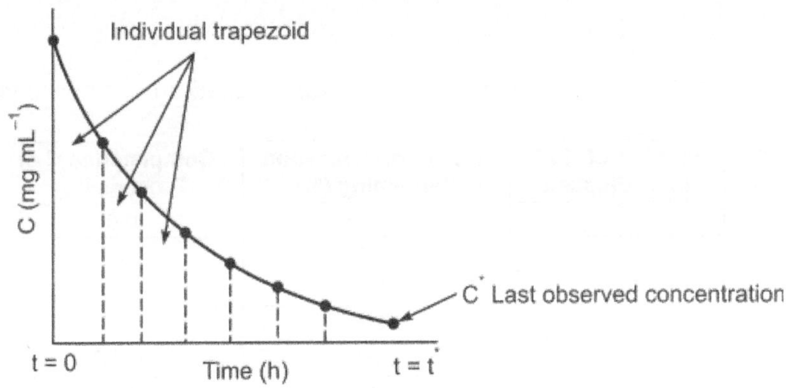

Fig. 6.3 Application of trapezoidal method to compute area under curve.

$$AUC_t^{\infty} = \frac{C^*}{K} \qquad .....(6.15)$$

where C* is the drug concentration at the last time point, t*.

The total area under the curve from t = 0 to t = ∝, AUC_0^{∞}, is given by

$$AUC_0^{\infty} = AUC_0^t + AUC_t^{\infty}$$

$$AUC_0^{\infty} = AUC_0^t + \frac{C^*}{K} \qquad .....(6.16)$$

The intensity and duration of a tissue response or antibacterial activity in most cases is usually a function of the concentration and persistence of the drug in the plasma, which indirectly is reflected by magnitude of AUC. An estimate of AUC is required to determine bioavailability, clearance, apparent volume of distribution, and other pharmacokinetic parameters.

Clearance

The rate of elimination of a drug from the body is directly proportional to the plasma concentration.

Rate of elimination (dX/dt) $\propto$ C_p, where C_p = plasma concentration

or
$$\frac{dX}{dt} = Cl_t . C_P \qquad .....(6.17)$$

where proportionality constant Cl_t is known as ***total body clearance.*** Total amount of drug eliminated from the body in infinite time is obtained by integrating the equation 6.17 with respect to time between t = 0 and t = '∞'.

$$\int_0^{\infty} dx = Cl_t \int_0^{\infty} C_p \, dt$$

Total amount eliminated

$$= Cl_t \, [AUC]_0^{\infty}$$

$\therefore$ Total body clearance,

$$Cl_t = \frac{\text{Total amount of drug eliminated}}{[AUC]_0^{\infty}}$$

In the case of I.V. injection (bolus), total drug eliminated is equal to the administered dose (X0).

$$Cl_t = \frac{X0 \text{ (I.V. dose)}}{[AUC]_0^{\infty}} \qquad .....(6.18)$$

But X_0 = Vd. C_0 and $[AUC]_0^{\infty} = C_0 / K$.

substituting these values in equations 6.18, we get

$$Cl_t = \frac{C_0 V_d}{C_0 / K} = V_d \, . \, K \qquad .....(6.19)$$

The units of Cl_t are volume/ unit time.

Clearence is defined as the volume of fluid cleared of the drug in a unit time and is expressed as ml / min or L / hr or ml/kg/min. It must be remembered that clearance is a hypothetical or fictive quantity, since the body rarely clears a drug completely from a specific volume of the body fluid.

For example, 50 mg of a drug was injected intravenously and the following pharmacokinetic parameters were estimated.

Vd = 5 liters, zero time concentration (C_0) = 10 mg/L and the first order elimination rate constant (K) = 0.2 hr^{-1}. Total body clearance (Cl_t) = Vd. K = 5 x 0.2 = 1 L/hr. It means the amount of the drug present in 1 L of body fluid (10 mg) is eliminated in one hour. So, the remaining 40mg of drug is present in 5 liters of the fluid, giving a concentration of 8 mg/L. In next one hour, 8 mg of the drug will be eliminated since clearance is 1 liter/hr. Total body clearance is the sum of all the separate clearances that contribute to drug elimination.

$$Cl_t = Cl_{metab} + Cl_{renal}, \text{ etc.,}$$

The concept of clearance can be applied to the whole body or to specific organs. The former application is convenient way to indicate the overall drug elimination, the later application is used to indicate the contribution of a specific organ to drug disappearance.

In order to calculate the total body clearance following extravascular administration of a drug that follows one compartment model, the amount of the drug absorbed from a given dose should be known. If 'F' is the fraction of the dose absorbed, following oral administration,

$$Cl_t = \frac{F\,X_0\text{ (oral)}}{[AUC]_0^\infty} \quad \text{.....(6.20)}$$

Clearance is a constant for a given drug since it is a product of two constants Vd and K. Therefore equations 6.18 and 6.20 can be equated and solved for the fraction of the dose absorbed.

$$\frac{X_0\text{ (I.V dose)}}{[AUC]_0^\infty\text{ I.V.}} = \frac{F\,X_0\text{ (oral)}}{[AUC]_0^\infty\text{ oral}} \quad \text{.....(6.21)}$$

$$F = \frac{X_0\text{ (I.V dose)}\,[AUC]_0^\infty\text{ oral}}{X_0\text{ (oral dose)}\,[AUC]_0^\infty\text{ I.V.}} \quad \text{.....(6.22)}$$

If the doses given by the I.V. route and the oral route of equal, then,

$$F = \frac{[AUC]_0^\infty\text{ oral}}{[AUC]_0^\infty\text{ I.V}} \quad \text{.....(6.23)}$$

If the areas under the curve obtained following administration of equal doses of a drug by I.V. and the mouth are equal, the value of 'F' will be 1. i.e. the drug is completely absorbed. F values less than unity indicate an incomplete absorption of the drug.

Scheme 6.1.2 I.V. Bolus - Unchanged Drug in Urine

Drug in the blood may exist as free- (i.e.,unbound drug) and as bound-drug (i.e., bound to plasma proteins, cellular components etc., or within the blood cells). There exists a dynamic equilibrium between free and bound drug. Its only free drug that is available for urinary excretion. Before understanding the kinetics of urinary excretion of drugs, it is necessary to understand the processes involved in urinary excretion of drugs and the factors influencing such processes.

The mammalian kidney is composed of many units called **nephrons** which are the basic units involved in the excretion of drugs or other substances. Fig. 6.4 shows the nephron structure with the sites for various processes occurring there.

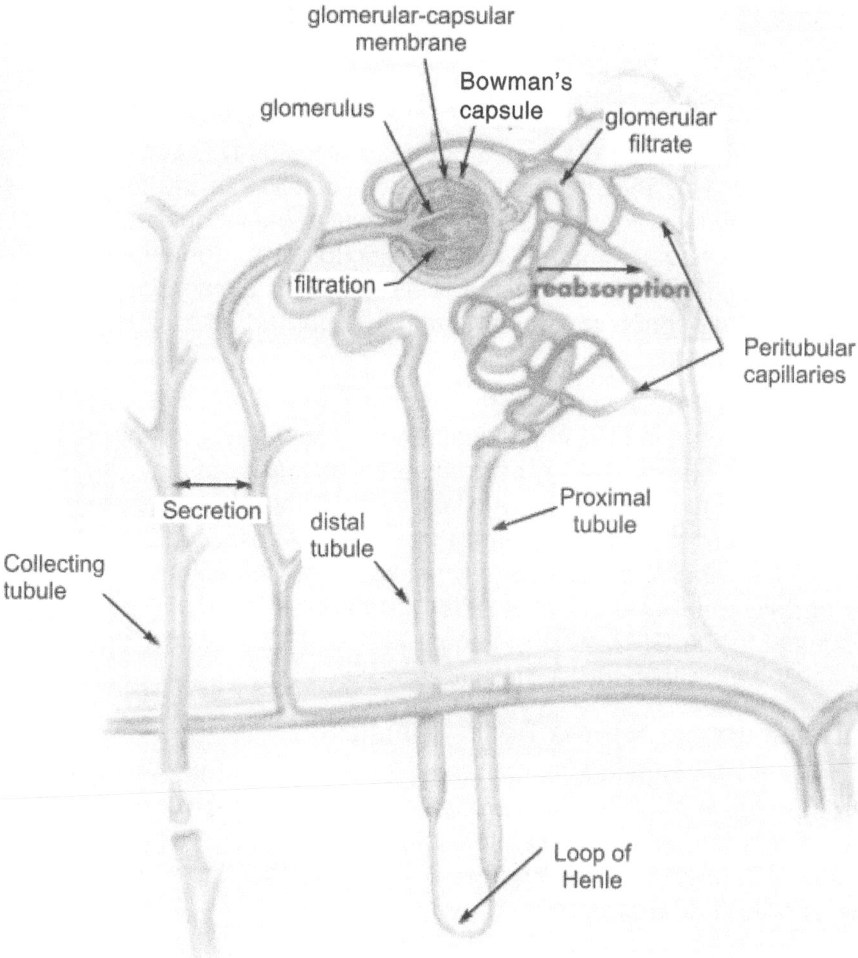

Fig. 6.4 Structure of nephron and formation of urine and excretion of drugs.

The kidney is supplied by blood via the renal artery, which subdivides into the interlobar arteries penetrating within the kidney and branching further into the afferent arterioles. Each afferent arteriole carries blood toward a single nephron into the glomerular portion of the nephron (*Bowman's capsule*). The filtration of blood occurs in the glomeruli in Bowman's capsule. From the capillaries (*glomerulus*) within Bowman's capsule, the blood flows out via the efferent arterioles and then into a second capillary network that surrounds the tubules (*peritubule capillaries* and *vasa recti*), including the loop of Henle, where some water is reabsorbed.

Excretion of an unchanged drug or its metabolite (s) in urine is influenced by the following processes.

1. Glomerular Filtration
2. Passive Transport across the Renal Tubule
3. Carrier mediated Transport Across the Renal tubule
4. Tubular Reabsorption.

Glomerular Filtration

Approximately 25% of the cardiac output goes to the kidneys, and 10% of this output to the kidneys is filtered by the glomerulus. The composition of the filtrate is same as that of the plasma with respect to water and low molecular weight solutes. Glomerular filtration separates gross particulate matter and such colloidal materials as proteins from the ultrafiltrate. Only the free drug in plasma is available for glomerular filtration and not the bound drug. The drug concentration in filtrate is equal to that in plasma water (free drug concentration in plasma).

The rate at which plasma water is filtered is called the **glomerular filtration rate** (GFR). The rate at which a drug is filtered is equal to the concentration of the free drug in plasma multiplied by GFR. The GFR can be measured in intact animals and humans by the measurement of the excretion and plasma concentration of an ideal substance, which is eliminated by filtration only (i.e, the drug is neither reabsorbed nor secreted), such as inulin or creatinine. Inulin, a fructose polymer of molecular weight 5200, appears to meet all criteria and its renal clearance provides an index of GFR. Therefore, the clearance of inulin is equal to the GFR, which is equal to 125–130 mL/min. The value for the GFR correlates fairly well with body surface area.

Passive Transport Across the Renal Tubule

Passive transport of exogenous compounds such as drugs, in the renal tubule involves a simple diffusion along a concentration gradient between plasma and urine. This concentration gradient is the driving force for drug diffusion. The rate of movement of a drug molecule is also governed by the diffusivity of the molecule through the tubular membrane and its features,

- the membrane/aqueous phase partition coefficient for the molecule,
- the thickness of the membrane at the site of diffusion, and
- the area of the membrane through which the molecule passes.

Biological membranes, being lipid in nature, are more permeable to lipid soluble substances, and transmembrane diffusion depends in part on the lipid solubility of the diffusing compound. In the case of acids and bases, the unionized species exhibit a greater lipid solubility than the ionized species. Most of the times, the unionized species are either the sole diffusing species or the more rapidly diffusing species. The rate of diffusion of a diffusing species is governed by the concentration gradient across the membrane and the pKa of the compound. In the specific case of passive diffusion across the renal tubular membrane, the concentration gradient depends on urinary pH since intracellular and blood pH are essentially constant.

Carrier Mediated Transport Across the Renal Tubule

The rate of transfer of a drug or substance across a biological membrane is higher in a carrier mediated transport than in simple diffusion. Carrier mediated transport includes active transport and facilitated diffusion.

Active Transport

The term active transport is usually applied only to those systems in which a substance is transported across a biological membrane against a concentration gradient (movement of substance from a region of low concentration to a region of higher concentration) at the expense of energy derived from cell metabolism.

The existence of active transport (active secretion) in the renal tubule transport system is well documented for organic acids and bases. Organic acids and bases are transported by a separate and specific active transport system. Probenicid and N^1-metheylnicotinamide are the examples of the organic anion transport system and organic cationic system, respectively. Neither of the systems have any high specificity. Substances transported by the same system compete with each other. Probenicid is used as a classic inhibitor of the organic anion transport system and its ability to inhibit the secretion of penicillin is taken as an advantage to prolong the duration of the action of penicillin. N^1-methylnicotinamide is a classic example of an organic base that is actively transported by the renal tubule.

For a drug that is excreted solely by glomerular filtration, the elimination half-life may change markedly in accordance with the binding affinity of the drug for plasma proteins. In contrast, drug protein binding has very little effect on the elimination half-life of the drug excreted mostly by active secretion. Because drug protein binding is reversible, drug bound to plasma protein rapidly dissociates as free drug is secreted by the kidneys. For example, some of the penicillins are extensively protein bound, but their elimination half-lives are short due to rapid elimination by active secretion.

Facilitated Diffusion

Facilitated diffusion is also a carrier mediated transport system, differing from active transport in that the drug moves along a concentration gradient (i.e., moves from a region of a high drug concentration to a region of a low drug concentration). Therefore, this system does not require an energy input. However, because this system is carrier mediated, it is saturable, structurally selective and shows competition kinetics for drugs of similar structure.

Tubular Reabsorption

The drug molecules transported into the urine by several mechanisms may again reach plasma by a tubular reabsorption of the drug molecules. The tubular reabsorption of drug molecules may be due to a passive transport and/or carrier mediated transport.

The amount of a substance excreted by the kidney is equal to the amount filtered by the glomerulus plus the net amount transferred by the renal tubules (difference between the amount of drug excreted into urine and the amount of drug reabsorbed).

If a drug is completely reabsorbed (eg, glucose), then the value for the clearance of the drug is approximately zero. For drugs that are partially reabsorbed, clearance values are less than the GFR of 125–130 mL/min. The reabsorption of drugs that are acids or weak bases is influenced by the pH of the fluid in the renal tubule (ie, urine pH) and the pK_a of the drug.

Kinetics of Urinary Excretion

Glomerular filtration and diffusion across the renal tubule are generally first-order processes so that the rate of transfer of a drug is related to the amount of the drug present in plasma, which is in turn related to the amount of the drug present in the body. Carrier mediated transport processes can also be approximated by the first-order process provided that the drug concentration achieved by a given dose does not saturate the transport systems. Hence, the urinary excretion of a drug can be explained by the apparent first-order process. It should be possible to write a simple differential equation for appearance of a drug in urine and to relate this to the amount of the drug in the plasma.

The concentration of a drug in tubular urine is usually influenced by changes in urine volume. It is therefore more relevant to consider the ***excretion rate*** of a drug rather than its concentration in urine.

It is often feasible to determine the elimination kinetics of a drug from its urinary excretion data. This frequently requires that at least some of the drug is excreted unchanged. Consider a drug that is eliminated from the body partly by renal excretion and partly by extra renal processes such as biotransformation, biliary excretion etc.

Scheme 6.1.2

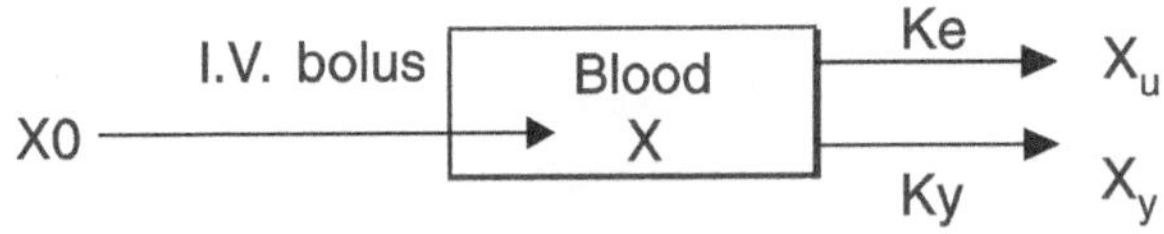

X0 = I.V. dose

Where X is the amount of the drug in the body at any time t. X_u and X_y are the cumulative amount of the drug excreted into the urine and cumulative amount of drug eliminated by all extra renal pathways, respectively. Ke is the urinary excretion rate constant and Ky is the sum of all other apparent first-order rate constants for drug elimination by non-renal pathways. Therefore, the overall elimination rate constant K is the sum of the individual rate constants that characterize the parallel elimination processes.

$$K = Ke + Ky \quad .....(6.24)$$

1. **Excretion Rate Method:** Since urinary excretion of a drug follows the first-order kinetics, the rate of appearance of the unchanged drug in urine is proportional to the amount of the drug in the body. The urinary excretion rate of the intact drug, dXu/dt, can be defined as,

$$dXu/dt \ \alpha \ X \quad .....(6.25)$$

$$dXu/dt = Ke\ X \quad .....(6.26)$$

X is the amount of the drug in the body at any time t. But we know that in I.V. bolus, the unchanged drug in blood is given equation 6.6.

$$X = X0\ .\ e^{-Kt}$$

Substituting the value of X in equation 6.26,

$$dXu\ /\ dt = Ke\ X0\ e^{-Kt} \quad .....(6.27)$$

Applying logarithms to the equation 6.27, we get

$$\log\ (dXu/dt) = \log\ k_e\ X0 - Kt\ /\ 2.303 \quad .....(6.28)$$

The term dXu/dt is called instantaneous rate of excretion. The excretion rates are determined experimentally by estimating the amount of the drug excreted in a given time period. The average excretion rate in this time period is ΔXu/Δt. The assumption is that the ΔXu/Δt closely approximates dXu/dt at the mid point of urine collection period (t'). The validity of this assumption, however, depends upon the relative collection periods and the drug half-life. It is important to remember that urinary excretion rates must be plotted against the mid points of the urine collection period and not at the beginning or end of these periods. As such,

$$\log\ (\Delta Xu/\Delta t) = \log\ Ke\ X0 - Kt'/\ 2.303 \quad .....(6.29)$$

Therefore, a plot of log (ΔXu/Δt) versus t' yields a straight line with a slope of -K / 2.303 (Fig. 6.5). This is the same slope as is obtained from semilogarithmic plot of plasma concentration of drug versus time. Thus, the elimination rate constant, K, of a drug can be obtained from either plasma drug concentration-time data or urinary excretion data. It must be remembered that the slope of the log excretion rate versus t' is a function of the elimination rate constant, K, and not of the urinary excretion rate constant, Ke. The intercept is equal to log KeX0.

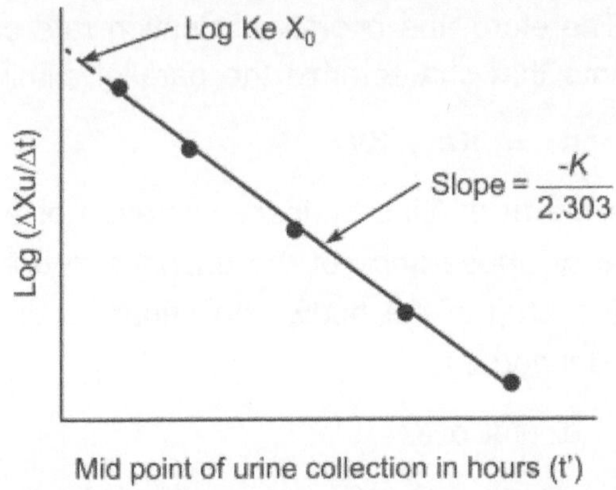

Fig. 6.5 log excretion rate versus mid point of urine collection (t').

The general format of urinary data processing is provided in Table 6.3. The method is known as **Excretion Rate Method** and the other method used to describe urinary kinetics is **Sigma-minus method.**

Calculation of Pharmacokinetic Parameters by Excretion Rate Method

The urinary excretion rate-time data obtained following I.V. bolus are first processed and a semilog plot of ($\Delta Xu/\Delta t$) versus t' (the mid point of urine collection) gives a straight line with a slope of -K / 2.303 (Fig. 6.5 and Table 6.3). The over all elimination rate constant, K can be calculated from the slope.

$$\text{Slope} = -K / 2.303$$

$$\therefore \quad K = \text{Slope} \times 2.303$$

Table 6.3 Urine Data Obtained Following an I.V. Bolus Dose.

Time (hr)	Urine volume (ml)	Concentration of unchanged drug (mg/ml)	Amount of drug excreted [illegible]X_u (mg)	[illegible] (hr)	[illegible] (mg/hr)	t' (hrs)
0	250	0	0			
0.25	280	0.5714	160	0.25	640	0.125
0.50	300	0.4666	140	0.25	560	0.375
1.0	350	0.5714	200	0.50	400	0.750
2.0	450	0.555	250	1.00	250	1.50
4.0	480	0.3917	188	2.00	94	3.0
6.0	360	0.1278	46	2.00	23	5.0

The intercept obtained by extending the straight line is equal to log KeX0. Since the dose administered is known, the urinary excretion rate constant, Ke, can be calculated.

Biological half-life of the drug is calculated using K, value.

$$t_{1/2} = 0.693 / K$$

2. **Sigma - Minus Method :** Another method used to analyze urinary excretion data is sigma-minus method, which requires an accurate assessment of the total amount of the drug or metabolite excreted in the urine. Figure 6.6 shows the amount remaining in the blood and amount being eliminated via urine following IV bolus. The main advantage of this method is that this does not has the assumption that dXu / dt ≈ DXu/Dt.

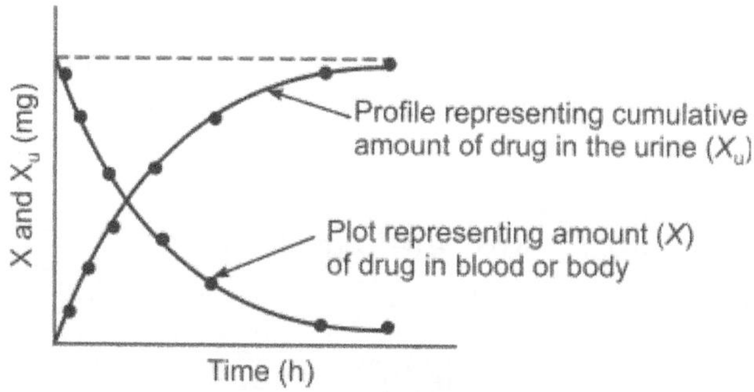

Fig 6.6 Profile exhibiting amount of drug remaining in the blood and amount of drug being excreted via urine following intravenous bolus.

The following mathematical treatment is required to get the usual equation of the sigma-minus method.

The rate of excretion of the drug in urine is proportional to the amount of the drug in blood,

$$dXu/dt = Ke\ X \qquad .....(6.30)$$

$X = X0\ e^{-Kt}$ as per equation 6.6, substituting X, value in equation 6.30, we get

$$dXu/dt = Ke\ X0\ e^{-kt} \qquad .....(6.31)$$

Integrating the equation 6.31 with respect to time between the limits of t = 0 to t = t.

$$\int_0^t dXu = \int_0^t KeX_0\ e(-Kt)dt$$

$$|Xu|_0^t = KeX_0 \frac{|e^{-Kt}|_0^t}{-K}$$

$$Xu^t - Xu^0 = KeX_0 \left| \frac{e^{-Kt}}{-Kt} + \frac{e^0}{K} \right| \qquad \text{but } e^0 = 1$$

Xu^t is the cumulative amount of drug excreted into urine to time 't' and Xu^0 is the cumulative amount of the drug excreted to zero time, which is equal to zero

$$\therefore \quad Xu^t - 0 = KeX_0 \left| \frac{1}{K} + \frac{e^{0-Kt}}{K} \right|$$

$$Xu^t = \frac{Ke\,X_0}{K}(1 - e^{-Kt}) \qquad .....(6.32)$$

The total amount of unchanged drug that will be excreted in urine with a dose of X0 to time $\propto$ can be obtained by integrating equation 6.31, between limits t = 0 to t = $\propto$.

$$\int_0^\infty dXu = \int_0^\infty KeX_0\, e(-Kt)dt$$

$$|Xu|_0^\infty = KeX_0 \frac{\left|e^{-Kt}\right|_0^\infty}{-K}$$

$$Xu^\infty - 0 = KeX_0 \left| \frac{e^{-K\infty}}{-K} + \frac{e^0}{K} \right| \quad \text{but } e^\propto = 0;\ e^0 = 1$$

$$Xu^\infty = KeX_0 \left| 0 + \frac{1}{K} \right|$$

$$Xu^\infty = \frac{KeX_0}{K} \qquad .....(6.33)$$

For a drug eliminated totally by renal excretion, K equals Ke, and therefore, the amount eliminated equals to X0, the administered dose.

Substituting $X_u^\propto$ in equation 6.32 instead of Ke X0 / K, we get:

$$Xu^t = Xu^\infty(1 - e^{-Kt}) \qquad .....(6.34)$$

By subtracting both the sides of equation 6.34 from X_u^∞, we get

$$Xu^\infty - Xu^t = Xu^\infty - [Xu^\infty(1 - e^{-Kt})]$$

$$Xu^\infty - Xu^t = Xu^\infty - Xu^\infty + Xu^\infty\, e^{-Kt}$$

$$Xu^\infty - Xu^t = Xu^\infty\, e^{-Kt} \qquad .....(6.35)$$

Applying logarithms to equation 6.35

$$\log\,(Xu^\infty - Xu^t) = \log Xu^\infty - \frac{Kt}{2.303} \qquad .....(6.36)$$

The symbol Σ (sigma) is used to denote the summation and X_u^∞ is the sum of the amounts of the drug excreted in infinite time. A value of X_u^t is subtracted at every time point from X_u^∞ and hence this method is called sigma-minus method.

A plot of the logarithm of the amount of the drug to be excreted versus time is linear and the slope is - K / 2.303 (Fig. 6.7) that is, the same slope as a plot of log plasma concentration versus t or of a plot of log $(\Delta X_u / \Delta t)$ versus t'.

Wherever possible, urine collection should be carried for a period of time equal to at least 7 half-lives of the drug in order to determine X_u^∞. This presents considerable practical difficulties if the drug has a long half-life.

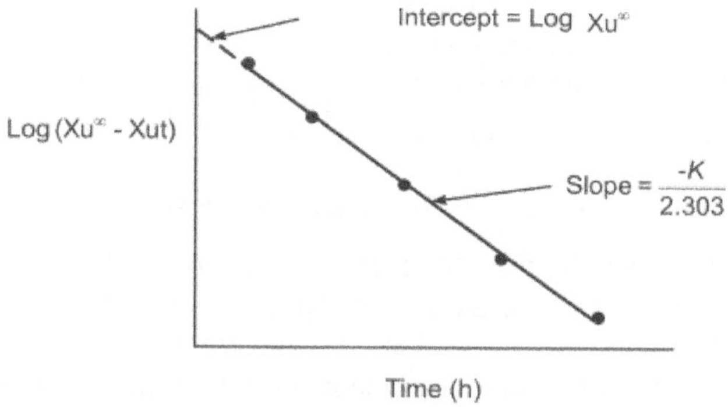

Fig. 6.7 Sigma-minus method of the amount of the drug remaining to be excreted method for the calculation of the elimination rate constant according to Equation 6.36.

This problem does not arise when log $(\Delta X_u / \Delta t)$ versus t' is used, since urine need to be collected for only 3 or 4 half lives to obtain a reasonable estimation of the elimination rate constant and also every urine sample need not have to be collected, since to determine one point on a rate plot requires the collection of two consecutive time samples only.

Calculation of Pharmacokinetic Parameters by Sigma-Minus Method :

A plot of log $(X_u^\alpha - X_u^t)$ versus t gives a straight line with a slope of -K / 2.303. Hence, the overall elimination rate constant, K is calculated from the slope.

$$\text{Slope} = -K / 2.303$$

$$K = \text{Slope} \times 2.303$$

The biological half-life of the drug $(t_{1/2})$ is estimated using the equation.

$$t_{1/2} = 0.693 \mid K$$

The intercept obtained by extending the line is equal to log X_u^∞. The value of I.V. dose (X0) and X_u^∞ are known. Using equation X_u^∞ = Ke X0 / K, the value of Ke is calculated.

$$Ke = \frac{K X_u^\alpha}{X0} \qquad .....(6.37)$$

Comparison of Excretion Rate Method and Sigma-Minus Method :

	Excretion Rate Method		Sigma-Minus Method
1.	dXu / dt is assumed to be equal to DXu / Dt	1.	Such assumption is not required
2.	More number of samples with short time intervals	2.	Less number of samples at convenient time intervals.
3.	Useful for drugs with long half-lives	3.	Not suitable for drug with long half-lives.
4.	Any urine sample losses do not affect the method.	4.	Sample loss means, the whole experiment is a failure
5.	This method is used for multiple doses also.	5.	It is not useful for a multiple dose study.
6.	This method requires the collection of urine samples for 3 or 4 half-lives of the drug.	6.	This method requires collection of urine samples for 7 half-lives of the drug for an accurate assessment.

Renal Excretion as a fraction of Total Elimination

An important pharmacokinetic parameter is the fraction of the amount of the drug entering the general circulation that is excreted unchanged, fe. In case of I.V. bolus, fe is a fraction of I.V. dose excreted unchanged in urine. It is a quantitative measure of the contribution of renal excretion to the overall drug elimination. Knowing 'fe' aids in establishing appropriate modifications in the usual dosage regimen of a drug for patients with varying degrees of renal function. Among drugs the value of 'fe' ranges between 0 and 1.0. When an 'fe'value is low, urinary excretion is a minor pathway of drug elimination. Occasionally, renal excretion is the only route of elimination, in which case the values of 'fe' is 1.0. By definition the difference, (1-fe), is the fraction of the amount entering the circulation that is eliminated by extra-renal mechanisms, usually metabolism.

An estimate of 'fe' is most readily obtained from the cumulative urinary excretion data, following I.V. administration, since by definition.

$$fe = \frac{\text{Total drug excreted unchanged}}{\text{I.V. Dose}} = \frac{X_u^{\infty}}{X0} \qquad .....(6.38)$$

In practice, care should be taken to ensure a complete urinary recovery (i.e., collect urine for at least 5 half-lives of the drug).

Problems in Obtaining Valid Urinary Excretion Data

Certain factors can make it difficult to obtain a valid urinary excretion data. Some of these factors are as follows:

1. A significant fraction of the unchanged drug must be excreted in the urine.
2. Frequent sampling is necessary for obtaining data for a pharmacokinetic analysis.

3. Collection of urine samples has to be made till almost all the drug is excreted. In practice, approximately seven elimination half-lives are needed for 99% of the drug to be eliminated. A graph of the cumulative amount of the drug excreted versus time will yield a curve that approaches an asymptote at "infinite" time.
4. Variations in urinary pH and volume may cause a significant variation in urinary excretion rates.
5. The assay technique employed for the estimation of the unchanged drug must be highly specific and must not have any interference due to metabolites that have a similar chemical structure.

Renal Clearance

The kinetics of urinary excretion of a drug may be characterized not only by the excretion rate constant, Ke, but also by renal clearance value, CL_R. Analogous to total clearance, renal clearance is defined as a proportionality term between urinary excretion rate and plasma concentration

$$\frac{dXu}{dt} = CL_R.C \qquad .....(6.39)$$

i.e.,

$$CL_R = \frac{dXu/dt}{C} \qquad .....(6.40)$$

Renal clearance, like total clearance, has units of flow, usually milliliters/minutes or liters/hour. In practice, renal clearance is estimated by dividing the average urinary excretion rate, $\Delta Xu/\Delta t$, by the plasma concentration of the drug, C, at the mid point of urine collection period, t'.

$$CL_R = \frac{dXu/dt}{C \text{ at } t'} \qquad .....(6.41)$$

But we know that $\Delta Xu/\Delta t = Ke\ X$, hence

$$CL_R = \frac{Ke\ X}{C \text{ at } t'} \qquad .....(6.42)$$

But $X/C = Vd$

Therefore, $CL_R = Ke.Vd \qquad .....(6.43)$

Renal clearance is equal to the product of the renal excretion rate constant, Ke, and the apparent volume of distribution, Vd.

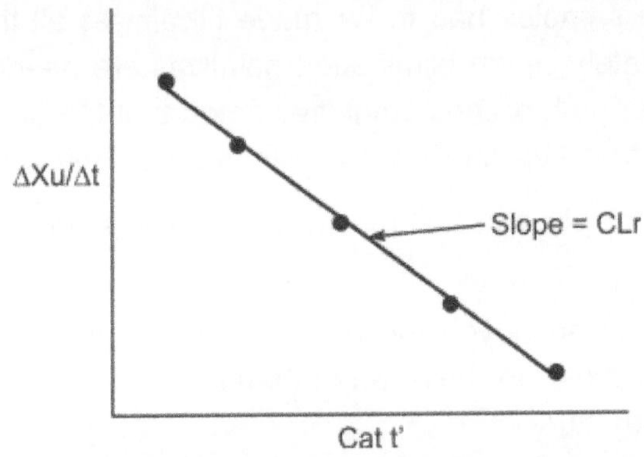

Fig. 6.8 A plot of urinary excretion rate versus the plasma concentration of the drug at the mid point of time interval for urine collection.

According to equation 6.41, a plot of excretion rate ($\Delta Xu/\Delta t$) versus plasma concentration at the mid point of the urine collection period in linear with a slope equal to renal clearance (Fig. 6.8). As mentioned previously, the urinary excretion rates determined experimentally ($\Delta Xu/\Delta t$) are not instantaneous rates (dXu/dt) but average rates over a period of time and therefore the validity of the method depends on the relative magnitudes of the urine collection periods and drug half-life.

A second approach to the calculation of renal clearance involves urine and plasma samples being taken simultaneously rather than plasma being taken at the mid point of urine collection. According to equation 6.39.

$$dXu/dt = CL_R \,.\, C, \quad \text{but} \quad CL_R = Ke \,.\, Vd$$

substituting Ke Vd for CL_R

$$dXu/dt = Ke\ Vd \,.\, C. \qquad .....(6.44)$$

If t_1 and t_2 are the time points at which urine and plasma samples are collected, integration of equation 6.44 over the time interval t_1 to t_2 yields.

$$\int_{t1}^{t2} dXu = KeVd \int_{t1}^{t2} C.dt$$

$$\left|Xu\right|_{t1}^{t2} = KeVd \int_{t1}^{t2} C.dt \qquad .....(6.45)$$

where $\left| Xu \right|_{t1}^{t2}$ is the amount of the unmetabolized drug eliminated in the urine during the time interval t_1 to t_2 and the area under the plasma concentration-time curve during the same interval (Fig. 6.9).

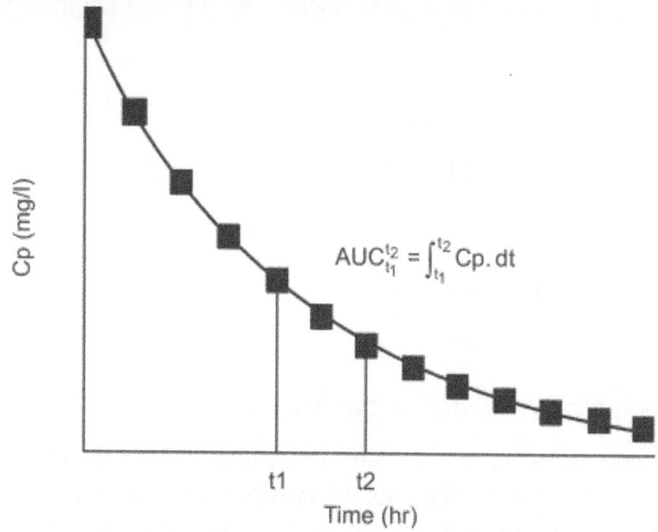

Fig 6.9 Area under the curve of plasma drug concentration-time curve between t1 and t2.

Integration of equation 6.44 from time zero to infinity and rearrangement of the integrated equation yields an expression for the average renal clearance over the entire time period from time zero to infinity.

$$\int_0^\infty dXu = KeVd \int_0^\infty C.dt$$

$$|Xu|_0^\infty = KeVd \int_0^\infty C.dt$$

$$Xu^\infty - 0 = KeVd \int_0^\infty C.dt$$

$$Xu^\infty = KeVd \int_0^\infty C.dt \quad .....(6.46)$$

or

$$KeVd = CL_R = \frac{X_u^\infty}{\int_0^\infty C.dt} = \frac{X_u^\infty}{[AUC]_0^\infty} \quad .....(6.47)$$

A relationship analogous to the average renal clearance (Equation 6.47), can be developed for the total body clearance, Cl_t, of a drug from equation 6.47

$$Vd = \frac{Xu^\infty}{Ke\int_0^\infty C.dt} \quad .....(6.48)$$

But we know that X_u^∞ = Ke X0/K or X_u^∞/Ke = X0 / K substituting X0/K for X_u^∞/Ke, we get.

$$Vd = \frac{X0}{K\int_0^\infty C.dt} \qquad .....(6.49)$$

and

$$VdK = \frac{X0}{\int_0^\infty C.dt} \qquad .....(6.50)$$

where, the product of Vd and K is the total body clearance Cl_t.

Equation 6.49 can be used for the determination of Vd. Equation 6.49 is applicable not only to the one compartment model but also to some multiple compartment linear systems. This can be used for any route of administration provided that the fraction of the dose absorbed is known.

I.V. Bolus - Metabolite in Blood/Plasma

The moment a drug injected into the systemic circulation, it is subjected to elimination by all possible pathways of elimination, such as renal excretion, metabolism, biliary secretion, etc. However, the fraction of the dose eliminated by all other processes except renal excretion and metabolism are, in general, negligible. Hence, the elimination of most drugs from the body involves the processes of both metabolism (biotransformation) and excretion of unchanged drugs in urine. The overall elimination rate constant, K, is the sum of the first order rate constants of metabolism, K_f, and the first order rate constant of excretion (Ke).

$$K = Ke + K_f \qquad .....(6.51)$$

Because a drug may be biotransformed into several metabolites (metabolite 1, metabolite 2, metabolite 3, etc.), the metabolism rate constant, ki, is the sum of the rate constants for the formation of each metabolite.

$$K_f = K_{f1} + K_{f2} + K_{f3} + \text{———} + K_{fn} \qquad .....(6.52)$$

The relationship in this equation assumes that the process of metabolism is the first order and that the substrate (drug) concentration is very low. Drug concentrations at therapeutic plasma levels for most drugs are much lower than the Michaelis-Menten constant and do not saturate the enzymes involved in metabolism. Hence, drug elimination by metabolism may be considered to follow the first order kinetics.

For example, a drug may be metabolized by two pathways to form two major metabolites. The elimination of the drug is represented in Fig. 6.10. The metabolites formed may be excreted in urine or may be further metabolized to form other metabolites.

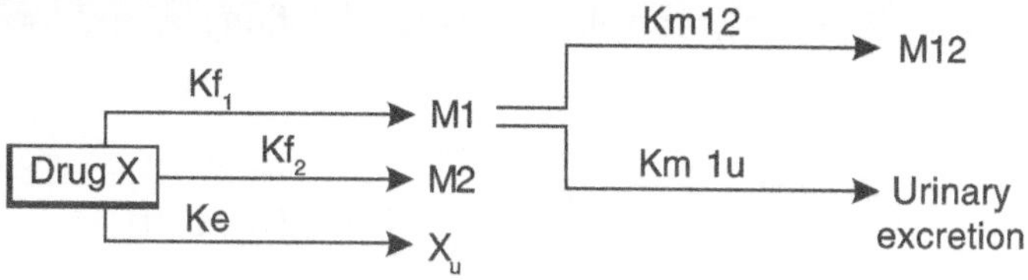

Fig. 6.10 Model for a drug that has 2 major metabolites and is also eliminated by renal excretion.

Scheme 6.1.3 I.V. Bolus - Metabolite in Blood/Plasma

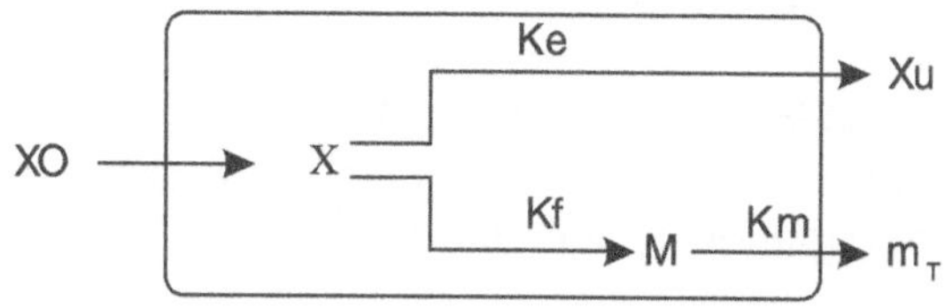

X0 = I.V. dose,

X = Amount of drug in blood at any time 't'.

Ke = Excretion rate constant

Xu = Cumulative amount of the unchanged drug excreted in urine.

M is the amount of a metabolite formed in the body, and M_T is the total amount of the metabolite eliminated by renal, biliary pathway as well as by further metabolism.

The rate constants K_f and Km are the representative first-order rate constants for metabolite formation and elimination, respectively. The time course of metabolite levels in the body is a function of the rates of formation and elimination of the drug. i.e. the difference between the rate of formation of the metabolite in the body and its rate of elimination. A differential equation may be written for the rate of change of metabolite,

$$\frac{dm}{dt} = K_f X - Km\ M \qquad .....(6.53)$$

But we know that $X = X0.\ e^{-Kt}$. Substituting X value in equation 6.53,

$$\frac{dm}{dt} = K_f\ X0\ e^{-Kt} - Km\ M \qquad .....(6.54)$$

Rearranging equation 6.54 and multiplying it with e^{Kmt},

$$\frac{dm}{dt} e^{Kmt} + Km\ M.\ e^{Kmt} = K_f\ X0.\ e^{-(K-Km)t} \qquad .....(6.55)$$

Integrating equation 6.55 between time zero and infinity and simplifying the resultant equation,

$$M\ e^{Kmt} = K_f\ X0\ ()\ \frac{e^{-(K-Km)t}}{-(K-Km)} + \frac{e^{0}}{(K-Km)}$$

$$M\ e^{Kmt} = \frac{K_f\ X0}{(K-Km)}\ [1 - e^{-(K-Km)t}] \qquad .....(6.56)$$

Dividing the above equation throughout by e^{Kmt}, we get

$$M = \frac{K_f\ X0}{(K-Km)}\ [e^{-Kmt} - e^{-Kt}] \qquad .....(6.57)$$

Equation 6.57 permits calculation of the amount of a metabolite in the body at any time after I.V. injection of a dose of a drug. Dividing both the sides of the equation 6.57 by the apparent volume of distribution of the metabolite, Vm, yields

$$\frac{M}{Vm} = \frac{K_f\ X0}{Vm\,(K-Km)}\ [e^{-Kmt} - e^{-Kt}]$$

The term M/Vm is equal to the concentration of the metabolite in plasma (Cm). It should be remembered that Vm is different from the apparent volume of distribution of the drug, Vd. The equation that describes metabolite plasma drug concentration-time profile is:

$$Cm = \frac{K_f\ X0}{Vm\,(K-Km)}\ [e^{-kmt} - e^{-kt}] \qquad .....(6.58)$$

In order to use the equation 6.58 for calculation of various pharmacokinetic parameters of the drug, the relative values of the over all elimination rate constant, K and elimination rate constant of metabolite, Km, are to be considered. Remember that Km is concerned with a metabolite and K is concerned with the parent drug. Three possible situations may arise, which have to be dealt separately.

Case 1. Km is greater than K

Case 2. K is greater than Km

Case 3. K = Km

Case 1: Km is greater than K: For most of the drugs the value of Km is greater than K. At one time the general assumption was that Km is always greater than K, since metabolites were considered to be more polar and more readily eliminated from the body than the parent drug. This assumption may be true when polar conjugates such as glucouronides, sulfates, glycine conjugates are the major metabolites formed. However, metabolites formed from acetylation and/or oxidation of the drug may actually be more lipophilic than the parent drug.

When Km is several times greater than K, the term e^{-Kmt} will approach to zero, while e^{-Kt} still have a finite value after some time. Neglecting the term e^{-Kmt} in equation 6.58, the equation may be written as,

$$Cm = \frac{K_f\, X0}{Vm\,(K - Km)} e^{-Kt} \quad .....(6.59)$$

which when written in logarithmic form becomes,

$$\log Cm = \log \left[\frac{K_f\, X0}{Vm\,(K - Km)}\right] - Kt/2.303 \quad ....(6.60)$$

Equation 6.58 is a biexponential equation which is the net result of metabolite formation and elimination. As the time increases after I.V. injection, the drug concentration in blood becomes negligible and hence, metabolite formation is ceased. Only the elimination of the metabolite takes place from that time point, and hence equation 6.58 is reduced to a mono exponential equation 6.59.

The metabolite concentration in the blood increases as the time increases to certain value and then falls. A plot of the log plasma concentration of metabolite versus time will eventually become linear and parallel to the line of the plasma concentration of drug versus time i.e., the slope of the both lines is equal to -K/2.303, as shown in Fig. 6.11.

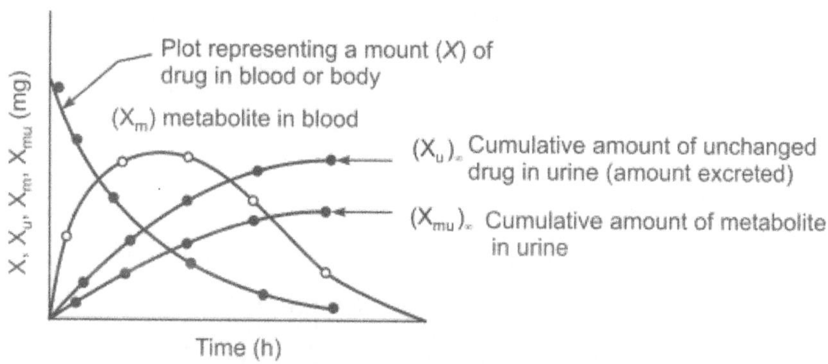

Fig 6.11 Curves obtained by plotting log drug and metabolite concentration vs time in blood as well as urine.

Case 2. K is Greater than Km: If K is several times larger than Km, metabolite levels in plasma will decline more slowly than the levels of the unchanged drug. In this instance, e^{-Kt} term becomes negligible but e^{-Kmt} still will have a finite value and the equation 6.58 may be written as,

$$\text{Log } Cm = \text{Log}\left[\frac{K_f\, X0}{Vm\,(K - Km)}\right] - \frac{Kmt}{2.303} \quad .....(6.61)$$

The slope of the terminal linear portion of the plot log Cm versus time is equal to – Km/2.303.

Case 3. Km is Equal to K: In either instance (i.e., when Km > K or when K > Km) the closer the K and Km values, the more is the difficult to delinear the linear segment of the curve. It means, that by simply following the metabolite levels in the plasma as a function of time and obtaining the linear portion of the curve we do not know whether the slope yields Km or K.

To resolve the dilemma, either the apparent first order elimination rate constant of the drug, K, must be known, or in some limited circumstances the metabolite can be administered as such and its elimination rate constant, Km, determined. Regardless which rate constant (K or Km) is determined from the terminal linear segment of the curve, the other rate constant can be estimated by the method of residuals or peeling of technique (for details see Appendix - III).

Scheme 6.1.4 I.V. Bolus - Metabolite in Urine

Urinary excretion data for a metabolite may be explored to determine the elimination kinetics of the parent drug. Figure 6.11 shows the profile of drug and its metabolite in the blood and their excretion via urinary route. Important points to be considered in pharmacokinetic analysis of urine data are discussed in scheme 6.1.4.

Scheme 6.1.4

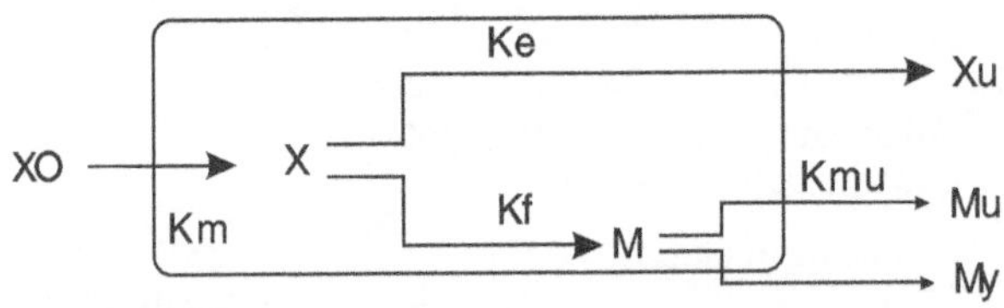

X0	=	I.V. dose
X	=	Among of drug present in the body at any time t
Xu	=	Cumulative amount of drug excreted into urine to time t
M	=	Amount of metabolite in the body at any time t.
Mu	=	Cumulative amount of metabolite eliminated by renal excretion
My	=	Cumulative amount of metabolite eliminated by all other processes (i.e., biliaryfurther metabolism etc.,)
Ke	=	Urinary excretion rate constant
K_f	=	Rate constant involved in the formation of the metabolite from the drug.
Kmu	=	Urinary excretion rate constant of metabolite
Kmy	=	Sum of the rate constants of the processes involved in metabolite elimination other than renal excretion.
Km	=	Overall elimination rate constant of the metabolite.

Urinary excretion and metabolism eliminate the drug. Both urinary excretion and other routes of elimination eliminate the metabolite formed. The elimination rate constant, Km, is the sum of urinary excretion rate constant, Kmu and sum of all other rate constants, Kmy.

$$Km = Kmu + Kmy \qquad .....(6.62)$$

Excretion Rate Method

The differential equation describing the appearance of the metabolite in urine is given by

$$\frac{dmu}{dt} = Kmu \,.\, M \qquad .....(6.63)$$

where, dmu/dt is the rate of urinary excretion of the metabolite. In practice, average excretion rate, $\Delta mu/\Delta t$, is used.

$$\frac{\Delta mu}{\Delta t} = Kmu \,.\, M \qquad .....(6.64)$$

But the amount of the metabolite in the body, M, at any time t is given by the equation 6.57.

$$M = \frac{K_f \, X0}{(K - Km)} \, (e^{-Kmt} - e^{-Kt})$$

Substituting M values in equation 6.64,

$$\frac{\Delta Mu}{\Delta t} = \frac{Kmu \; K_f \; X0}{(K - Km)} \, (e^{-Kmt'} - e^{-Kt'}) \qquad .....(6.65)$$

t′ = mid-point of the urine collection period.

In general Km is assumed to be several times greater than K and hence after some time t, the value of $e^{-Kmt'}$ becomes negligible, but e^{-Kt} will have a finite value. So equation 6.65 reduces to:

$$\frac{\Delta Mu}{\Delta t} = \frac{Kmu \; K_f \; X0}{(K - Km)} \, e^{-Kt'} \qquad .....(6.66)$$

$$\log \left[\frac{\Delta Mu}{\Delta t}\right] = \log \left[\frac{Kmu \, K_f \; X0}{(K - Km)}\right] - \frac{Kt'}{2.303} \qquad .....(6.67)$$

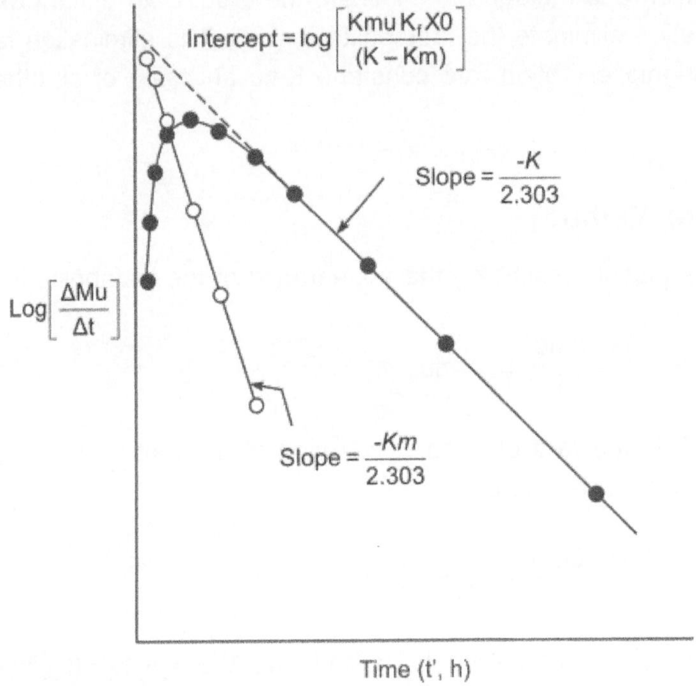

Fig. 6.12 Application of method of residuals for computing excretion parameters.

A plot of the log urinary excretion rate of the metabolite versus mid point of urine collection t′ gives a curve initially and it eventually becomes linear (Fig. 6.12). The terminal linear portion of the plot gives a slope equal to -K/2.303 from which elimination rate constant of the drug and its biological half-life can be estimated. The elimination rate constant of the metabolite and its biological half-life are estimated from the residual line obtained by the method of residuals (for details see Appendix-III). The above method is called Excretion Rate Method.

Sigma-Minus method

The urinary data obtained for the metabolite can be analyzed by another method called Sigma-Minus Method. According to Equation 6.63

$$\frac{dmu}{dt} = Kmu\ M$$

where dmu/dt = instantaneous rate of excretion (excretion rate over a small period of time). According to Equation 6.57, M is equals to:

$$M = \frac{K_f\ X0}{(K - Km)}\ (e^{-Kmt} - e^{-Kt})$$

Substituting M value in equation 6.63, we get

$$\frac{dMu}{dt} = \frac{Kmu\,K_f\,X0}{(K-Km)}\,(e^{-Kmt} - e^{-Kt}) \quad .....(6.68)$$

Integration of equation 6.68 between the limits of t = 0 to t = t yields.

$$\int_0^t dmu = [Kmu.\ K_f\ X0/(K\text{-}Km)] \int_0^t (e^{-kmt} - e^{-kt}).dt \quad .....(6.69)$$

$$Mu^t - 0 = \frac{Kmu\,Kf\,Xo}{(K-Km)} \quad .....(6.70)$$

On further simplification,

$$Mu^t = Kmu\ K_f\ Xo\left[\frac{1}{Kkm} + \frac{e^{-kmt}}{Km\,(Km-K)} - \frac{e^{-kt}}{K\,(Km-K)}\right] \quad ....(6.71)$$

Rearranging the above equation 6.71.

$$Mu^t = \frac{Kmu\,Kf\,XO}{KKm}\,[1 + \frac{1}{(Km-K)}\,(K.\ e^{-kmt} - Km.\ e^{-kt})] \quad .....(6.72)$$

At time = ∞, M_u^t becomes M_u^∞, the total amount of the metabolite excreted into urine in infinite time. Setting the time limit to ∞, equation 6.72, can be written as:

$$Mu^\infty = \frac{Kmu\,K_f\,X0}{KKm} \quad .....(6.73)$$

Substituting $M_{u\infty}$ in Equation 6.72

$$Mu^t = Mu^\infty\,[1 + \frac{1}{(Km-K)}\,(K.\ e^{-Kmt} - Km.\ e^{-Kt})] \quad .....(6.74)$$

Subtracting both the sides of Equation 6.74 from M_u^∞ and simplifying the resultant equation,

$$Mu^\infty - Mu^t = \frac{Mu^\infty}{(Km-K)}\,(Km\ e^{-Kmt} - K\ e^{-Kt}) \quad .....(6.75)$$

The term $(M_u^\infty - M_u^t)$ represents the amount of the metabolite to be excreted from that time point. If Km is several times greater than K, then, after some time equation 6.75 reduces to:

$$Mu^\infty - Mu^t = \frac{Mu^\infty}{(Km-K)}\,(Km.\ e^{-Kt}) \quad .....(6.76)$$

Applying logarithms,

$$\log\ (Mu^{\infty} - Mu^{t}) = \log\left[\frac{Km\,Mu^{\infty}}{(Km-K)}\right] - \left[\frac{Km\,Mu^{\infty}}{(Km-K)}\right] Kt\ /\ 2.303$$

.....(6.77)

A plot of log (Mu^{∞} – Mu^{t}) versus time gives a curve, the slope of the terminal linear portion of which is equal to – K/2.303 (Fig. 6.13). By applying the method of residuals Km is estimated (for details see Appendix - III).

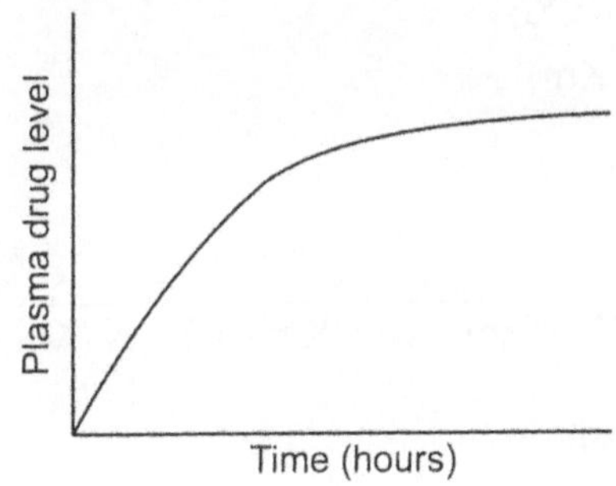

Fig. 6.13 Plasma drug level-time curve for constant intravenous infusion.

Application of the method of residual in both instances will enable the estimation of Km, the apparent first order elimination rate constant of the metabolite. If, however, K is greater than Km, the value of Km can be determined from the slope of the terminal linear phases of the plots and K, can be determined from the slopes of the residual lines. Without prior knowledge of the relative values of K and Km, it is not possible to solve the equation. In general it is assumed that Km>>K, because metabolites are more polar than their parent drug.

PRACTICE PROBLEMS

1. A single dose of a drug was given to a 50 kg person at a dose level of 10 mg/kg. Blood and urine samples were collected periodically and the unchanged drug (parent drug) content in the samples was estimated. Calculate all possible pharmacokinetic parameters using the data given below.

(i) Blood Data

Time (hrs)	Drug level in Blood (C) (μg / ml)	Log C
1	20.00	1.3010
3	11.30	1.0531
5	7.00	0.8451
7	4.30	0.6335
10	2.00	0.3010

(ii) Urine Data

Time of collection (hrs)	Volume of urine (ml)	Concentration of unchanged drug in urine (μg / ml)
2	120	1330
4	180	500
6	89	630
8	340	100
12	178	180
24	950	20

Solution :

1. Blood Data: The equation that describes the blood concentration time data is

$$\log C = \text{Log } C0 - \frac{Kt}{2.303}$$

Step 1: Plot the blood levels of the drug versus time data on a semi-logarithmic graph paper taking time on X-axis and concentration of drug in blood on logarithmic axis. An alternative method is to convert blood concentration of the drug into a log concentration and then a plot of log C versus time can be made on ordinary graph paper.

Step 2: Make the best fit of points to give a straight line. Extend the straight line to cut the Y-axis, to give the initial concentration of the drug, C0 (i.e. zero time concentration of drug in blood).

Note: When log C vs time plot is made, the intercept is equal to log C0. Therefore, C0 will be the anti-log of the intercept.

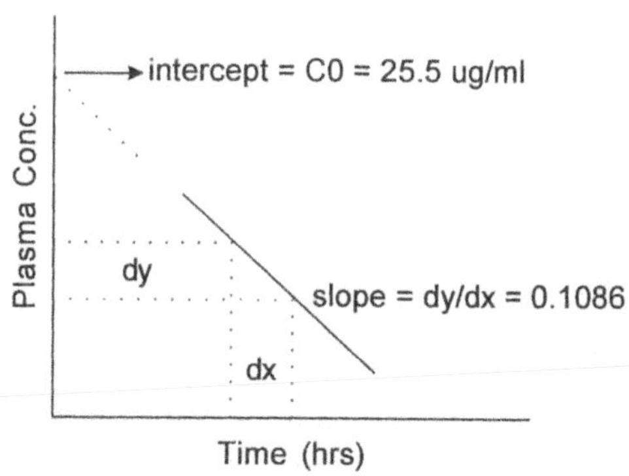

Step 3: Find out the slope of the line as shown in the figure. The slope is equal to K/ 2.303. Therefore the elimination rate constant,

$$K = \text{slope} \times 2.303 = 0.1086 \times 2.303 = 0.25 \text{ hr}^{-1}.$$

Elimination rate constant (K) = 0.25 hr^{-1}.

Step 4: Biological half-life ($t_{1/2}$)

Biological half-life ($t_{1/2}$) = 0.693/K = 0.693/0.25 = 2.772 hrs

Step 5: Volume of distribution (Vd)

The volume of distribution of the drug,

$$Vd = \frac{X_0}{C_0} = \frac{\text{I.V. dose}}{\text{C0}}$$

$$Vd = \frac{50,00,000}{25.5} = 19607.8 \text{ ml} = 19.6798 \text{ L}$$

Step 6: Area under the curve (AUC): Area under the blood concentration-time curve is calculated by the trapezoidal rule.

$$AUC_0^t = \frac{1}{2}(C_0 + C_1)(t_1 - t_0) + \frac{1}{2}(C_1 + C_2)(t_2 - t_1) + \text{.........} + \frac{1}{2}(C_{n-1} + C_n)(t_n - t_{n-1})$$

$$\text{Therefore, } AUC_0^t = \frac{1}{2}(25.5 + 20.0)(1 - 0) + \frac{1}{2}(20 + 11.3)(3 - 1) + \frac{1}{2}(11.3 + 7.0)(5 - 3) + \frac{1}{2}(7.0 + 4.3)(7 - 5) + \frac{1}{2}(4.3 + 2.0)(10 - 7)$$

$$= 22.75 + 31.3 + 18.3 + 11.3 + 9.45 = 93.1 \text{ mg-hr/ml}$$

$$AUC_t^{\infty} = C^*/K = 2.0 / 0.25 = 8 \ \mu\text{g-hr/ml}$$

where C* is the drug concentration in blood at the last time point, t*

Total AUC = $AUC_0^{\infty} = AUC_0^t + AUC_{t^*}^{\infty}$ = 93.1 + 8.0 = 101.1 ug-hr/ml

AUC_0^{∞} based on integration method

$$= C_0/K = \frac{25.5}{0.25} = 102 \text{ mg-hr/ml}$$

Step 7: Total body clearance, Cl_t,

Total Body clearance, Cl_t = Vd . K

$$= 19.6078 \times 0.25 = 4.9 \text{ Liters / hr}$$

Step 8: Volume of distribution based on clearance

$$Vd = \frac{CL_t}{K} = \frac{4.9}{0.25} = 19.6 \text{ liters.}$$

$$Vd \text{ per kg} = \frac{19.6}{50} = 0.392 \text{ liters/kg.}$$

(ii) Urine Data: The urine data obtained can be analysed by two methods namely *excretion rate method* and *sigma-minus method.*

Excretion Rate Method: The equation that describes the excretion rate versus time data is

$$\log \frac{\Delta Xu}{\Delta t} = \log Ke\ X0 - Kt'/2.303$$

Step 1: Step up the following table.

Time (hr)	Amount of drug excreted in the time interval ΔXu, (mg) (volume of urine x conc of drug in urine)	Urine collection period Δt (hrs) $(t_n - t_{n-1})$	Excretion rate $\Delta Xu/\Delta t$ (mg/hrs)	Mid point urine collection periodt' (hrs) $(t_n + t_{n-1})/2$
0	-	-	-	-
2	159.60	2	79.8	1
4	90.00	2	45.0	3
6	56.07	2	28.0	5
8	34.00	2	17.0	7
12	32.04	4	8.0	10
24	19.00	12	1.58	18

Step 2: Plot the excretion rate versus t' (mid point of urine collection) on a semilogarithmic graph paper or log ($\Delta Xu/\Delta t$) versus t' on an ordinary Cartesian graph paper. Make the best fit of the points to give a straight line.

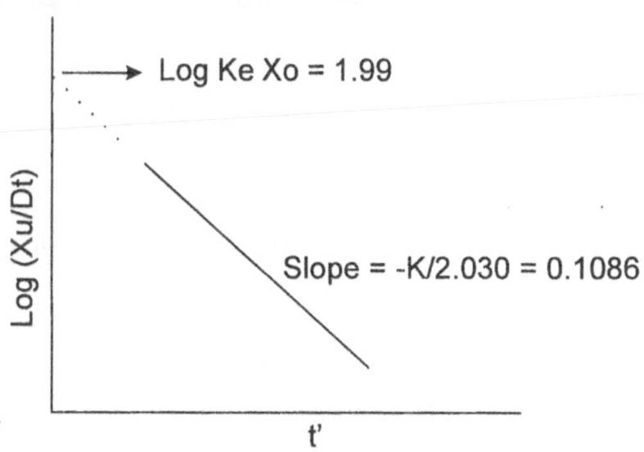

Step 3: Extend the straight line to obtain the intercept on Y-axis. Intercept = log KeX0 = 1.99

Therefore, $\quad Ke\ X0 = \text{anti-log } 1.99 = 97.6675.$

$$Ke = \frac{99.6675}{500} = 0.195\ hr^{-1}$$

Step 4 : *Overall elimination rate constant, K.*

Calculate the slope.

Slope $= -K/2.303 = 1.086$

Therefore, $\quad K = 1.086 \times 2.303 = 0.25\ hr^{-1}$

Step 5 : *Biological half life ($t_{1/2}$)*

$$t_{1/2} = 0.693 / K = 0.693 / 0.25 = 2.772 \text{ hrs.}$$

Step 6 : *Fraction of dose excreted unchanged,* fe.

$$fe = \frac{Ke}{K} = \frac{0.195}{0.25} = 0.78$$

Using the plasma and urine data obtained from a single study, the renal clearance can be calculated

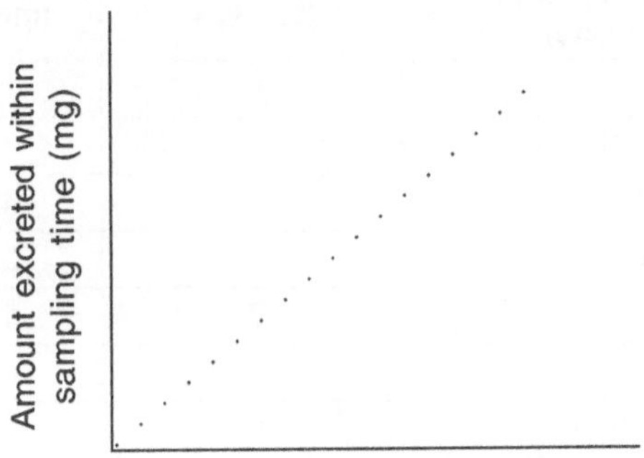

I. A plot of the amount excreted versus the area under the curve of the blood data gives a straight line with a slope equal to the renal clearance.

II. Renal clearance $CL_R = Ke.\ Vd$

$$= 0.195 \times 19.6 = 3.83\ L/hr$$

Sigma - Minus Method:

The equation that describes the amount of the unchaged drug to be excreted versus time data is

$$\log (X_u^{\infty} - x_u^{t}) = \text{Log } X_u^{\infty} - Kt / 2.303$$

Step 1 : Set up the table as shown below

Processing of urine data for sigma minus method

Time (hrs)	Amount excreted (mg) excreted (X_u^t)	Cumulative amount	$X_u\mu - X_u^t$
2	159.60	159.60	231.1
4	90.00	249.6	141.11
6	56.07	305.67	85.04
8	34.00	339.67	51.04
12	32.04	371.71	19.00
24	19.00 $X_u^\infty = 390.71$	390.71	0

Step 2: Plot log $(X_u^\infty - X_u^t)$ versus time data on a graph paper. Make the best fit of the points to give a straight line.

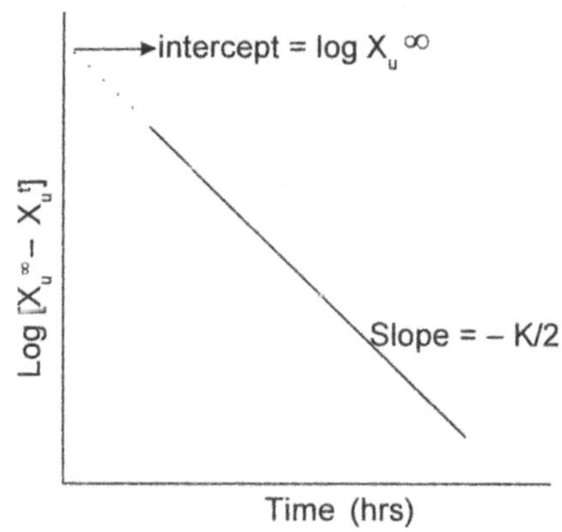

Step 3: *Elimination rate constant* : The slope of the line is equal to -K/2.303. Elimination rate constant is obtained from the slope.

$$K = 2.303 \times 0.108 = 0.25 \text{ hr}^{-1}$$

Step 4 : *Excretion rate constant*, Ke can obtained from $X_u^\propto$ value.

$$X_u^\propto = \frac{Ke\ X0}{K}$$

$$Ke = \frac{K.X_u^\infty}{X0} = \frac{0.25 \times 390.71}{500} = 0.195 \text{ hr}^{-1}$$

Using the plasma and urine data obtained from a single study, renal clearance can be calculated.

$$X_u^{\infty} = CL_R \int_0^{\infty} C.dt = CL_R\ [AUC]_0^{\infty}$$

$$CL_R = \frac{X_u^{\infty}}{[AUC]_0^{\infty}} = \frac{390.71}{93.9} = 4.16 \text{ liters / hr.}$$

2. A new drug was given in a single intravenous dose of 200 mg to an 80 - kg male. After 6 hrs, the blood concentration of the drug was found to be 1.5 mg/100 ml of the blood. Assuming that the apparent volume of distribution, Vd is 10% body weight, compute the total amount of the drug in the body fluids after 6 hrs. What is the half-life of this drug ?

$$\text{I.V. dose} = X0 = 200 \text{ mg}$$

$$Vd = 10\% \text{ of body weight} = 0.1\ (80 \text{ kg}) = 8000 \text{ ml}$$

At 6 hrs, $C = 1.5$ mg/100 ml

Drug in body at any time t, $X = Vd\ .\ C$

$$= 80000 \times \frac{1.5}{100} = 120 \text{ mg}$$

$$\log X = \log X0 - Kt / 2.303$$

$$\log 120 = \log 200 - K\ .\ \frac{6}{2.303}$$

$$\therefore \quad K = (\log 200 - \log 120) \times \frac{2.303}{6}$$

$$= (2.3010 - 2.07918) \times 0.3838$$

$$K = 0.2218 \times 0.3838 = 0.08513 \text{ hr}^{-1}$$

$$t_{1/2} = 0.693 / K = 0.693 / 0.08513 = 8.14 \text{ hours}$$

3. A long acting pencillin has a half-life of 21 days. How long will it take for the drug concentration in the blood to drop to 90% of its initial value ?

$$K = 0.693 / t_{1/2} = \frac{0.693}{21} = 0.033 \text{ day}^{-1}$$

Initial concentration, $C0 = 100\%$ and the final concentration, $C = 90\ \%$

$\text{Log}\ (C0/C) = Kt / 2.303$

$$t = \frac{2.303}{K} \log \frac{C0}{C} = \frac{2.303}{0.038} \times \log \frac{100}{90} = 3.19 \text{ days.}$$

6.2 I.V. Infusion - Unchanged drug in Blood/Plasma

I.V. drug solutions may be given either as a bolus dose or infused slowly at a constant rate (zero-order rate). Drugs are given by I.V. infusion for the precise control of the plasma drug levels, as per the needs of the patient. For drugs with a narrow therapeutic window, plasma drug levels can be maintained without many fluctuations by I.V. infusion. Many drugs can be administered with I.V. fluids, including electrolytes and nutrients. Another important advantage with I.V. infusion is that the duration of drug therapy may be maintained for a longer time and may be terminated when desired.

During I.V. infusion, the drug concentration slowly increases as the time proceeds and reaches a steady state concentration or plateau level (Fig. 6.14). The rate of drug infusion into the body is a zero order process i.e., drug reaches blood at a constant rate, K0. At the steady state, the rate of the drug leaving the body is equal to the rate of the drug (infusion rate) entering the body. This drug level is maintained as long as the infusion is continued.

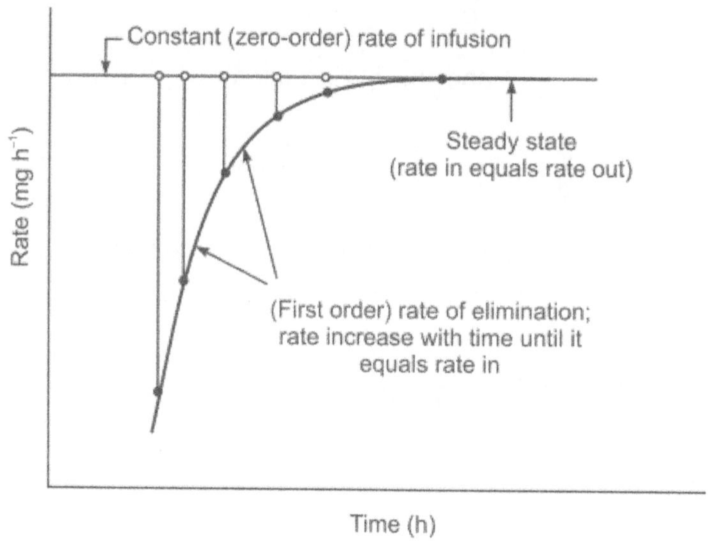

Fig. 6.14 Graphical presentation of dosing by intravenous infusion.

Scheme 6.2.1

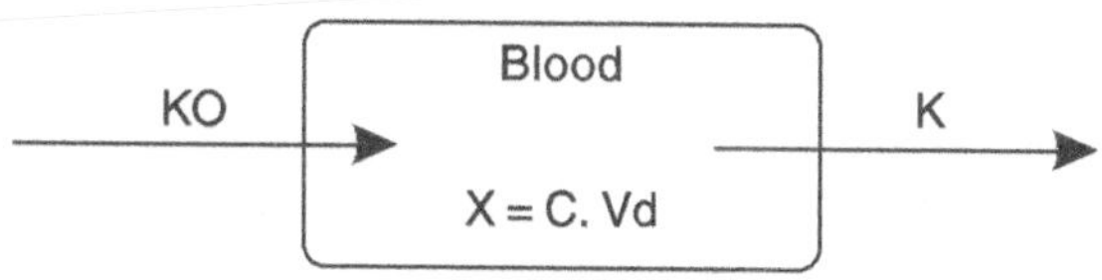

Where, K0 = infusion rate (zero order) mg/hr. All other symbols are as defined previously. In this scheme the drug enters the body by the zero order process and leaves the body by the first order process. The change in the amount of the drug in the body at any time (dX/dt) during the infusion is the rate of input minus the rate of output.

$$\frac{dX}{dt} = K0 - KX \quad .....(6.78)$$

Dividing the entire equation by the volume of distribution of the drug, Vd, we get the following equation.

$$\frac{dX/Vd}{dt} = \frac{K0}{Vd} = \frac{KX}{Vd} \quad .....(6.79)$$

But $X/Vd = C$

Therefore, $$\frac{dC}{dt} = \frac{K0}{Vd} - KC \quad .....(6.80)$$

Rearranging equation 6.80 and multiplying it with e^{kt}, we get

$$\frac{dC}{dt} e^{Kt} + KC\, e^{Kt} = \frac{K0}{Vd} e^{Kt} \quad .....(6.81)$$

Integrating equation 6.81 between the limits of t = zero to t = t, and on simplification of the resultant equation, we get the following equation,

$$C\, e^{Kt} = \frac{K0}{Vd} \left(\frac{e^{Kt}}{K} - \frac{1}{K}\right) \quad .....(6.82)$$

Dividing equation 6.82 by e^{kt} and simplifying the resultant equation is 6.83,

$$C = \frac{K0}{Vd\,K} (1 - e^{-Kt}) \quad .....(6.83)$$

Equation 6.83 describes the plasma concentration of drug-time profile during I.V. infusion. Since the product of Vd and C is equal to the amount of the drug in the body at any time, we can write it as follows,

$$X = \frac{K0}{K} (1 - e^{-Kt}) \quad .....(6.84)$$

Theoretically, a steady state level is reached after an infinitely long infusion time. In clinical practice, the plasma drug level within the 95% to 99% of plateau level is considered to be steady state level. Mathematically it can be shown that after I.V. infusion of the drug for 5 half-lives the plasma drug concentration is between 95% and 99% of steady-state drug level.

The steady state drug concentration in plasma can be determined from equation 6.83 by setting the time equal to infinity (i.e. by recognizing that the term e^{-kt} approaches zero).

$$Css = K0 / Vd.K \qquad .....(6.85)$$

Where, Css = steady state drug concentration in plasma since Vd and K are considered to be constant for a drug, the Css is directly proportional to the infusion rate of the drug, K0.

An increase in the rate of infusion will not shorten the time to reach the steady state drug concentration. If the drug is given at a higher rate, a higher steady state drug level will be obtained, but the time to reach steady state is the same. Therefore the infusion rate decides the steady-state drug concentration, and biological half-life of the drug determines the time to reach that level.

Another method of developing the equation for the steady state level of the drug is based on the fact that at the steady state, the rate of input is equal to rate of output (i.e. the rate of change of drug concentration (dC/dt) at the steady state level is zero).

According to equation 6.80

$$\frac{dC}{dt} = \frac{K0}{Vd} - K.C$$

at steady state dC/dt = 0.

$$K0/Vd - K\ Css = 0$$

$$K0/Vd = K\ Css$$

$$Css = K0/Vd.K \qquad .....(6.86)$$

This equation shows that the steady state concentration (Css) is dependent on the volume of distribution, the elimination rate constant, and the infusion rate. Altering any one of these factors can affect the steady state concentration.

Equation that describes the plasma drug concentration at any time during I.V. infusion can be obtained in terms of Css, by substituting Css for K0/Vd K in Equation 6.83.

$$C = Css\ (1 - e^{-Kt}) \qquad .....(6.87)$$

Calculation of Elimination Half-life of a Drug in Patient by I.V. Infusion Method

In practice, before starting an I.V. infusion, an appropriate infusion rate (K0) is generally calculated from Equation 6.85 using literature values for Css, K Vd and Cl_t (total body clearance). Two plasma samples are taken, one before reaching the steady state to get C and the second near the theoretical time for the steady state to get Css. The equation used to calculate the half-life of a drug can be derived as shown under;

$$C = Css\ (1 - e^{-Kt})$$

$$C = Css - Css.\ e^{-Kt}$$

$$Css\ \ e^{-Kt} = Css - C$$

$$e^{-Kt} = \frac{Css - C}{Css}$$

Rearranging and taking the logarithms on both sides,

$$\log\left(\frac{Css - C}{Css}\right) = -\frac{kt}{2.303}$$

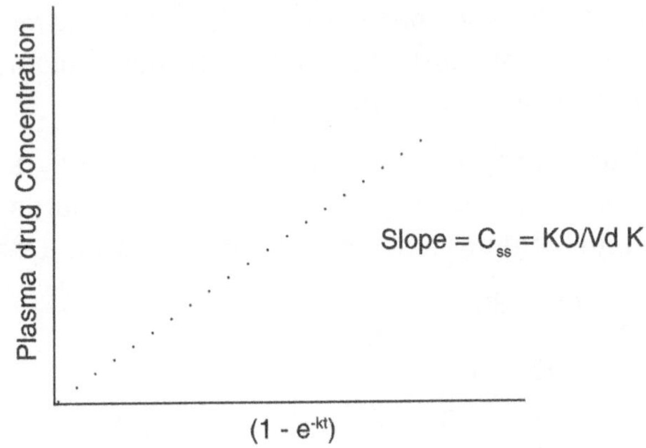

Fig. 6.15 Plasma concentration versus $(1-e^{-kt})$ curve for constant intravenous infusion.

$$K = \frac{2.303}{t} \log\left(\frac{Css - C}{Css}\right) \quad .....(6.88)$$

The elimination half-life ($t_{1/2}$) of the drug = 0.693/K. The elimination half-life calculated confirms that whether the second sample was taken at a steady state or not. Even though the estimated half-life is not an accurate value, it helps in deciding the new rate of infusion.

A plot of the plasma concentration versus $(1-e^{-Kt})$ will yield a straight line with a slope of (K0/Vd K) or (Css), from which Vd can be calculated if the elimination rate constant K, is known (Fig. 6.15)

Post infusion - Plasma concentration of Drug

The rate of change in plasma concentration after stopping the infusion can be expressed by the following differential equation,

$$\frac{dC}{dt} = -KC \quad .....(6.89)$$

Where, C = the plasma concentration of the drug when I.V. infusion is stopped. If the infusion is stopped after reaching plateau level, then C is nothing but Css. Whether the infusion is stopped before the steady state or after the steady-state is reached, plasma drug concentrations decline exponentially with the slope equal to -K/2.303. Therefore, for a case where infusion stopped after reaching steady – state the equation is the following,

$$\frac{dC}{dt} = -\, KCss \qquad .....(6.90)$$

Integrating the equation and rearranging the resulting equation gives,

$$C = Css.\ e^{-Kt^*} \qquad .....(6.91)$$

t* = post infusion time

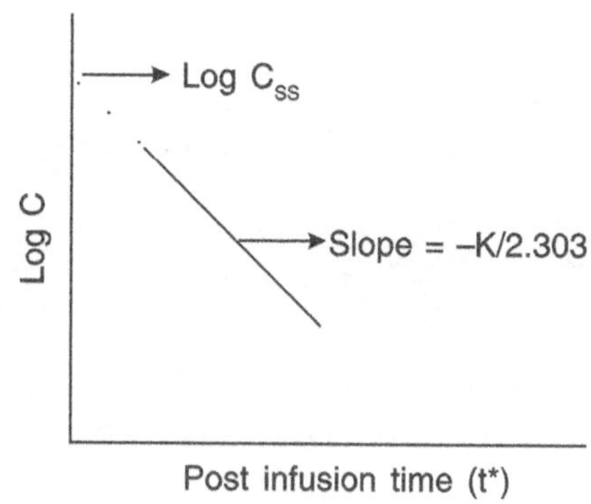

Fig. 6.16 Plasma concentration versus post infusion time (t*).

Taking logarithms of both the sides,

$$\log C = \log Css - Kt^* / 2.303 \qquad ....(6.92)$$

A plot of the logarithm of the post infusion plasma concentrations of a drug versus time will yield a straight line with the slope of -K/2.303 from which the apparent elimination rate constant can be calculated (Fig. 6.16). The intercept obtained by extending the line is equal to log Css.

If the infusion is stopped before reaching steady-state level, the post infusion concentration of the drug in plasma is calculated using the following equation.

$$C = [\frac{K0}{VdK}\ (1 - e^{-Kt})]\ \ (e^{-Kt^*})] \qquad .....(6.93)$$

t = length of time of infusion period and t* = length of time after infusion is stopped.

6.2.2 I.V. Infusion - Unchanged Drug in Urine

Drug elimination kinetics can also be determined from the urinary excretion data of the unchanged drug following intravenous infusion. The rate of appearance of the unchanged drug in urine is proportional to the amount of the unchanged drug in the body. Hence, a differential equation for the rate of appearance of the unchanged drug in urine can be written as,

$$\frac{dXu}{dt} = Ke\ X \qquad .....(6.94)$$

Where dXu/dt is the instantaneous rate of excretion of the drug, Ke is the excretion rate constant and X is the amount of the drug in the body at any time. But according to equation 6.84,

$$X = \frac{K0}{K}(1 - e^{-Kt})$$

Substituting X values in Equation 6.94,

$$\frac{dXu}{dt} = \frac{Ke\,K0}{K}(1 - e^{-Kt}) \qquad .....(6.95)$$

Integrating Equation 6.95 between the limits of t = 0 to t = t results in an equation that describes cumulative excretion of unchanged drug versus time data,

$$\int_0^t dXu = (Ke\ K0)/K \int_0^t (dt - e^{-Kt}.dt)$$

$$X_u^t - 0 = \frac{Ke\,K0}{K}\left[t - \left(\frac{e^{-Kt}}{-K} + \frac{1}{K}\right)\right]$$

$$X_u^t = \frac{Ke\,K0}{K}t - \frac{Ke\,K0}{K^2} + \frac{Ke\,K0}{K^2}.e^{-Kt}$$

$$X_u^t = \frac{Ke\,K0}{K}t - \frac{Ke\,K0}{K^2}(1 - e^{-Kt}) \qquad .....(6.96)$$

The steady-state level is reached after 5 half-lives of the drug, the term e^{-kt} approaches zero and equation 6.96 reduces to,

$$X_u^t = \frac{Ke\,K0}{K}t - \frac{Ke\,K0}{K^2} \qquad .....(6.97)$$

or

$$X_u^t = \frac{Ke\,K0}{K}\left(t - \frac{1}{K}\right) \qquad .....(6.98)$$

According to Equation 6.98, a plot of the cumulative amount of the drug excreted versus time should be curve until the steady-state is reached and becomes linear after steady-state level (Fig. 6.17). It should be remembered that at the steady-state the amount of the drug in the body remains constant so that the rate of excretion of drug is also constant. From the Fig. 6.17 it can be observed that extrapolation of the linear segment of the curve to $X_u = 0$ yields an intercept of 1/K. The slope of this linis KeK0/K. Therefore, the apparent elimination rate constant of the drug, can be estimated from intercept and the excretion rate constant, Ke from the slope since K0 is known.

From equation 6.96, we can write

$$X_u^t = \frac{Ke\,K0}{K}\left[t - \frac{1}{K}\left(1 - e^{-Kt}\right)\right] \qquad .....(6.99)$$

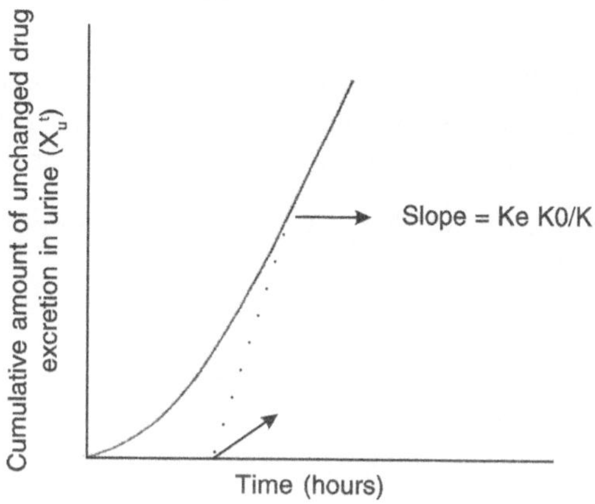

Fig. 6.17 Cumulative amount of unchanged drug excreted in urine versus time curve for constant intravenous infusion.

If the overall elimination rate constant, K of a drug is known, a plot of X_u^t versus $[t - 1/K(1-e^{-Kt})]$ will give a straight line, the slope of which is KeK0/K. Therefore, a knowledge of the infusion rate constant, K0 and K will enable the estimation of Ke from this plot. This type of plot does not require infusion to the steady-state.

6.3 Simultaneous Intravenous Injection and Infusion - Unchanged Drug in Blood/Plasma

Since the time required to attain Css will be quite long for a drug with a long half-life, it is often convenient in such cases to administer an intravenous loading dose to attain immediately the desired drug concentration. This drug concentration can be maintained by infusion.

I.V. Loading Dose: A simple method of calculating the loading dose is to use the values of the steady-state drug concentration, Css and the volume of distribution of the drug Vd, from literature. The dose of the drug required to attain Css is equal to the product of Css and Vd.

$$\text{I.V. loading dose (X0)} = \text{Css. Vd} \qquad .....(6.100)$$

According to Equation 6.85 Css.Vd = K0/K. Therefore,

$$X0 = Css.Vd = K0/K \qquad .....(6.101)$$

The loading dose can also be calculated from the values of the infusion rate, K0 and the over all elimination rate constant, K.

Infusion Rate

The infusion rate of a drug, K0 required to maintain the steady-state level is given by

$$K0 = Css.Vd.K = X0 \,.\, K \qquad .....(6.102)$$

Scheme 6.3

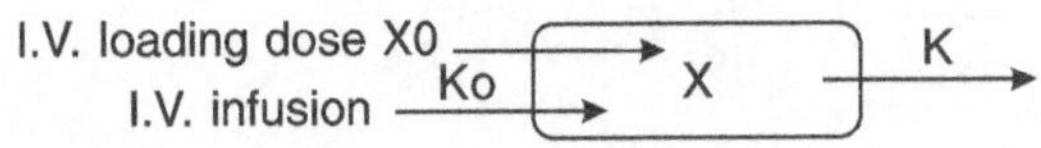

The equation describing the time course of the amount of the drug in the body following a simultaneous injection of an intravenous loading dose and initiation of infusion is the sum of the two equations describing these two processes individually.

We know that the amount of the drug in the body for a one compartment model after an I.V. bolus dose is described by,

$$X_1 = X0 \ e^{-Kt} \qquad .....(6.103)$$

And the amount of the drug by infusion at the rate of K0 is:

$$X_2 = \frac{K0}{K}(1 - e^{-Kt}) \qquad .....(6.104)$$

Now, the sum of equations 6.103 and 6.104 will give an equation that describes the time course of the amount of the drug in the body following a simultaneous I.V. injection and infusion.

$$X = X_1 + X_2$$

$$X = X0 \ e^{-Kt} + \frac{K0}{K}(1 - e^{-Kt}) \qquad .....(6.105)$$

But X0 = K0/K (according to Equation 6.101). Substituting, K0/K for X0,

$$X = \frac{K0}{K} e^{-Kt} + \frac{K0}{K}(1 - e^{-Kt}) \qquad .....(6.106)$$

or

$$X = \frac{K0}{K} e^{-Kt} + \frac{K0}{K} - \frac{K0}{K} e^{-Kt}$$

$$X = \frac{K0}{K} \qquad .....(6.107)$$

K0/K is equal to the amount of the drug in the body at any time following a simultaneous administration of I.V. bolus and infusion, which is nothing but an I.V. loading dose, X0.

It means I.V. loading dose brings the plasma drug concentration to a steady-state level (Css) and the infusion maintains this concentration.

According to Equation 6.101,

$$X0 = Css.\ Vd = \frac{K0}{K}$$

Therefore, $Css = K0/Vd\ K$ .....(6.108)

Following an intravenous loading dose and simultaneous infusion the plasma drug concentration remains constant from time zero until the infusion is stopped.

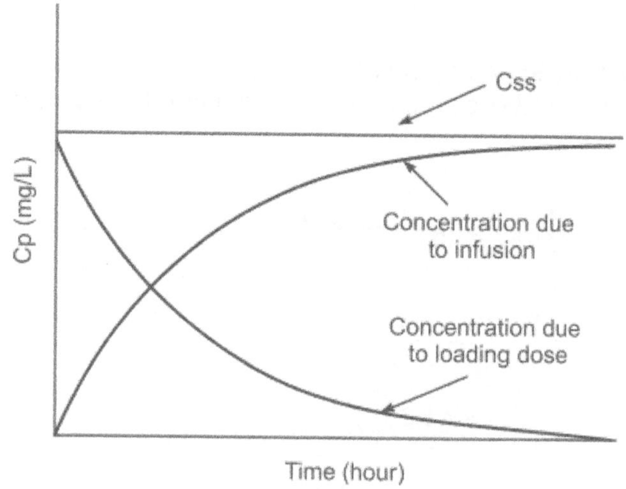

Fig. 6.18 Simultaneous administration of loading dose by IV bolus and maintenance dose by IV infusion.

Fig. 6.18 shows the pattern of graph that will be obtained with different loading doses with a constant infusion rate. An ideal situation is observed when an accurate loading dose is administered. When loading dose is large, the plasma concentration of the drug will be greater than Css initially, and decline slowly to steady-state levels. If the loading dose is low, the plasma concentrations will increase slowly to the steady-state levels.

6.4 Simultaneous I.V.injection and I.V. infusion - unchanged drug in urine

Scheme 6.4

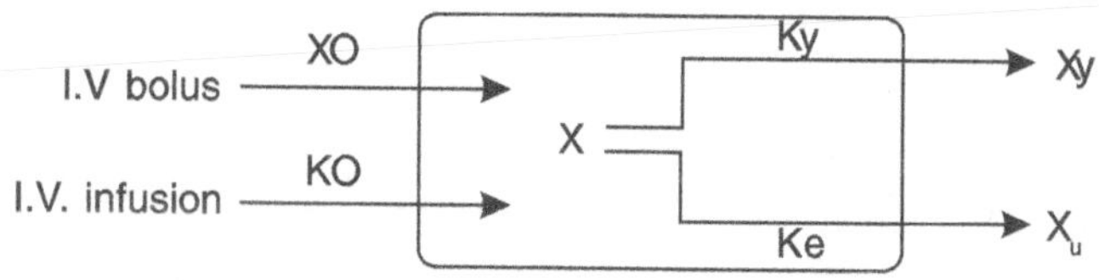

K = Ke + Ky, where K = overall eliminaiton rate constant, Ke = first order urinary excretion rate constant and Ky = sum of all the rate constants involved in drug eliminaiton other than renal excretion.

The rate of appearance of the unchanged drug in urine is proportional to the amount of the drug present in the body at any time.

$$\frac{dX_u}{dt} = Ke\ X \quad .....(6.109)$$

Where, X is the amount of the drug present in the body at any time following a simultaneous administration of an I.V. loading dose and infusion, which is equal to K0/K (Equation 6.108).

Therefore,
$$\frac{dX_u}{dt} = \frac{Ke\,K0}{K} \quad .....(6.110)$$

An equation that describes the cumulative amount of the unchanged drug excreted in urine, X_u^c versus time can be developed by integrating the Equation 6.110 between the limits of t = 0 and t = t.

$$\int_0^t dX_u = (Ke\ K0)/K \int_0^t dt$$

$$X_u^t - 0 = \frac{Ke\,K0}{K}\ |t - 0|$$

$$Xu^t = \frac{Ke\,K0}{K}\ t \quad .....(6.111)$$

Equation 6.111 is a straight line equation in the form of y = bx, where b is the slope of the line.

A plot of the cumulative amount of the drug excreted versus time (Fig. 6.19) will yield a straight line passing through the origin with a slope of KeK0/K. Knowledge of the values of K0 and K enables us to calculate the excretion rate constant, Ke, from the slope.

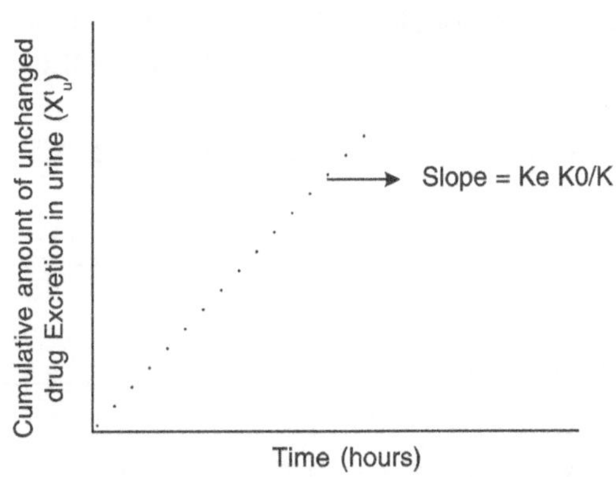

Fig. 6.19 Cumulative amount of unchanged drug in urine (Xut) versus time curve for simultaenous I.V. bolus and I.V. infusion.

According to Equation 6.110,

$$dX_u/dt = \frac{Ke\,K0}{K} \text{ but } \frac{K0}{K} = Css.\ Vd \text{ (from Equation 6.101)}$$

$$\therefore \quad \frac{dX_u}{dt} = Ke\ Vd.\ Css \qquad \text{.....(6.112)}$$

Integrating of equation 6.112 between the limits of t = 0 and t = t results.

$$\int_0^t Xu = Ke\ Vd \int_0^t Css.\ dt$$

$$X_u^t = Ke\ Vd \int_0^t Css.\ dt\ X \qquad \text{.....(6.113)}$$

$$X_u^t = Ke\ Vd\ [AUC]_0^t \qquad \text{.....(6.114)}$$

Where Ke.Vd is equal to renal clearance, CL_R and $[AUC]_0^t$ is the area under the plasma concentration-time curve from time zero to t. A plot of X_u^t versus AUC yields a straight line with a slope equal to Ke.Vd, the renal clearance. Simultaneous sampling of plasma and urine samples enables us to estimate the renal clearance of the drug and to assess the renal function of the patient based on the literature values.

Practice problems :

1. A drug has a volume of distribution of 12 L and a K of 0.18 hr^{-1}. A steady state concentration (Css) of 12 mg/ml is desired.
   (a) What is the infusion rate needed to maintain this concentration ?
   (b) How long it takes to achieve 90% and 99% of the Css ?
   (c) If the elimination rate constant, K, in a patient with a renal impairment is 0.1 hr^{-1}, what is the infusion rate required to maintain the same Css in this patient?

Solution :

(a) Equation 6.85 can be rewritten as

$$K0 = Css.\ Vd.\ K$$

Therefore:

infusion rate

$$\begin{aligned} K0 &= 12 \times 12000 \times 0.18 \\ &= 25290 \text{ mg/hr} \\ &= 25.29 \text{ mg/hr} \end{aligned}$$

(b) According to equation 6.87

$$C = Css\ (1 - e^{-Kt})$$

Now, C = 90% of Css, therefore, we can write,

$$90\% \text{ of Css} = \text{Css}\,(1-e^{-Kt})$$

$$0.9\,.\,\text{Css} = \text{Css}\,(1-e^{-Kt})$$

$$0.9 = 1 - e^{-Kt}$$

or $$e^{-Kt} = 1 - 0.9 = 0.1$$

Taking the natural logarithm of both sides - Kt = ln 0.1

$$t_{90\%} = \frac{\ln 0.1}{-K}\quad t = \frac{\ln 0.1}{0.18} = 12.788 \text{ hrs}$$

In terms of $t_{1/2}$ (0.693 / K = 3.85 hrs),

$$t_{90\%} = \frac{12.788}{3.5} = 3.32\ t_{1/2}$$

Similarly, $$t_{99\%} = \frac{\ln 0.01}{-K} = \frac{\ln 0.01}{0.18} = 25.58 \text{ hrs} = 6.645\ t_{1/2}$$

(c) The elimination rate constant of the patient is 0.1 hr^{-1}

The infusion rate for this patient to maintain the steady - state concentration of 12 mg/ml is

$$K0 = \text{Css.Vd}\,.\,K = 12 \times 1200 \times 0.1 = 14400 = 14.4 \text{ mg/hr}$$

When the elimination rate constant decreases, then the infusion rate must decrease proportionately to maintain the same Css. However, because the elimination rate constant is smaller (i.e., the elimination half-life is longer), the time to reach Css will be longer.

The $t_{90\%}$ for this patient is 23.02 hrs, and $t_{99\%}$ = is 46.05 hrs.

2. A patient is given an antibiotic having $t_{1/2}$ of 4 hrs by constant I.V. infusion at a rate of 3 mg/hr. At the end of 36 hours, the plasma drug concentration is 2.2 mg/L. Calculate the total body clearance, CL_t for this antibiotic. What is the volume of distribution, Vd, of the drug ?

Solution : Equation 6.85 can be rewritten as

$$\text{Vd.K} = \frac{K0}{\text{Css}} = CL_t$$

The plasma sample is taken after 36 hrs of infusion, which time represents 9 times $t_{1/2}$. Therefore, the plasma drug concentration approximates the Css.

$$CL_t = \frac{K0}{\text{Css}} = \frac{3\,\text{mg/hr}}{2.2\,\text{mg/L}} = 1.363 \text{ L / hr} = 1363 \text{ ml/hr}$$

Volume of distribution,

$$Vd = \frac{CL_t}{K} = \frac{1363}{(0.693/4)} \qquad = 7870.9 \text{ ml}$$

$$= 7.871 \text{ Liters}$$

3. A pateint is given an I.V. infusion of an antibiotic at an infusion rate of 26 mg/hr. Blood samples are taken at 10 and 28 hours and plasma drug concentrations are 10 and 11.9 mg/ml, respectively. The antibiotic has an elimination half-life of 3 to 5 hrs in the general population. Estimate the elimination half-life of the drug in this patient.

Solution :

The second plasma sample is taken at 28 hours, i.e., 28/5 = 5.6 half-lives after infusion. The plasma drug concentration in the second sample is more than 95% of the true plasma steady-state drug concentration assuming the highest half-life observed in the general population.

Equation 6.88 can be used to estimate the elimination rate constant and the biological half-life of the drug in the patient.

$$K = \frac{2.303}{t} \log \frac{Css - C}{Css} \qquad .....(6.88)$$

$$K = \frac{2.303}{10} \log \frac{11.9 - 10}{11.9}$$

$$K = 0.1835 \text{ hr}^{-1}$$

$$\text{Biological half-life} = \frac{0.693}{K} = \frac{0.693}{0.18} = 3.776 \text{ hrs}$$

Since $Css = \frac{0.693}{K} = \frac{0.693}{0.18}$, Vd can be calculated.

Assuming $Css = 11.9$ mg/ml

$$Vd = \frac{K0}{Css\,K} = \frac{26}{11.9 \times 0.1835} = 12 \text{ Liters}$$

4. A drug whose K = 0.02 hr^{-1} and Vd = 20 liters is infused to a patient at a rate of 3 mg/hr for 8 hrs. What is the concentration of the drug in the body 2 hours after the cessation of the infusion.

Solution :

Method 1 : Equation 6.93 should be used to solve this problem.

$$C = [\frac{K0}{Vd\,K}]\ (1 - e^{-Kt})\ \ (e^{-Kt^*})$$

Where, t = infustion time = 8 hrs

t* = Post infusion time = 2hrs

$$C = [\frac{3}{20\times0.02}] (1 - e^{-0.02 \times 8}) \quad (e^{-0.02 \times 2})$$

$$= \frac{3}{20\times0.02} \times 0.1479 \quad \times \; 0.96$$

$$C = 1.065 \text{ mg/L}$$

Method 2 : Calculate the concentration of the drug in plasma after 8 hours of infusion using eqation 6.87.

$$C = \frac{K0}{Vd\,K} (1 - e^{-Kt})$$

$$C = \frac{3}{20\times0.02} (1 - e^{-0.02 \times 8}) \quad = \quad 1.1089 \text{ mg/L}$$

Now, treating this concentration of the drug in plasma as initial concentration, calculate the drug plasma level, after 2 hours.

$$C = C0 \,.\, e^{-Kt^*} = 1.1089 \times e^{-0.02 \times 2}$$

$$C = 1.065 \text{ mg/L}$$

The two methods should give the same answer.

5. What is the concentration of a drug after 8 hours after administration of a loading dose of 100 mg and simultaneous infusion of 20 mg/hr (the drug has a $t_{1/2}$ of 3hrs and a volume of distribution 100 L) ?

Solution : $K = 0.693 / 3 = 0.231 \text{ hr}^{-1}$

$$C = \frac{X0}{Vd} \cdot e^{-Kt} + \frac{K0}{Vd\,K} (1 - e^{-Kt})$$

$$= \frac{100}{100} \cdot e^{-0.231 \times 8} + \frac{20}{100\times0.231} (1 - e^{-0.231 \times 8})$$

$$= 0.1576 + 0.7294$$

$$C = 0.887 \text{ mg/L}$$

6. A doctor wants to maintain 2 mg/L of plasma drug level in a patient by administering a loading dose and simultaneously I.V. infusion to get Css of 2 mg/L. If the drug has an elimination rate constant, K = 0.1 hr^{-1} and Vd = 15 L, what is the required loading dose and what is the required infusion rate?

$$Css = \frac{K0}{Vd.K} = 2 \text{ mg/ml}$$

$$\therefore \quad K0 = Css.\, Vd \,.\, K = 3 \text{ mg/hr}$$

Infusion rate = 3 mg/hr

$$\text{Loading dose} = \frac{K0}{K} = \frac{3}{0.1} = 30 \text{ mg}$$

7. An adult male patient (52 years, 70 kg) is to be given an antibiotic by I.V. infusion. According to the literature, the antibiotic has an elimination half-life of 2 hours, Vd of 0.9 L/Kg, and is effective at a plasma drug concentration of 10 mg/L. The drug is supplied in 5ml ampoules containing 200 mg/ml.

   (a) Recommend a starting infusion rate in mg/hour and ml/hour.

Solution :

The effective concentration of the drug in plasma is 10 mg/L. This drug level has to be maintained by infusion, i.e., Css = 10 mg/L

$$\text{Infusion rate, } K0 = Css. Vd. K$$

$$= (10 \text{ mg/L}) \ (0.9 \text{ L/kg x } 70 \text{ kg}) \ \left(\frac{0.693}{2}\right) \text{ hrs}$$

$$= 218.3 \text{ mg/hr}$$

Because the drug is supplied at a concentration of 200 mg/ml,

$$K0 = \frac{218.3}{200} = 1.09 \text{ ml/hr.}$$

8. An adult male asthmatic patient (78 kg, 48 years old) with a history of heavy smoking is given an I.V. infusion of aminophylline at a rate of 0.5 mg/kg per hour. A loading dose of 6 mg/Kg was given by I.V. bolus injection just prior to the start of the infusion. At 2 hours after the start of the infusion, the plasma theophylline concentration is measured and found to contain 5.8 mg/ml. The apparent Vd for theophylline is 0.45 L/Kg. Aminophylline is the ethylenediamine salt of theophylline and contains 80% of theophylline base.

   Because the patient is responding poorly to the aminophylline therapy, the physician wants to increase the plasma theophylline concentration in the patient to 10 mg/ml. What dosage recommondation would you give to the physician ? would you recommend another loading dose ?

Solution :

If no loading dose is given and the infusion rate is increased, the time to reach the steady-state plasma drug concentrations will be about 4 to 5 $t_{1/2}$ to reach 95% of the Css. Therefore, a second loading dose should be recommended to rapidly increase the plasma theophylline concentration to 10 mg/ml. The infusion rate must also be increased to maintain this desired Css.

The calculation of the loading dose, X0, must consider the present plasma theophylline concentration.

$$X0 = \frac{Vd\,(C_{desired} - C_{present})}{(S)(F)}$$

Where, S is the salt form of the drug and F is the fraction of the drug bioavailable. For aminophylline S is equal to 0.80 and for an I.V. bolus injection F is equal to 1.

$$X0 = \frac{(0.45\,L/kg)\,(78\,kg)\,(10 - 5.8\,mg/L)}{[0.80\,(1)]}$$

$$Xo = 184.3 \text{ mg aminophylline}$$

The I.V. injusion rate may be calculated after an estimation of the patient's clearance, CL_t. Because a loading dose and an I.V. infusion of 0.5 mg/hr per kg is given to the patient, the plasma theophyline concentration of 5.8 mg/L is at steady-state Css. Total clearance may be estimated by:

$$CL_t = Vd.\,K = \frac{K0}{Css} = \frac{(0.5\,mg/Kg\,per\,hr)\,(78\,Kg)}{5.8\,mg/L}$$

$$= 6.72 \text{ L/hr or } 1.44 \text{ ml/min/Kg}$$

The usual CL_t for adult, non-smoking patients with uncomplicated asthma is approximately 0.65 ml/min/Kg. Heavy smoking is known to increase the CL_t of theophylline

The new I.V. infusion rate, K0', is calculated by

$$K0' = Css\ desired\ .CL_t$$

$$= (10\ mg/L)\ (6.72\ L/hr) = 67.2\ mg/hr$$

or 0.86 mg/hr per kg.

6.5 Extravascular Administration

6.5.1 Pharmacokinetics of Drug Absorption

Extravascular

In extravascular administration, a drug undergoes the process of absorption before it reaches systemic circulation. The absorption of a drug from the gastrointestinal (GI) tract or any other extravascular site is dependent on the following:

1. Physicochemical properties of the drug
2. Physicochemical properties of dosage form and
3. Anatomy and physiology of the absorption site.

Oral route of administration of a drug is used to develop equations, which are representative of the extravsacular routes of administration of a drug. The absorption of a drug at the absorption site is assumed to follow the first order kinetics. Most of the drugs are absorbed by a passive diffusion process which follows the first order kinetics. Absorption of drugs by active transport can be approximated by the first order kinetics at the concentration of the drug well below the concentration required to saturate the process (Fig. 6.20). Other mechanisms of absorption (facilitated diffusion, pore transport, vesicular transport and Ion-pair transport) contribute very little for transport of drugs. Unless a drug is proved to be absorbed exclusively by a particular mechanism which can not be explained by the first order kinetics, it is generally assumed that the drug absorption follows the first order process.

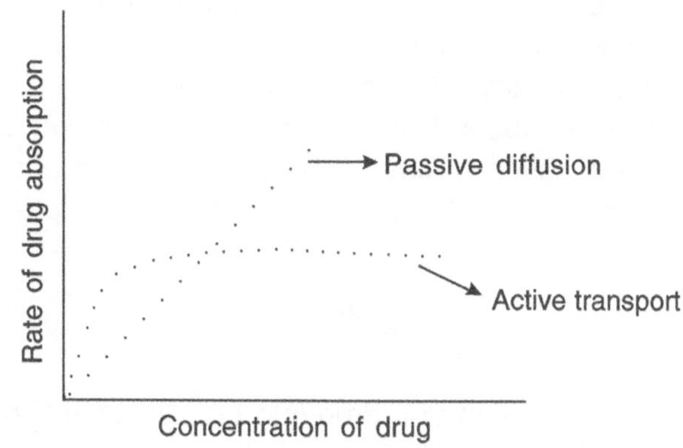

Fig. 6.20 Relation between the rate of absorption of drug & drug concentration at the site of absorption.

The rate of change of the amount of the drug (dX/dt) in the body following extravascular administration is equal to the difference between the rate of absorption (dXa/dt) and the rate of elimination (dXe/dt).

$$\frac{dX}{dt} = \frac{dXa}{dt} - \frac{dXe}{dt} \quad .....(6.115)$$

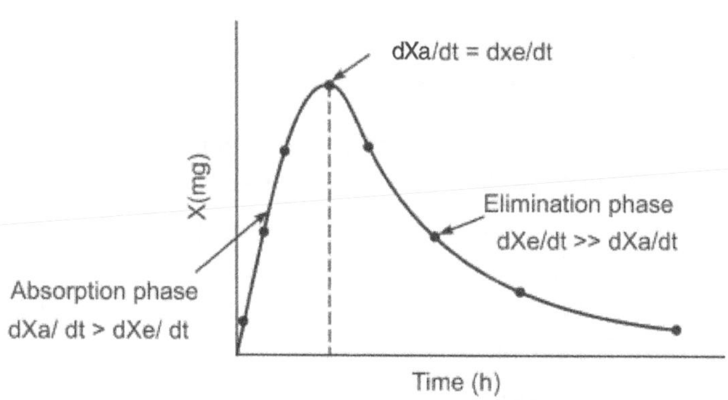

Fig. 6.21 Various phases of a drug plasma level vs time curve for a drug given in a single oral dose.

It should be noted that rate of a process depends on the amount of the drug available for such a process at a given time and is equal to the product of rate constant and the amount of the drug at a given time. Hence, the rate of a process changes with time since the amount of the drug changes with time.

Fig. 6.21 shows the plasma drug level-time curve obtained following a single oral dose of a drug. The curve can be divided into various parts based on relative magnitudes of the rate of absorption and rate of elimination at different time points.

1. **Absorption Phase :** Drugs, through dosage forms, are most frequently administered extravascularly and the majority of them are intended to act systemically; for this reason, absorption is a prerequisite for pharmacological effects. Delays or drug loss during absorption may contribute to variability in drug response and, occasionally, may result in a failure of drug therapy. After the oral administration of a drug, the whole dose of the drug is available for absorption at zero time. The amount of the drug at the absorption site declines as a function of time. Hence, during the absorption phase of a plasma level-time curve (Fig. 6.21), the rate of drug absorption is greater than the rate of drug elimination.

$$\frac{dXa}{dt} > \frac{dXe}{dt} \qquad .....(6.116)$$

2. **Plateau Phase :** Absorption of a drug into the systemic circulation gradually increases the plasma level of the drug as long as the absorption rate is greater than the elimination rate. The gradual increase of the drug level in plasma increases the rate of elimination of drug, dXe/dt, as a function of time. It means that the rate of absorption of drug decreases with time, while the rate of elimination of drug increases with time. Eventually, at a particular time the rate of absorption of the drug and the rate of elimination of drug will become equal. The time at which this occurs is called **time of peak drug concentration** (t_p or t_{max}) in plasma and the concentration is known as **peak concentration** or **maximum plasma drug concentration** (C_{max}), following a single oral dose of the drug. At t_p, the rate of absorption = rate of elimination

$$\frac{dXa}{dt} = \frac{dXe}{dt} \qquad .....(6.117)$$

   During this phase the rate of change of the amount of the drug in the body (dX/dt) is equal to zero. Theoritically, this phase will exist momentarily.

3. **Post Absorption Phase:** Immediately after the plateau phase, the rate of elimination of the drug is faster than the rate of absorption, as represented by the post absorption phase in Fig. 6.21. During this phase the drug levels decline slowly since the absorption of the drug is still in progress.

$$\frac{dXa}{dt} < \frac{dXe}{dt} \qquad .....(6.118)$$

4. **Elimination Phase :** When the drug at the absorption site becomes depleted, the rate of drug absorption approaches zero, or dXa/dt = 0. The **elimination phase** of the curve then represents only the elimination of the drug from the body, which is usually a first order process. Therefore, the rate of change in the amount of the drug in the body during the elimination phase is described by the first order process.

$$\frac{dXe}{dt} = -K\,X \qquad .....(6.119)$$

X = Amount of drug in the body at any time
K = Overall elimination rate constant.

6.5.2 Oral Administration of Drug - Unchanged Drug in Blood/Plasma

The following scheme is used to understand the concept of first order absorption and elimination process in developing equations that describe the time course of drug levels in the body following oral administration.

Scheme 6.5.2

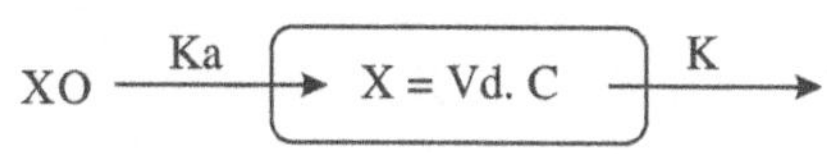

Where, X0 is an oral dose of the drug administered, X is the amount of the drug in the body at any time which is equal to the product of the volume of distribution of the drug and the plasma drug concentration. Ka and K are the first order rate constants of drug absorption and elimination processes, respectively.

For a drug that enters the body by an apparent first order absorption process, and is eliminated by a first order process and distributes in the body according to one compartment model, the following differential equation applies.
Rate of change in drug amount in the body = Rate of drug absorption - Rate of drug elimination .....(6.120)

$$\frac{dX}{dt} = \frac{dXa}{dt} - \frac{dXe}{dt} \qquad .....(6.121)$$

$$\frac{dX}{dt} = Ka\,Xa - KX \qquad .....(6.122)$$

Where Xa is the amount of the drug available at the absorption site at any time.

Let us assume that 'F' is the fraction of the oral dose (X0) that will be absorbed ultimately. At time zero, FX0 amount is available for absorption and it declines as a function of time. Therefore,

$$Xa^{o} = F\,X0 \qquad .....(6.123)$$

Xa^0 = amount of drug available for absorption at t = 0. The rate of disappearance of the drug from the gastrointestinal tract is described by,

$$\frac{dXa}{dt} = -\,Ka\,Xa \qquad .....(6.124)$$

Integration of Equation 6.124 between the limits of t = 0 and t = t, yields the following

$$\int_0^t (dXa/Xa) = -Ka \int_0^t dt$$

$$| \ln Xa|_o^t = -Ka\ |t|_o^t$$

$$\ln Xa - \ln Xa^o = -Kat$$

$$\ln Xa = \ln Xa^o - Kat \quad .....(6.125)$$

But we know that $Xa^o = F\ X0$

$$\ln Xa = \ln F\ X0 - Kat \quad .....(6.126)$$

Equation 6.126 can be written in an exponential form as :

$$Xa = FX0\ .\ e^{-Kat} \quad .....(6.127)$$

The differential equation for the amount of the drug in plasma, is given by eqn. 6.122

$$\frac{dX}{dt} = Ka\ Xa - K\ X$$

but $Xa = F\ X0\ e^{-Kt}$

$$\frac{dX}{dt} = Ka\ F\ X0\ \ e^{-Kat} - K\ X \quad .....(6.128)$$

$$\frac{dX}{dt} + K\ X = Ka\ F\ X0\ \ e^{-Kat} \quad .....(6.129)$$

Multiply Equation 6.129 with e^{Kt} and rearranging it.

$$\frac{dX}{dt}\ e^{Kt} + K\ X\ e^{Kt} = Ka\ F\ X0\ e^{-(Ka-K)t}$$

$$dX\ \ e^{Kt} + K\ X\ e^{Kt}\ dt = Ka\ F\ X0\ \ e^{-(Ka-K)t}\ \ dt \quad .....(6.130)$$

Integrating equation 6.130 between limits t = 0 and t = t

$$\int_0^t (dX\ \ e^{Kt} + K\ X\ e^{Kt}\ \ dt) = Ka\ F\ X0 \int_0^t e^{-(Ka-K)}\ dt$$

$$X\ e^{Kt} = Ka\ F\ X0\ [\frac{e^{-(Ka-K)t}}{-(Ka-K)} + \frac{1}{(Ka-K)}]$$

$$X\ e^{Kt} = \frac{Ka\ F\ X0}{(Ka-K)}\ [1 - e^{-(Ka-K)t}] \quad .....(6.131)$$

Dividing equation 6.131 but e^{Kt}, we get

$$X = \frac{Ka\,F\,X0}{(Ka - K)}\left[\frac{1}{e^{Kt}} - \frac{e^{-(Ka-K)}}{e^{Kt}}\right]$$

$$X = \frac{Ka\,F\,X0}{(Ka - K)}\left(e^{-Kt} - e^{-Kat}\right) \qquad .....(6.132)$$

Equation 6.132 describes the time course of the amount of the drug in the body. But plasma drug concentration - time data is used in pharmacokinetic study. Dividing equation 6.132 by the volume of distribution of drug (Vd),

$$\frac{X}{Vd} = C = \frac{Ka\,F\,X0}{Vd\,(Ka - K)}\left(e^{-Kt} - e^{-Kat}\right) \qquad .....(6.133)$$

Equation 6.133 describes the time course of the drug concentration in plasma following the oral route of administration. A survey of the literature indicates that for most drugs administered in readily available dosage forms, the absorption rate constant (Ka) is significantly larger than the elimination rate constant (K). Exceptions to this general observations are also found in the literature, which will be discussed later in this chapter. If Ka is much larger than K (a good rule is that it must be at least five times larger), the second exponential (e^{-Kat}) in equation 6.133 will approach zero much more rapidly that the first exponential term (e^{-Kt}). And at larger values of t, equation 6.133 will reduce to,

$$C = \frac{Ka\,F\,X0}{Vd\,(Ka - K)}\,e^{-Kt} \qquad .....(6.134)$$

Equation 6.134 explains the elimination phase (i.e. the time when absorption no longer occurs) of the plasma drug concentration-time curve (Fig. 6.22). Equation 6.134 can be written in common logarithms as :

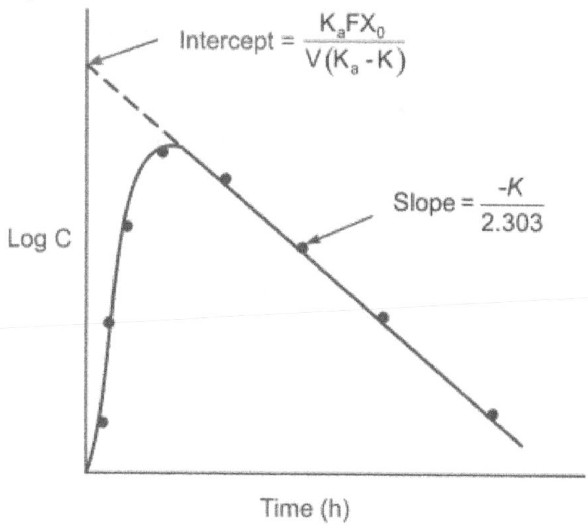

Fig. 6.22 Semilogarithmic plasma drug concentration vs time curve after single oral dose administration.

$$\log C = \log \left[\frac{Ka\, F\, X0}{Vd\,(Ka - K)}\right] - K\, t/2.303 \qquad .....(6.135)$$

A plot of the log of the plasma drug concentration versus time yields a bioexponential curve initially and becomes linear during the elimination phase, which is described by Equation 6.135 (Fig. 6.22). The slope of the terminal linear portion of the graph is equal to -K/2.303 and the intercept is equal to log Ka F X0/Vd (Ka-K). Hence, the value of the elimination rate constant, K can be obtained from the slope of the terminal linear portion and elimination of the half-life of the drug is given by 0.693/K.

Determination of Absorption Rate Constant From Oral Data

1. **Method of Residuals:** The time course of drug concentration in plasma following an oral administration of a drug is given by Equation 6.133. The value of Ka is obtained by using the following procedure.
   (a) Plot the drug concentration versus time on semilog paper with the concentration values on the logarithmic axis.
   (b) Calculate the slope of the terminal linear portion of the graph. From the slope calculate, 'K' and the elimination half-life.
   (c) Extend the terminal linear portion of the graph to cut Y-axis. The intercept is equal to Ka F X0/Vd (Ka-K).
   (d) Apply the method of residuals (for details see Appendix-III) to obtain residual concentration time data and plot the data on the same graph paper to obtain residual line Fig. 6.23. The slope of the residual line is equal to -Ka/2.303. Calculate the absorption rate constant, Ka, and absorption half-life, which is equal to 0.693/Ka.

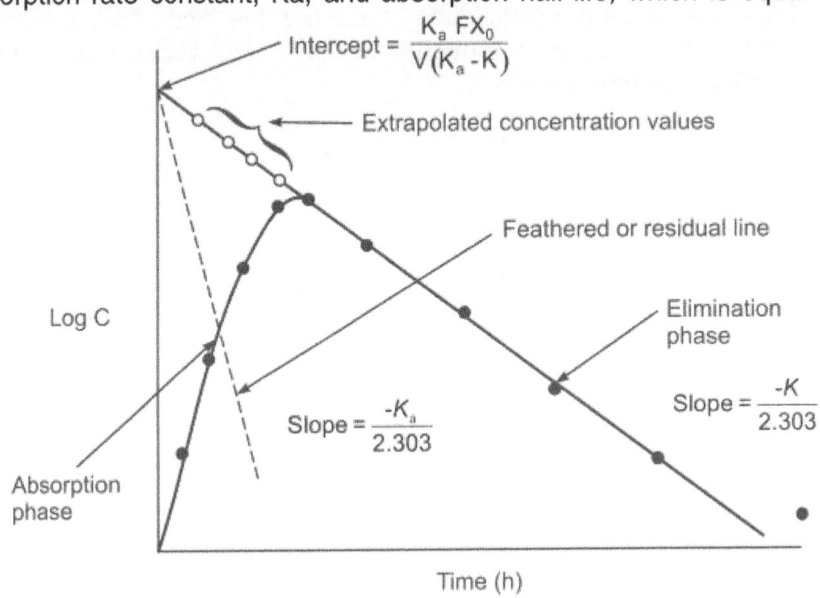

Fig. 6.23 Semilogarithmic plot showing calculation of absorption rate constant by method of residuals.

2. **Wagner-Nelson Method :** In the method of residuals, the absorption process is assumed to be of the first order kinetics. This assumption is valid for solutions and rapidly dissolving dosage forms, where the absorption process itself is rate determining. In cases where the release of the drug from the dosage form is rate limiting, the kinetics are often zero-order, mixed zero and first order, or even more complex processes.

The Wagner-Nelson method of calculation does not require a model assumption concerning the absorption process. It does require the assumption that (1) the body behaves as a single homogeneous compartment, and (2) drug elimination obeys the first order kinetics.

Derivation : For any extravascular drug administration, the mass balance equation can be written as the amount administered equals the amount absorbed (A) plus the amount unabsorbed, (Aun), that is the amount of the drug remained at the absorption site.

$$X0 = A + Aun \quad \text{.....(6.136)}$$

The amount absorbed (A) to any time t, is equal to the sum of the amount of the drug in body (X) and the amount of the drug eliminated from the body to time, t (Xe).

$$A = X + Xe \quad \text{.....(6.137)}$$

Taking the derivative with respect to time yields

$$\frac{dA}{dt} = \frac{dX}{dt} + \frac{dXe}{dt} \quad \text{.....(6.138)}$$

But $X = Vd\ C$, hence

$$\frac{dX}{dt} = Vd\ \frac{dC}{dt} \quad \text{.....(6.139)}$$

and $dXe / dt = KX$ but $X = Vd\ C$

Therefore, $$\frac{dXe}{dt} = K\ Vd\ C \quad \text{.....(6.140)}$$

Therefore, $$\frac{dA}{dt} = Vd.\ \frac{dC}{dt} + K\ Vd\ C \quad \text{.....(6.141)}$$

$$dA = Vd\ dC + K\ Vd\ C\ dt \quad \text{.....(6.142)}$$

Integrating equation 6.142 between limits of t = 0 to t = t gives,

$$\int_0^t dA = Vd \int_0^t dC + K\ Vd \int_0^t C\ dt$$

$$A_t - A_o = Vd\ |\ C_t - C_o\ |\ + K\ Vd \int_0^t C.\ dt \quad \text{.....(6.143)}$$

A0 = amount of drug absorbed at t = 0 is equal to zero and the concentration of the drug in the body at t = 0 also equal to zero. So,

$$A_t = Vd\ Ct + K\ Vd \int_0^t C\ dt \qquad .....(6.144)$$

Rearranging the equation 6.144,

$$\frac{At}{Vd} = C_t + K \int_0^t C\ dt \qquad .....(6.145)$$

Where At/Vd is the amount of the drug absorbed up to time t divided by the volume of distribution.

Ct = The plasma (serum or blood) concentration at time t

$\int_0^t C\ dt\ C\ dt$ = The area under the plasma (serum or blood) concentration versus time curve up to time t.

Integrating equation 6.142 between the limits of t = 0 to t = ∞ and rearranging the resultant equation, gives the following

$$\int_0^\infty dA = Vd \int_0^\infty dC + KVd \int_0^\infty C.\ dt$$

$$A\infty = Vd\ (C_\infty - C_0) + K\ Vd \int_0^\infty C.dt \quad \text{but} \quad C_\infty = 0\ C_0 = 0$$

Therefore, $$A\infty = K\ Vd \int_0^\infty C.\ dt. \qquad .....(6.146)$$

or $$\frac{A\infty}{Vd} = K \int_0^\infty C.\ dt \qquad .....(6.147)$$

Where, $A\infty/Vd$ = the total amount of the drug absorbed from the dosage form up to infinite time divided by the volume of distribution of the drug.

$\int_0^\infty C.dt$ = The area under the entire plasma (serum or blood) concentration versus time curve.

The fraction of the drug absorbed at any time is obtained when Equation 6.145 is divided by Equation 6.147.

$$(At/Vd)/(A_\infty/Vd) = (Ct + K\int_0^t C.\,dt)/(K\int_0^\infty Cdt) \qquad \text{.....(6.148)}$$

$$At/A_\infty = (Ct + K\int_0^t Cdt)/(K\int_0^\infty Cdt) \qquad \text{.....(6.149)}$$

The fraction unabsorbed at any time t is

$$\left(1-\frac{At}{A\infty}\right) = [1-(Ct+K\int_0^t Cdt/K\int_0^\infty Cdt)] \qquad \text{.....(6.150)}$$

$$100\left(1-\frac{At}{A\infty}\right) = 100\,[1-(Ct+K\int_0^t Cdt/K\int_0^\infty Cdt)] \qquad \text{.....(6.151)}$$

The percent unabsorbed at any time t can be calculated using Equation 6.151. If a plot of percent-unabsorbed drug versus time gives a straight line then the absorption process is zero-order. A semi-logarithmic plot of the percent unabsorbed versus time yields a straight line, then the absorption process is said to follow the first-order kinetics. The slope of the straight line is equal to -Ka/2.303 (Fig. 6.24).

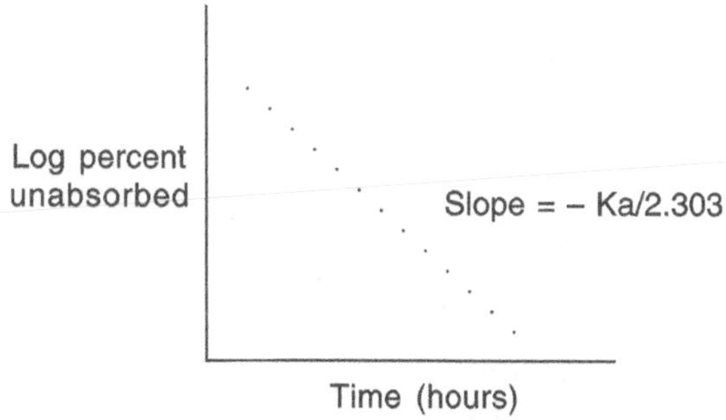

Fig. 6.24 Logarithm of the percent unabsorbed versus time plot showing the first-order absorption process.

The Wagner-Nelson method allows us to understand the absorption kinetics without any prior assumption. This method is also useful for studying the mechanism of release of drugs from dosage forms *in vivo*. In general the absorption process itself usually obeys the first order kinetics, whereas the dissolution of capsules, tablets, especially sustained release dosage forms, often must be described by more complex kinetic mechanisms.

Determination of C_{max} and t_p

Maximum plasma concentration, $\mathbf{C_{max}}$, following a single oral dose of a drug occurs at the plateau of the plasma concentration-time curve. The time needed to reach the maximum concentration is called peak time, t_p. The time needed to reach $\mathbf{C_{max}}$ is independent of the dose and is dependent on the rate constants for absorption (Ka) and elimination (K). At the maximum concentration, some times called peak concentration, the rate of drug absorption is equal to the rate of drug elimination. Therefore, the rate of concentration change, dC/dt, is equal to zero.

The rate of concentration change can be obtained by differentiating equation 6.133, as follows,

$$C = \frac{Ka\,F\,X0}{Vd\,(Ka - K)} \left(e^{-Kt} - e^{-Kat}\right)$$

Which when differentiated with respect to time,

$$\frac{dC}{dt} = \frac{-K\,Ka\,F\,X0}{Vd\,(Ka - K)}\,e^{-Kt} + \frac{Ka^2\,F\,X0}{Vd\,(Ka - K)}\,e^{-Kat} \qquad .....(6.152)$$

When the plasma concentration reaches C_{max} at time t_p, dC/dt = 0, therefore

$$\frac{K\,Ka\,F\,X0}{Vd\,(Ka - K)}\,e^{-Ktp} = \frac{Ka^2\,F\,X0}{Vd\,(Ka - K)}\,e^{-Ka\,tp}$$

Which can be simplified to,

$$K\,e^{-Ktp} = Ka\,e^{-Katp} \qquad .....(6.153)$$

or

$$\frac{Ka}{K} = \frac{e^{-Ktp}}{e^{-Katp}}$$

In common logarithms:

$$\log \frac{Ka}{K} = \frac{-Kt_p}{2.303} + \frac{Kat_p}{2.303}$$

therefore,

$$t_p = \frac{2.303}{(Ka - K)} \log \frac{Ka}{K} \qquad .....(6.154)$$

As explained earlier, t_p, is dependent only on the rate constants Ka and K.

The maximum concentration of the drug in plasma occurs at t_p, hence, by substituting t_p for t in Equation 6.133, we get equation

$$C_{max} = \frac{Ka\,F\,X0}{Vd\,(Ka - K)} \left(e^{-Ktp} - e^{-Katp}\right) \qquad .....(6.155)$$

However, a much simpler expression can be obtained from Equation 6.155, by substituting e^{-Katp} equal to K/Ka e^{-Ktp} according to Equation 6.153,

$$C_{max} = \frac{Ka\,F\,X0}{Vd\,(Ka - K)} \left(e^{-Ktp} - \frac{Ka}{K}\, e^{-Ktp}\right) \qquad .....(6.156)$$

$$= \frac{Ka\,F\,X0\,e^{-Ktp}}{Vd\,(Ka - K)} \left(1 - \frac{Ka}{K}\right)$$

$$= \frac{Ka\,F\,X0}{Vd\,(Ka - K)}\,\frac{(Ka - K)}{Ka}\, e^{-Ktp}$$

$$C_{max} = \frac{F\,X0}{Vd}\, e^{-Ktp} \qquad .....(6.157)$$

Therefore C_{max} observed following the first order input is a function of the fraction of the dose entering the body, the apparent volume of distribution, and the apparent first order absorption and elimination rate constants.

Volume of distribution (Vd)

For a drug administered by the oral, or any other extravascular, route of administration, the apparent volume of distribution cannot be calculated from plasma drug concentration data alone. The reason is that the value of F (the fraction of administered dose that reaches the general circulation) is not known.

Extrapolation of the terminal linear portion of the semilog plot of the plasma drug concentration versus time Fig. 6.23 gives an intercept equal to the following,

$$\text{Intercept (I)} = \frac{Ka\,F\,X0}{Vd\,(Ka - K)} \qquad .....(6.158)$$

or

$$Vd = \frac{Ka\,F\,X0}{I\,(Ka - K)} \qquad .....(6.159)$$

If the fraction of the dose absorbed is equal to unity (i.e., F = 1) then

$$Vd = \frac{Ka\,X0}{I\,(Ka - K)} \qquad .....(6.160)$$

An estimate of Vd, can be made from Equation 6.160, since all other terms in the equation are known. If the value of F is known, equation 6.159 can be used to estimate the volume of distribution, Vd.

A more satisfactory method for determining the volume of distribution following the first order absorption is obtained by integrating equation 6.133, between t = 0 to t = ∞,

$$\int_0^\infty C\,dt = [(Ka\ F\ X0)/Vd\ (Ka\text{-}K)] \int_0^\infty (e^{-Kt} - e^{-Kat})\,dt$$

$$\int_0^\infty Cdt = [AUC]_0^\infty$$

$$[AUC]_0^\infty = \frac{Ka\,F\,X0}{Vd\,(Ka-K)} \left[\left|\frac{e^{-Kt}}{-K_1}\right|_0^\infty - \left|\frac{e^{-Kat}}{-K_a}\right|_0^\infty \right]$$

$$[AUC]_0^\infty = \frac{Ka\,F\,X0}{Vd\,(Ka-K)} \left(\frac{1}{K} - \frac{1}{Ka}\right) \qquad .....(6.161)$$

where $\frac{Ka\,F\,X0}{Vd\,(Ka-K)}$ = I, the zero time intercept.

Equation 6.161 readily permits the estimation of the area under the plasma concentration-time curve, since the values of Ka, K and zero time intercept, I are known.

Further simplification of Equation 6.161 yields,

$$[AUC]_0^\infty = \frac{Ka\,F\,X0}{Vd\,K\,(Ka-K)} - \frac{Ka\,F\,X0}{Vd\,Ka\,(Ka-K)}$$

$$= \frac{Ka\,F\,X0 - K\,F\,X0}{Vd\,K\,(Ka-K)}$$

$$[AUC]_0^\infty = \frac{F\,X0}{Vd\,K}\,\frac{(Ka-K)}{(Ka-K)} = \frac{F\,X0}{Vd\,K} \qquad .....(6.162)$$

Which is an equation for the total area under the plasma drug concentration-time curve from t = 0 to t = ∞ after a first order absorption. Rearrangement of Equation 6.162 results,

$$Vd = \frac{F\,X0}{K[AUC]_0^\infty} \qquad .....(6.163)$$

Equation 6.163, enables the calculation of the apparent volume of distribution of a drug from the plasma drug concentration-time data obtained following the first order absorption.

Lag Time

In some instances absorption of the drug after a single oral dose does not start immediately due to such physiological factors as stomach-emptying time and intestinal mobility or due to formulation itself. The time delay prior to the commencement of the first order drug absorption is known as **lag time** (t_l).

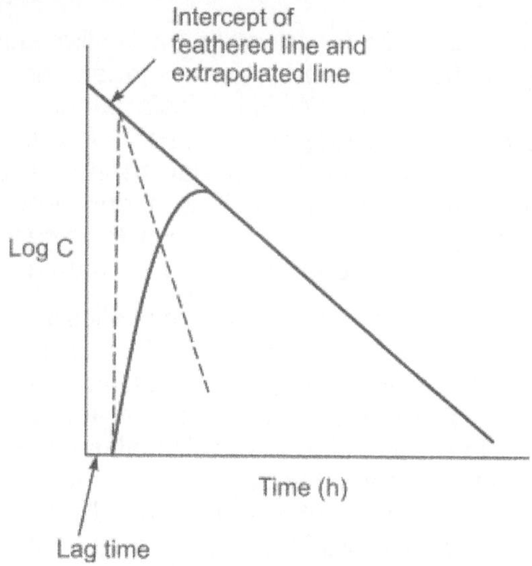

Fig 6.25 Semilogarithmic graph between plasma drug concentration versus time showing lag time.

Irrespective of the relative magnitudes of the constants for absorption and elimination, the same intercept on the log concentration axis [log KaFX0/Vd Ka-K] should be obtained on extrapolation of the terminal exponential phase and the residual line to time zero. Interaction of these two lines at some point in time greater than t = 0 suggests that there is a lag time (t_l) before absorption. The time at which two lines intersect is used to find out lag time. A perpendicular drawn on to X-axis from the point of intersection of the lines gives the lag time (Fig. 6.25).

The lag time, t_l, represents the beginning of drug absorption and a more appropriate equation that can adequately describe the curve in Fig. 6.25 can be obtained by subtracting the lag time from each time point, as shown in Equation 6.164.

$$C = \frac{Ka\,F\,X0}{Vd\,(Ka - K)}\,(e^{-K(t-t_e)} - e^{-Ka(t-t_e)}) \qquad .....(6.164)$$

Where Ka F X0/Vd(Ka-K) is the y value at the point of intersection of the lines in Fig. 6.24.

A second expression that describes the curve in Fig. 6.24 can be written without considering the lag time.

$$C = B.e^{-Kt} - A.e^{-Kat} \qquad .....(6.165)$$

Where, A and B represent the intercepts on Y-axis after extrapolation of the lines for absorption and elimination, respectively.

Flip-flop of Ka and K

The estimation of the rate constants for absorption and elimination by method of residuals is based on the assumption that Ka >> K. Hence, the terminal phase of the plasma level time curve represents elimination (from which K is calculated) and the residual line obtained by feathering plasma level-time curve represents absorption (from which Ka is calculated). If K >> Ka, then the values of Ka and K are obtained in a reverse way. i.e. Ka from the terminal phase and K from the residual line. This phenomenon is called **flip-flop** of the absorption and elimination rate constants. The only way to be sure of estimates is to compare the K calculated from oral administration with K from intravenous data.

Most of the drugs observed to have flip-flop characteristics are drugs with a fast elimination (i.e. K > Ka). The absorption rate constant for a given drug can change as a result of changing the formulation, the dosage form (tablet, suspension and capsule) or the extravascular route of drug administration (oral, intramuscular, subcutaneous, etc.). Administration of a drug with or without food will also influence the absorption rate constant for the same drug administered orally through the same formulation of the same dosage form. Drug absorption of most drug solutions or rapidly dissolving products are essentially complete or at least half completed within an hour (i.e. absorption half life is 0.5 to 1 hour, corresponding to a Ka of 1.38 hr^{-1} to 0.69 hr^{-1}). Because most of the drugs used orally have longer elimination half-lives, the assumption of using a smaller rate constant (i.e. the terminal phase of plasma level-time curve) as an elimination rate constant is generally correct.

The larger the elimination rate constant (K > 0.69 hr^{-1}) of a drug, the greater is the chance for the flip-flop of Ka and K. The flip-flop of Ka and K has been noted for isoproterenol which has an oral half life of only a few minutes (i.e. K >> 0.69 hr^{-1}). The flip-flop of Ka and K has been reported for salicyluric acid which has K much larger than Ka.

Special Case where Ka = K

A situation may occur in theory where the absorption rate constant and elimination rate constant of a drug are equal. For such a situation an equation that describes the time course of drug concentration in plasma can be developed using Equation 6.130.

$$\int_0^t dX\, e^{Kt} + K\, X\, e^{Kt} \int_0^t dt = Ka\, F\, X0 \int_0^t e^{-(Ka-K)t}\, dt \qquad .....(6.130)$$

Since Ka = K, we can write Ka = K = K'.

Substituting K' for K and Ka in Equation 6.130.

$$\int_0^t dX\, e^{K't} + K'\, X\, e^{K't} \int_0^t dt = K'\, F\, X0 \int_0^t e^{-(K'-K')t}.\, dt \qquad .....(6.166)$$

$$X\, e^{K't} = K'\, F\, X0 \int_0^t e^0\, dt \qquad .....(6.167)$$

$$X\, e^{K't} = K'\, F\, X0\, t \qquad .....(6.168)$$

$$X = K'\, F\, X0\, t\, e^{-K't} \qquad .....(6.169)$$

In concentration terms,

$$C = \frac{K' F X0}{Vd} \Big|_0^t t.\ e^{-K't} \quad .....(6.170)$$

In logarithmic form,

$$\log C = \log \left[\frac{K' F X0}{Vd}\right] - \frac{K' t}{2.303} \quad .....(6.171)$$

A plot of log C versus time will be a curve from time zero to infinity, because 't' is present in intercept value which is a variable.

The rate of change in plasma drug concentration, dC/dt can be obtained by differentiating equation 6.170 with respect to time using formula differentiation of

$$U.V. = \frac{du}{dy} V + \frac{dv}{dy} U.$$

$$\frac{dC}{dt} = \frac{K' F X0}{Vd} e^{-K't} - \frac{K'^2 F X0}{Vd} t\ e^{-K't} \quad .....(6.172)$$

At C_{max}, dC/dt = 0 and time is equal to t_p. Therefore

$$\frac{K' F X0}{Vd} e^{-K'tp} = \frac{K'^2 F X0}{Vd} t_p\ e^{-K'tp}$$

$$t_p = \frac{1}{K'} \quad .....(6.173)$$

Substitution of t_p for t in Equation 6.170 yields an equation for C_{max}.

$$C_{max} = \frac{K' F X0}{Vd} t_p\ e^{-K'tp} \quad .....(6.174)$$

but $t_p = 1/K'$

$$C_{max} = \frac{K' F X0}{Vd} \frac{1}{K'} e^{-K'\ 1/K'}$$

$$C_{max} = (FX0/Vd)\ e^{-1} = 0.3679\ FX0/Vd \quad .....(6.175)$$

C_{max} is dependent only on the fraction of the dose absorbed and the volume of distribution.

6.5.3 Oral Administration of Drug - Unchanged Drug in Urine

Urinary excretion data obtained following the first order input into a one compartment model can be treated in the same manner as when a drug is administered intravenously. The reader is advised to refer to the urinary kinetics of the drug following I.V. bolus to understand the factors affecting urinary excretion of drugs.

Scheme 6.5.3

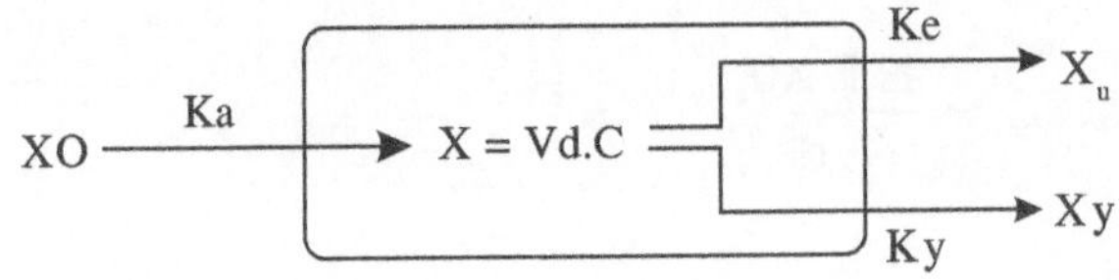

Where, all the terms are as defined previously.

Excretion Rate Method

The amount of the unchanged drug excreted in urine is only dependent on the amount of unchanged drug in the body. The rate of urinary excretion of the unchanged drug is given by,

$$\frac{dXu}{dt} = Ke\ X \qquad .....(6.176)$$

but
$$X = \frac{Ka\,F\,X0}{(Ka - K)}\left(e^{-Kt} - e^{-Kat}\right)$$

Substituting X value in 6.176

$$\frac{dXu}{dt} = \frac{Ke\,Ka\,F\,X0}{(Ka - K)}\left(e^{-Kt} - e^{-Kat}\right) \qquad .....(6.177)$$

Because the rate of urinary drug excretion, dXu/dt can not be determined directly, ΔXu/Δt is used, which is the average rate of urinary drug excretion at the mid point of urine collection period (t'). Therefore,

$$\frac{\Delta Xu}{\Delta t} = \frac{Ke\,Ka\,F\,X0}{(Ka - K)}\left(e^{-Kt'} - e^{-Kat'}\right) \qquad .....(6.178)$$

Where in t' = mid-point of urine collection period. In practice, ΔXu/Δt is assumed to be equal to dXu/dt and is valid if the urinary sampling time intervals are short.

If Ka >> K, the term $e^{-Kat'}$ in equation 6.178 will approach to zero after some time (after post absorption phase) but the term $e^{-Kt'}$ still has some finite value. Therefore, after some time, Equation 6.178 becomes,

$$\frac{\Delta Xu}{\Delta t} = \frac{Ke\,Ka\,F\,X0}{(Ka - K)}\left(e^{-Kt'}\right) \qquad .....(6.179)$$

In logarithmic form,

$$\log \frac{\Delta Xu}{\Delta t} = \log \left[\frac{Ke\,Ka\,F\,X0}{(Ka - K)}\right] - \frac{Kt'}{2.303} \qquad .....(6.180)$$

A plot of (ΔXu/Δt) versus the mid point of urine collection period will yield a curve (Fig. 6.26a) identical in appearance to the plasma level-time curve (Fig. 6.26b)

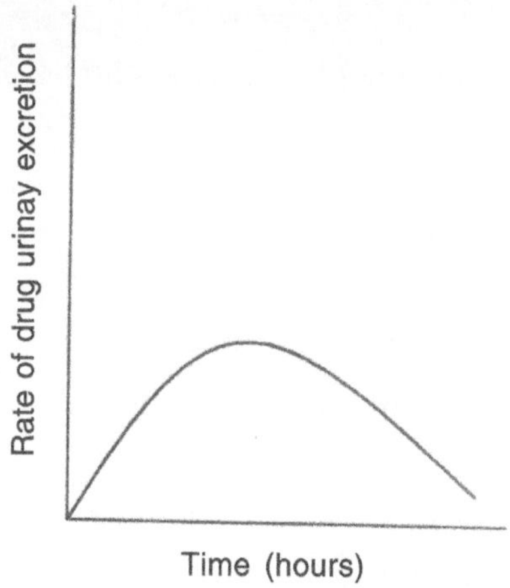

Fig. 6.26 (A) Rate of urinary drug excretion versus time plot following a single oral dose.

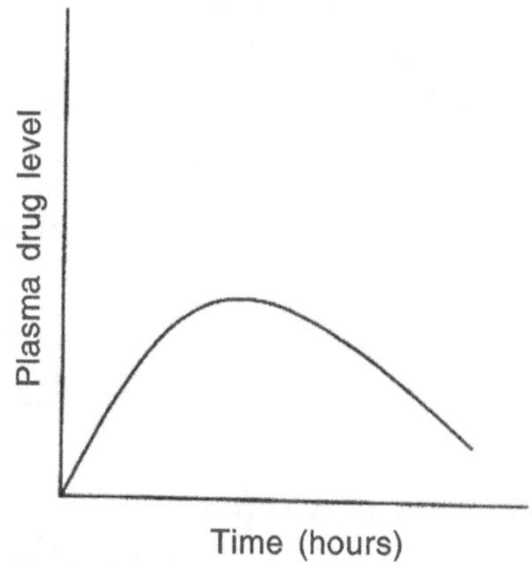

Fig. 6.26 (B) Plasma drug level versus time plot following a single oral dose.

A plot of log ($\Delta Xu/\Delta t$) versus t' is used to calculate the pharmacokinetic parameters (Fig. 6.27), also the slope of the terminal linear portion of the plot is equal to -K/2.303. The absorption rate constant, Ka is calculated from the slope of the residual line obtained by the method of residuals. The intercepts of both the lines are equal (i.e. log Ke Ka F X0/(Ka-K). If the fraction of the dose absorbed, F and the oral dose, X0 are known, Ke can be calculated from the intercept.

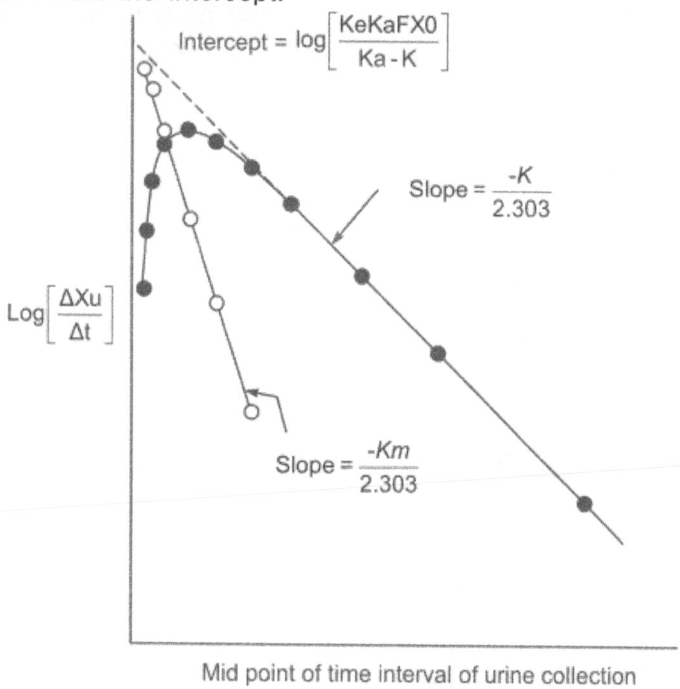

Fig. 6.27 Computation of rate constants from plot of rate of drug excreted in urine vs mid time points of urine collection period.

Sigma-Minus Method

Cumulative amount of the unchanged drug excreted in urine upto any time can be obtained by integrating Equation 6.177 between t = 0 to t = t.

$$\int_0^t dXu = \int_0^t [(Ke\ Ka\ F\ X0)/(Ka - K)](e^{-Kt} - e^{-Kat})\ dt$$

$$X_u^t - X_u^o = \frac{Ke\,Ka\,F\,X0}{(Ka - K)}\left[\frac{e^{-Kt}}{-K} + \frac{1}{K} - \left(\frac{e^{-Kat}}{-Ka} + \frac{1}{Ka}\right)\right] \qquad .....(6.181)$$

Xu^o = cumulative amount of drug excreted in urine at t = 0 is equal to zero. Simplifying Equation 6.181, we get

$$Xu^t = \frac{Ke\,FX0}{K} + \frac{Ke\,Ka\,FX0}{(Ka - K)}\left(\frac{e^{-Kat}}{Ka} - \frac{e^{-Kt}}{K}\right) \qquad .....(6.182)$$

A plot of Xu^t versus time will give the urinary excretion curve described in Fig. 6.27. When the total drug has been excreted, i.e., at t = ∞, Equation 6.182 reduces to,

$$Xu^{\infty} = \frac{Ke\,F\,X0}{K} \qquad .....(6.183)$$

Where in Xu^{∞} is the total amount of the unchanged drug excreted in urine in infinite time.

An equation that describes the amount of the drug to be excreted versus time (Fig. 6.28) can be developed from Equations 6.182 and 6.183.

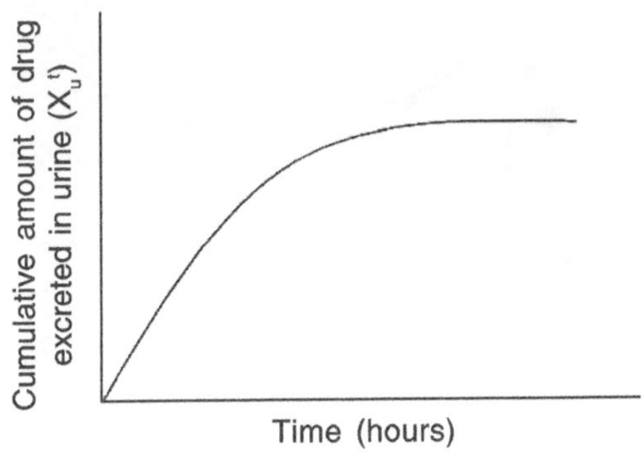

Fig. 6.28 Cumulative amount of drug excreted in urine versus time plot.

$$Xu^{\infty} - Xu^t = \frac{Xu^{\infty}}{(Ka - K)}\,(Ka.e^{-Kt} - K.\ e^{-Kat}) \qquad .....(6.184)$$

A plot of log (Xu^{∞} - Xu^t) versus time is used to calculate the pharmacokinetic parameters (Fig. 6.29). The slope of the terminal linear portion of the graph is equal to -K/2.303. A residual line can be obtained by the method of residuals, the slope of which is equal to -Ka/2.303.

Since, X_u^∞ = Ke F X0/K, Ke can be calculated if F and X0 are known.

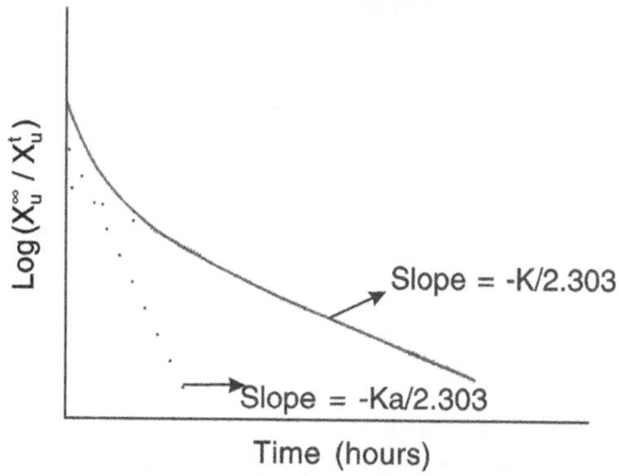

Fig. 6.29 Log (X_u^∞ / X_u^t) versus time plot.

Practice Problems

1. A 59 Kg male received 2 mg/kg of an antibiotic orally. The following plasma concentration versus time data is obtained. Assume that the drug follows one compartment open model and is completely absorbed. Calculate the following
   (a) Estimation rate constant (K) and biological half-life ($t_{1/2}$)
   (b) Absorption rate constant (Ka) and absorption half-life
   (c) Volume of distribution, Vd
   (d) t_{max} or t_p and C_{max}
   (e) AUC

Time (hrs)	Plasma concentration (mg/ml)
0.25	2.2
0.5	3.8
0.75	5.0
1.0	5.8
1.5	6.8
2.0	7.1
2.5	7.1
3.0	6.9
4.0	6.2
6.0	4.8
8.0	3.5
12.0	1.9
18.0	0.8
24.0	0.3

(a) Plot plasma concentration versus time data on a semi-logarithmic paper. Find out the terminal linear portion of the graph. The slope of this line is - K/2.303.

Slope = 0.0669

$K = 0.0669 \times 2.303 = 0.154\ hr^{-1}$

$$\text{Biological half-life} = \frac{0.693}{K} = \frac{0.693}{0.154} = 4.5 \text{ hrs.}$$

(b) Extrapolate the terminal linear portion to cut Y-axis. Measure the plasma concentration on the extrapolated line at sampling times. Calculate the difference between the concentrations on the extrapolated line and practical data. These concentrations are called "Residual plasma concentrations". Plot a graph on the same paper taking the residual concentrations on a log scale and time on an ordinary scale. Fit the data points to yield a straight line, the slope of which is equal to -Ka/2.303.

Time (hrs)	Observed plasma Conc (μg/ml)	Extrapolated plasma Conc (μg/ml)	Residual plasma Conc. (μg/ml)
0.25	2.2	11.4	9.2
0.5	3.8	10.9	7.1
0.75	5.0	10.6	5.6
1.0	5.8	10.1	4.3
1.5	6.8	9.4	2.6
2.0	7.1	8.7	1.6
2.5	7.1	8.1	1.0
3.0	6.9	7.5	0.6
4.0	6.2	6.4	0.2
6.0	4.8	4.8	—
8.0	3.5	3.5	—
12.0	1.9	1.9	—
18.0	0.8	0.8	—
24.0	0.3	0.3	—

Slope = 0.43

Absorption rate constant (Ka) =

$\text{slope} \times 2.303 = 0.43 \times 2.303 = 0.99\ hr^{-1}$

Absorption half-life

$$= \frac{0.693}{Ka} = \frac{0.693}{0.99} = 0.7 \text{ hrs.}$$

(c) Read the value of the intercept obtained by extrapolating the terminal linear portion of the graph.

Intercept = 11.8 μg/ml

Therefore, $$11.8 = \frac{Ka\,F\,X0}{Vd(Ka - K)}$$

The drug is completely absorbed,

so F = 1 and X0 = 2 mg/Kg x 59 Kg = 118 mg

Volume of distribution

$$(Vd) = \frac{0.99 \times 1 \times 118 mg}{11.8(0.99 - 0.154)}$$

$$= \frac{116.92}{9.8648} = 11.842 \text{ Liters}$$

(d) Time at which peak concentration occurs (tp) or t_{max}

$$= \frac{2.303}{(Ka - K)} \log \frac{Ka}{K}$$

$$= \frac{2.303}{(0.99 - 0.154)} \log \frac{0.99}{0.154} = 2.226 \text{ hrs}$$

Maximum plasma concentration, C_{max}

$$C_{max} = .\frac{FX0}{Vd}\ e^{-Ktp} = \frac{1 \times 118}{11.842} \times e^{-0.154 \times 2.226}$$

= 7.1 μg/ml

(e) AUC

$$AUC_0^t = \frac{1}{2}(C_0 + C_1)(t_1 - t_0) + \frac{1}{2}(C_1 + C_2)(t_2 - t_1) + \ldots\ldots + \frac{1}{2}(C_{n-1} + C_n)(t_n - t_{n-1})$$

$$AUC = \frac{1}{2}(0 + 2.2)(0.25 - 0) + \frac{1}{2}(2.2 + 3.8)(0.5 - 0.25) + \frac{1}{2}(3.8 + 5)(0.75 - 0.5) + \ldots\ldots. + \frac{1}{2}(0.8 + 0.3)(24 - 18) = 65.20 \ \mu gh/ml$$

$$AUC_t^{\infty} = C^*/K = 0.3/0.154 = 1.95 \ \mu g\text{-}hr/ml$$

$$AUC_t^{\infty} = 65.20 + 1.95 = 66.3 \ \mu g\text{-}hr/ml$$

2. A drug is injected intramuscularly to a healthy volunteer and the following plasma concentration of the drug versus time data obtained. Calculate the absorption rate constant and state the order of the absorption process.

Time (hrs)	Plasma Drug concentration (mg/ml)
0.25	0.6
0.50	1.2
0.75	1.8
1.0	2.3
1.5	3.4
2.0	4.3
3.0	6.0
6.0	5.6
12.0	2.3
18.0	0.9
24.0	0.4

Solution :

The order of the absorption process can be assessed with the Wagner-Nelson method. Therefore, the Wagner-Nelson method should be used here for the calculation of the absorption rate constant.

The equation used is

$$\frac{At}{Vd} = C_t + K \int_0^t C.\, dt \qquad .....(6.185)$$

Step 1. A semilog plot of plasma drug concentration versus time should be made. The slope of the terminal linear portion of the graph is equal to -K/2.303

$$\text{Slope} = 0.0651$$

$$K = 0.651 \times 2.303 = 0.15 \text{ hr}^{-1}$$

Biological half-life

$$(t_{1/2}) = \frac{0.693}{0.15} = 4.62 \text{ hrs}$$

Construct the following table :

Time (hrs)	Plasma Drug Conc. (μg/ml)	$\int_0^t C.dt$	$K\int_0^t C.dt$	$\frac{At}{Vd}$	$\frac{A\infty}{Vd}-\frac{At}{Vd}$
0.25	0.6	0.1	0.02	0.62	9.38
0.50	1.2	0.3	0.05	1.25	8.75
0.75	1.8	0.7	0.11	1.91	8.09
1.0	2.3	1.2	0.18	2.48	7.52
1.5	3.4	2.6	0.39	3.79	6.21
2.0	4.3	4.5	0.68	4.98	5.02
3.0	6.0	9.7	1.46	7.46	2.54
6.0	5.6	27.1	4.07	9.67	0.33
12.0	2.3	50.8	7.62	9.92	0.08
18.0	0.9	60.4	9.06	9.96	0.04
24.0	0.4	64.3	9.645	10.0*	

$$\frac{A\infty}{Vd} = 10.0$$

The above table shows the steps involved in carrying out the Wagner-Nelson calculation.

The third column ($\int_0^t C.\,dt$) shows the area under the C versus time curve calculated sequentially from t = 0 to each of the time points using the trapezoidal rule. The fourth column ($K\int_0^t C.dt$) shows each of the preceding areas multiplied by K. The fifth column (At/Vd) shows the sums of the values indicated in the second and fourth columns according to equation 6.145. A∞/Vd is the maximum value in the fifth column (i.e., 10.00). The sixth column shows the residual between A∞/Vd and each sequential value of At/ Vd in the fifth column. Now plot the values in sixth column versus time and log of values in sixth column versus time. If the absorption process obeyed first-order kinetics, a semilog plot will be a straight line with a slope of -Ka/2.303. If the absorption process follows zero order kinetics, the regular Cartesian plot will yield a straight line with the slope equal to the zero order rate constant. *In this case, a straight line is obtained with the cartesian plot. Hence, the absorption process follows zero order kinetics.* The zero order rate constant is equal to 25 mg/hr. This example illustrates the usefulness of the Wagner-Nelson calculation for studying the mechanism of release of drugs from dosage forms *in vivo*. Drug absorption from a solution follows the first order process and deviations from it indicates release characters of the dosage forms.

Likely Questions

1. What do you mean by one compartment open model?
2. What are the assumptions made in developing equations for a one compartment model? How do you justify the assumptions?
3. What are required for developing mathematical equations that describe drug concentration in body-time profile?
4. Derive an equation that describes the time course of the drug level in the blood following I.V. administration (bolus).
5. What is an apparent volume of distribution?
6. What are the factors responsible for non-homogenous distribution of a drug in its volume of distribution?
7. What do you mean by apparent first-order elimination rate constant?
8. Prove that $t_{1/2} = 0.693/K$.
9. How do you calculate plasma clearance and total body clearance?
10. What is GFR? What are the ideal characters of a substance used to estimate the GFR?
11. What are the factors that govern the passive transport of drugs across the renal tubule?
12. Write about the active transport of drugs across the renal tubule.
13. With the help of a neat sheme, derive an equation that describes the urinary excretion rate-time data following I.V.bolus administration of a drug.
14. How do you calculate pharmacokinetic parameters by Sigma-Minus method, following I.V.bolus administration of a drug?
15. Compare and contrast Excretion Rate method and Sigma-Minus method.
16. What are the problems encountered in obtaining a valid urinary excretion data?
17. What is renal clearance? How do you estimate it?
18. Give an equation that describes the plasma metabolite concentration-time data following I.V.bolus administration. What happens when the metabolite elimination rate constant (Km) is much more greater than the overall elimination rate constant (K)?
19. Draw a scheme for urinary excretion of metabolite following I.V.blolus administration of a drug.
20. What are the advantages of administering a drug by a constant rate I.V. infusion?
21. How do you calculate the half-life of a drug in a patient by I.V. infusion method?

22. Derive an equation that describes the unchanged drug excretion in urine following I.V.infusion.
23. Simultaneous I.V.injection and infusion are used for an immediate therapeutic effect. Explain.
24. What are the various phases of a plasma drug level-time curve following oral administration?
25. How do you determine the absorption rate constant by the method of residuals?
26. What are the advantages of the Wagner-Nelson method over method of residuals in estimating absorption rate constant?
27. Derive the equations for t_p and C_{max}.
28. How do you estimate the *lag time* for an orally administered drug?
29. What is the "flip-flop" of Ka and K?
30. Give the equations used for urinary Excretion Rate and Sigma-Minus method following oral administration of a drug.
31. A dose of 325 mg of a new drug is injected intravenously to a healthy volunteer and the following blood data was obtained. Assume that the drug follows one compartment open model and calculate all possible pharmacokinetic parameters.

Time (hrs)	Concentration
2	18.3
4	10.1
6	5.8
8	3.3
10	1.8
12	1.0
16	0.31
20	0.12

32. The following plasma data is obtained after a I.V. bolus dose of 184 mg of ceftriaxone, a semisynethetic cephalosporin antibiotic. Estimate all possible pharmacokinetic parameters.

Time (hrs)	Concentration (mg/L)
1	137
6	120
12	103
24	76
48	42
72	23
96	12
144	3.7

33. Plasma concentrations of cocaine after a single I.V. dose of 33 mg in a 75 Kg male are given below

Time (hrs)	Concentration (mg/L)
0.16	170
0.5	122
1.0	74
1.5	45
2.0	28
2.5	17
3.0	10

Calculate all possible pharmacokinetic parameters.

34. A single I.V. dose of 1 gram of a new drug is given to a healthy male volunteer. The following urine data is obtained. Calculate the possible pharmacokinetic parameters by the Excreted Rate Method and Sigma-Minus Method.

Time (hrs)	Cumulative amount of unchanged drug excreted in urine X_u^t (mg)
0.25	160
0.50	300
1.00	500
2.00	750
4.00	938
6.00	984

35. Plasma concentrations following I.V. and oral administration of 500 mg of an antibiotic to a subject are given below.

Time (hrs)		0.33	0.5	0.67	1	1.5	2	4	6	10
Plasma concentration (mg/L)	I.V	14.7	12.6	11.0	-	9.0	8.2	7.9	6.6	6.2
	Oral	-	2.4	-	3.8	4.2	4.6	8.1	5.8	5.1

Time	16	24	32	48
I.V.	4.6	3.2	2.3	1.2
Oral	4.1	3.0	2.3	1.3

(a) From a semilogarthmic plot of the plasma concentrations, estimate the elimination the half-life of the antitbiotic in the subject

(b) Calculate the total AUC following I.V. and oral administration.

(c) From the I.V. data, estimate the clearance and volume of distribution of the antibiotic.

(d) Calculate the oral bioavailability of the drug.

36. A pharmacokinetinetist gives griseofulvin orally, 0.5 g of a micronized drug formulation and, on another occasion intravenously, 100 mg to volunteers. The plasma concentration time data obtained in one subject are given below.

Time(hrs)	Plasma concentration of griseofulvin (mg/L) I.V.bolus	Oral route
1	1.4	0.4
2	1.1	0.95
3	0.98	1.15
4	0.90	1.15
5	0.80	1.05
7	-	1.20
8	0.68	1.20
12	0.55	0.90
24	0.37	1.05
28	-	0.90
32	0.24	0.85
35	-	0.80
48	0.14	0.50

From appropriate plots and calculations, what can be concluded from these data with respect :

(a) Rate of absorption of griseofulvin with time on oral administration in this individual?

(b) Completeness of absorption ?

37. A scientist measures phenytoin concentrations after the administration of sodium phenytoin intramuscularly (500 mg) and intravenously (250 mg). The average data obtained in 12 subjects, each of whom received both treatments, are listed below.

Time (hrs)	Route	0	1	2	4	6	8	12	24	48	72	96	120
Plasma Phenytoin	I.M.	0	3.0	3.2	3.5	3.2	3.6	3.8	4.1	3.2	1.6	0.8	0.4
Concentration (mg/L)	I.V.	5.6	5.4	5.2	4.9	-	3.9	3.2	2.2	0.88	0.42	-	-

(a) Estimate the bioavailability of phenytoin from the I.M. Site based on the areas of comparisions.

(b) From an appropriate plot of the data, comment on the process limiting the decline of the plasma phenytoin concentration following I.M. administration.

38. A 50 kg woman is given a single I.V. dose of an antibacterial drug at a dose level of 6 mg/kg. Blood samples are taken at various time intervals. The concentration of the drug (C) is determined in the plasma fraction of each blood sample and the following data were obtained :

Time (hrs)	0.25	0.50	1.00	3.00	6.00	12.00	18.00
C (mg/ml)	8.21	7.87	7.23	5.15	3.09	1.11	0.40

(a) What are the values of Vd, K and t1/2 for this drug ?

(b) This antibacterial agent is not effective at a plasma concentration of less than 2.5 mg/ml. What is the duration of activity for this drug ?

(c) How long would it take for a 99% of this drug to be eliminated ?

(d) If the dose of the antibiotic are doubled exactly, what be the increase in duration of activity.

39. A new drug was given in a single intravenous dose of 300 mg to a 80-kg male. After 4 hrs, the plasma concentration of drug is found to be 1.52 mg/100 ml. Assuming that the apparent Vd is 12% of body weight, compute the total amount of the drug in the body fluids after 4 hrs. What is the half-life of this drug ?

40. A new antibiotic drug is given in a single intravenous bolus of 4 mg/kg to 5 healthy male adults ranging in age from 23 to 38 years (average weight 75 kg). The plasma level-time curve for this drug fits into a one-compartment model. The equation of the curve that best fits the data is

$$C = 78\ e^{-0.46t}$$

Determine the following (assume units of micrograms per milli liter for C and hours for t):

(a) What is the t1/2 ?

(b) What is the Vd ?

(c) What is the plasma level of the drug after 4 hrs?

(d) How much drug is left in the body after 4 hrs?

(e) Predict what body water compartment this drug might occupy and explain why you make this prediction ?

(f) Assuming the drug is no longer effective when levels decline to less that 2 mg/ml, when would you administer the next dose ?

41. A single intravenous injection containing 400 mg of an antibiotic is given to an adult (58 years, 52 kg) for a specific injection. The elimination rate constant is 0.576 hr^{-1} and apparent volume of distribution is 0.15 L/Kg. Assuming the drug is eliminated

by first-order kinetics and may be described by a one-compartment model, calculate the following

(a) The C0

(b) The amount of the drug in the body at 6 hrs after the dose is given

(c) The time for the drug to decline to 1.8 mg/ml (the minimum inhibitory concentration)

42. A drug has an elimination half life of 4 hrs and follows first-order kinetics. If a single 300mg dose is given to an adult male patient (68 kg) by I.V. bolus injection, what percent of the dose is lost in 24 hours ?

43. A drug has an elimination half-life of 8 hrs and follows first order elimination kinetics. If a single 600 mg-dose is given to an adult female patient (62 kg) by a rapid I.V. injection, what percent of the dose is eliminated in 24 hrs ? Assuming the apparent volume of distribution, Vd is 400 ml/kg, what is the expected plasma drug concentration at 24 hrs postdose ?

44. An antibiotic is administered to a male adult suffering from urinary tract infection by an I.V. bolus injection (300 mg). The patient is instructed to empty his bladder prior to being medicated and to save his urine specimens for analysis. The urine samples are analysed for drug content. The drug assays gave the following results

Time (hrs)	Amount of Drug in Urine (mg)
0	0
4	100
8	26

Assuming first-order elimination, calculate the elimination half-life for the antibiotic in this patient.

Suggested Readings

1. Gibaldi, M., Perrier, D. Pharmacokinetics 2nd Edn. Informa Health care, NY, 2007.

2. Jambhekar, S.S., Breen, P.J. Basic Pharmacokinetics, Pharmaceutical Press Inc., UK 2009.

3. Rowland, M., Tozer, T.N. Clinical Pharmacokinetics, Concepts and Applications., 3rd Edn. A lea and Febriger, Philadelphia, 1994.

4. Shargel, L., Wu-Poug, S., Yu, A.B.C. Applied Bio Pharmaceutics and Pharmacokinetics. 5th Ed. Mc Graw-Hill Publishers, USA. 2005.

7

Multi-Compartment Models

Multi-Compartment Models

In one compartment open model, drug distributes only in the central compartment (i.e. blood and highly perfused tissue) and this distribution is assumed to occur instantaneously. Following I.V. bolus, if a drug distributes to some tissue which are not highly perfused with blood, the distribution of the drug to tissue may take a longer time to establish equilibrium between the central compartment and the tissue (Peripheral compartment). During this time the drug levels in the central compartment will fall because of two reasons. 1. Distribution of the drug from the central compartment to peripheral compartment 2. Elimination of the drug from the central compartment by all possible pathways of elimination. It means the decrease in drug levels in the central compartment can be described by biexponential equation. This part of the plasma level time curve is called *distribution phase* (Fig.7.1). Once an equilibrium is established between the amount of the drug present in the central compartment and that of the pheripheral compartment, a decline in the plasma level takes place mono exponentially. This decline is only because of elimination of the drug from the body and is called *elimination phase* (Fig.7.1).

The more the number of peripheral compartments that will equilibrate with the central compartment at different rates, the more will be the exponentials in the equation that describe the plasma level-time curve. After equilibration of the drug within these peripheral tissues, the elimination of the drug follows first-order kinetics.

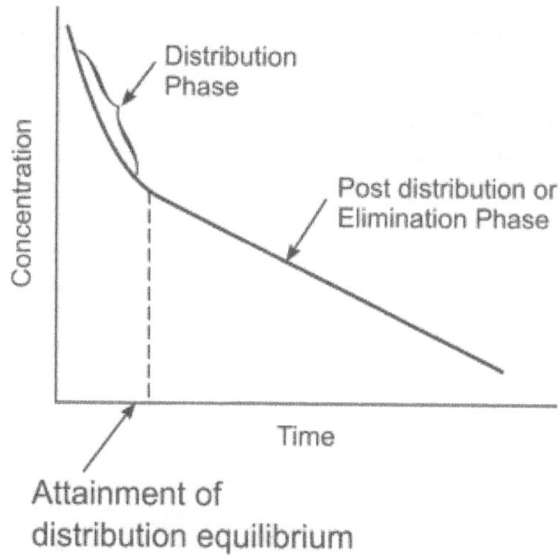

Fig. 7.1 Log plasma drug concentration-time curve for a single I.V. bolus administration of drug that follows a two compartment open model.

A drug will concentrate in a tissue in accordance with the affinity of the drug for that particular tissue. For example, lipid-soluble drugs tend to accumulate in fat tissues. Drugs that bind proteins may be more concentrated in the plasma, because protein-bound drugs do not diffuse into the tissues. Drugs may also bind with tissue proteins and other macromolecules, such as DNA and melanin.

7.1 Two Compartment Open Model

The following points should be considered in developing the equations for a two compartment open model :

1. In this model, the drug distributes into two compartments, *the central compartment* (compartment 1) and the tissue or *peripheral compartment* (compartment 2). The central compartment consists of blood, extracellular fluid, and highly perfused tissues where the drug distributes rapidly. The tissue or peripheral compartment, contains tissues in which the drug equilibrates slowly.
2. Drug transfer between the two compartments is assumed to take place by a first-order process.
3. There are three possible types of two compartment systems (Fig. 7.2). They differ in that whether the elimination of the drug occurs from central compartment (Model 1), peripheral compartment (Model 2) or both (Model 3). Model 1 is most often used and describes the plasma level-time curve observed in Fig. 7.1. Drug elimination is presumed to occur from the central compartment, because the major sites of drug elimination (renal excretion and hepatic drug metabolism) occur in organs such as kidney and liver which are highly perfused with blood. However, other models may be used if information about the elimination of a particular drug is known.

4. Elimination of the drug from the body is assumed to follow first order kinetics.
5. The concentration of the drug in a compartment is assumed to be uniform in its volume of distribution.
6. Two compartment model assumes that at t = 0 there is no drug in the tissue compartment. After an I.V. dose, drug levels in the tissue compartment will first increase, reach maximum and then decline (Fig. 7.3).

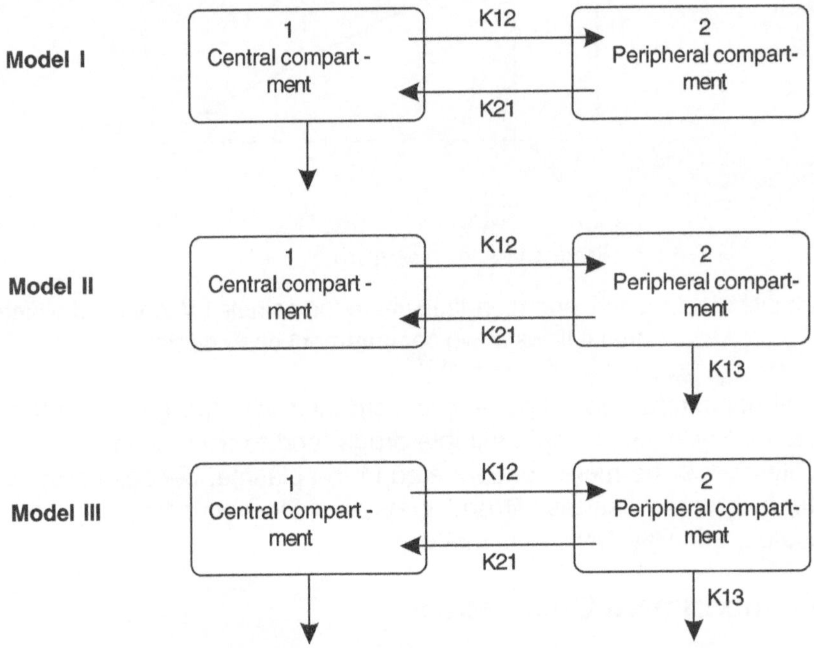

Fig. 7.2 Possible models of two compartment open model.

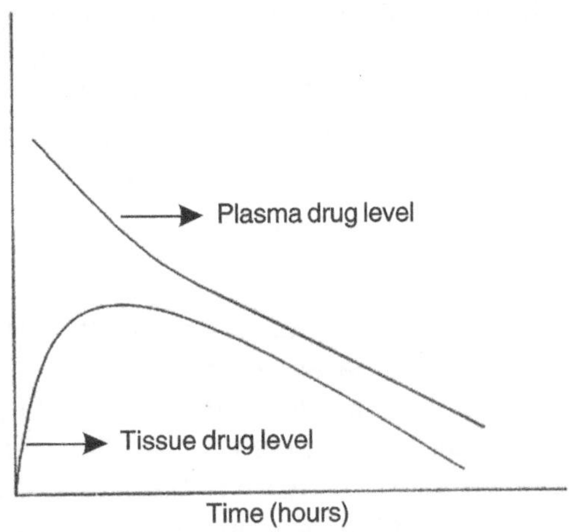

Fig. 7.3 Relationships between tissue and plasma drug levels for a two compartment open model following intravenous injection.

7.1.1 I.V. Bolus - Uncharged Drug in Blood/plasma

In practice, samples of blood are taken from the central compartment at different time intervals and analyzed for the drug content. The drug plasma level-time curve represents an initial *distributive phase*, during which the drug is diffused into the peripheral compartment till an equilibrium is attained, followed by an *elimination phase* during which the drug elimination can be described monoexponentially.

Scheme: 7.1.1

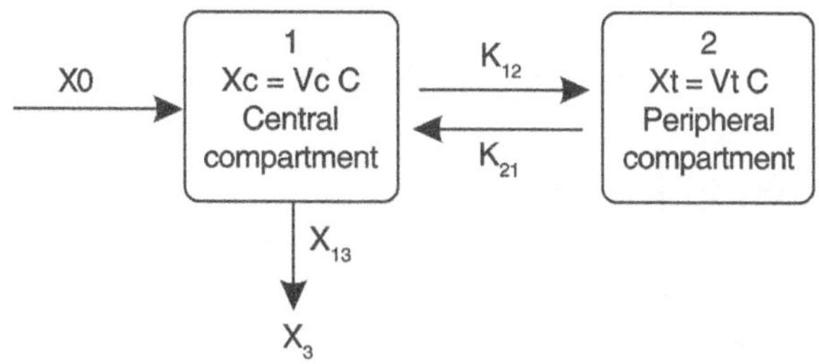

Where :

X0 = I.V. dose given as bolus

Xc = Amount of the drug in the central compartment at any time (compartment 1)

Xt = Amount of the drug in the tissue compartment at any time (compartment 2)

X_3 = Amount of drug eliminated to time t.

Vc = Volume of distribution of drug in the central compartment

Vt = Volume of distribution of the drug in the tissue compartment.

C = Concentration of the drug in the central compartment at any time

Ct = Concentration of the drug in the tissue compartment at any time.

The rate constants K_{12} and K_{21} represent the first-order rate transfer constants for the movement of the drug from compartment 1 to compartment 2 (K_{12}) and from compartment 2 to compartment 1 (K_{21}). The transfer constants are some times called *microconstants*, and their values can not be estimated directly. K_{13} is the elimination rate constant (sum of all rate constants involved in the elimination of the drug from the central compartment).

Equations that describe the time course of drug concentration in the central compartment and tissue compartment following I.V. bolus can be developed as described below.

According to mass balance equation,

$$X0 = Xc + Xt + X_3 \qquad .....(7.1)$$

The rate of change in the amount of the drug in central compartment is the net balance of rate of input (K_{21} Xt) and output (K_{12} Xc and K_{13} Xc).

$$\frac{dXc}{dt} = K_{21} X_t - K_{21} X_c - K_{13} X_c \qquad .....(7.2)$$

$$\frac{dXc}{dt} = K_{21} Xt - (K_{12} + K_{13}) Xc \qquad .....(7.3)$$

The differential equation describing the rate of change of drug levels in tissue compartment is

$$\frac{dXt}{dt} = K_{12}\, Xc - K_{21}\, Xt \qquad .....(7.4)$$

The rate of elimination of drug from central compartment is given by,

$$\frac{dX_3}{dt} = K_{13}\, Xc \qquad .....(7.5)$$

Integrating Equation 7.5 between t = 0 and t = t, we get

$$\int_0^t dX_3 = \int_0^t K_{13}\, X_c.dt$$

$$X_3 = K_{13} \int_0^t Xc.dt \qquad .....(7.6)$$

Substitute the X_3 value in Equation 7.1.

$$X0 = Xc + X_t + X_{13} \int_0^t Xc\, dt \qquad .....(7.7)$$

Re-write the Equation 7.7 for X_t.

$$X_t = X0 - Xc - K_{13} \int_0^t Xc\, dt \qquad .....(7.8)$$

Substitute the value of X_t in Equation 7.3.

$$\frac{dX_C}{dt} = K_{21}\, (X0 - Xc - K_{13} \int_0^t Xc\, dt) - (K_{12} + K_{13})\, Xc \qquad .....(7.9)$$

Differentiating Equation 7.9 with respect to time,

$$\frac{d^2\, Xc}{dt^2} = K_{21}\, (0 - \frac{dXc}{dt} - K_{13}\, Xc) - (K_{12} + K_{13}) \frac{dXc}{dt}$$

$$\frac{d^2\, Xc}{dt^2} = K_{21} \frac{dXc}{dt} - K_{21}\, K_{13}\, Xc - (K_{12} + K_{13}) \frac{dXc}{dt} \qquad .....(7.10)$$

$$\frac{d^2\, Xc}{dt^2} = -\, (K_{21} + K_{12} + K_{13}) \frac{dXc}{dt} - K_{21}\, K_{13}\, Xc \qquad .....(7.11)$$

$$\frac{d^2\, Xc}{dt^2} + (K_{21} + K_{12} + K_{13}) \frac{dXc}{dt} + K_{21}\, K_{13}\, Xc = 0 \qquad .....(7.12)$$

Let us define that

$$K_{21} + K_{12} + K_{13} = a + b \qquad .....(7.13)$$

and

$$K_{21}\ K_{13} = ab \qquad .....(7.14)$$

Now,

$$\frac{d^2\ Xc}{dt^2} + (\alpha + \beta)\ \frac{dXc}{dt} + \alpha\beta\ Xc = 0 \qquad .....(7.15)$$

Equation 7.15 is in the form of a quadratic equation a $x^2 + bx + c = 0$. Therefore, integration of Equation 7.15 yields a biexponential curve in the form of,

$$Xc = A'\ e^{-m1\ t} + B'\ e^{-m2\ t} \qquad .....(7.16)$$

The constants m_1 and m_2 are roots of the quadratic equation. The roots of the quadratic equation 7.15, can be calculated using the equation.

$$m_1 \text{ or } m_2 = \frac{-b \pm \sqrt{b^2 - 4ac}}{2a} \qquad .....(7.17)$$

m_1 or m_2 of Equation 7.15,

$$= \frac{-\alpha + \beta \pm \sqrt{(\alpha+\beta)^2 - 4\alpha\beta}}{2}$$

$$= \frac{-\alpha + \beta \pm \sqrt{(\alpha-\beta)^2}}{2}$$

$$= \frac{-\alpha + \beta + \alpha - \beta}{2}$$

$$= \frac{-2\beta}{2} = -\beta$$

another root is

$$= \frac{-\alpha - \beta - (\alpha - \beta)}{2} = \frac{-2\alpha}{2} = -\alpha$$

Let us define that $\alpha > \beta$, now.

$$Xc = A'\ e^{-\alpha t} + B'\ e^{-\beta t} \qquad .....(7.18)$$

Equation 7.18 describes, the amount of the drug in the central compartment time data. The values of A' and B' have to be found to get an equation that describes the time course of drug levels in the central compartment and tissue compartment.

Differentiating Equation 7.18 with respect to time.

$$\frac{dXc}{dt} = -\alpha\ A'\ e^{-\alpha t} - \beta\ B'.\ e^{-\beta t} \qquad ....(7.19)$$

At time zero, t = 0 and the Equation 7.19 becomes.

$$\frac{dXc}{dt} = -\alpha A' \ e^0 - \beta B'. e^0 = -\alpha A' - \beta B' \quad .....(7.20)$$

According to Equation 7.3,

$$\frac{dXc}{dt} = K_{21} Xt - (K_{12} + K_{13}) Xc$$

At t = 0, X_t will be equal to zero and Xc is nothing but I.V. dose, X0 and hence,

$$\frac{dXc}{dt} = 0 - X0 (K_{12} + K_{13}) = - X0 (K_{12} + K_{13}) \quad .....(7.21)$$

Now, equating equation, 7.20 and 7.21 is

$$- \alpha A' - \beta B' = - X0 (K_{12} + K_{13}) \quad .....(7.22)$$

But according to Equation 7.18

$$Xc = A' e^{-\alpha t} + B' e^{-\beta t}$$

At t = 0, $X0 = A' + B'$ .....(7.23)

Hence, $A' = X0 - B'$ and $B' = X0 - A'$ .....(7.24)

Substituting the value of A' in Equation 7.22

$$- \alpha(X0 - B') - \beta B' = - X0 (K_{12} + K_{13}) \quad .....(7.25)$$

Solving Equation 7.25 for B', we get

$$B' = \frac{X0(\alpha - K_{12} - K_{13})}{(\alpha - \beta)} \quad .....(7.26)$$

The assumption made as per Equation. 7.13 is that

$$(\alpha + \beta) = K_{21} + K_{12} + K_{13}$$

Therefore, $K_{21} - \beta = \alpha - K_{12} - K_{13}$ .....(7.27)

Substituting $(K_{21} - \beta)$ in place of a-$K_{12} - K_{13}$ in Equation 7.26

$$B' = \frac{X0(K_{21} - \beta)}{(\alpha - \beta)} \quad .....(7.28)$$

Substituting $A' = X_0 - B'$ in Equation 7.22, A' value can be derived

$$A' = \frac{X0(\alpha - K_{21})}{(\alpha - \beta)} \quad .....(7.29)$$

Substituting A' and B' values in Equation 7.18, we get

$$Xc = \frac{X0(\alpha - K_{21})}{(\alpha - \beta)} e^{-\alpha t} + \frac{X0(K_{21} - \beta)}{(\alpha - \beta)} e^{-\beta t} \quad .....(7.30)$$

Although the drug concentration in the central compartment is obviously not homogeneous, by assuming that the ratio of drug concentration in the various tissue and plasma is constant, a linear relationship exists between the drug concentration in plasma and the amount of the drug in the central compartment.

$$Xc = Vc.\ C \quad .....(7.31)$$

Where, Vc is the apparent volume of distribution of the drug in the central compartment. This relationship enables the conversion of Equation 7.30 from amount-time to a concentration-time equation, which can be expressed as,

$$C = \frac{X0(\alpha - K_{21})}{Vc(\alpha - \beta)} e^{-\alpha t} + \frac{X0(K_{21} - \beta)}{Vc(\alpha - \beta)} e^{-\beta t} \quad .....(7.32)$$

or in simpler form,

$$C = A\ e^{-\alpha t} + B\ e^{-\beta t} \quad .....(7.33)$$

where $A = \frac{X0(\alpha - K_{21})}{Vc(\alpha - \beta)}$ and $B = \frac{X0(K_{21} - \beta)}{Vc(\alpha - \beta)}$ .....(7.34)

A plot of the logarithm of plasma drug concentration versus time according to Equation 7.33 will yield a biexponential curve. The constant α is by definition larger than β and hence, at some time, t the term $A.e^{-\alpha t}$ will approach zero, while $B.e^{-\beta t}$ still has a definite value. It mean after the distribution phase, the equation 7.33 reduces to

$$C = B\ e^{-\beta t} \quad .....(7.35)$$

or $\log C = \log B - \beta t / 2.303$ .....(7.36)

Equations 7.35 and 7.36 describe the plasma drug-level time data during the elimination phase.

A plot of the log plasma drug level versus time can be used to estimate various pharmacokinetic parameters as shown in Fig. 7.4 An estimate of β can be made from the slope of the terminal linear portion (Slope = $-\beta t/ 2.303$) and the biological half-life ($t_{1/2}$) can be determined employing the following relationship.

$$t_{1/2} = 0.693/\beta \quad .....(7.37)$$

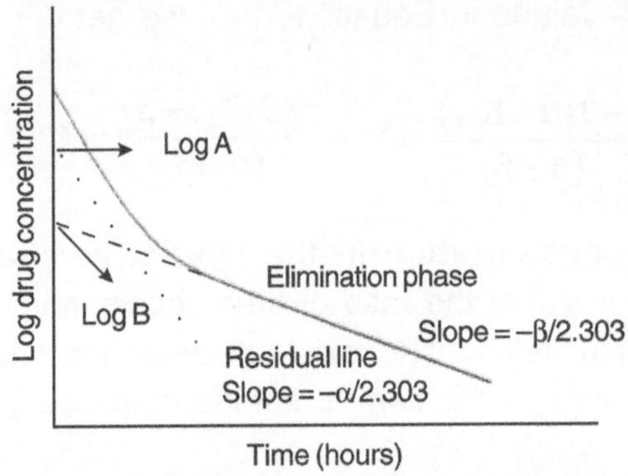

Fig. 7.4 A plot of log plasma drug concentration versus time. The rate constants and intercepts are determined by the method of residuals.

The zero time intercept obtained by extrapolation of the terminal linear phase is log B. Application of the method of residuals may be carried out by subtracting the plasma drug level on the curve from the plasma drug level on the extended line at the same time point to obtain residual concentration-time data. A plot of residual concentration versus time gives a residual line with a slope = -α/2.303 and an intercept = log A.

The constants A, B, α and β may be obtained graphically as explained above or with the aid of a digital computer. Once these experimental constants are obtained, the pharmacokinetic parameters, Vc, K_{12}, K_{13} and K_{21} can be generated by considering the following relationship.

1. Vc

$$\frac{X0}{Vc} = C0 = A + B \qquad .....(7.38)$$

Therefore,

$$Vc = \frac{X0}{(A+B)} = \frac{X0}{C0} = \frac{\text{I.V. dose}}{A+B} \qquad .....(7.39)$$

2. K_{21}

We know that

$$A = \frac{X0\,(\alpha - K_{21})}{Vc\,(\alpha - \beta)} \quad \text{but} \quad \frac{X0}{Vc} = A + B$$

$$A = \frac{(A+B)(\alpha - K_{21})}{(\alpha - \beta)} \qquad .....(7.40)$$

Solving Equation 7.40 for K_{21}, we get

$$K_{21} = \frac{B\alpha + A\beta}{A+B} \qquad .....(7.41)$$

3. K_{13}

By definition $\alpha\beta = K_{13}K_{21}$,

or $K_{13} = \alpha\beta/K_{21}$ .....(7.42)

Substituting K_{21} value in Equation 7.42, we get

$$K_{13} = \frac{(A+B)\alpha\beta}{(B\alpha + A\beta)} \quad .....(7.43)$$

4. K_{12} : By definition $(\alpha + \beta) = K_{12} + K_{13} + K_{21}$. Substituting K_{21} and K_{13} values in the above equation and solving it for K_{12} we get

$$K_{12} = \frac{AB(\alpha+\beta)^2}{(A+B)(B\alpha+A\beta)} \quad .....(7.44)$$

Drug levels in tissue or peripheral compartment

The differential equation that describes the rate of change in the amount of the drug in the tissue compartment is,

$$\frac{dXt}{dt} = K_{12}\,Xc - K_{21}\,X_t \quad .....(7.45)$$

$$\frac{dXt}{dt} + K_{21}\,X_t = K_{12}\,Xc \quad .....(7.46)$$

But we know that:

$$Xc = \frac{X0\,(\alpha - K_{21})}{Vc\,(\alpha-\beta)}\,1\,e^{-\alpha t} + \frac{X0\,(K_{21} - \beta)}{(\alpha - \beta)}\,e^{-\beta t}$$

or

$$Xc = \frac{X0}{(\alpha-\beta)}\,[(\alpha - K_{21})\,e^{-\alpha t} + (K_{21} - \beta)\,e^{-\beta t}] \quad .....(7.47)$$

Substituting Xc in Equation 7.46 :

$$\frac{dXt}{dt} + K_{21}\,X_t = \frac{K_{12}\,X_0}{(\alpha-\beta)}\,[(\alpha-K_{21})e^{-\alpha t} + (K_{21} - \beta)\,e^{-\beta t}] \quad .....(7.48)$$

Multiplying both the sides of Equation 7.48 with e^{K21t}

$$\frac{dXt}{dt}\,e^{K_{21}t} + K_{21}\,X_t\,.\,e^{K_{21}t} = \frac{K_{12}\,X0}{(\alpha-\beta)}$$

$$[(\alpha-K_{21})e^{-(\alpha-K21)t} + (K_{21} - \beta)\,e^{-(\beta-K21)t}] \quad .....(7.49)$$

Integrating the Equation 7.49 between t = 0 to t = t,

$$Xt\ e^{K_{21}t} = \frac{K_{12}\ X0}{(\alpha - \beta)}\ \{[(\alpha - K_{21})\ (\frac{e^{-(\alpha - K_{21})t}}{-(\alpha - K_{21})} + \frac{1}{(\alpha - K_{21})})] +$$

$$[(K_{21} - \beta)\ (\frac{e^{-(\beta - K_{21})t}}{-(\beta - K_{21})} + \frac{1}{(\beta - K_{21})})]\} \qquad .....(7.50)$$

Further simplification of Equation 7.50 yields,

$$Xt = \frac{K_{12}\ X0}{(\alpha - \beta)}\ (e^{-\beta t} - e^{-\alpha t}) \qquad .....(7.51)$$

Equation 7.51 describes the time course of the amount of the drug in the peripheral compartment following I.V. bolus. It is obvious from Equation 7.51 that after a sufficiently long time (post distribution phase), the term $e^{-\alpha t}$ approaches zero and Equation 7.51 reduces to,

$$Xt = \frac{K_{12}\ X0}{(\alpha - \beta)}\ e^{-\beta t} \qquad .....(7.52)$$

Hence, the slope of the terminal exponential phase equals to - β/2.303. Therefore, in the post distribution phase the plasma and tissue compartment levels decline in parallel. Fig. 7.5 depicts the drug levels in two compartments after an I.V. injection of the drug and the influence of the distribution of drug.

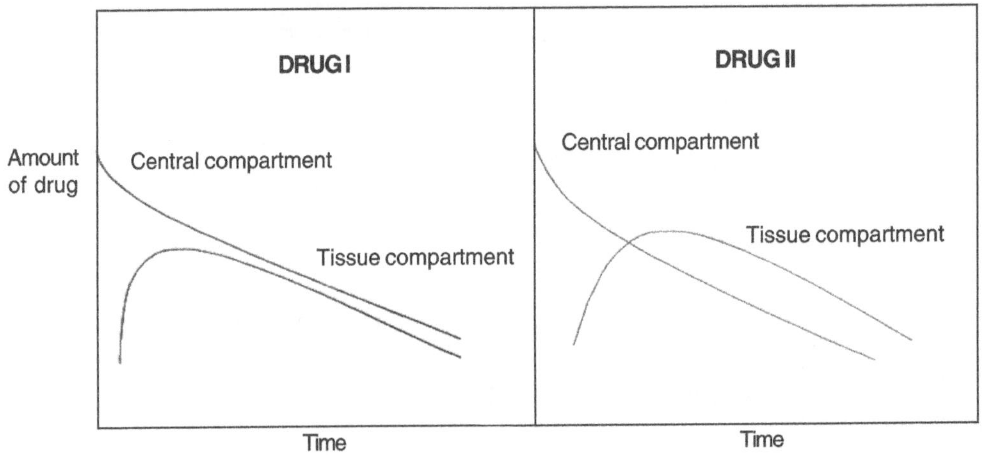

Fig. 7.5 Drug levels in central and tissue compartments-time curves. Drug II is having more affinity to tissue compartment than Drug I.

Equation 7.51 may be useful in determining the relationship between pharmacological action and the tissue levels of the drug. It must be kept in mind, however, that such relationships are only approximations. The hypothetical "tissue" levels of a drug may not accurately reflect the concentration of the drug at the site of action even though the site of action may be a part of the tissue compartment.

It is assumed that the drug in the tissue compartment distributes uniformly in its volume of distribution, V_t, then Equation 7.51 can be written in concentration terms.

$$C_t = \frac{K_{12}\, X0}{Vt(\alpha - \beta)}\left(e^{-\beta t} - e^{-\alpha t}\right) \qquad .....(7.53)$$

Apparent Volumes of Distribution

Even though the volume of distribution is fictive, it provides not only some insight into distribution but also importantly relates to the rate of clearance of the drug from plasma. In multiple compartments we may consider mathematically hypothetical volumes, such as the volume of the central compartment and the volume of the tissue or peripheral compartment.

In a two-compartment open model, the determination of the volume of distribution, Vd is complicated by 1. the slow attainment of a distribution equilibrium; and 2. the volume of distribution is changing continually during the distribution phase.

Hence, Vd should be estimated by such methods that cancel the distributive factors or Vd should be estimated during the post distribution phase. There are several volumes of distribution that may be considered for a drug that follows a two compartment open model.

Volume of Distribution of the Central Compartment

The Volume of distribution of the central compartment, Vc, is an important parameter to understand distribution pattern of the drug in the body, to estimate drug clearance and to describe the time course of plasma drug levels because the central compartment is usually the sampling compartment.

At time zero, the total drug injected is in the central compartment. Hence Vc is the ratio of I.V. dose and plasma drug concentration at t = 0 i.e., C0.

$$Vc = \text{I.V. Dose} / C0 \qquad .....(7.54)$$

C0, can be estimated from equation

$$C = A.e^{-\alpha t} + B.e^{-\beta t}, \text{ at } t = 0$$

$$Co = A + B \qquad .....(7.55)$$

Therefore, $$Vc = X0 / A + B \qquad .....(7.56)$$

A and B are estimated from the plasma drug level - time graph by the method of residuals.

Alternatively, the volume of the central compartment may be calculated from $[AUC]_0^\alpha$ in a manner similar to the calculation for the apparent Vd in the one-compartment model. For one compartment model,

$$[AUC]_0^\infty = X0/Vd\ K \quad .....(7.57)$$

In contrast, $[AUC]_0^\infty$ for a two-compartment model is

$$[AUC]_0^\infty = X0/K_{13}\ Vc \quad .....(7.58)$$

Rearrangement of this equation yields

$$Vc = \frac{X0}{K_{13}\ [AUC]_0^\alpha} \quad .....(7.59)$$

Apparent volume of distribution at steady state

The apparent volume of distribution at the steady state V_d^{ss}, is equal to the total drug in the body at the steady state divided by the plasma drug concentration at that time.

$$V_d^{ss} = \frac{\text{Total drug in the body at steady state}}{\text{Plasma drug concentration}}$$

Total drug in the body = Amount of the drug in the central compartment (Xc) + Amount of drug in the tissue compartment (Xt).

Therefore, $$V_d^{ss} = \frac{Xc + Xt}{C} \quad .....(7.60)$$

At steady state condition the rate of drug entry into the tissue compartment from the central compartment is equal to the rate of drug exit from the tissue compartment into the central compartment. This steady-state condition may exist for a moment, theoretically, following I.V. bolus. Hence, at the steady state condition.

$$K_{12}\ Xc = K_{21}\ Xt \quad .....(7.61)$$

$$Xt = \frac{K_{12}\ Xc}{K_{21}} \quad .....(7.62)$$

but $$Xc = Vc.\ C \quad .....(7.63)$$

Therefore,

$$Xt = \frac{K_{12}\ Vc\ C}{K_{21}} \quad .....(7.64)$$

Substituting Xc and Xt in Equation. 7.60

$$V_d^{ss} = Vc + \frac{Vc\ C + (K_{12}\ Vc\ C)/K_{21}}{C} \quad .....(7.65)$$

which reduces to $$V_d^{ss} = Vc + \frac{K_{12}}{K_{21}}\ Vc \quad .....(7.66)$$

Equation 7.66 is useful in calculating V_d^{ss}, which is a function of transfer constants, K_{12} and K_{21}, which represent the rate constants of the drug into and out of the tissue compartment, respectively.

Volume of distribution by area

In this method, the value of β is used to calculate the volume of distribution V_d^{β}. The designation V_d^{β} indicates the method of calculation. The rationale for the method is the valid assumption that plasma and tissue concentrations decline in parallel during the post distributive phase. It means that the distribution ratio of the drug between the two compartments is constant during the elimination phase. Therefore, total body clearance (V_d^{β}. β) is equal to drug clearance from the central compartment (Vc. K_{13}).

$$Vd^{\beta}\ \beta = K_{13}\ Vc \qquad .....(7.67)$$

$$Vd^{\beta} = \frac{K_{13}\ Vc}{\beta} \qquad .....(7.68)$$

The method is shown to yield the same values for Vd as one based on area.

$$Vd^{area} = \frac{Dose}{[AUC]_0^{\alpha}} = \frac{X0}{\beta\,[AUC]_0^{\alpha}} = V_d^{\beta} \qquad .....(7.69)$$

$[AUC]_0^{\infty}$ can be obtained by integrating the equation $C = A\ e^{-\alpha t} + B\ e^{-\beta t}$ with respect to time between the limits of t = 0 and t = ∞.

$$\int_0^{\infty} C\ dt = A\int_0^{\infty} e^{-\alpha t} + B\int_0^{\infty} e^{-\beta t}$$

$$[AUC]_0^{\infty} = A\ (0 + 1/\alpha) + B\ (0 + 1/\beta)$$

$$[AUC]_0^{\infty} = A/\alpha + B/\beta \qquad .....(7.70)$$

$$Vd^{area} = \frac{X0}{\beta(A/\alpha + B/\beta)} \qquad .....(7.71)$$

This method can also be applied for extravascular administration of drugs.

$$Vd^{area} = \frac{F\ X0}{\beta\,[AUC]_0^{\alpha}} \qquad .....(7.72)$$

Where F = fraction of the dose absorbed.

Volume of Distribution by Extrapolation (V_d^{exp})

The extrapolated volume of distribution V_d^{exp} is calculated by the following equation

$$V_d^{exp} = \frac{X0}{B} \qquad .....(7.73)$$

Where B is the intercept of Y-axis obtained by extrapolating the terminal linear portion of the log drug plasma level-time graph.

But $$B = \frac{X0\,(K_{21} - \beta)}{Vc\,(\alpha - \beta)}$$ according to Equation 7.34

Substituting B values in Equation 7.73, we get.

$$V_d^{exp} = Vc.\ \frac{(\alpha - \beta)}{(K_{21} - \beta)} \qquad .....(7.74)$$

The equation shows that a change in the distribution of a drug, which is observed by a change in the value of Vc, will be reflected in a change in V_d^{exp}. The method does not take into account the effect of the process K_{21} to limit the size of the tissue compartment.

Significance of the volumes of Distribution

The value of V_d^{area} or V_d^{β} are the most correct approximation of Vd to apply to the post distribution phase. V_d^{area} and V_d^{β} are affected by changes in the overall elimination rate and by changes in total body clearance of the drug. After the drug is distributed, the total amount of the drug in the body during the elimination phase is calculated by using V_d^{β}.

In contrast, V_d^{ss} is not affected by changes in drug elimination. V_d^{ss} reflects the true distributional volume changes and not changes due to drug elimination. The volume of distribution of central compartment, Vc, is useful in the calculation of drug clearance. V_d^{exp} over estimates the volume of distribution of drug. By magnitude, these volumes of distribution rank as follows:

$$V_d^{exp} > V_d^{area} \text{ or } V_d\beta > V_d^{ss} > Vc$$

Clearance

The definition and concept of clearance can be found in Chapter 3. The definition of clearance applies whether the elimination occurs in one or multi-compartment system, hence, clearance is model independent. However, mathematical identities of clearance do depend on the model.

In a two compartment model, the elimination rate constant (K_{13}) represents the elimination of the drug from the central compartment, where as β represents drug elimination from the entire body after the diffusable drug has established an equilibrium. Hence, total body clearance, CL_t is given by

$$CL_t = \beta \, V_d^{area} \qquad .....(7.75)$$

But

$$V_d^{area} = \frac{\text{I.V. dose}}{\beta(A/\alpha + B/\beta)}$$

Therefore,

$$CL_t = \frac{X0}{\beta(A/\alpha + B/\beta)} \cdot \beta = \frac{X0}{\beta(A/\alpha + B/\beta)} \qquad .....(7.76)$$

However, if the elimination of the drug occurs only from the central compartment, the product of the volume of central compartment, Vc, and the elimination rate constant gives the total clearance.

$$CL_t = Vc. \, K_{13} \qquad .....(7.77)$$

7.1.2 I.V. Bolus - Unchanged Drug in Urine

It is possible to obtain pharmacokinetics of a drug from urinary excretion data that follows a two-compartment open model following an I.V. Bolus. The elimination of the drug from the body in such cases is by the parallel renal and extra-renal elimination processes.

Scheme 7.1.2

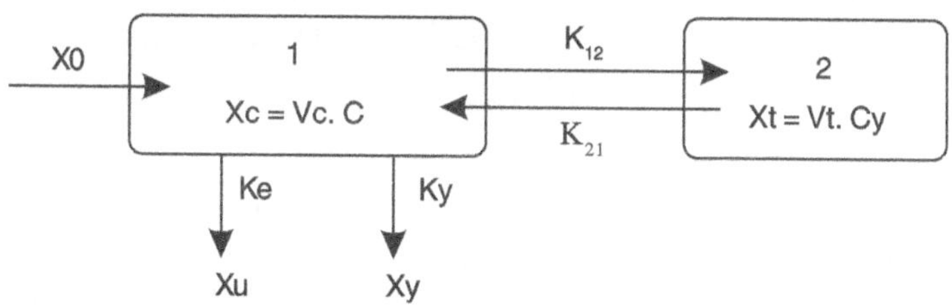

Where:

Ke = Urinary excretion rate constant for unchanged drug.

Ky = Sum of the rate constants of all the processes involved in the elimination of drug other than renal excretion.

Xu = Cumulative amount of the unchanged drug excreted in urine to any time.

Xy = Cumulative amount of drug eliminated by all other routes other than renal to any time.

All other symbols are as defined previously. The over all elimination rate constant from the central compartment, K_{13} is the sum of the individual rate constants which characterize the parallel elimination processes.

$$K_{13} = Ke + Ky \qquad .....(7.78)$$

The excretion rate of an unchanged drug, dXu/dt can be defined as

$$dXu/dt = Ke \, Xc \qquad .....(7.79)$$

But we know from Equation 7.30, that

$$Xc = \frac{X0}{(\alpha - \beta)} [(\alpha - K_{21}).e^{-\alpha t} + (K_{21} - \beta).e^{-\beta t}]$$

Substituting Xc value in 7.79

$$dXu/dt = \frac{Ke\ X0}{(\alpha - \beta)} [(\alpha - K_{21}).e^{-\alpha t} + (K_{21} - \beta).e^{-\beta t}] \quad .....(7.80)$$

or $$dXu/dt = \frac{Ke\ X0}{(\alpha - \beta)} (\alpha - K_{21}).e^{-\alpha t} + \frac{Ke\ X0}{(\alpha - \beta)} (K_{21} - \beta).e^{-\beta t} \quad .....(7.81)$$

or $$dXu/dt = A'' e^{-\alpha t} + B'' e^{-\beta t} \quad .....(7.82)$$

Where $$A'' = \frac{Ke\ X0}{(\alpha - \beta)} (\alpha - K_{21}) \text{ and } B'' = \frac{Ke\ X0}{(\alpha - \beta)} (K_{21} - \beta) \quad .....(7.83)$$

dXu/dt is the instantaneous rate of excretion of the drug, which can not be determined experimentally. Hence, instead of dXu/dt, the average excretion rate, $\Delta Xu/\Delta t$, is used. $\Delta Xu/\Delta t$ approximates dXu/dt if the sampling intervals are short.

Therefore, $$\Delta Xu/\Delta t = A'' e^{-\alpha t'} + B'' e^{-\beta t'} \quad .....(7.84)$$

t'= mid-point of urine collection period.

Because $\alpha > \beta$, after some time following an I.V. bolus administration, the term $e^{-\alpha t}$ will approach to zero while the term $e^{-\beta t}$ still have a finite value and the equation reduces to,

$$\Delta Xu/\Delta t = B'' e^{-\beta t'} \quad .....(7.85)$$

It means after some time (i.e., after distribution phase) the biexponential equation 7.84 will be reduced to a monoexponential equation. Equation 7.85 describes the rate of urinary excretion of the drug during elimination phase of the plasma drug level-time plot.

A semilogarithmic plot of average excretion rate ($\Delta Xu/\Delta t$) versus time, according to Equation 7.84 will yield a biexponential curve. The value of β can be obtained from the slope ($-\beta/2.303$) of the terminal linear phase and B" is obtained by extrapolating the linear phase line to time zero (Fig. 7.6). Application of the method of residuals will yield a second linear segment with a slope of $-\alpha/2.303$ and zero-time intercept of A".

It must me emphasized that the slope of the terminal linear portion of the plot of log ($\Delta Xu/\Delta t$) versus t' is a function of the overall elimination rate constant β, and not of the urinary excretion rate constant, Ke. However, Ke can be calculated once the experimental constants A", B", α and β are determined.

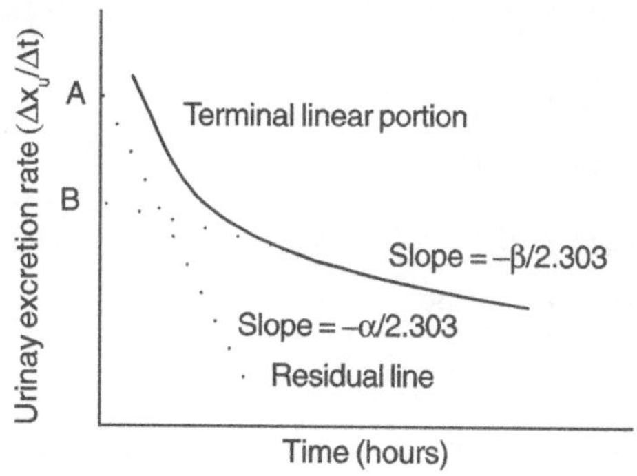

Fig. 7.6 Semi-logarithmic plot of urinary excretion rate versus time for a drug that follows two compartment open model following I.V. Bolus.

Taking the sum of A" and B" and expanding.

$$A'' + B'' = \frac{Ke\ X0}{(\alpha - \beta)}(\alpha - K_{21}) + \frac{Ke\ X0}{(\alpha - \beta)}(K_{21} - \beta)$$

$$= \frac{Ke\ X0\ \alpha - Ke\ X0\ K_{21} + Ke\ X0\ K_{21} - Ke\ X0\ \beta}{(\alpha - \beta)}$$

$$A'' + B'' = \frac{Ke\ X0\ (\alpha - \beta)}{(\alpha - \beta)}$$

$$A'' + B'' = Ke\ X0 \quad .....(7.86)$$

Therefore, $$Ke = \frac{A'' + B''}{X0} \quad .....(7.87)$$

Therefore, knowing the intravenous dose, A" and B", the urinary excretion rate constant of the unchanged drug can be determined. The other pharmacokinetic parameters K_{12}, K_{13} and K_{21} can be calculated with the following equations.

$$B'' = \frac{Ke\ X0}{(\alpha - \beta)}\ (K_{21} - \beta)$$

Therefore, $$K_{21} = \frac{B''(\alpha + \beta)}{Ke\ X0} + \beta \quad .....(7.88)$$

or $$K_{21} = \frac{B''\alpha + A''\beta}{A'' + B''} \quad .....(7.89)$$

Since $Ke\ \ X0 = A'' + B''$

Similarly we can get,

$$K_{13} = \frac{\alpha\beta(B'' + A'')}{B''\alpha + A''\beta} \quad .....(7.90)$$

or $$K_{12} = (\alpha + \beta) - K_{21} - K_{13} \quad .....(7.91)$$

Since, $$(\alpha + \beta) = K_{12} + K_{13} + K_{21}$$

Renal Clearance

To obtain a renal clearance for a drug demonstrating two compartment kinetics with metabolism and excretion, the following equation is used.

$$CL_R = Ke\ Vc \quad .....(7.92)$$

For many drugs the total amount of the unchanged drug, X_u^∞, excreted in urine may be obtained by direct assay of urine samples. The ratio of X_u^∞ to the I.V. dose (in case of extravascular administration), fraction of dose absorbed, (F X0) is equal to the fraction of the drug excreted unchanged in the urine.

Fraction of the drug excreted unchanged in the urine =

$$fe = \frac{X_u^\alpha}{X0} \quad .....(7.93)$$

By integrating Equation 7.80 between limits of t = 0 to t = ∞, and simplifying the resultant equation,

$$\int_0^\infty dXu = \left[\frac{Ke\ X0}{(\alpha - \beta)}(\alpha - K_{21})e^{-\alpha t} + \frac{Ke\ X0}{(\alpha - \beta)}(K_{21} - \beta)e^{-\beta t}\right]$$

$$X_u^\infty = \frac{Ke\ K_{21}\ X0}{\alpha\beta} \quad .....(7.94)$$

But $$\alpha\beta = K_{13}K_{21}$$

Therefore, $$X_u^\infty = \frac{Ke\ K_{21}\ X0}{K_{13}\ K_{21}} = \frac{Ke\ X0}{K_{13}} \quad .....(7.95)$$

Substituting X_u^∞ value in Equation 7.93,

$$fe = \frac{Ke\ X0}{K_{13}} \cdot \frac{1}{X0} = \frac{Ke}{K_{13}} \quad .....(7.96)$$

Therefore, 'fe' is nothing but the ratio of Ke to K_{13}

Renal clearance may be determined from the fraction of the unchanged drug excreted in the urine and the total body clearance, CL_t.

$$CL_R = fe \cdot CL_t \quad .....(7.97)$$

or

$$CL_R = \frac{Ke}{K_{13}} \cdot CL_t \quad .....(7.98)$$

Total body clearance of the drug can be obtained using Equations 7.99 and 7.100, depending on the elimination processes involved in drug elimination.

$$CL_t = K_{13}\, Vc \quad .....(7.99)$$

or

$$CL_t = \beta \cdot V_d^{\beta} \quad .....(7.100)$$

7.1.3 I.V. Infusion - Unchanged Drug in Blood / Plasma

Drugs are administered by I.V. infusion to maintain drug levels in plasma for a desired time. Plasma concentration of the drug versus time data of certain drugs can not be explained with a simple one compartment open model. Many drugs given by I.V. infusion follow two compartment kinetics. Plasma drug levels increase slowly to a stable level following an I.V. infusion. The time needed to reach a steady-state blood level depends entirely on the half-life of the drug. This point has been explained under one-compartment model.

Scheme 7.1.3

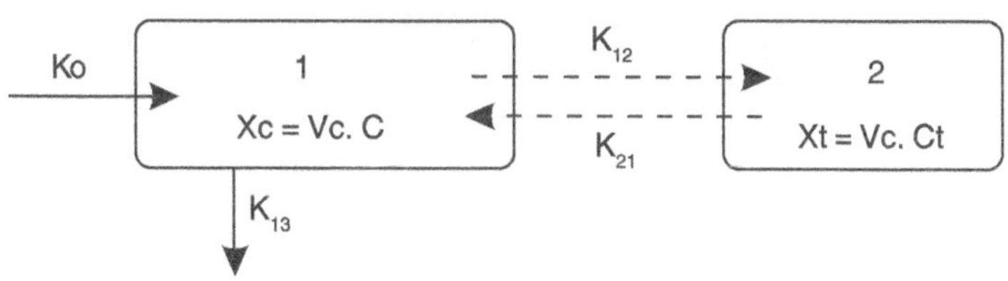

Where, K0 is the constant infusion rate (mg/hr). The rate of input is a zero order process. Three important processes are to be considered in deriving an equation that describes the plasma drug level-time profile following I.V. infusion.

1. **Input:** Drug is infused at a constant rate, K0. The zero-order kinetics govern this process.
2. **Distribution of Drug:** The drug entering the central compartment is distributed to the tissue compartment till the steady state is reached.
3. **Elimination of Drug:** Drug in the central compartment is eliminated by an apparent first order process.

The net result of the above processes is that the drug level builds up slowly in the body till a steady-state level is reached.

The rate of change of the drug level in the central compartment is given by

$$\frac{dc}{dt} = K0 + K_{21}\, Ct - (K_{12} + K_{13})\, C \quad .....(7.101)$$

Solving Equation 7.101 for drug concentration in blood, we get

$$C = \frac{K0}{Vc\,K_{13}}\left[1 - \frac{(K_{13} - \beta)}{(\alpha - \beta)} e^{-\alpha t} - \frac{(\alpha - K_{13})}{(\alpha - \beta)} e^{-\beta t}\right] \qquad .....(7.102)$$

Equation 7.102 describes the time course of drug concentration in plasma with I.V. infusion. At the steady-state, i.e., when t = ∝, Equation 7.102 reduces to

$$C = \frac{K0}{Vc\,K_{13}} \qquad .....(7.103)$$

Equation 7.103 can be rearranged to give an equation which can be used to calculate the infusion rate required to attain the desired Css.

$$K0 = Css.\ Vc.\ K_{13} \qquad .....(7.104)$$

Hence, using the mean values of the terms in the right hand side of equation 7.104 from the literature, the required infusion rate can be calculated. If the infusion is stopped after attaining the steady-state level, the fall in the drug plasma levels can be described by a mono exponential equation (Fig. 7.7).

$$C = Css.\ e^{-\beta t} \qquad .....(7.105)$$

or

$$C = \frac{K0}{Vc\,K_{13}} e^{-\beta t} \qquad .....(7.106)$$

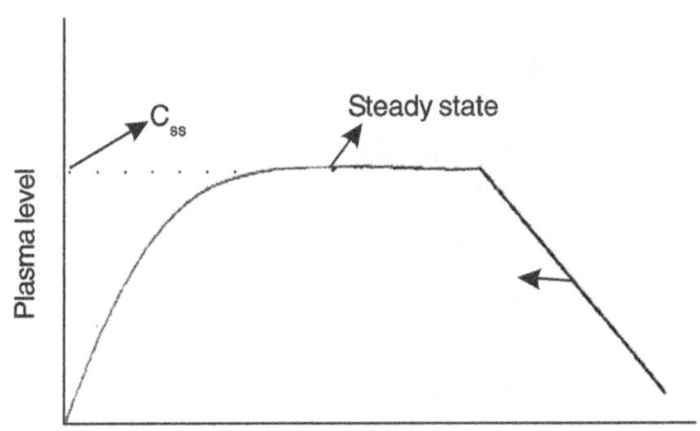

Fig. 7.7 Plasma – Drug levels vs. time graph for infusion administration

7.1.4 Infusion Plus Loading Dose - Unchanged Drug in Blood/Plasma

The time needed to reach a steady-state level with I.V. infusion alone is too long. It is desirable to rapidly attain the steady state in many pharmacokinetic studies, such as renal clearance studies, as well as in the therapy of certain diseases. Hence, a loading dose to attain the steady-state level is given and I.V. infusion is started simultaneously to maintain the steady-state level. For drugs that follow a one compartment model, rapid I.V. injection (loading dose) and a simultaneous I.V. infusion will establish the steady-state level "instantaneously". The plasma concentration of the drug would be the same from time zero upto the time the infusion ceases. But, for drugs that follow a two-compartment pharmacokinetic model, the drug distributes slowly into the extravascular tissues. Thus, the equilibrium between the drug levels of the central compartment and that of the tissue compartment is not immediate. Therefore, rapid I.V. injection of a loading dose results in high plasma drug levels initially, which decrease slowly to a steady-state level. Therefore, a loading dose produces an initial blood level either slightly higher or lower than the steady-state blood level depending upon the loading dose administered (Fig.7.8).

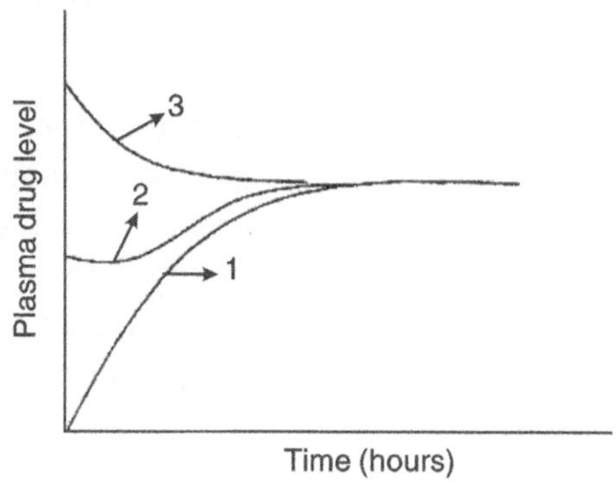

Fig. 7.8 Plasma drug concentration after various loading doses and constant infusion for a drug that follows a two-compartment open model. 1. Without loading dose; 2. Loading dose less than Css Vc; 3. Loading dose equal to Css Vc.

In practice loading dose is calculated by rearranging the Equation 7.103.

$$\text{Loading dose} = \quad Css.\ Vc. = \frac{K0}{Vc\,K_{13}} \qquad .....(7.107)$$

The differential equation for I.V. infusion is given by,

$$\frac{dc}{dt} = K0 - (K_{12} + K_{13})C + K_{21}\ Ct \qquad .....(7.108)$$

The equation that describes the plasma drug level-time data can be obtained by the addition of equations that describe I.V. bolus and I.V. infusion cases individually.

$$C = \frac{X0}{Vc(\alpha-\beta)}\ [(\alpha - K_{21})\ e^{-\alpha t} + (K_{21} - \beta)\ e^{-\beta t}] + \frac{K0}{Vc\,K_{13}}$$

$$[1 - \frac{(K_{13} - \beta)}{(\alpha - \beta)}\ e^{-\alpha t} - \frac{(\alpha - K_{13})}{(\alpha - \beta)}\ e^{-\beta t}] \qquad .....(7.109)$$

7.1.5 Oral route of administration - Unchanged drug in Blood/Plasma

It is possible to estimate various pharmacokinetics of a drug that follows a two-compartment open model after an extravascular administration of the drug.

Scheme 7.1.5

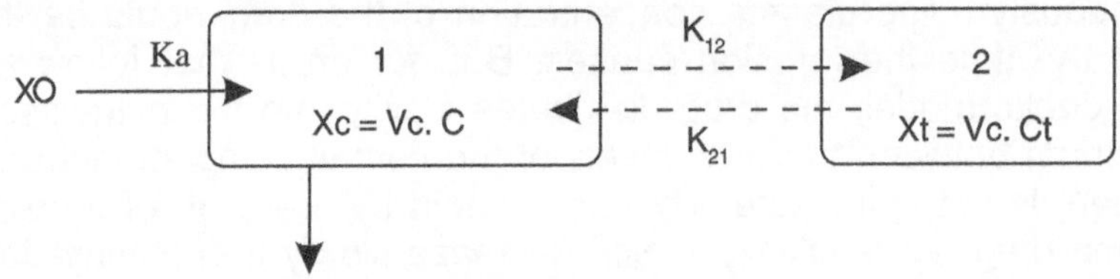

Where, Ka is the first order absorption rate constant and all other symbols are as defined earlier. After an extravascular administration into a two compartment system, there are three first-order processes occurring simultaneously: absorption, distribution and elimination.

As long as the drug enters the central compartment by absorption process, it undergoes distribution and elimination simultaneously. After the cessation of absorption, distribution process occurs for some time till an equilibrium is established, after which only the elimination of the drug occurs. It means the plasma concentration of the drug depends initially on three processes (three exponentials), then on two processes of distribution and elimination (two exponentials) and finally on elimination process only (mono exponential).

The equation that describes the time course of drug concentration in the central compartment is given by

$$C = A \, . \, e^{-\alpha t} + B. \, e^{-\beta t} - C0 \; e^{-Kat} \qquad .....(7.110)$$

At time zero, $0 = A\,e^{o} + B\,e^{o} - C0 \; e^{o} = A + B - C0$ .....(7.111)

or $A + B = C0$ .....(7.112)

Where, $A = \frac{X0}{Vc} \frac{(\alpha - K_{21})}{(\alpha - \beta)}$ and $B = \frac{X0}{Vc} \frac{(K_{21} - \beta)}{(\alpha - \beta)}$

If 'F' is the fraction of the dose absorbed, then

$$A = \frac{FX0}{Vc} \frac{(\alpha - K_{21})}{(\alpha - \beta)} \qquad .....(7.113)$$

$$B = \frac{FX0}{Vc} \frac{(K_{21} - \beta)}{(\alpha - \beta)} \qquad .....(7.114)$$

According to Equation 7.110, semilogarthmic plot of plasma drug concentration versus time gives a complex curve which is triexponential initially, becomes biexponential after some time (post absorptive phase) and finally gives a straight line (after distribution phase) whose slope is equal to – β/2.303 (Fig. 7.9). The method of residuals is used to resolve

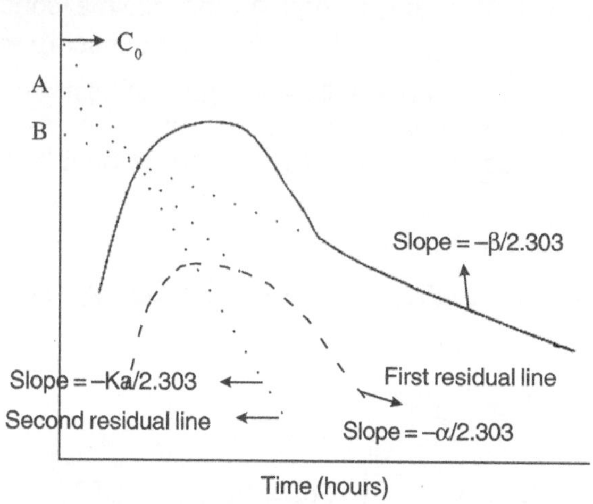

Fig. 7.9 Resolution of absorption, distribution and elimination components of a drug concentration-time curve of a drug with two-compartment kinetics by method of residuals.

the exponents. The steps involved are summarized below (Fig. 7.9).

1. Plot plasma drug level-time data on a semilogarithmic graph.
2. Locate and extend the terminal linear portion of the curve, to cut Y-axis. The slope of this line is equal to $-\beta/2.303$ and the intercept = B.
3. Apply the method of residuals between the actual curve and extended line to obtain the first residual concentration - time data. Plot the first residual concentration-time data on the same graph paper. The slope of the terminal linear portion of this curve is equal to $-\alpha/2.303$. Intercept obtained by extending this line is equal to A.
4. A second residual line representing the absorption phase is obtained by substracting the absorption segment of the first residual curve from the extrapolated line to give the second residual line slope -Ka/2.303 and intercept C0.

By this way, the parameters α, β, Ka, A, B and C0 are estimated. Other pharmacokinetic parameters can be calculated using the equations described under I.V. bolus. This method is not useful for the formulations that release the drug slowly.

It should be remembered that in order to resolve the data by the method of residuals, sufficient data points should be present in all the phases of drug absorption, distribution and elimination.

Determination of Ka by Loo-Riegelman Method

Loo and Reigelman method is useful in determining the absorption rate constant, Ka from plasma concentration-time data of a drug that follows a two compartment model. The percent of drug unabsorbed versus time plot is utilized in this method. The main advantage of this method is that there is no limitation on the order of the absorption process. The main disadvantage of this method is that it requires the plasma concentration time data after I.V. bolus and oral administration to obtain all the necessary kinetic constants.

The amount of the drug absorbed following oral administration of the drug that follows a two compartment model is equal to the sum of the amounts of the drug in the central compartment (Xc), tissue compartment (Xt) and the amount of the drug eliminated by all possible routes.

$$Ab = Xc + Xt + X_3 \quad .....(7.115)$$

However, the terms in Equation 7.115 can also be expressed as:

$$Xc = Vc.\ C \quad .....(7.116)$$

$$Xt = Vt.\ Ct \quad .....(7.117)$$

$$X_3 = Vc.K_{13} \int_0^t C.dt = Vc\ K_{13}\ [AUC]_0^t \quad .....(7.118)$$

Substituting the values of Xc and X_3 into Equation 7.115, we get

$$Ab = Vc.C + Xt + Vc\ K_{13}\ [AUC]_0^t \quad .....(7.119)$$

Dividing Equation 7.119 by Vc, we obtain

$$\frac{Ab}{Vc} = C + \frac{Xt}{Vc} + K_{13}\ [AUC]_0^t \quad .....(7.120)$$

Setting the value of t = ∞, this equation becomes

$$\frac{Ab}{Vc} = 0 + 0 + K_{13}\ [AUC]_0^t = K_{13}\ [AUC]_0^\infty \quad .....(7.121)$$

Where, $Ab^\propto$ is the amount of the drug that will be ultimately absorbed from the dosage form. It means that the ratio of $Ab^\propto$ to the dose is the fraction of the dose absorbed, F.

$$F = Ab^\propto / X0 \quad .....(7.122)$$

The fraction of the dose absorbed at any time in comparison with $Ab^\propto$ can be obtained by dividing the Equation 7.120 by Equation 7.121.

$$\frac{Ab}{Ab^\alpha} = \frac{C + Xt/Vc + K_{13}[AUC]_0^t}{K_{13}[AUC]_0^\alpha} \quad .....(7.123)$$

or

$$\frac{Ab}{Ab^\alpha} = \frac{C + Ct + K_{13}[AUC]_0^t}{K_{13}[AUC]_0^\alpha} \quad .....(7.124)$$

Where, Ct = Xt/Vc = apparent tissue concentration, A plot of the fraction of the dose unabsorbed [1-(Ab/Abα)] versus time gives a straight line with the slope -Ka/2.303 from which the value of the absorption rate constant is obtained (Fig. 7.10).

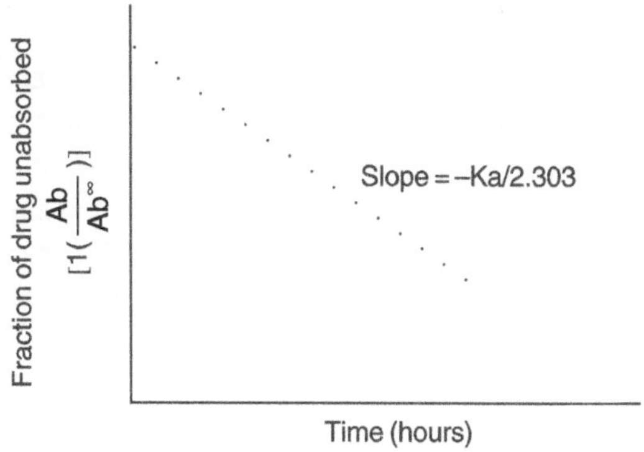

Fig. 7.10 A plot of the fraction of the drug unabsorbed $[1-(Ab/Ab^{\infty})]$ versus time used to determine the absorption rate constant by Loo-Riegelman method for a drug that follows a two-compartment model.

The values of C and $K[AUC]_0^t$ can be obtained from the plasma drug level versus time plot. The values for Ct can be approximated by the Loo-Riegelman method using equation.

$$(Ct)_{tn} = K_{12}\ \Delta C\ \Delta t + \frac{K_{12}}{K_{21}}\ (C)\ t_{n-1}\ (1 - e^{-K21\Delta t}) + (Ct)\ t_{n-1}\ (1 - e^{-K21\Delta t}) \quad .....(7.125)$$

Where:

Ct	=	Apparent tissue concentration
tn	=	Time of sampling for sample n
tn-1	=	Time of sampling for the sampling point proceeding sample n
(C) tn-1	=	concentration of drug at central compartment for sample n-1
DC	=	Concentration difference at central compartment between two sampling times.
Dt	=	Time difference between two sampling times.

For example, plasma is sampled at times zero and t = 0.5 hours, and corresponding concentrations of the drug in the central compartment are zero and 2 ug/ml.

Then, $(Ct)_{tn}$ = 2 ug/ml and $(C)_{tn-1}$ = 0, DC = 2 ug/ml, Dt = 0.5 hours

As mentioned previously, the drug must be administered intravenously for the estimation of distribution and elimination rate constants. Then only the estimation of absorption rate can be made by Loo-Riegelman method. For drugs that can not be given by I.V. route, Ka can not be calculated by the Loo-Riegelman method.

Method of "Inspection" in comparing the absorption rate of drug from different dosage forms

When the aim of a study is to know whether the absorption rates of a drug from different formulations are the same or different, the method of inspection may be sufficient. There is no need to calculate absorption rate constants accurately for this purpose. The peak-time (t_p), in the plasma concentration versus time curve provides a convenient measure of the absorption rate. For example, when different formulations containing the same drug are all found to be absorbed completely and all give plasma peak at the same time, it can be safely concluded that drug absorption from all the formulations is at the same rate.

Significance of Absorption Rate Constant

Many processes contribute to the overall absorption process of a drug given by oral route. For example, a tablet is administered orally, it has to undergo processes such as disintegration, dissolution before the drug is available for absorption. Biological factors like G.I. motility, pH, blood flow to the GIT, and transport of the drug across the capillary membranes and into the circulation also influence absorption process. The rate of drug absorption is the net result of all the processes mentioned above.

The drug absorption process may be zero order, first order, or a complex process that can not easily be quantitated. For many dosage forms that release the drug immediately, the absorption process is first order due to the physical nature of drug diffusion. The certain control-released drug products, the rate of drug absorption may be more appropriately described by the zero order rate constant.

The estimation of Ka is useful in designing a proper multiple-dosage regimen. Prediction of peak and trough plasma drug levels following multiple dosing of a drug is possible if Ka and K values are known.

7.1.6 Oral Route of Administration - Unchanged Drug in Urine

Scheme 7.1.6

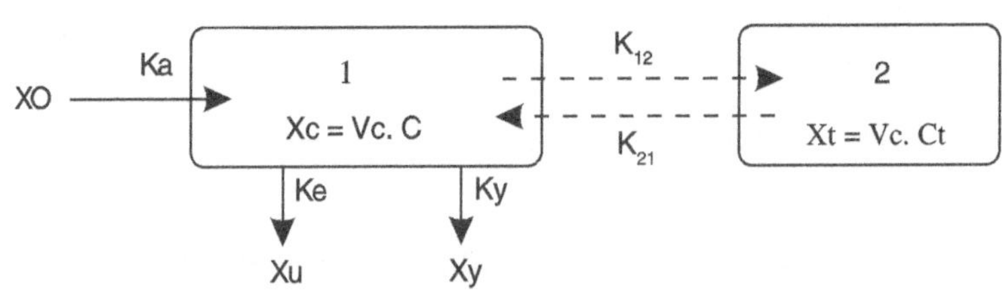

Where Ke is the urinary excretion rate constant and Xu is the cumulative amount of the drug excreted in urine, while Ky is the sum of elimination rate constants of all the processes involved in the elimination of drug other than renal route and Xy is the cumulative amount of the drug excreted by other processes. All other terms are as defined previously. The elimination rate constant, K_{13} is the sum of Ke and Ky.

$$K_{13} = Ke + Ky \qquad .....(7.126)$$

The rate of appearance of unchanged drug in urine is given by:

$$\frac{dXu}{dt} = Ke\ Xc \qquad .....(7.127)$$

but Xc = Vc.C, therefore

$$\frac{dX}{dt} = Ke\ Vc\ .\ C \qquad .....(7.128)$$

Where, Ke Vc is the renal clearance of the drug. According to Equation 7.110

$$C = A.e^{-\alpha t} + B\ e^{-\beta t} - C0\ e^{-K\alpha t}$$

Substituting for C in equation 7.128,

$$\frac{dXu}{dt} = Ke\ Vc.A.\ e^{-\alpha t} + Ke\ Vc.\ B\ e^{-\beta t} - Ke\ Vc\ C0\ e^{-K\alpha t} \qquad .....(7.129)$$

or

$$\frac{dXu}{dt} = A'.e^{-\alpha t} + B'\ e^{-\beta t} - C0'\ e^{-K\alpha t} \qquad .....(7.130)$$

dXu/dt is known as an instantaneous rate of excretion. In practice, we use average urinary excretion rate, $\Delta Xu/\Delta t$, at the mid-point of urine collection period (t'). Hence, $\Delta Xu/\Delta t$ approximates dXu/dt at t' if the urine sampling intervals are short.

$$\frac{\Delta Xu}{\Delta t} = A'.\ e^{-\alpha t} + B'\ e^{-\beta t} - C0'\ e^{-K\alpha t} \qquad .....(7.131)$$

Where, t' is the mid-point of urine collection period. Equation 7.131 can be subjected to the method of residuals as described under plasma concentration time data, to obtain the values of α, β, Ka, A', B' and C0'.

It is assumed that the rate constant involved are first-order rate constants and elimination of the drug occurs from the central compartment.

Practice Problems

1. A dose of 100 mg of a drug is administered by rapid intravenous injection to a 70 kg healthy adult male. Blood samples are taken periodically after the administration of the drug and plasma fraction of each sample is assayed. The following data are obtained:

Time (hrs)	0.25	0.50	1.0	1.50	2.0	4.0	8.0	12.0	16.0
Plasma Conc. (mg/ml)	43	32	20	14	11	6.5	2.8	1.2	0.52

Assume that the drug follows a two-compartment model and calculate all possible phamracokinetic parameters.

Solution :

The equation that describes the time-course of drug concentration in plasma following I.V. bolus for a drug that follows a two-compartment open model is

$$C = \frac{X0}{Vc\,(\alpha - \beta)}[(\alpha - K_{21})\,e^{-\alpha t} + (K_{21} - \beta)e^{-\beta t}]$$

or $$C = A \,.\, e^{-\alpha t} + B.\, e^{-\beta t}$$

Step 1. A semilogarithmic plot of plasma concentration versus t should be made. The terminal linear portion is used to calculate β.

$$\text{Slope} = \frac{-\beta}{2.303}$$

$$\text{Slope} = 0.091$$

Elimination rate constant, $\beta = 0.091 \times 2.303 = 0.21\ hr^{-1}$

$$\text{Elimination half-life} = \frac{0.693}{\beta} = \frac{0.639}{0.21} = 3.3\text{hrs.}$$

Step 2. Extrapolate the terminal linear portion to cut Y-axis.

$$\text{The intercept, } B = \frac{X0\,(K21 - \beta)}{Vc\,(\alpha - \beta)} = 15\ mg/ml.$$

3. Apply the method of residuals and set up the following table.

Time (hrs)	Observed plasma level (C)	Exprapolated plasma level (C_p)	Residual plasma concentration ($Cr = C_p$)
0.25	43.0	14.5	28.5
0.50	32.0	13.5	18.5
1.0	20.0	12.3	7.7
1.5	14.0	11.0	3.0
2.0	11.0	10.0	1.0
4.0	6.5		
8.0	2.8		
12.0	1.2		
16.0	0.50		

Plot residual plasma concentration versus time on the same paper to obtain a residual line, the slope of which is equal to - α/2.303 and intercept = A.

$$\text{Slope} = -\alpha/2.303 = 0.782$$

$$\alpha = 0.782 \times 2.303 = 1.8\ hr^{-1}$$

Intercept, $A = 45\ \mu g/ml.$

Step 4. Now, the equation that relates plasma drug concentration and time can be written as below

$$C = 45\ \mu g/ml \times e^{-1.8\,t} + 15\ \mu g/ml \times e^{-0.21\,t}$$

The other rate constants involved in the equation can be calculated.

$$K_{21} = \frac{B\alpha + A\beta}{A+B} = \frac{(15\times1.8)+(45\times0.21)}{(45+15)} = 0.61\ hr^{-1}$$

$$K_{13} = \frac{(A+B)\alpha\beta}{B\alpha + A\beta} = \frac{(45+15)+(1.8\times0.21)}{(15\times1.8)+(45\times0.21)} = 0.622\ hr^{-1}$$

$$K_{12} = \frac{AB\,(\alpha-\beta)^2}{(A+B)\,(B\alpha+A\beta)} = \frac{(45\times15)+(1.8-0.21)^2}{(45+15)+(15\times1.8+45\times0.21)} = 0.780\ hr^{-1}$$

Step 5. Volume of distribution of the central compartment, Vc.

$$A + B = C0 = \frac{X0}{Vc}$$

Therefore $$Vc = \frac{X0}{C0} = \frac{IV\ dose}{(A+B)} = \frac{100\ mg}{(45+15)}$$

$$Vc = \frac{100\,000\ \mu g}{60\ \mu g/mL} = 1666.7\ ml$$

Vc according to the equation,

$$Vc = \frac{X0}{K_{13}\ [AUC]^{\alpha}{}_{0}} = \frac{100mg}{0.622\times92.52} = \frac{100\,000\ \mu g}{57.55\ \mu g/mL}$$

$$Vc = 1737.7\ ml$$

* See next point for AUC_0^∞.

Step 6. Area Under the Curve: Are under the curve is calculated by the Trapezoidal rule.

$$AUC_0^t = \frac{1}{2}(C_0 + C_2)\ (t_1 - t_0) + \frac{1}{2}\ (C_1 + C_2)\ (t_2 - t_1) + \ldots\ldots + \frac{1}{2}\ (C_{n-1} + C_n)\ (t_n - t_{n-1})$$

$$AUC_0^t = \frac{1}{2}(0 + 43)\ (0.25) + \frac{1}{2}\ (43 + 32)\ (0.25) + \frac{1}{2}\ (32 + 20)\ (0.5) + \frac{1}{2}\ (20 + 14)$$

$$(0.5) + \frac{1}{2}\ (14 + 11)\ (0.5) + \frac{1}{2}\ (11 + 6.5)\ (2) + \frac{1}{2}\ (6.5 + 2.8)\ (4) + \frac{1}{2}\ (2.8 + 1.2)$$

$$(4) + \frac{1}{2}\ (1.2 + 0.52)\ (4)$$

$$= 5.375 + 9.375 + 13 + 8.5 + 6.25 + 17.5 + 18.6 + 8 + 3.44 = 90.04\ \mu g\text{-}hr/ml$$

$$AUC_0^t = 90.04 \ \mu g\text{-hr/ml}$$

$$AUC_t^\infty = \frac{C^*}{\beta} = 2.476 \ \mu g\text{-hr/ml}$$

$$AUC_0^\infty = 90.04 + 2.476 = 92.52 \ \mu g\text{-hr/ml}$$

Step 7. Drug levels in tissue or peripheral compartment

$$X_t = \frac{K_{12}\ X0}{(\alpha - \beta)} (e^{-\beta t} - e^{-\infty t})$$

The amount of the drug in the tissue compartment at any time 't' after I.V. bolus injection can be estimated using the above equation.

For example the amount of the drug in the tissue compartment after 4 hours is the following :

$$X_t = \frac{0.78 \times 100}{(1.8 - 0.21)} (e^{-0.21 \times 4} - e^{-1.8 \times 4})$$

$$= 49.06\ (0.431) = 21.16 \text{ mg.}$$

The amount of the drug in the central compartment after 4 hrs

$$= V_c .C = 1.6667 \text{ ml x } 6.5 \text{ mg/ml} = 10.83 \text{ mg.}$$

The total amount of the drug in the body after 4 hrs

$$= Xc + X_t = 10.83 \text{ mg} + 21.16 \text{ mg} = 31.99 \text{ mg.}$$

Volume at steady state,

$$V_d^{ss} = \frac{\text{Total drug in the body at steady state}}{\text{Plasma drug concentration}}$$

$$= \frac{31.99}{6.5} = 4.92 \text{ L}$$

$$V_d\beta = \frac{K_{13}\ Vc}{\beta} = \frac{0.622 \times 1666.67}{0.21} = 4.94 \text{ L}$$

$$V_d^{area} = \frac{X0}{\beta\,[AUC]_0^{\alpha}} = \frac{100}{0.21 \times 92.52} = 5.15 \text{ L}$$

$$V_d^{exp} = \frac{Vc\,(\alpha - \beta)}{(K_{21} - \beta)} = \frac{1666.7\text{ml}\,(1.8 - 0.21)}{(0.61 - 0.21)} = \frac{1.666.7 \times 1.59}{0.4} \quad 6.63 \text{ L}$$

ist of Pharmacokinetic Parameters Estimated From the Data:

1. $A = 45\ \mu g/ml$
2. $B = 15\ \mu g/ml$
3. $\alpha = 1.8\ hr^{-1}$
4. $\beta = 0.21\ hr^{-1}$
5. $CO = 60\ \mu g/ml$
6. $t_{1/2} = 3.3$ hrs
7. $K_{21} = 0.61\ hr^{-1}$
8. $K_{13} = 0.622\ hr^{-1}$
9. $K_{12} = 0.78\ hr^{-1}$
10. $AUC_0^{\alpha} = 92.52\ \mu g\text{-}ml/hr$
11. $V_c = 1666.7$ ml
    $V_c = 1737.7$ ml (area method)
12. X_t at 4 hrs = 21.16 mg
13. X_c at 4 hrs = 10mg
14. Volumes of distributuion.
    $V_d^{ss} = 4.92$ L $V_d b = 4.94$ L
    $V_d^{area} = 5.15$ L $V_d^{exp} = 6.63$ L

General ranking of these volumes of distribution is as below:

$$Vd^{exp} > Vd^{area} \text{ or } Vba > V_d^{ss} > Vc$$

$$6.63 \text{ L} > 5.15\text{L or } 4.94\text{L} > 4.92\text{L} > 1.667\text{L}$$

7.2 Three Compartment Open Model

The kinetics of certain drugs can be best explained by a three compartment model. The distribution of drug is very rapid in the central compartment, less rapid in one of the tissue compartments (2nd compartment) and very slow in the deep tissue compartment (3rd compartment). In other words, the time required for the equilibration of the drug in tissue comparment 2 is less than that of deep tissue compartment 3. Poorly perfused tissues such as bone and fat represent the third compartment. The deep tissue compartment may also represent a tightly bound drug in the tissue.

Scheme 7.2

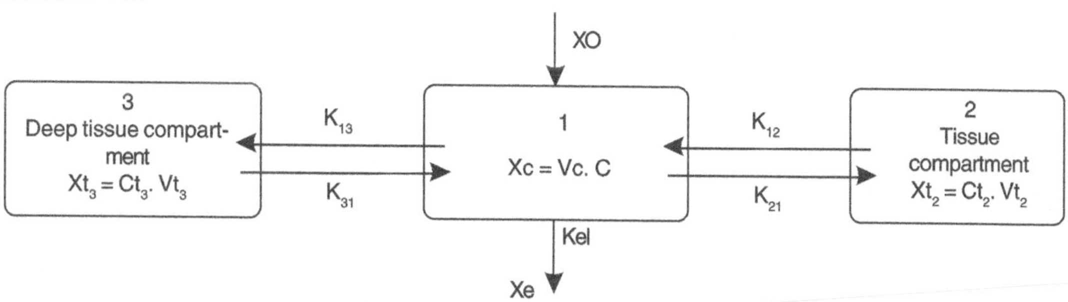

Where; X0 = I.V. dose (bolus)

Kel is the elimination rate constant

K_{12}, K_{21}, K_{13} and K_{31} are the first order rate constants representing the rate processes of drug movement from one compartment to the other.

X, V and C represent the amount of the drug, and the volume of distribution and concentration of the drug in each compartment. Subscripts C, t_2 and t_3 represent the central compartment, tissue compartment 2 and tissue compartment 3, respectively.

The differential equation that describes the rate of change of drug concentration in the central compartment following I.V. bolus is,

$$\frac{dc}{dt} = K_{21}\,Xt_2 + K_{31}\,Xt_3 - (K_{12} + K_{13} + Kel)\,Xc \qquad .....(7.132)$$

A solution of the above differential equation describing the rate of flow of the drug into and out of the central compartment gives the following equation.

$$C = A.e^{-at} + B.e^{-bt} + C\,e^{-ct} \qquad .....(7.133)$$

Where, C is the drug concentration in plasma at any time after I.V. injection.

A, B, and C can be calculated by extrapolating the lines obtained by method of residuals, on Y-axis. A, B and C are the Y intercepts of extrapolated lines for the central, tissue and deep tissue compartments, respectively, and a, b and c are the first order rate constants for the central, tissue and deep tissue compartments, respectively. The parameters in equation 7.133 may be resolved by the method of residuals or computers. Equation 7.133 represents a triexponential curve which becomes biexponential after an equilibrium between the drug levels in the central compartment and tissue compartment 2 has been established, and finally becomes monoexponential after an equilibrium between the drug levels in the central compartment and deep tissue compartment 3 has been established.

A semilogarithmic plot of drug levels in plasma versus time results in a curve, the slope of the terminal linear portion of which is -c/2.303 and the intercept obtained by extrapolating it is C (Fig. 7.11). Substraction of concentration of the drug on the extrapolated line from the actual concentrations give residual drug concentration versus time data. A plot of residual concentration versus time data gives a curve with a terminal linear portion. The slope of the terminal linear portion of the residual curve is equal to –b/2.303 and extrapolation of this line on to Y-axis gives a value for B. Application of the method of residuals between the extrapolated B line and the first residual curve, yields a straight line with the slope of -a/2.303 and intercept A.

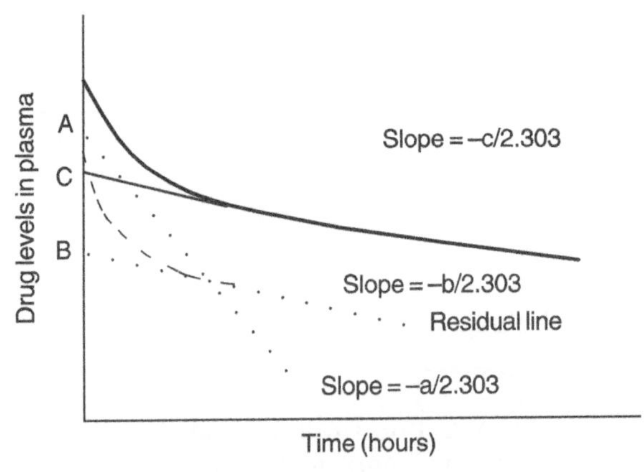

Fig. 7.11 Semi-logarithmic plot of drug concentration in plasma versus time curve for a three compartment open model. Estimation of rate constants and intercepts by the method of residuals.

The volume of distribution of the drug in the central compartment is calculated by equation

$$Vc = \frac{X0}{A+B+C} \quad .....(7.134)$$

The elimination rate constant, Kel, can be calculated with the following equation.

$$Kel = \frac{(A+B+C)\,abc}{Abc+Bac+Cab} \quad .....(7.135)$$

Area under the curve from time zero to infinity is obtained by integrating equation 7.133 between the limits of t = 0 and t = ∞, with respect to time,

$$\int_0^\infty C\,dt = \int_0^\infty A\,e^{-at} + \int_0^\infty B\,.\,e^{-bt} + \int_0^\infty C.e^{-ct} \quad .....(7.136)$$

$$[AUC]_0^\infty = \frac{A}{a} + \frac{B}{b} + \frac{C}{c} \quad .....(7.137)$$

Likely Questions

1. What are the factors that determine the number of compartments for a given drug?
2. What are the important points to be considered in developing equations for a *two* compartment open model?
3. Give the equation for drug concentration in the central compartment-time data and tissue drug level-time data.
4. How do you estimate the volume of distribution of the central compartment?
5. What is the siginificance of different volumes of distribution?
6. Write a note on total body clearance of two compartment open model.
7. How do you calculate the infusion rate required to achieve the desired C_{ss}?
8. What are the steps to be followed to resolve the various exponents by the Method of Residuals?
9. Write about the Loo-Riegelman method used for the determination of absorption rate constant from plasma drug concentration-time data of a drug that follows a two compartment open model.
10. An antibiotic is given intravenously (bolus) to a patient weighing 65-kg. A dose of 650 mg is injected and plasma samples are collected at different time intervals. The samples are analyzed for drug content and the drug levels in plasma were found to decline biexponentially. The following data are obtained.

Suggested Readings

1. Gibaldi, M.; Perrier, D. Drug elimination and apparent volume of distribution in multi compartment systems. J. Pharma. Sci. 60 952-954 (1972).
2. Gibaldi, M.; Perrier, D. Pharmacokinetics. 2nd Edn. Informa health care NY, 2007.
3. Perrier, D.; Gibaldi, M, Relationship between plasma or serum drug concentration and amount of drug in the body at steady state upon multiple dosing. J. Pharmacokin. and Pharmawdynamics . 1, 17-22 (1973).
4. Shargel, L.; wu-Pong, S.; Y_u, A.B.C. Applied Biopharmaceutics & Pharmacokinetics Fifth Edn. Mc Craw-Hill Publishers, USA. 2005.

8

Multiple-Dose Regimens

Drugs are infrequently used in single doses to produce an acute effect, the way aspirin is used to relieve a headache. More often, drugs are administered in successive doses to produce a chronic or prolonged effect, the way NSAIDs are used to relieve the pain and inflammation of arthritis. The goal in the design of dosage regimens is to achieve and maintain drug concentrations in plasma or at the site of action that are both safe and effective. Maximum safe concentration (MTC) and minimum therapeutic concentration (MEC) are schematically illustrated in Fig. 8.1. Toxicity would results if doses are administered too frequently, whereas, effectiveness would be lost if the dosage rate are too infrequent. The two main parameters that can be adjusted in developing a proper dosage regimen are (1) the size of the dose of the drugs and (2) the frequency of drug administration (τ) - that is, the time interval between doses.

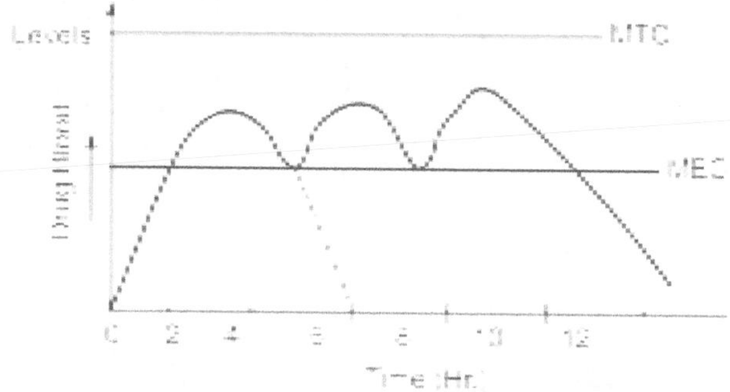

Fig. 8.1 Plasma drug concentration vs. time profile upon multiple oral administration indicating maximum tolerable conc. (MTC) and minimum effective conc. (MEC)

8.1 Drug Accumulation

When drugs are administered on a multiple dose regimen, each dose (after the first) is administered before the preceding doses are completely eliminated. The peak plasma level (highest plasma concentration), following the administration of second and each succeeding dose of a drug, is higher than the peak concentration following the administration of the first dose.This results in a phenomenon known as ***accumulation***, where the amount of the drug in the body (represented by plasma concentration) builds up as successive doses are administered. Figure 8.2 shows the drug accumulation occurring with multiple dosing.

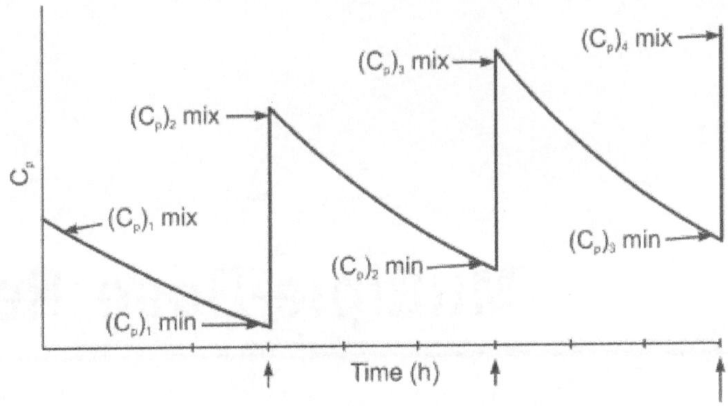

Fig. 8.2 Drug plasma level –time graph showing accumulation occurring after every dosing.

Following the administration of a number of doses (theoretically an infinite number of doses, and practically greater than seven or eight doses) of a suitable but identical size and at a suitable but identical dosing interval, the condition is reached where the administration of a chosen dose (X0) and dosing interval (τ) will provide, at steady state, all concentrations within the therapeutic range of a drug (Figure 8.3). ***Steady state*** is achieved at a time when, under a given dosage regimen, the mass (amount) of drug administered (for intravenous) or absorbed (for extravascular route), is equal to the mass (amount) of drug eliminated over a dosing

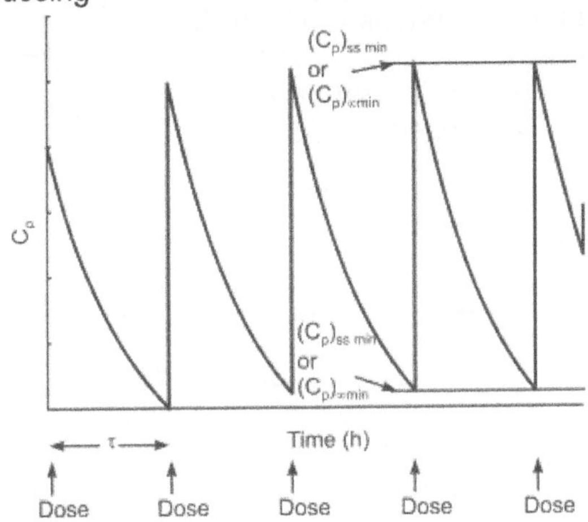

Fig. 8.3 Drug plasma level –time graph showing steady state attainment after few dosing intervals.

Table 8.1 Drug accumulation during multiple dose regimen.

Dose = 10 mg Dosing interval = $t_{1/2}$ of the drug

Frequency No. **No. of Half-lives**	**No. of doses** 1	2	3	4	5	6	7	8	
0	100 max	—							
1	50 min	150							
2		75	175						
3			87.5	187.5					
4				93.8	193.8				
5					96.88	196.88			
6						98.44	198.44		
7							99.22	199.22	max
8								99.61	min

To appreciate the phenomenon of accumulation, consider what happens when a 100 mg dose is given intravenously (bolus) at every elimination half-life ($t_{1/2}$). The amounts in the body just after each dose and just before the next dose can readily be calculated; these values correspond to the maximum (A_{max}) and minimum (A_{min}) amounts obtained within each dosing interval. A_{max} and A_{min} for first dose are 100mg and 50mg respectively. The maximum amount of the drug in the body in the second dosing interval, $A_{2,max}$ (150 mg) is the dose (100mg) plus the amount remaining from the previous dose (50mg). The minimum amount of the drug in the second dosing $A_{2,min}$, is 75 mg. Table 8.1 shows the maximum and minimum amounts in the dosing intervals. It can be seen from the table that after seven doses of the drug, at an interval equal to the drug half-life, the maximum and minimum amounts in the body become fairly constant. This is called steady-state level. In this example, the maximum and minimum amounts in the body at the steady state are 200 mg and 100 mg, respectively. It means the amount of the drug lost during dosing interval at the steady-state is equal to the administered dose.

The prediction of the amount of the drug in the body following repeated doses of a drug in the above is example based on the assumption that its elimination half-life is constant throughout the dosage regimen.

As repetitive equal doses are given at a constant frequency, the plasma level–time curve plateaus and a steady state is obtained. At steady state, the plasma drug levels fluctuate between C^{∞}_{max} and C^{∞}_{min}. Once steady state is obtained, C^{∞}_{max} and C^{∞}_{min} are constant and remain unchanged from dose to dose. The C^{∞}_{max} is important in determining drug safety. The C^{∞}_{max} should always remain below the minimum toxic concentration (MTC). The C^{∞}_{max} is also a good indication of drug accumulation. If a drug produces the same C^{∞}_{max} at steady state, compared with the $(C_{n=1})_{max}$ after the first dose, then there is no drug accumulation. If $C^{\infty}{}_{max}$ is much larger than $(C_{n=1})_{max}$, then there is significant accumulation during the multiple-dose regimen. Accumulation is affected by the elimination half-life of the drug and the dosing interval. The index for measuring drug accumulation *R* is

$$R = \frac{(C^{\infty})_{max}}{(C_{n=1})_{max}} \quad .....(8.1)$$

Substituting for C_{max} at first and steady state, we get

$$R = \frac{X0/Vd\left[1/(1-e^{-K\tau})\right]}{X_0/Vd} = \frac{1}{1-e^{-kt}}$$

Equation 8.2 shows that drug accumulation measured with the *R* index depends on the elimination constant and the dosing interval and is independent of the dose. For a drug given in repetitive oral doses, the time required to reach steady state is dependent on the elimination half-life of the drug and is independent of the size of the dose, the length of the dosing interval, and the number of doses.

Principle of Superposition

An acceptable plasma concentration profile at the steady state can be devised with the aid of pharmacokinetic parameters derived from single dose experiments based on the principle of ***superposition.*** The principle of superposition assumes that early doses of a drug do not affect the pharmacokinetics of subsequent doses. The basic assumptions are that the drug is eliminated by first order kinetics and that the pharmacokinetics of the drug after a single dose (first dose) are not altered for multiple doses. Therefore, the blood levels after the second, third or nth dose will overlay or superimpose the blood level attained after the (n-1)th dose. In addition, $[AUC]_0^{\infty}$ following the administration of a single dose equals the $[AUC]_{t1}^{t2}$ during a dosing interval at steady state (Fig. 8.4).

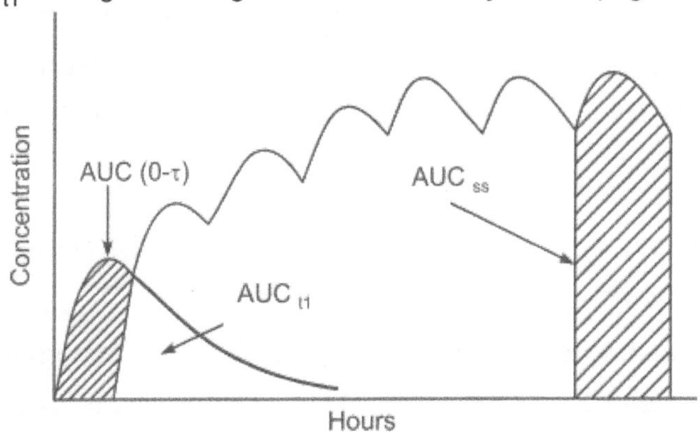

Fig. 8.4 Simulated data showing blood levels after administration of multiple doses and accumulation of blood levels when equal doses are given at equal time intervals.

The principle of superposition can be used to predict the drug levels in plasma after multiple doses using the plasma concentration-time data obtained after a single dose, as shown in Table-8.2. The drug levels in plasma versus time data obtained with a single dose is used to predict the drug levels in plasma after multiple doses at an interval of 4 hours each. The drug concentration-time data obtained with a single dose is repeated for each dose from the time it is administrated (see Table 8.2). Thus, the predicted plasma drug concentration would be the total drug concentration obtained by adding the residual drug concentration obtained after each previous dose. Because the superposition principle is an overlay method, it may be used to predict drug concentrations after multiple doses given at equal and unequal dosage intervals. Further, if the dose or dosage interval of the drug is altered, the time required for the drug to reach steady state is the same, but the final steady- state plasma level changes proportionately.

An equation for the estimation of the time to reach one-half of the steady-state plasma levels or the accumulation half-life

$$\text{Accumulation } t_{1/2} = t_{1/2}\left(1 + 3.3 \log \frac{Ka}{Ka - K}\right) \quad .....(8.3)$$

For IV administration, K_a is very rapid (approaches ∞); K is very small in comparison to K_a and can be omitted in the denominator of Equation 8.3. Therefore Equation reduces to

$$\text{Accumulation } t_{1/2} = t_{1/2}\left(1 + 3.3 \log \frac{Ka}{Ka}\right)$$

Because Ka/Ka=1 and log 1=0, the accumulation t1/2 of a drug administered intravenously is the elimination t1/2 of the drug. From this relationship, the time to reach 50% steady state drug concentration is dependent on the elimination t1/2 and not on the dose or dosage interval.

From a clinical viewpoint, the time needed to reach 90% of the steady-state plasma concentration is 3.3 times the elimination half-life, whereas the time required to reach 99% of the steady-state plasma concentration is 6.6 times the elimination half-life

There are situations where the superposition principle can not be applied. In these cases, the pharmacokinetics of the drug change after multiple dosing due to various factors, including changing pathophysiology in the patient, saturation of the drug carrier system, saturated protein binding, saturated active secretion, enzyme induction, and enzyme inhibition.

8.2 Repetitive Intravenous Injections - One Compartment Open Model

Calculation of plasma drug concentrations following repetitive doses of a drug using superposition principle requires preparation of a list of plasma drug concentrations for each dose as shown in Table 8.2. It is possible to develop equations that describe drug concentration in plasma versus time profile for repetitive injection of a drug that follows one compartment open model.

Table 8.2 Predicted Plasma Drug Concentration for Multiple Dose Regimen using Superposition Principle*.

Dose Number	Time (hours)	Plasma drug level (ug/ml)	Doses				Total
		1	2	3	4	5	
1	0	0					0
	1	21.0					21.0
	2	22.3					22.3
	3	19.8					19.8
2	4	16.9	0				16.9
	5	17.3	21.0				35.3
	6	12.0	22.3				34.3
	7	10.1	19.8				29.9
3	8	8.5	16.9	0			25.4
	9	7.15	17.3	21.0			42.5
	10	6.01	12.0	22.3			40.3
	11	5.06	10.1	19.8			35.0
4	12	7.25	8.50	16.9	0		29.7
	13	3.58	7.15	17.3	21.0		46.0
	14	3.01	6.01	12.0	22.3		43.3
	15	2.53	5.06	10.1	19.8		37.5
5	16	2.13	7.25	8.50	16.9	0	31.8
	17	1.79	3.58	7.15	17.3	21.0	47.8
	18	1.51	3.01	6.01	12.0	22.3	44.8
	19	1.27	2.53	5.06	10.1	19.8	38.8
	20	1.07	2.13	7.25	8.50	16.9	32.9

* A single oral dose of 350 mg was given and the plasma drug concentration were measured 0 - 20 hours. The same plasma drug concentrations are assumed to occur after doses 2-5. The total plasma drug concentration is the sum of the plasma drug concentration due to each dose.

Let us consider that a drug was repeatedly injected intravenously a dose of X0 with a dosing interval of t hours. The maximum concentration of the drug in plasma following a rapid IV injection is equal to the dose divided by volume of distribution of the drug.

$$C0 = X0 / Vd \qquad .....(8.4)$$

The concentration of the drug in plasma at any time t is given by,

$$C = C0\ e^{-Kt} \qquad .....(8.5)$$

Where, K is the overall elimination rate constant.

The concentration of the drug in plasma at the end of the first dosing interval, τ, is given by

$$C_1t = C_1^0.e^{-K\tau} \qquad .....(8.6)$$

Where C_1^{τ} = concentration of the drug in plasma at the end of the first dosing interval of τ.

C_1^0 = Zero time concentration for first dose.

The zero time concentration of the drug in plasma following the second dose will be

$$C_2^0 = C_1^{\tau} + C_1^0 \quad .....(8.7)$$

but $C_1^{\tau} = C_1^0 . e^{K\tau}$

Therefore, $$C_2^0 = C_1^0 e^{-K\tau} + C_1^0 \quad .....(8.8)$$

Let $r = e^{-K\tau}$ then, Equation 8.8 can be written as

$$C_2^0 = C_1^0 r + C_1^0 \quad .....(8.9)$$

The drug concentration in plasma at the end of the second dosing interval is given by

$$C_2\tau = C_2^0 . e^{-K\tau} = (C_1^0 r + C_1^0) r \quad .....(8.10)$$

Now, this procedure can be used for finding zero time concentration (maximum drug concentration in plasma) and drug concentration at the end of dosing interval (minimum drug concentration in plasma) for each dose of the drug.

$$C_3^0 = C_2\tau + C_1^0 = (C_1^0 r + C_1^0) r + C_1^0 \quad .....(8.11)$$

$$C_3\tau = C_3^0 r = [(C_1^0 r + C_1^0) r + C_1^0] r \quad .....(8.12)$$

Therefore, the plasma concentrations at the beginning and end of the nth dosing interval are given by the following series :

$$\text{Beginning} = C_1^0 + C_1^0 r + C_1^0 r^2 + \text{.............} + C_1^0 r^{(n-1)} \quad .....(8.13)$$

$$\text{End} = C_1^0 r + C_1^0 r^2 + C_1^0 r^3 + \text{............} + C_1^0 r^n \quad .....(8.14)$$

Since, r is always smaller than 1, r^n becomes smaller as n increases. Therefore, the high power terms in Equations 8.13 and 8.14 become negligible as n increases, and additional doses do not change the value of C_n^0 or $C_n\tau$ significantly. This explains why the plasma concentrations reach a plateau instead of continuing to rise as more doses are given.

When, $n = \infty$, Equations 8.13 and 8.14 become

$$C_{max} = \frac{C_1^0}{1-r} = \frac{X_0}{Vd(1-e^{-K\tau})} \quad .....(8.15)$$

$$C_{min} = C_{max} . r = \frac{C_1^0 r}{1-r} \quad .....(8.16)$$

Hence, C_{max} and C_{min} are defined as the plasma concentration at the beginning and end, respectively, of the nth dosing interval after the plateau has been reached (i.e., $n = \infty$). The term $Cmax^{\infty}$ represents the maximum plasma concentration of a drug in the body at the steady-state condition (i.e. following the administration of many doses). Thus, the maximum and minimum plasma concentrations on the plateau of a repetitive I.V. dosing regimen can be calculated if the dosing interval (τ), the overall elimination rate constant (K), and the initial plasma concentration (C0) are known.

An average steady state plateau drug concentration, C_{ave}, is obtained by dividing AUC for a dosing period by the dosing interval.

$$Cav = \frac{[AUC]_{t1}^{t2}}{\tau} \quad .....(8.17)$$

It should be remembered that C_{ave} is not the arithmetic mean of C_{max} and C_{min} because plasma drug concentrations decline exponentially. The $[AUC]_{t1}^{t2}$ is related to the dose (X0) divided by the total body clearance (Vd.K).

$$[AUC]_{t1}^{t2} = \frac{X0}{Vd.K} \quad .....(8.18)$$

Therefore, $$C_{ave} = \frac{X0}{VdK\tau} \quad .....(8.19)$$

Equations can also be expressed in terms of the amount of the drug in the body at the steady state.

$$X_{max} = \frac{X0}{1-r} \quad .....(8.20)$$

$$X_{min} = X_{max}\ r = \frac{X0.r}{1-r} \quad .....(8.21)$$

$$X_{ave} = \frac{X0}{K\tau} \quad .....(8.22)$$

Where, X_{max}, X_{min} and X_{ave} are the maximum, minimum and average amount of the drug in the body at the steady-state.

It is some time desirable to know the plasma drug concentration at any time after the administration of n doses of a drug. The general expression for calculating this plasma drug concentration is

$$C_n^t = C0\ \left(\frac{1-e^{-nK\tau}}{1-e^{-K\tau}}\right)\ e^{-Kt} \quad .....(8.23)$$

Where n is the number of doses given and τ is the time after the nth dose.

At steady-state $e^{-nk\tau}$ approaches zero and Equation 8.23 reduces to

$$C_n^{\infty} = C0\left(\frac{1}{1-e^{-K\tau}}\right)e^{-Kt} \quad .....(8.24)$$

Where C_n^{∞} is the steady-state drug concentration at time t, after the dose.

8.3 Repetitive Extravascular Dosing - One Compartment Open Model

Although the equations become considerably more complex than for the I.V. case, C_{max}, C_{min} and C_{ave} can be calculated when the drug is administered by an extravascular route. The basic assumptions made in developing the equations for the extravascular route are:

1. Drug absorption and elimination processes follow first order kinetics.
2. The pharmacokinetic parameters such as Ka, K, Vd and the fraction of the dose absorbed, (F) remain constant during multiple-dosing.

The equation describing the plasma drug concentration-time profile following a single dose of extravascular administration of the drug is given by

$$C = \frac{Ka\,FX0}{Vd\,(Ka - K)}\,(e^{-Kt} - e^{-Kat}) \qquad .....(8.25)$$

If n fixed doses of the drug (X0) are administered at fixed time intervals (t), the plasma concentrations following the 'nth' dose are given by

$$C_n^{\ t} = \frac{KaF\,X0}{Vd\,(Ka - K)}\left[\left(\frac{1 - e^{-nK\tau}}{1 - e^{-K\tau}}\,e^{-Kt} - \frac{1 - e^{-nKa\tau}}{1 - e^{-Ka\tau}}\right)e^{-Kat}\right] \qquad .....(8.26)$$

Where $C_n^{\ t}$ is the concentration of the drug at time t, after nth dosing. When n is large (i.e., when the plasma concentrations reach a plateau), the terms $e^{-nK\tau}$ and $e^{-nka\tau}$ becomes negligible and Equation 8.26 simplifies to,

$$C_n^{\ \infty} = \frac{KaF\,X0}{Vd\,(Ka - K)}\left[\left(\frac{1}{1 - e^{-K\tau}}\right)e^{-Kt} - \left(\frac{1}{1 - e^{-Ka\tau}}\right)e^{-Kat}\right] \qquad .....(8.27)$$

Equation 8.27 can be used to calculate the C_{max} and C_{min} values on the plasma concentration plateau by substituting values for t which correspond to the "peaks" and "valleys" in the C versus t curve.

The term t_p (peak concentration of drug in plasma after single dose) is given as

$$t_p = \frac{2.303}{(Ka - K)}\log\frac{Ka}{K}$$

The time at which a maximum plasma concentration of drug at steady state occurs (t_p') can be obtained by differentiating the Equation 8.27 with respect to time and setting the resultant equal to 0.

$$\frac{dC_n^{\infty}}{dt} = \frac{Ka\,F\,X0}{Vd\,(Ka - K)}\left[\left(\frac{Ka\,e^{-Kat}}{1 - e^{-Ka\tau}}\right) - \left(\frac{Ke^{-Kt}}{1 - e^{-K\tau}}\right)\right]$$

When $t = t_p'$,

$$\frac{Ka\,e^{-Ka\,t_p'}}{1 - e^{-Ka\tau}} = \frac{Ke - Kt_p'}{1 - e^{-K\tau}} \qquad .....(8.28)$$

Rearranging the above equation, we get

$$t_p' = \frac{2.303}{(Ka-K)} \log\left[\frac{Ka(1-e^{-K\tau})}{K(1-e^{-Ka\tau})}\right]$$

Thus, if t = tp (the time of the peak concentration of drug in plasma), Equation 8.27 gives C_{max}.

$$C_{max} = \frac{Ka\,F\,X0}{Vd\,(Ka-K)}\left[\left(\frac{1}{1-e^{-K\tau}}\right)e^{-Kt_p'} - \left(\frac{1}{1-e^{-Ka\tau}}\right)e^{-Ka\,t_p'}\right] \qquad .....(8.29)$$

From Equation 8.28, we get

$$e^{-Kat_p'} = \frac{K(1-e^{-ka\tau})}{Ka\,(1-e^{-K\tau})}\,e^{-Kt_p'}$$

Substituting in Equation 8.29 and solving, we get

$$C_{max} = \frac{F\,X0}{Vd}\left[\left(\frac{1}{1-e^{-K\tau}}\right)e^{-Kt_p'}\right] \qquad .....(8.30)$$

If t = τ (the time at which another dose is to be given), Equation 8.27 gives C_{min}.

$$C_{min} = \frac{Ka\,F\,X0}{Vd\,(Ka-K)}\left[\left(\frac{1}{1-e^{-K\tau}}\right)e^{-K\tau} - \left(\frac{1}{1-e^{-Ka\tau}}\right)e^{-Ka\tau}\right] \qquad .....(8.31)$$

In the post absorptive phase, $e^{-Ka\,\tau}$ will become zero, therefore, the Equation for Cmin becomes

$$C_{min} = \frac{Ka\,FX0}{Vd\,(Ka-k)}\left[\left(\frac{1}{1-e^{-kz}}\right)e^{-Kt}\right]$$

The mean plasma level at steady-state C_{ave} is obtained using the similar method employed for repeat I.V. injections.

$$C_{ave} = \frac{[AUC]_{t_1}^{t_2}}{\tau} \qquad .....(8.32)$$

or $$C_{ave} = \frac{FX0}{Vd.K\tau} \qquad .....(8.33)$$

Since $$[AUC]_{t_1}^{t_2} = \frac{FX0}{Vd.K}$$

8.4 Multiple Dosage Regimen - Loading Dose

As discussed earlier, the time required for the drug to accumulate to a steady state plasma level is dependent mainly on its elimination half-life. The time need to reach 95% C_{ave}

is approximately 5 half-lives of the drug. For a drug with a half-life of 5 hours, it would take approximately 25 hours to reach 95% of C_{ave}.

In order to initiate a immediate therapeutic effect, an initial dose also called loading dose, or priming dose, is administered to achieve C_{ave}. Thereafter, a maintenance dose is given to maintain C_{ave} so that the therapeutic effect is also maintained.

I.V. injections

According to equation 8.22

$$Xa\nu = \frac{X0}{K\tau} = Ca\nu \, . \, Vd \quad .....(8.34)$$

Where, X0 is I.V. dose, τ is dosing interval, Vd is the volume of distribution of the drug and K is the elimination rate constant. Therefore, we should administer a loading dose X* just before the administration of the maintenance dose, X0. The amount present in the body is equal to X0/Kτ. The amount of the drug present in the body after t = τ, following an I.V. dose of X* is, X_{ave}.

$$X_{ave} = X^* \, . \, e^{-K\tau} \quad .....(8.35)$$

The amount of the drug eliminated during this period must be supplied in the form of a maintenance dose, X0.

The amount of the drug eliminated from a loading dose in time τ, is equal to the difference between the loading dose (X*) and the amount remained in the body after τ (X_{ave}).

Amount of the drug eliminated

$$= X^* - X_{ave} \quad .....(8.36)$$

$$= X^* - X^* \, e^{-K\tau}$$

$$= X^* (1 - e^{-K\tau}) \quad .....(8.37)$$

The amount of the drug eliminated should be equal to the maintenance dose, X0, to maintain the steady-state level. Therefore.

Maintenance dose,

$$X0 = X^* (1-e^{K\tau}) \quad .....(8.38)$$

and loading dose,

$$X^* = \frac{X0}{(1-e^{-K\tau})} \quad .....(8.39)$$

In practice, the C_{ave} value for a particular drug is known. The elimination rate constant (K), volume of distribution (Vd) and dosing interval are taken from the literature to calculate the loading dose (X*), using the following equation.

$$\text{Loading dose } X^* = X_{ave}/e^{-K\tau} = C_{ave} \, Vd/ \, e^{-K\tau} \quad .....(8.40)$$

Maintenance dose can be calculated using Equation 8.38.

The ratio of loading to maintenance dose depends on the dosing interval and the half-life of the ***dose ratio*** as described below.

$$\text{Dose ratio} = \frac{X^*}{X0}$$

For extremely rapid absorption, dose ratio is also known as accumulation index, R, as given below

$$\text{Dose ratio} = \frac{1}{(1-e^{-k\tau})} \qquad .....(8.41)$$

Extravascular Dosing

In case of extravascular dosing, the fraction of the dose absorbed, F, should be taken into consideration while calculating the loading dose.

$$\text{Loading dose} = X^* = \text{loading dose} = X^* = \frac{Ca\nu\,.\,Vd/e^{-K\tau}}{F} \qquad .....(8.42)$$

Maintenance dose,

$$X0 = X^*\,(1 - e^{-K\tau}) \qquad .....(8.43)$$

8.5 Multiple Dose Regimen - Two Compartment Open Model

Equations can be developed for determining the average concentration of the drug in the central compartment, following I.V. bolus and extravascular dosing of a drug that follows a two compartment open model similar to that of one compartment model. However, more complex equations result which are difficult to follow for the nonspecialist. However, one compartment equations modified in minor ways apply to two-compartment systems with reasonable accuracy, when the distribution phase after one dose is approximately complete before the next dose is administered. Under these conditions, β may be substituted for K and V_d^{area} for Vd, to adopt one compartment equations to two-compartment systems for rough approximations of the two compartment parameters and plasma concentrations.

For I.V. injections,

$$C_{ave} = \frac{X0}{\beta V_d^{area} T} \qquad .....(8.44)$$

$$\text{Loading dose} = C_{ave}\, V_d^{area}/\, e^{-\beta t} \qquad .....(8.45)$$

For extravascular dosing:

$$C_{ave} = \frac{F\,X0}{\beta V_d^{area} \tau} \qquad .....(8.46)$$

$$\text{Loading dose} = \frac{C_{ave}\, V_d^{area}/e^{-\beta\tau}}{F} \qquad .....(8.47)$$

The accumulation or dose ratio of the drug R, is the ratio of loading and maintenance doses.

$$R_I \text{ Dose Ratio} = \frac{X^*}{X0} = \frac{1}{(1-e^{-\beta\tau})} \qquad .....(8.48)$$

The rate at which the steady state is attained depends almost entirely on β. It takes approximately 5 half-lives of the drug to reach the plateau level. Using β in place of K in the equations developed for one compartment model allows us to calculate the various pharmacokinetic parameters of the two-compartment system at the plateau level.

Practice Problem

1. A subject receives 1000 mg every 6 hours by repetitive I.V. injections of an antibiotic with an elimination of half-life of 3 hours. Assume that the drug is distributed according to a one compartment open model and the volume of distribution is 20 L. Find the maximum, minimum and average plasma drug level. What are the loading and maintenance doses for this case?

Solution :

Dosing interval, $\tau = 6$ hours

The biological half-life

$(t_{1/2}) = 3$ hours

Therefore, $K = 0.693/t_{1/2} = 0.693/3 = 0.231\ hr^{-1}$

According to Equation 8.12,

$C_{max} = C_1^0 /(1-R)$

Where, $C_1^0 = I.V.dose/V_d = 1000/20 = 50$ mg/L

$r = e^{-K\tau} = e^{-(0.231)\,(6)} = 0.25$

$C_{max} = 50/(1 - 0.25) = 66.67$ mg/L

According to Equation 8.16,

$C_{min} = C_{max}\ r.$

Therefore, $C_{min} = (66.67)\ (0.25) = 16.67$ mg/L

According to Equation 8.19,

$C_{ave} = I.V.dose/(V_d\ K\ \tau)$

$= 1000/(20)(0.231)(6) = 36.1$ mg/L

Loading doe, $X^* = C_{ave}\ V_d/e^{-K\tau}$ 8.40

$= (36.1)(20)/e^{-(0.231)\,(6)} = 2887.15$ mg

Maintenance dose $= X^*\ (1- e^{-K\tau})$ 8.38

$= 2887.15(1 - e^{-(0.231)\,(6)} = 2165.15$ mg

2. A male patient is given orally 250 mg of tetracycline Hcl every 8 hours. The antibiotic absorption rate constant is $0.9 hr^{-1}$ and the biological half-life is 10 hours. If the fraction of the dose absorbed is 0.75 and the volume of distribution is 121.5 liters, Calculate C_{max}, C_{min} and C_{ave} at steady-state. Find out the loading dose and maintenance dose for this case.

Solution :

Biological half-life= 10hours.

Hence, $K = 0.693/10 = 0.0693\ hr^{-1}$

Dosing interval, $\tau = 8$ hours

Volume of distribution,

$V_d = 121.5$ liters

Fraction of dose absorbed,

$F = 0.75$

Absorption rate constant,

$Ka = 0.9 hr^{-1}$

According to Equation ,

$t_p = 2.303/(Ka-K) \log (Ka/K)$

$= 2.303/(0.9 - 0.0693) \log(0.9/0.0693)$

$= 3.087$ hours

$$C_{max} = \frac{Ka\,F\,X0}{Vd\,(Ka-K)}\left[\left(\frac{1}{1-e^{-K\tau}}\right)e^{-Kt_p'} - \left(\frac{1}{1-e^{-Ka\tau}}\right)e^{-Ka\,t_p'}\right] \quad .....(8.29)$$

$$C_{max} = \frac{(0.9)\,(0.75)\,(250)}{121.5\,(0.9-0.0693)}\left[\left(\frac{1}{1-e^{-0.0693\times8}}\right)e^{-0.0693\times3.087} - \left(\frac{1}{1-e^{-0.9\times8}}\right)e^{-0.9\times3.087}\right]$$

$= 3.0675$ mg/L

$$C_{min} = \frac{Ka\,F\,X0}{Vd\,(Ka-K)}\left[\left(\frac{1}{1-e^{-K\tau}}\right)e^{-K\tau} - \left(\frac{1}{1-e^{-Ka\tau}}\right)e^{-Ka\tau}\right] \quad .....(8.31)$$

$= 2.24$ mg/L

$C_{ave} = F\,X0/V_d\,K\tau = (0.75)\,(250)/(121.5)(0.0693)(8) = 2.78$ mg/L

$$\text{Loading dose} = X^* = \frac{Ca\nu.Vd/e^{-K\tau}}{F} \quad .....(8.42)$$

$$\text{Loading dose,} \quad X^* = \frac{2.78\times121.5/e^{-0.0693\times8}}{0.75} = 784\,mg$$

Maintenance dose $= X^*\,(1 - e^{-K\tau})$

$= 784\,[1 - e^{-(0.0693)(8)}] = 333.65$ mg

Likely Questions

1. Why the drugs are administered in multiple-doses?
2. Explain the phenomenon of drug accumulation.
3. What do you mean by the principle of superposition?
4. Give the equation for calculating C_{max}, C_{min} and C_{ave} following repeated I.V injections.
5. Give the equations for calculating a loading dose and a maintenance dose for repeated extravascular administration.
6. A drug has an average elimination half-life of approximately 2 hours and an apparent volume of distribution of 20% of body weight. The drug is administered to a woman weighing 50-kg at a dose of 1 mg/kg every 8 hours by multiple I.V. injections. Calculate,
   (a) C_{max}
   (b) C_{min} and
   (c) C_{ave}.
7. The elimination half-life of an antibiotic is 3 hours and the apparent volume of distribution is 20% of body weight. The therapeutic window for this drug is from 2 to 10 μg/ml. Adverse toxicity is often observed at drug concentration above 15 μg/ml. The drug is given by multiple I.V. bolus injections.
   (a) Calculate the dose for an adult male patient (52 years, 82-kg) to be given every 8 hours.
   (b) Calculate the expected C_{min} and C_{ave}.
   (c) Comment on the adequacy of your dosage regimen.
8. What is the loading dose for an antibiotic ($K = 0.23\ hr^{-1}$) with a maintenance dose of 200 mg every 3 hours?

Suggested Readings

1. Gibaldi, M.; Perrier, D. Pharmacokinetics. 2nd edn. Informa Healthcare, NY, 2007.
2. Jambhekar, S.S., Breen, P.J. Basic Pharmacokinetics, Pharmaceutical Press Inc, UK. 2009.
3. Notari, R.E. Biopharmaceutics and Clinical Pharmacokinetics. 4th edn. Marcel Dekker Inc., NY. 1987.
4. Ronland, M., Tozen, T.N. Clinical Pharmacokinetics. Concepts and Applications. 3rd edn. Lea & Febrigen, USA. 1994.
5. Shargel, L., Wu - Pong, S., Yu, A.B.C. Applied Biopharmaceutics & Pharmacokinetics. fifth ed". Mc Graw - Hill Publishers, USA, 2005.

9

Nonlinear Pharmacokinetics

9.1 Introduction

The pharmacokinetic parameters of most drugs are not expected to change when different doses are administered or when the drug is given through different routes of administration or as single or multiple doses. Or in other words plasma concentration and the amount of a drug and its metabolites excreted in urine at any given time all increase in direct proportion to its dose, when the drug is administered in either a single dose, or in multiple doses.

Generally five pharmacokinetic parameters F (fraction absorbed), Ka (absorption rate constant), Vd (volume of distribution), CL_R (renal clearance) and CL_h (hepatic clearance) defines and summarize the time-course of a drug in the body and are generally linear or dose dependent (i.e. that if the dose is increased, the plasma concentration or area under the plasma concentration-time curve (AUC) will be increased proportionally, as demonstrated in Fig.1. The superposition principle is based on the above points. When superposition occurs, the pharmacokinetics of a drug is said to be dose- independent or linear.

The kinetics (*e.g.* clearance and volume of distribution) of these molecules are said to be linear or dose-independent, and this is a characteristic of first-order kinetics.

However, for some drugs, the principle of superposition may not hold good. For example, when the dose of phenytoin is increased by 50 percent in a patient from 300 mg/day to 450 mg/day, the average steady state concentration may increase by as much as ten fold. This dramatic increase in the concentration is due to the nonlinear pharmacokinetics of phenytoin. For these drugs (drugs with nonlinear kinetics or dose-dependent kinetics), the kinetic parameters, such as F (fraction absorbed), Ka (absorption rate constant), Vd (volume of distribution), CL_R (renal clearance) and CL_h (hepatic clearance), vary depending on the administered dose. The pharmacokinetics of such drugs are said to be *dose-dependent*. When there is a lack of superposition on administering a drug on *separate occasions* or a lack of predictability following *repeated* or *continuous dosing*, based on a single-dose data, the drug is said to show *time-dependent* kinetics. Although relatively uncommon, they occur frequently enough in drug therapy to warrant a special consideration. Besides there are certain cases of route dependent pharmacokinetics as well.

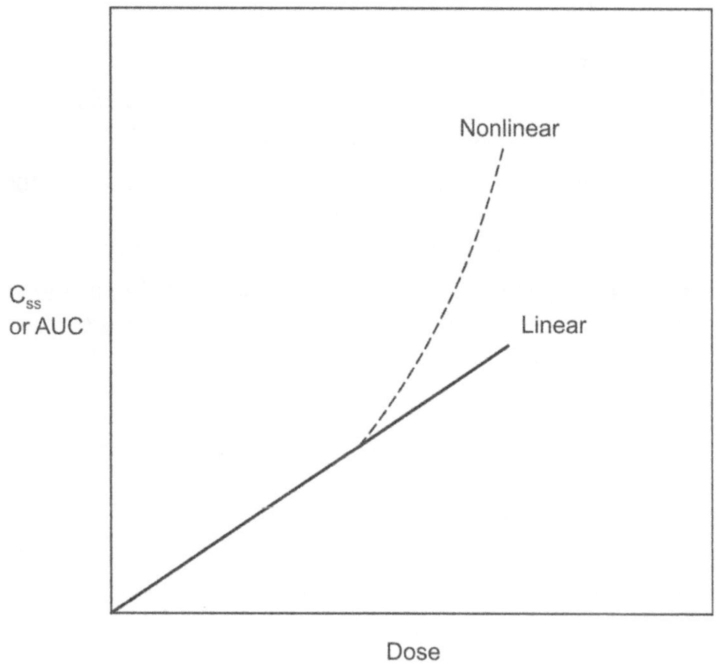

Fig. 9.1 The qualitative relationship between the steady-state plasma concentration (CSS) or area under the plasma concentration-time curve (AUC) and the administered dose for drugs with linear (solid line) and nonlinear (dashed line) pharmacokinetics.

This dependency is because one or more of the kinetic processes of the drug (absorption, distribution, and/or elimination) may be via a process other than simple first-order kinetics. For these drugs, the relationship between the AUC or CSS and dose is not linear (Fig 9.1). Additionally, different doses of these drugs may not result in parallel plasma concentration-time courses expected for drugs with linear pharmacokinetics. For example, for drugs with nonlinear metabolism, the initial decline in the plasma concentrations may be slower at higher doses, compared with that after the administration of the lower doses (Fig 9.2). This means that the rate of elimination is not directly proportional to the plasma concentration for these drugs.

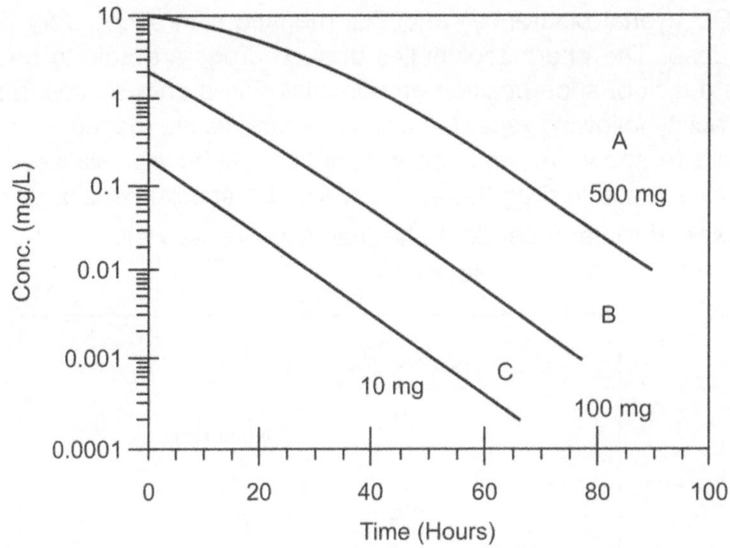

Fig. 9.2 The simulated plasma concentration-time courses of a drug after the intravenous administration of 3 different doses. Average pharmacokinetic parameters of phenytoin (volume of distribution of 50 L, Vmax of 500 mg/day, and Ku of 4 mg/L) were used for the simulation).

Fig. 9.2 shows the plasma level time curves for a drug that exhibits saturable kinetics. When a large dose is given as an I.V. bolus, the elimination of a drug is slow initially and become rapid at lower plasma concentrations (curve A). With a small dose of drug apparent first-order kinetics are observed, because no saturation occur (curve B). Curve C is generated based on the kinetic parameters derived from curve B, by a dose twice that for curve B (equal to the dose used for curve A). Curve C under-estimates the drug concentration as well as the duration of action.

Both dose-dependent and time-dependent kinetic behaviors can easily be quantified and predicted. The first step in evaluating this behavior is to identify its occurrence, and the subsequent steps involve determining the parameters affected and the likely mechanism(s) of nonlinearity. There are many potential causes of dose and time dependencies. Table 9.1 lists examples of the representative causes together with the pharmacokinetic parameters affected.

In order to determine whether a drug is following dose-dependent kinetics or not, the drug is given at various dose levels and a plasma level-time curve is obtained for each dose. The curves should exhibit parallel slopes if the drug follows a dose-independent kinetics. Alternatively, a plot of the areas under the plasma level-time curves at various doses should be linear (Fig. 9.1).

Table 9.1 Representative Causes of Dose and Time Dependent kinetics and Selected Drug Examples

Cause	Example	Parameter	Affected[a]
1. Gastrointestinal absorption			
a) Saturable transport in the gut wall	Amoxycillin	F	↓
b) Drug comparatively insoluble	Griesofulvin	F	↓
c) Saturable gut wall or hepatic metabolism on the first pass	Nicardipine	F	↑
d) Saturable gastric or GI decomposition	Some pencillins	F	↑
2. Distribution			
a) Saturable protein binding	Naproxen	Vd	↑
b) Saturable tissue binding	Naproxen	Vd	↓
3. Renal excretion			
a) Active secretion (saturable)	Penicillin G	CL_R	↓
b) Active reabsorption (saturable)	Ascorbic acid	CL_R	↑
c) Change in urine pH	Salicyclic acid	CL_R	↓
d) Saturable plasma protein binding	Disopyramide	CL_R	↑
e) Nephrotoxicity[b]	Aminoglycosides	CL_R	↓
f) Increase in urine flow[b]	Theophylline	CL_R	↑
4. Hepatic metabolism			
a) Capacity limited metabolism	Phenytoin	CL_H	↓
b) Enzyme induction[b]	Carbamazepine	CL_H	↑
c) Hepatotoxicity[b]	Acetaminophen	CL_H	↓
d) Saturable plasma protein binding	Prednisdone	CL_H	↑
e) Decreased hepatic blow flow	propranolol	CL_H	↓
f) Inhibition by metabolite[b]	Lidocaine	CL_H	↓
	Diazepam	CL_H	↓

[a] Direction of change; - increase, ↓decrease on increasing dose
[b] time dependent as well as dose dependent.

Sources of Nonlinearity

As mentioned, nonlinearity may be at different kinetic levels of absorption, distribution and/or elimination or in other words many a times the reason for non-linearity is the saturation of a particular process involved in drug absorption, distribution, metabolism and/or elimination. These processes can be explained by the apparent first order kinetics at low doses of a drug, but they become saturated or capacity limited at higher doses.

For example, the extent of absorption of amoxicillin decreases with an increase in dose. For distribution, plasma protein binding of disopyramide is saturable at therapeutic concentrations, resulting in an increase in the volume of distribution with an increase in dose of the drug. As for nonlinearity in renal excretion, it has been shown that the antibacterial agent dicloxacillin has saturable active secretion in the kidneys, resulting in a decrease in renal clearance with an increase in dose. For metabolism, both phenytoin and ethanol have saturable metabolism which means an increase in the dose would result in a decrease in hepatic clearance and a more than proportionate increase in the drug AUC.

Absorption related nonlinearity

Characteristics of Drug Transport

Most of the drugs are transported by passive diffusion. That is, the membrane itself does not actively participate in the transfer process but instead it simply provides a physical barrier for drug movement.

The characteristics of passive transport are:

1. Drug molecules move from a region of relatively high concentration to one of relatively low Concentration.
2. The rate of transfer is proportional to the concentration gradient between the compartments involved in the transfer.
3. The transfer process achieves equilibrium with respect to drug concentration and transfer process ceases at equilibrium.
4. When a drug can exist in both ionized and unionized form, equilibrium exists only with respect to the unionized form.

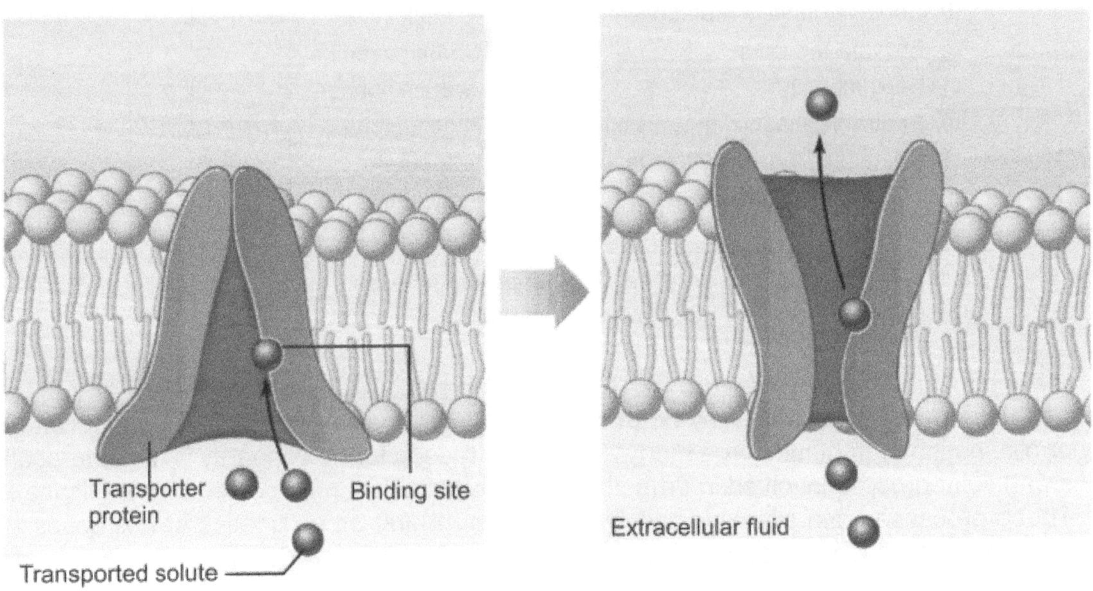

Fig. 9.3 Passive transport.

However, transport of certain drugs, such as amoxicillin across the gut wall and secretion of some drugs, such as penicillin G, into the renal tubule involves an active transport mechanism. Figure 9.4 illustrates the active transport mechanism. The drug molecule in compartment A (periplasm) is picked up by the enzyme at the surface of the membrane. The drug-enzyme complex then moves across the membrane and the drug is discharged to compartment B (cytoplasm) at the membrane surface open to B. The enzyme then returns to the surface of the membrane of the compartment A for the transport of another drug molecule.

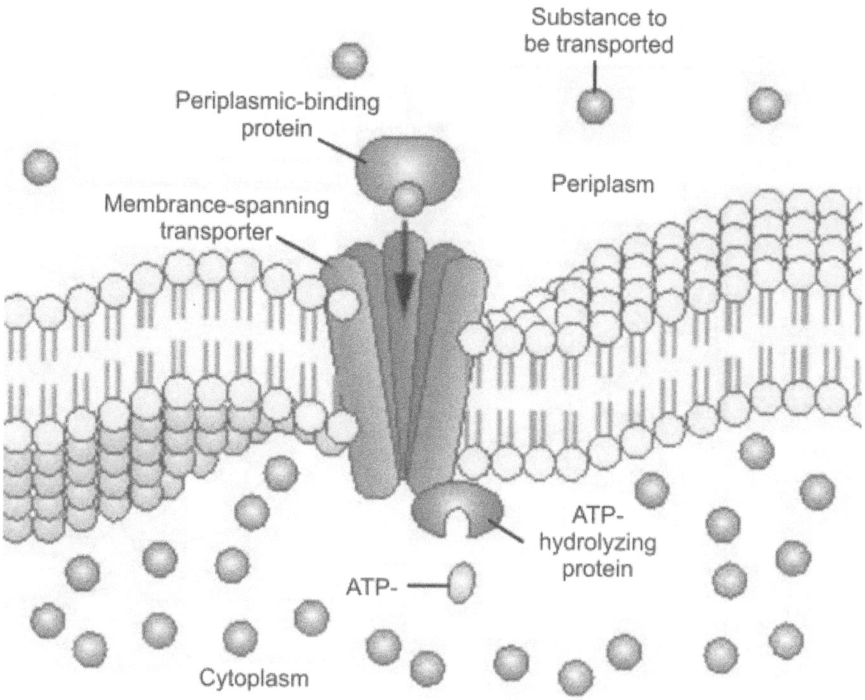

Fig. 9.4 illustrates the active transport mechanism.

Characteristics of Active transport:

1. This process consumes energy.
2. This process can be poisoned with some chemicals such as fluorides, dinitrophenol etc.
3. Unlike any passive transport, an active transfer process can work against the concentration gradient.
4. The system is structure specific and hence there exists a competition between the compounds of similar chemical structure.

5. Since there are a finite number of carriers or enzymes available, the system is *capacity limited*. If the total number of transferable molecules exceeds the number of enzyme sites available for transfer, the system will be *saturated*. Here the enzyme system will be working at its full capacity and the transfer of a drug may thus occur at a constant rate until the concentration of the drug falls below that of the capacity limit of the enzyme system.

Eg: 1 UK-294,315 (a human _1-adrenoceptor antagonist) appears to be extensively absorbed in humans, with only a small proportion of [^{14}C] UK-294,315 excreted unchanged in feces after oral administration, accounting for approximately 14% of the dose. Assuming no metabolism by gut microflora, the extent of absorption of UK-294,315 in humans is therefore estimated to be at least 86%. However, a nonproportional relationship between dose and oral absorption parameters was observed in clinical studies. In humans, the shape of the pharmacokinetic profile changed dramatically from a flat, prolonged profile at lower doses to a sharp peak with rapid decline in concentrations at higher doses (Fig. 9.5).

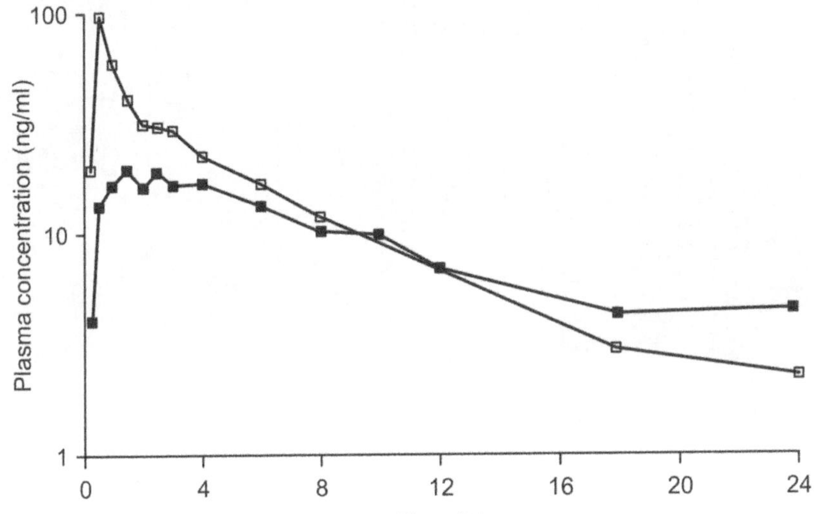

Fig. 9.5 Mean pharmacokinetic profiles after oral administration of UK-294,315 in solution to man at doses of 3 mg (solid) and 100 mg (hole).

A decrease in Tmax from 3.8 to 0.5 h was observed with increasing dose (1–100 mg), which is indicative of slower absorption at lower doses (Fig. 9.6), in contrast to the good intrinsic membrane permeability of the compound. At doses 30 mg in humans, T_{max} of approximately 0.5 h was consistently observed, suggesting saturation of the limiting process had occurred. The decrease in T_{max} was accompanied by a superproportional increase in Cmax as dose increased from 1 to 50 mg.

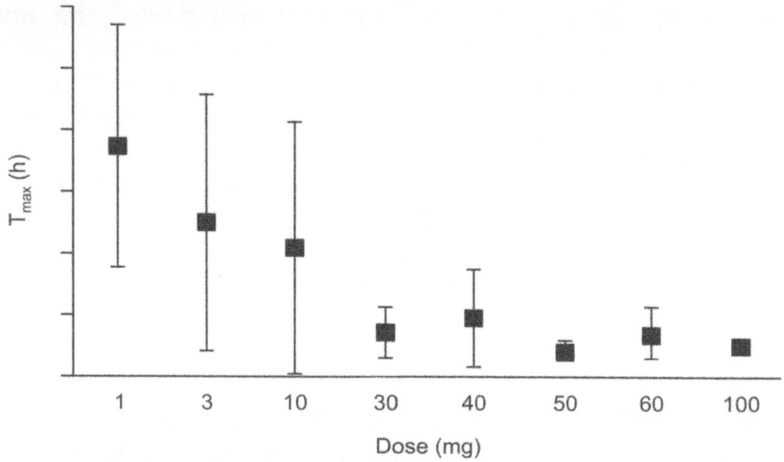

Fig. 9.6 Mean T_{max} versus dose after administration of single oral solution doses of UK-294,315 to healthy volunteers.

However, increases in C_{max} became dose-proportional from 50 to 100 mg, in line with changes in T_{max}, again suggesting saturation of a process that was limiting absorption rate at lower doses. Regardless of the nonlinearity observed in C_{max} and T_{max}, systemic exposure (AUC0-T) was dose-proportional across the whole dose range. Therefore, saturation of first-pass metabolism is unlikely to contribute significantly to the nonlinearity observed in the oral disposition of UK-294,315, where rate but not extent of absorption is affected at the lower end of the dose range.

Amoxicillin

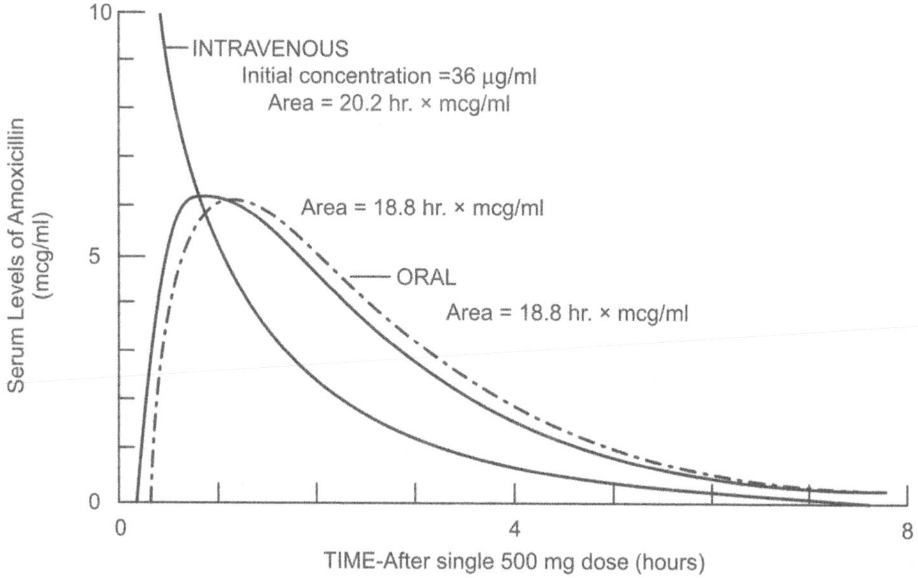

Fig 9.7 Amoxicillin pharmacokinetic data.

Amoxicillin was studied in normal subjects after intravenous, oral, and intramuscular administration of 250-, 500-, and 1,000-mg doses. Serum drug levels were analyzed using a two-compartment open model, as well as area under the curve (AUC) and urinary recovery. The variations of these pharmacokinetic parameters were then examined using the three-way analysis of variance and linear regression equations. These results confirmed nearly complete oral absorption: AUC was 93% of intravenous absorption, and urinary recovery was 86%. The intramuscular administration of amoxicillin results in complete and reliable absorption with peak drug levels, AUCs, and urinary recovery equivalent to oral dosage. The absorption of lyophilized amoxicillin after intramuscular injection resulted in an AUC that was 92% of intravenous absorption and urinary recovery of 91%. The peak serum levels, time to peak, and other pharmacokinetic parameters for intramuscular injection were nearly identical to those for oral administration. Kinetics of both intramuscular and oral administration exhibited dose-dependent absorption (absorption rate constant, 1.3/h for 250 mg and 0.7/h for 1,000 mg). This resulted in relatively later and lower peak serum levels for increasing dose. Total absorption, however, showed no dose dependence, as indicated by urinary recovery and AUC, which changed by less than 10%.

Saturable Enzymatic Elimination Processes

Many of the elimination processes such as active secretion, active reabsorption, drug metabolism involve enzymes. The limited number of enzyme molecules involved in the process leads to a saturable condition at high concentrations of substrate (drugs). Enzymatic elimination can be represented by:

$$E + D \underset{K_d}{\overset{K_f}{\rightleftharpoons}} ED \xrightarrow{K_2} E + P \qquad .....(9.1)$$

Where, E is the enzyme, D is the drug, ED is the enzyme drug complex and P represent product. K_f , K_d and K_2 are the rate constant of the processes.

In the usual treatment where the enzyme substrate complex is assumed to be in a steady - state then the reaction rate or velocity v, is defined as in

$$v = K_2 \text{ Eo } C/Km + C \qquad .....(9.2)$$

where, $Km = (K_2 + K_d)/K_f$

K_2 and K_d account for enzyme and drug complex dissociation where as K_f is the enzyme-drug complex formation rate constant.

The enzyme concentration Eo, is considered to be constant and equal to the initial concentration, since the concentration of enzyme-drug complex in equation 9.1 would be negligible in the steady state. The concentration of the drug (C) available for the process will decide the velocity rate. A plot of velocity rate, v of the process versus the concentration of the drug gives a curve, which attains a constant velocity at higher concentrations of the drug (Fig. 9.8). At this point, C >> Km and equation 9.2 becomes.

$$V_{max} = K_2 \text{ Eo} \qquad .....(9.3)$$

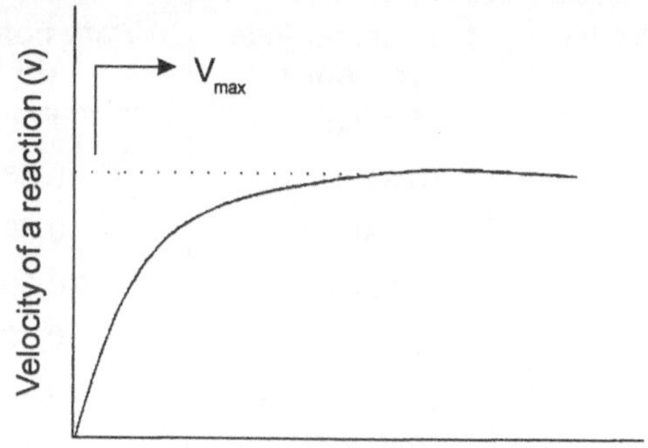

Fig. 9.8 Effect of drug concentration on the velocity of an enzymatic reaction.

It means the rate of the reaction is concentration dependent up to a certain drug concentration (first order process) beyond which the rate of reaction is constant or independent of drug concentration (zero-order process, saturation or capacity limited process). The maximum velocity, V_{max}, possible with the system is constant. Substituting the value of V_{max} in Equation 9.2,

$$v = V_{max}\ C/Km + C \quad .....(9.4)$$

This is the equation developed by Michalis-Menton for a saturable enzymatic process. Km is the Michaelis constant, and is equal to the drug concentration at half of the maximum velocity of a process (i.e. at 1/2 V_{max}).

Table 9.2 Effect of Drug Concentration on the Elimination Rate* and Rate Constant**

Drug concentration (mg/ml)	Elimination Rate (μg/ml per hr)	Rate constant (hr^{-1})
0.001	0.00128	1.28
0.002	0.00256	1.28
0.003	0.00384	1.28
0.004	0.00511	1.28
0.005	0.00638	1.28
0.006	0.0016	1.27
0.008	0.016	1.27
0.01	0.0126	1.26
0.02	0.0250	1.25
0.03	0.0369	1.23
0.04	0.0486	1.22
0.05	0.0600	1.20
0.06	0.0710	1.18
0.1	0.1125	1.13

Table 9.2 Contd...

Drug concentration (mg/ml)	Elimination Rate (μg/ml per hr)	Rate constant (hr^{-1})
0.2	0.2000	1.00
0.4	0.3272	0.82
0.8	0.4800	0.60
1.0	0.5294	0.53
2.0	0.6666	0.33
7.0	0.7659	0.19
6.0	0.8059	0.13
10.0	0.8411	0.08
15.0	0.8598	0.06
20.0	0.8695	0.04
25.0	0.8754	0.045
30.0	0.8794	0.03
40.0	0.8845	0.02
45.0	0.8862	0.02
50.0	0.8875	0.02

* Km = 0.7 mg/ml V_{max} = 0.9 mg/ml/hr

** The ratio of the elimination rate to the concentration is equal to the rate constant. If C is the concentration of a drug in plasma, then:

$$\text{Elimination Rate} = -\frac{dC}{dt} = \frac{V_{max}\,C}{Km + C} \qquad .....(9.5)$$

The values for Km and V_{max} are dependent on the nature of the drug and the enzymatic process involved.

It is possible to generate the elimination rate of a drug using Equation 9.5, if Km and V_{max} are known. Elimination rates of a drug at different concentrations with a Km of 0.7 μg/ml and V_{max} of 0.9 mg/ml/ per hour are calculated and presented in Table 9.2. based on the data generated from Equation 9.5. Table 9.2 shows how enzymatic drug elimination can change from a linear process to a non-linear process to a zero order process depending on drug concentration. When the drug concentration, C, is small in relation to Km $C \leq 0.005$ μg/ml, Table 9.2, The rate of elimination becomes a first-order process. This is evident since the rate constant values are constant (1.28 hr^{-1}) at drug concentrations below 0.005 μg/ml. Mathematically, when C << Km, the value of C in the denominator of Equation 9.2 is negligible when compared to Km value. Hence,

$$-\frac{dC}{dt} = \frac{V_{max}\,C}{Km} \qquad .....(9.6)$$

or

$$\frac{dC}{dt} = K'\,C \qquad .....(9.7)$$

Where K' is the first-order rate constant, which can be calculated from Equation 9.6

$$K' = V_{max}/Km = \frac{0.9}{0.7} = \sim 1.28 \text{ hr}^{-1}$$

The value of K' obtained is equal to that shown in Table 9.2 at drug concentration below 0.005 µg/ml. Accordingly, $t_{1/2}$ due to enzymatic elimination can be calculated.

$$t_{1/2} = 0.693/1.28 = 0.54 \text{ hr.}$$

At drug concentrations 0.008 to 20 µg/ml, the enzyme system is not saturated and the rate of elimination is a mixed or nonlinear process. This can be observed with changing values of the rate constant. At higher concentrations, 40 µg/ml or above, the elimination rate approaches a maximum velocity (V_{max}) of approximately 0.9 mg/ml per hour. Now, the process can be explained by the zero order process. At this point, C >> Km and hence, Km value can be neglected in the denominator of Equation 9.2, and the equation becomes,

$$-\frac{dC}{dt} = \frac{V_{max}\,C}{C} = V_{max} = K0 \qquad .....(9.8)$$

where K0 is the zero order rate constant.

Determination of Km and V_{max}

In enzymatic kinetic work, the classic Michaelis-Menton equation (Equation 9.4),

$$v = V_{max}\, C/\, Km + C$$

relating the reaction rate, v and substrate concentration, C is used to determine V_{max} and Km. In order to estimate V_{max} and Km values, the velocity of the reaction (v) at various concentration levels of drug (C) are determined either by *in vitro* experiments or *in vivo* experiments at constant enzyme levels.

The following three linear equations obtained by rearranging Equation 9.4 are widely employed in enzyme kinetics

$$\frac{1}{v} = \frac{1}{C}\,\frac{Km}{V_{max}} + \frac{1}{V_{max}} \qquad .....(9.9)$$

$$\frac{C}{v} = \frac{1}{V_{max}}\,C + \frac{Km}{V_{max}} \qquad .....(9.10)$$

$$v = -\,Km.\,\frac{v}{C} + V_{max} \qquad .....(9.11)$$

According to equation 9.9, a plot of 1/v versus 1/C gives a straight line with the slope of Km/V_{max} and the intercept equal to $1/V_{max}$. Table 9.3 shows the data used in Fig. 9.5. This plot is known as Lineweaver-Burk plot (double reciprocal plot), in which the data points are clustered.

Table 9.3 Velocity of an Enzymatic Reaction at Different Concentrations of Substrate (Drug). Data Has Been Processed for Graphic Determination of V_{max} and Km.

Exp.No.	C μg/ml	v (μg/ml/min)	1/v (ml/μgmin)	1/C (ml/μg)	C/v (min^{-1})	v/C (min)
1	0.5	0.416	2.404	2.00	1.202	0.832
2	1.0	0.455	2.197	1.00	2.198	0.455
3	1.5	0.469	2.132	0.66	3.198	0.313
4	2.0	0.476	2.100	0.50	4.202	0.238
5	2.5	0.481	2.079	0.40	5.196	0.192
6	3.0	0.484	2.066	0.33	6.198	0.161

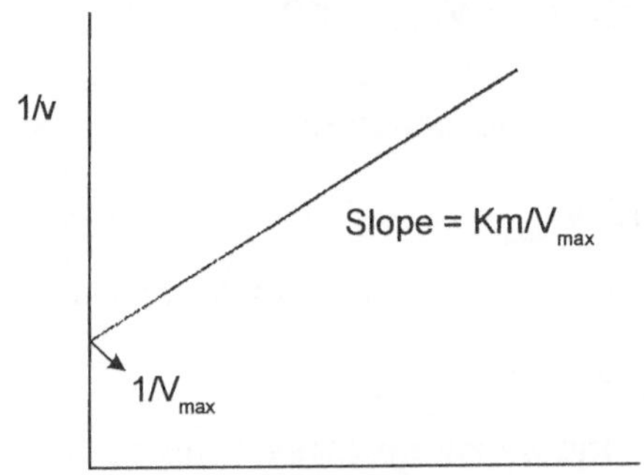

Fig. 9.9 Plot of 1/v versus 1/C for determining Km and Vmax values.

According to equation 9.10 a plot of C/v versus C gives a straight line with the slope equal to $1/V_{max}$ and intercept equal to Km/V_{max} (Fig. 9.9). A plot of v versus v/C would yield a straight-line with a slope of -Km and an intercept of V_{max} (Fig. 9.10)

A comparison of the above three methods reveals that the Lineweaver-Burk plot (Equation 9.9) is far inferior to the other two methods. It was found that the plot of v (ordinate) against v/C (abscissa) produced estimates of Km and V_{max} which were more reliable than those obtained by the other two equations. The different capacities of the three equations to provide reliable estimates of Km and V_{max} was due to the fact that the experimental error (s) normally inherent in the measurement of v would be magnified in equations 9.9 and 9.10 by the presence of v in its reciprocal form.

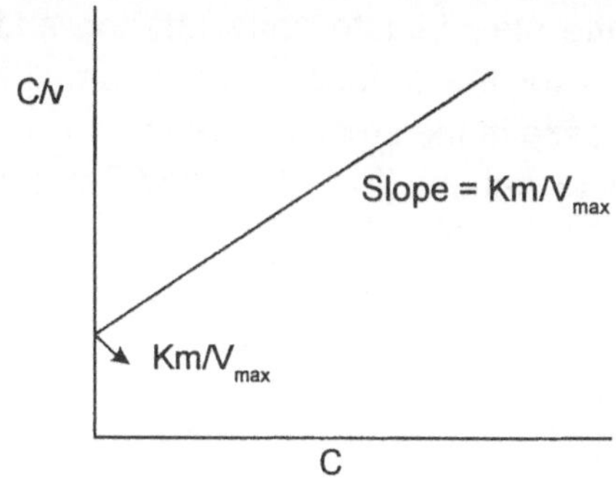

Fig. 9.10 Plot of C/v versus C for determining Km and Vmax.

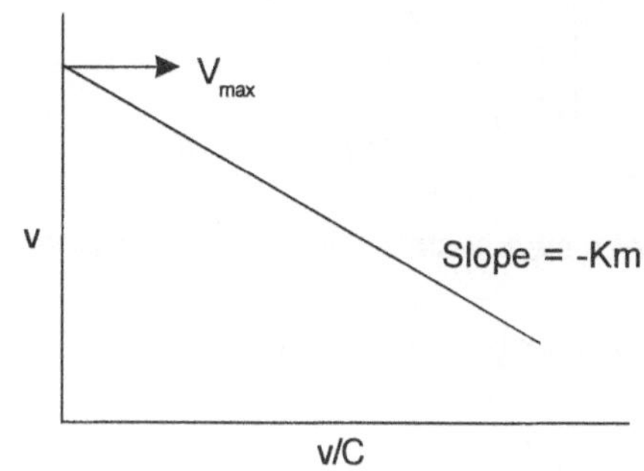

Fig. 9.11 Plot of V versus v/C for determining Km and V_{max}.

Table 9.4 Calculated Steady-State Phenytoin Serum Concentrations With Different Daily Doses of Phenytoin*.

Daily dose (D) (mg/day)	Steady state serum concentration (C_{ss}) (mg/l)
100	1.00
150	1.71
200	2.67
250	4.00
300	6.00
350	9.33
400	16.00
450	36.00

* C_{ss} = Km D/(D_{max} – D); Km = 4 mg/L and D_{max} = 500 mg/day

Estimation of Km and V_{max} in patients

Therapeutic problems encountered with a capacity limited metabolism are classically exemplified by phenytoin. Typical V_{max} and Km values of this drug are 500 mg/day and 4 mg/L, respectively. These values vary widely from patient to patient. Consequently, the curvilinear relation between the steady-state concentration and maintenance dose poses practical therapeutic problems for the clinician since a small increase in dose results in a disproportionately large increase in the steady-state serum concentration (C_{ss}), the extent of which varies from patient to patient (Fig. 9.12 and Table 9.4).

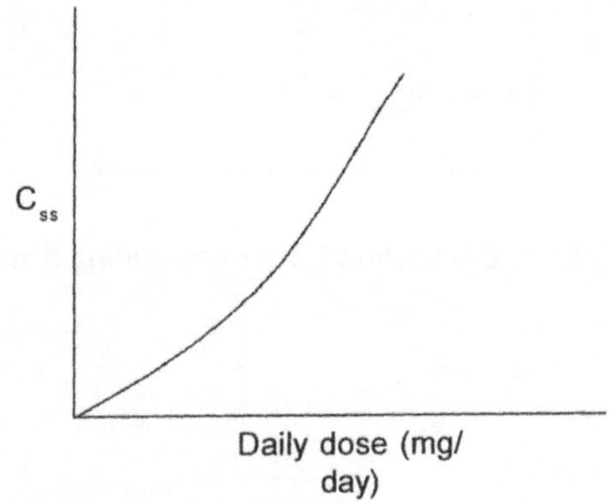

Fig. 9.12 The relation between steady-state serum concentration of phenytoin (C_{ss}) and daily dose.

Equation 9.4 may be rearranged in the form,

$$D = \frac{D_{max}\ C_{ss}}{Km + C_{ss}} \qquad .....(9.12)$$

or

$$C_{ss} = \frac{D\,Km}{D_{max} - D} \qquad .....(9.13)$$

Where, v is replaced by D (dose in mg/day) so that V_{max} becomes D_{max} (the theoretical maximum daily dose) Km being the steady-state serum concentration of phenytoin existing at half D_{max}.

Analogous to equations 9.9, 9.10 and 9.11, three linear forms of equation 9.13 can be written, each having C_{ss} (or its reciprocal) as the dependent variable.

$$\frac{1}{C_{ss}} = \frac{D_{max}}{Km}\ \frac{1}{D} - \frac{1}{Km} \qquad .....(9.14)$$

$$\frac{D}{C_{ss}} - \frac{1}{Km}\ D + \frac{D_{max}}{Km} \qquad .....(9.15)$$

$$C_{ss} = D_{max} \cdot \frac{C_{ss}}{D} - Km \qquad .....(9.16)$$

To determine Km and D_{max}, two doses of phenytoin are given at different times until a steady state is reached, the steady-state drug concentrations are then measured by assay. At the steady-state, the rate of elimination (v) is assumed to be the same as the rate of drug input, D (dose/day). Using the experimental values of D and C_{ss} the values of Km and D_{max} are determined using Equations 9.14, 9.15 and 9.16.

Example

The drug phenytoin is administered to a patient at dosing rates of 200 and 400 mg/day, on different occasions and the steady state serum concentrations found are 2.67 and 16.0 mg/L, respectively (Table 9.5). Find the Km and D_{max} for this patient. What would be the dose needed to achieve a steady state level of 10.0 mg/L ?

Solution :

Method 1: Using Equation 9.14

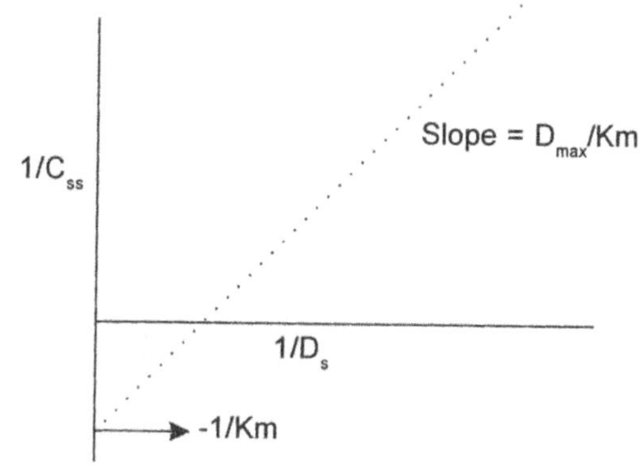

Fig. 9.13 Plot of $1/C_{ss}$ versus 1/D for the determination of Km and D_{max}.

Table 9.5 Steady-State Concentrations Achieved in a Patient at Different Dosing Rates. Data Has Been Processed for Graphic Determination of Km and D_{max}.

Dosing rate (D) (mg./day)	Steady state concentration (C_{ss}-mg/l)	$1/C_{ss}$	1/D	$C_{ss}D$	D/C_{ss}
200	2.67	0.3750	0.005	0.0134	77.91
400	16.00	0.0625	0.0025	0.040	25.00

According to Equation 9.14:

$$\frac{1}{C_{ss}} = \frac{D_{max}}{Km}\frac{1}{D} - \frac{1}{Km}$$

A plot of $1/C_{ss}$ versus 1/D yields a straight line with a slope of D_{max}/Km and an intercept of -1/Km (Fig. 9.13).

Method 2

Using Equation 9.15,

$$\frac{D}{C_{ss}} = -\frac{1}{Km} D + \frac{D_{max}}{Km} \quad .....(9.15)$$

A plot of D/C_{ss} versus D gives a straight line with a slope of -1/Km and an intercept of D_{max}/Km (Fig. 9.14)

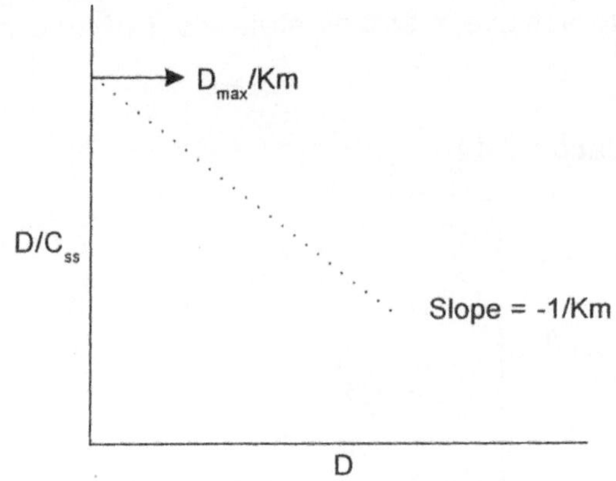

Fig. 9.14 Plot of D/C_{ss} versus D for the determination of K_m and D_{max}.

The slope obtained

$$= -0.25 = -1/Km$$

$$\therefore \quad Km = 1/0.25 = 4 mg/L$$

Intercept obtained from the graph

$$= D_{max}/Km = 125.$$

Therefore $\quad D_{max} = 125\ Km = 125 \times 4 = 500$ mg/day.

D/C_{ss} is nothing but clearance

Dose required to attain C_{ss} of 10 mg/L can be calculated from Equation 9.15, using the values of D_{max} and Km.

$$\frac{D}{10} = -\frac{1}{4} D + \frac{500}{4}$$

$$\frac{D}{10} + \frac{D}{4} = \frac{500}{4}$$

$$\frac{14D}{40} = \frac{500}{4}$$

$$D = \frac{40 \times 500}{14 \times 4} = 357.1 \text{ mg/day}$$

Method 3

A plot of C_{ss} versus C_{ss}/D, according to equation 9.16, yields a straight line with a slope of D_{max} and an intercept equal to -Km (Fig. 9.15).

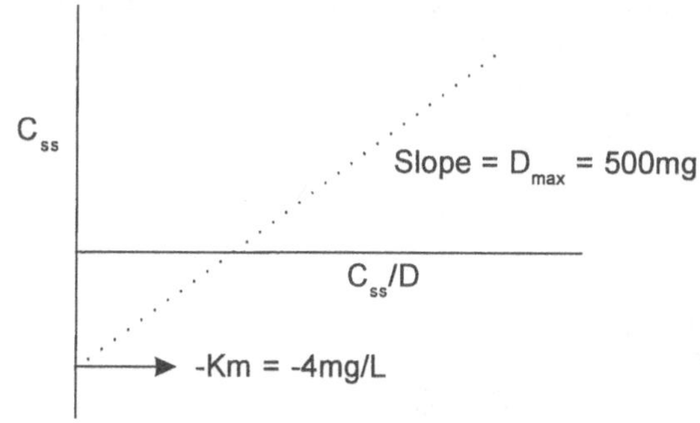

Fig. 9.15 Plot of C_{ss} versus C_{ss}/D for the determination of Km and D_{max}.

Dose required to achieve C_{ss} of 10 mg/L can be read from the graph. The value on X-axis corresponding to 10 mg/L is 0.028.

i.e., $C_{ss}/D = 0.028$

$$D = \frac{C_{ss}}{0.028} = \frac{10}{0.028} = 357.1 \text{ mg/day}$$

Method 4: The direct linear plot

This method allows for an estimation of phenytoin dose based on the steady state concentration resulting from one dose. This method is based on a statistically compiled nomogram that makes it possible to project a most likely dose for the patient.

The dose required to produce a desired steady-state concentration can be determined simply by drawing a straight line from the intersection point in the first quadrant to the desired absolute value on the negative part of the concentration axis. The point where this line cuts the dose axis gives the required dose. (Fig. 9.16).

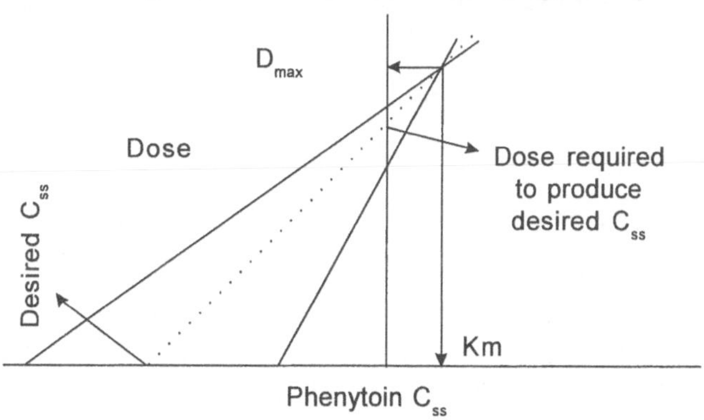

Fig. 9.16 Direct linear plot used for the determination of the dose required to achieve desired steady-state level in plasma.

Method 5: Direct method

When steady state concentrations of phenytoin are known only at two dose levels, there is no advantage of using the graphic method. Km and D_{max} can be calculated by solving two simultaneous equations formed by substituting C_{ss} and D (Equation 9.12) with C_1, D_1, C_2 and D_2. The equations contain two unknowns, Km and D_{max}, and may be solved easily.

$$D_1 = \frac{D_{max} \cdot C_1}{Km + C_1}$$

$$D_2 = \frac{D_{max} \cdot C_2}{Km + C_2}$$

Combining two equations yield equation 9.17.

$$Km = \frac{D_2 - D_1}{\frac{D_1}{C_1} - \frac{D_2}{C_2}} \quad \text{.....(9.17)}$$

Where, C_1 is steady state plasma concentration after dose 1, C_2 is steady state plasma concentration after dose 2, D_1 is the first dosing rate, and D_2 is the second dosing rate. To calculate Km and D_{max}, use Equation 9.17, with the values C_1 = 2.67 mg/L, C_2 = 16.0 mg/L, D_1 = 200 mg/day, and D_2 = 400 mg/day. The results are

$$Km = \frac{400 - 200}{\frac{200}{2.67} - \frac{400}{16}} = 4.00 \text{ mg/L}$$

Substitute Km into either of the two simultaneous equations to solve D_{max}.

$$200 = \frac{D_{max}\,(2.67)}{4.00 + 2.67}$$

$$D_{max} = 499.63 \text{ mg/day}$$

Using the values of Km and D_{max} the dose required to achieve steady state concentration of 10.0 mg/L can be calculated.

$$\text{Dose} = \frac{499.63 \times 10.0}{4.00 + 10.0} = 356.9 \text{ mg/L}$$

9.2 One Compartment Open Model - I.V. Bolus - Pharmacokinetics of Drug Eliminated by Capacity Limited Process

It is possible to develop an equation for a drug that follows one compartment open model with capacity limited elimination. The rate of elimination of a drug that follows a capacity limited or saturable process can be determined using Michaelis-Menten equation (Equation 9.5).

$$\frac{dC}{dt} = \frac{V_{max}\, C}{Km + C}$$

Integration of the above equation with respect to time gives

$$\frac{C0 - C}{t} = V_{max} - \frac{Km}{t} \ln \frac{C0}{C} \qquad .....(9.18)$$

Where, C0 is the zero time concentration of the drug in plasma following an I.V. bolus injection of dose X0 and C is the concentration of drug in plasma at time t.

Alternatively, the amount of the drug in the body after an I.V. bolus injection may be calculated by the following equation.

$$\frac{D_O - D_t}{t} = V_{max} - \frac{Km}{t} \ln \frac{D_o}{D_t} \qquad .....(9.19)$$

Where, D0 is the I.V. bolus dose, Dt is the amount of the drug in the body at any time, t. Equation 9.19 may be used to simulate the decline of the drug in the body after various size doses are given, provided the Km and Vmax of the drug are known.

In order to calculate the time for the dose of the drug to decline to a certain amount of the drug in the body, Equation 9.19 must be rearranged and solved for time t.

$$t = \frac{1}{V_{max}} (D_O - D_t + Km \log D_O/D_t) \qquad .....(9.20)$$

Using Equation 9.20, the time required to fall to a certain amount of the drug in the body following an I.V. bolus of 300 mg of drug with Km = 30 mg and V_{max} varied from 150 to 100 mg/hr is represented in Table 9.6. Similarly, data was generated for a drug keeping V_{max} = 150 mg/hr, Km = 30 mg and 60 mg to show the influence of Km on kinetics (Table 9.7). Effect V_{max} and Km are shown in Figures 9.17 and 9.18, respectively.

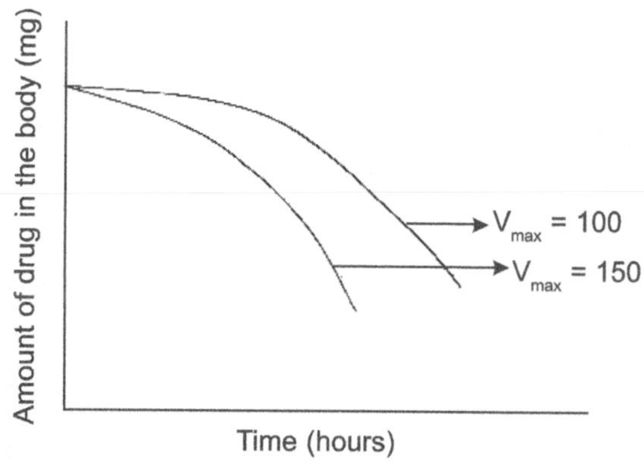

Fig. 9.17 Effect of Vmax on drug levels in the body (data from table 9.6).

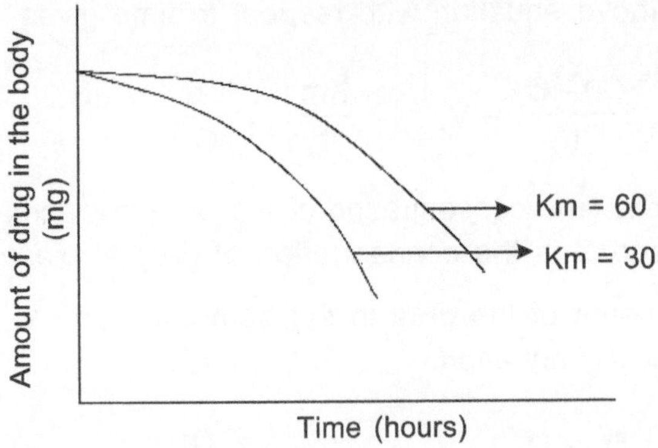

Fig. 9.18 Effect of Km on drug levels in the body (data from table 9.7).

Time required to bring the drug levels in the body to 20 mg is 2.4 and 2.6 hours with V_{max} 150 and 100 mg, respectively (Km is constant 30 mg) (Table 9.6). It means an increase in V_{max} increases the rate of elimination of the drug (time required to eliminate the drug decreases).

Table 9.6 Capacity Limited Pharmacokinetics: Effect of V_{max} on the Elimination of Drug.

Amount of Drug in body (mg)	Time for drug elimination (hr) V_{max} = 150	V_{max} =100
300	0	0
260	0.295	0.443
220	0.612	0.893
180	0.902	1.353
140	1.219	1.829
100	1.553	2.330
60	1.922	2.883
20	2.408	3.612

Km = 30 mg/L Dose = 300 mg

Table 9.7 Capacity Limited Pharmacokinetics: Effect of Km on the Elimination of Drug.

Amount of Drug in body (mg)	Time for drug elimination (hr) Km = 30mg/L	Km = 60 mg/L
300	0	0
260	0.295	0.324
220	0.612	0.657
180	0.902	1.004
140	1.219	1.372
100	1.553	1.773
60	1.922	2.244
20	2.408	2.949

V_{max} = 150 mg/hr Dose = 300mg

It can be seen from Table 9.7, that an increase in Km value increases the time required for the drug to come to a certain amount in body (the rate of elimination of the drug is decreased) at constant V_{max} for a given dose.

Equation 9.18 adequately describes the plasma concentration-time profiles of drugs that follow a one compartment open model with a capacity limited elimination. The mathematics needed to describe nonlinear pharmacokinetic behavior of drugs that follow a two compartment model and/or have both combined capacity limited and first-order kinetic profiles are very complex and have little practical application for dosage calculations and therapeutic drug monitoring.

Drug Clearance

The total body clearance of a drug that follows one compartment model and nonlinear kinetics according to Michaelis-Menton equation, is dependent on time and plasma concentration. It means, total body clearance changes with respect to time and plasma drug concentration. Within a certain drug concentration range, an average or *mean clearance* (Cl_{av}) may be determined for the given dose. The Cl_{av} is dose dependent since drug elimination follows Michaelis-Menton equation. Mean clearance, Cl_{av} can be obtained using the area under the curve for a given dose.

Area under the curve $[AUC]_0^{\infty}$

$$= \frac{F.Dose}{Clearance} \qquad .....(9.21)$$

or

$$Cl_{av} = \frac{F.Dose}{[AUC]_0^{\alpha}} \qquad .....(9.22)$$

F = Fraction of the dose absorbed. For I.V. bolus,

$$Cl_{av} = Dose/[AUC]_0^{\alpha} \qquad .....(9.23)$$

According to Michaelis-Mention equation,

$$\frac{dC}{dt} = \frac{V_{max}\ C}{Km + C} \qquad .....(9.24)$$

Inverting and rearranging equation 9.24 yields.

$$C.\ dt = \frac{Km}{V_{max}}\ dC + \frac{C}{V_{max}}\ dC \qquad .....(9.25)$$

Integration of equation 9.25 between the limits of t = 0 to t = ∝ results in the following equations

$$\int_0^{\infty} C.\ dt = (Km\ C0)/V_{max} + (C0^2)/2V_{max} \qquad .....(9.26)$$

$$\int_0^\infty C.dt = [AUC]_0^\infty = (C0/V_{max})\ [Km + C0/2] \qquad .....(9.27)$$

Mean clearance, Cl_{av} = Dose (D0)/$[AUC]_0^\infty$

$Cl_{av} = (Vd\ V_{max})/(Km+C0/2)$

Because C0 = D0/Vd,

$$Cl_{av} = (Vd.\ V_{max})/(Km + D0/2Vd) \qquad .....(9.28)$$

Alternatively, clearance (CL_t) can be calculated by dividing the small amount of the drug eliminated by the plasma drug concentration.

$$CL_t = \frac{Vd.\, dC/dt}{C} \qquad .....(9.29)$$

but dC/dt

$$= \frac{V_{max}\, C}{Km + C}$$

$$CL_t = Vd.\ \frac{V_{max}\, C}{Km + C} \times \frac{1}{C} = \frac{Vd.\ V_{max}}{Km + C} \qquad .....(9.30)$$

It means the clearance of a drug that follows nonlinear pharmacokinetics is dependent upon the plasma concentration C, Km and V_{max}.

Equation 9.28 calculates the average clearance (Cl_{av}) for the drug after a single I.V. bolus dose over the entire course of the drug in the body. For any time period, total body clearance may be calculated using the equation given below.

$$CL_t = \frac{dXe/dt}{C} \qquad .....(9.31)$$

Where, dxe/dt is the amount of the drug eliminated in a given time and C is the plasma drug level.

9.3 One Compartment Open Model - Pharmacokinetics of Drugs Eliminated by Nonlinear Processes

Equations can be developed for other routes of administration and mixed drug elimination (drug may be eliminated by both nonlinear and linear processes), for drug that follows a one compartment model. Absorption kinetics and elimination processes have to be considered in developing equations for extravascular administration of a drug.

Mixed Drug elimination

Drugs may be metabolized by several parallel processes to several different metabolites. Let us consider a drug that is metabolized by two parallel processes.

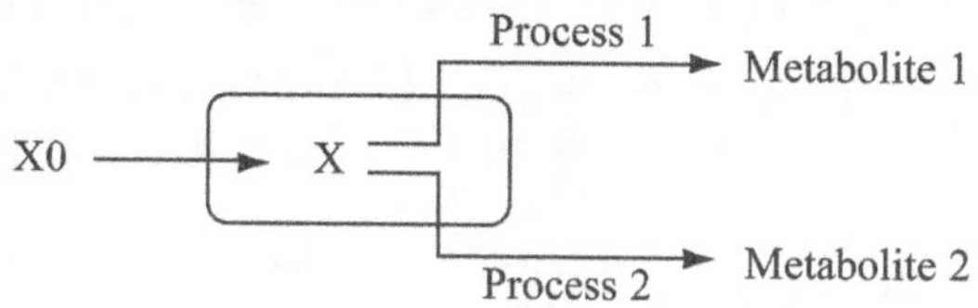

Enzymatic conversion of a drug into metabolite by process 1 is saturable. Hence, the rate of drug metabolism of process 1 follows the first order kinetics at a lower concentration, becomes mixed at a higher concentration and approaches zero order at a very high concentration of the drug.

Enzymatic conversion of a drug by process 2 is non-saturable at therapeutic concentrations of the drug and hence, the rate of drug metabolism by process 2 can be described by first-order kinetics.

For example, sodium salicylate is metabolized to both glucuronide and glycine conjugate (hippurate). The rate of formation of glycine conjugate is limited by the amount of glycine available. Thus, the rate of formation of glycine conjugate is capacity limited (nonlinear) whereas the rate of formation of glucuronide continues as a first-order process.

Following an I.V. bolus of a drug, the rate of change in drug concentration for a drug eliminated by both the first order kinetics and nonlinear kinetics (Michaelis-Menton kinetics) is given by

$$-\frac{dXe}{dt} = K\ C + \frac{V_{max}\ C}{Km + C} \quad .....(9.32)$$

Where, K is the first order rate constant representing the sum of all first-order rate constants for elimination. Therefore, the product of K and C is the rate of elimination of the drug by all first-order processes.

First-Order Absorption and Capacity Limited Elimination

The rate of change in the amount of a drug in the body following extravascular administration (e.g. oral administration) of the drug is equal to the rate of absorption minus the rate of elimination.

$$\frac{dX}{dt} = Ka\ Xa - \frac{V_{max}\ X}{Km + X} \quad .....(9.33)$$

Where, dX/dt is the rate of change in the amount of the drug in the body, Xa is the amount of the drug available at the absorption site, Ka is the first order absorption rate constant and X is the amount of the drug in body. Equation 9.33 can be written in concentration terms as

$$\frac{dC}{dt} = Ka\ Ca\ e^{-Kat} - \frac{V_{max}\ C}{Km + C} \quad .....(9.34)$$

Ca = concentration of drug at the absorption site.

If the elimination of a drug occurs by parallel processes consisting of both linear and nonlinear pharmacokinetics, Equation 9.34 may be extended to Equation 9.35.

$$\frac{dC}{dt} = Ka\ Ca\ e^{-Kat} - \frac{V_{max}\ C}{Km + C} - KC \qquad .....(9.35)$$

Where, K is the first order rate constant.

Zero-Order Input and Nonlinear Elimination

Drugs given as I.V. infusion represent a zero-order input in addition to certain sustained action dosage forms administered by extravascular routes. For drugs which enter the systemic circulation at a constant rate and eliminated by a nonlinear process, the equation that describes the rate of change in the plasma drug concentration is given by

$$\frac{dC}{dt} = \frac{K0}{Vd} - \frac{V_{max}\ C}{Km + C} \qquad .....(9.36)$$

Where, K0 is the zero-order rate constant and Vd is the apparent volume of distribution of the drug.

If the drug is eliminated by parallel pathways of both linear and nonlinear pharmacokinetics, the following equation may be used to calculate the rate of change in the plasma drug levels.

$$\frac{dC}{dt} = \frac{K0}{Vd} - \frac{V_{max}\ C}{Km + C} - K\ C \qquad .....(9.37)$$

Where, K is the overall first-order rate constant.

Nonlinear Absorption and Nonlinear Elimination

If both drug absorption and elimination processes are saturable at the therapeutic dose level, the following equation may be useful in estimating the rate of change in the plasma drug concentration.

$$\frac{dC}{dt} = \frac{(V_{max})_a\ Ca}{(Km)_a + Ca} - \frac{V_{max}\ C}{Km + C} \qquad .....(9.38)$$

Ca = Concentration of drug at the absorption site

C = Concentration of drug in plasma.

Where the first part of Equation 9.38 represent a capacity limited rate of absorption and the second part represent the nonlinear elimination of the drug.

9.4 Other Factors Responsible for Nonlinear Pharmacokinetics

There are other factors which contribute to nonlinear pharmacokinetics of a drug in addition to capacity limited absorption and elimination.

Solubility

Oral administration of relatively large doses of drugs with a low aqueous solubility may exhibit a dose dependent pharmacokinetics due to dissolution. Small doses can undergo dissolution during transit time though the G.I.T. and may be absorbed completely. When large doses are administered, the amount of the drug absorbed may not be proportional to the administered dose because of poor aqueous solubility, dissolution and a fixed transit time through the gastrointestinal tract. An example is griseofulvin (Fig. 9.19). For this sparingly soluble drug (aqueous solubility in 10 mg/l), bioavailability decreases as the dose is increased from 250 to 500 mg.

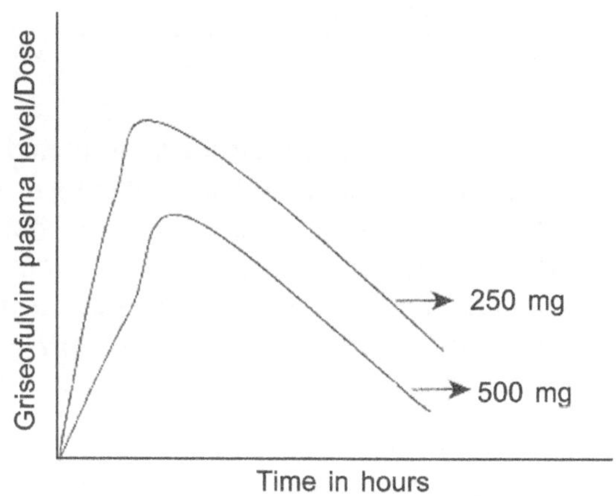

Fig. 9.19 Plasma concentration of griseofulvin, normalized to a dose, as a function of time following an oral administration of 250mg and 500mg of ultra micronized griseofulvin.

Table 9.8 Examples of Drug Showing Saturated First-Pass Metabolism in the Liver or Gut Wall After Oral Administration of Therapeutic Doses

Alprenolol	Propronolol
5-fluorouracil	Salicylamide
Nicardipine	Verapamil
Propoxyphene	

Saturable First-Pass Metabolism

Saturable first-pass metabolism occurs for a number of orally administered drugs that are highly extracted by the liver or intestinal tissue. Examples are listed in Table 9.8. For several of these drugs, dose dependence on bioavailability is observed without an apparent change in elimination half-life. This behavior can be understood by realizing that the amount of the drug reaching liver during absorption with low doses of the drug is not sufficient to saturate the enzymatic process and hence, the first-pass metabolism rate is proportional to the amount of the drug entering the liver (first-order process). With large doses of the drug, the amount of the drug entering the liver is greater than the metabolizing capacity of the enzymatic system and hence, a capacity limited first-pass metabolism (zero-order kinetics) is observed. Therefore, an increase in the dose above the saturable dose, increases the bioavailability of drugs that undergo the first-pass metabolism (Table 9.9).

Table 9.9 Saturable first-pass metabolism of nicardipine observed at steady state following oral doses of 10-40 mg per 8 hr.

Dose	Bioavailability
10	19%
20	22%
30	28%
40	38%

Saturability of plasma protein and tissue binding: A limited number of sites exist on plasma proteins. Table 9.10 shows the concentration of plasma proteins available for binding. Average plasma concentration of albumin is 43 g/L or 600 mM. At one binding site per albumin molecule, there is a limiting concentration of 600 mM for the bound drug. For a_1 acid glycoprotein, the limitation occurs at about 15 mM, a much lower concentration. The sites to which drugs bind in the tissue may be similarly limited. Consequently, the volume of distribution depends on drug concentrations, a *concentration-dependent* behavior.

Table 9.10 Representative Proteins to Which Drugs Bind in Plasma.

Protein	Molecular Weight (g/mole)	Normal concentrations g/L	μM
Albumin	67,000	35 - 50	500 - 700
α-acid glycoprotein	42,000	0.4 - 1.0	9 - 23
Lipoproteins Cortisol	2,00,000 - 24,00,000	Variable	Variable
binding globulin (transcortin)	53,000	0.03 - 0.07	0.6 - 1.4

For drugs that show a saturable binding to plasma proteins, the volume of distribution is expected to increase with the plasma concentration. This is because of the fact that unbound (free) drug concentration increases after saturation, which is available for distribution. Conversely, for drugs that show a saturability in biding to the tissues, the volume of distribution decreases as the plasma concentration is increased. Dose dependence in distribution may be difficult to identify and quantify unless plasma protein binding is measured. This is because of the dependence of drug distribution on the fraction of the drug unbound in plasma and the dependence of the half-life of the drug on both clearance and volume of distribution. Drugs that are protein bound must dissociate into a free or unbound form to be eliminated by glomerular filtration and by biotransformation. The nature and extent of drug-protein binding affects the magnitude of deviation from normal linear or the first-order elimination rate process.

Let us consider a hypothetical situation wherein two drugs are given by an I.V. bolus in equal doses. One drug is 90% protein bound whereas the other drug does not bind to the plasma protein and both are eliminated solely by glomerular filtration through the kidney.

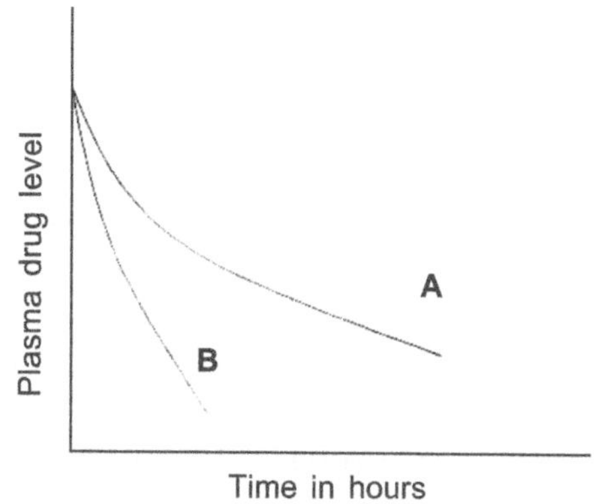

Fig. 9.20 Plasma drug level-time profile of two drugs given in equal doses. Curve A represents a drug 90% bound to plasma protein. Curve B represents a drug not bound to plasma protein.

The plasma concentration-time curves of two drugs are shown in Fig. 9.20. The protein-bound drug is more concentrated in plasma than the drug that is not protein-bound. Free drug concentration of protein-bound drug is low and hence, its elimination rate will be slow when compared with the drug that does not bind to plasma protein. Further, the protein-bound drug shows a nonlinear elimination whereas the drug that is not bound to the plasma protein shows a linear elimination (Fig. 9.20).

A careful examination of curve A reveals that the slope of the bound drug decreases gradually as the drug concentration decreases. It means that the free drug concentration decreases and bound-drug concentration increases as the total drug concentration in plasma decreases. In other words, the ratio of the bound-drug to free drug is not constant but increases at a low plasma concentration of the drug. Therefore, fitting the plasma concentration-time data of a protein-bound drug into a simple one compartment model without accounting for protein binding results in an erroneous estimation of volume of distribution and half-life. Apparently, a plot of plasma concentration of drug-time curve resemble a two compartment model. Some times, plasma data for drugs that are highly protein bound have been inappropriately fitted to two compartment models.

9.5 Drugs With Protein Binding - One Compartment Open Model

Drugs that bind to the plasma proteins exists in a bound form and free form. Only a free form of the drug is available for metabolism, excretion and is responsible for the observed pharmacological response. However, there exists an equilibrium between the bound drug and free drug in plasma. As the free drug concentration in plasma falls due to elimination, the equilibrium is disturbed and re-established by the dissociation of the protein - drug complex to release the free drug. However, the fraction of the bound drug is not constant throughout the concentration change, resulting a nonlinear elimination kinetics.

Let us consider a drug that binds to the plasma protein. At equilibrium,

$$P + Cf \underset{K_2}{\overset{K_1}{\rightleftharpoons}} PD \qquad .....(9.39)$$

Dissociation constant

$$Kd = K_2/K_1 = \frac{[PD]}{[P]\,Cf} \qquad .....(9.40)$$

Where:

[PD] = Concentration of drug-protein complex, which is also equal to the concentration of bound drug (Cb) or bound protein (Pb) at 1 : 1 binding condition.

[P] = Concentration of free protein or unbound protein.

Cf = concentration of free drug

Therefore the total protein concentration, Pt is given by

$$Pt = P + Pb \qquad .....(9.41)$$

Total drug concentration, Ct is given by

$$Ct = Cf + Cb \qquad .....(9.42)$$

Now, the dissociation constant, Kd, can be expressed as

$$Kd = \frac{Cb}{(Pt - Cb)\,Cf} \qquad .....(9.43)$$

Since $[Pt] - Cb = [P]$

Equation 9.43 can be rearranged as follows:

$$Cb = Ct - Cf = \frac{Pt\,Cf}{Kd + Cf} \qquad .....(9.44)$$

Equation 9.44 can be written as a quadratic equation ($ax^2 + bx + c = 0$)

$$-Cf^2 - (Pt + Kd - Ct)\,Cf + KdCt = 0 \qquad .....(9.45)$$

Solving for Cf, (root of quadratic equation)

$$Cf = \frac{1}{2}\,[-(P + Kd - Ct) + (P + Kd - Ct)^2 + 4\,KdCt \qquad .....(9.46)$$

The rate of drug elimination from the plasma is proportional to the free drug concentration (Cf) in plasma. Therefore,

$$\frac{dC}{dt} = -K.Cf \qquad .....(9.47)$$

where K is the elimination rate constant of the drug. Substituting the value of Cf, we get

$$\frac{dC}{dt} = -\frac{K}{2}[-(P + Kd - Ct) + (P + Kd - Ct)^2 + 4\,KdCt \qquad .....(9.48)$$

This equation is not easily integrated but could be solved by means of a numerical method.

Nonlinear elimination pharmacokinetics of a drug with protein binding is observed at higher doses, since the free drug in plasma is high and hence the elimination rate is also high, initially. At low doses, an apparent first order kinetics may be observed. As the dose of the drug is increased, the free drug concentration increases slowly. But at higher doses beyond the dose required to saturate protein binding, the free drug concentration increases abruptly and may precipitate the toxic effects. Therefore, in order to make sure that the patient receives a proper dose it is necessary to calculate the free drug concentration, taking the protein binding into consideration,

9.6 Time-Dependent Pharmacokinetics

The study of changes in response to drug administration or kinetics with the time of day, month, or year is an area called *chronopharmacology. Chronopharmacokinetics* describes the changes in drug absorption, distribution, and/or elimination due to normal physiological circadian rhythms. For example, diurnal variations in renal function, urine pH, α_1-acid glycoprotein concentration, gastrointestinal physiology (food and drink), and cardiac output all occur. An example of diurnal changes in absorption and distribution of verapamil is shown in Fig. 9.21. Note that administration in the evening produces a lower peak drug concentration and, as such, may produce less effect than does administration in the morning.

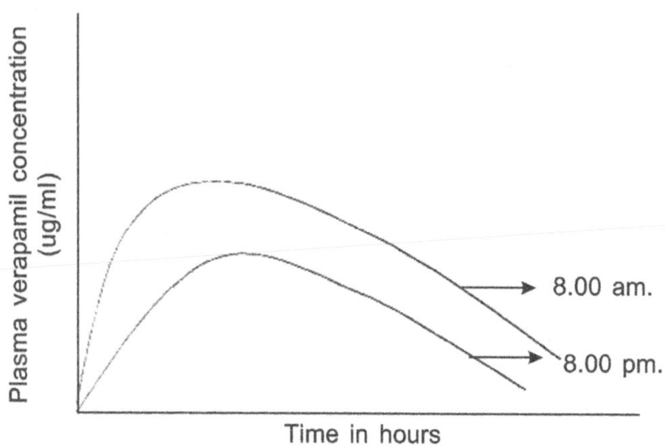

Fig. 9.21 Mean plasma verapamil concentration time profile for eight subjects, each given a single 80mg tablet of drug at 8.00 am. and 8.00 pm.

Drug Absorption, distribution, metabolism and elimination are influenced by many different physiological functions of the body which may vary with time of day. Thus, the pharmacokinetic parameters characterizing these different steps, conventionally considered to be constant in time, depend on the moment of drug administration. However, the time of day has to be regarded as an additional variable influencing the kinetics of a drug since many drugs are affected by time of administration and the activity or rest period of the human or animal.

Chronopharmacokinetics deals with the study of the temporal changes in absorption, distribution, metabolism and elimination and thus takes into account the influence of time of administration on these different steps. Temporal changes can be involved at each step of the sequence of pharmacokinetic processes: temporal variations in drug absorption from the gastro-intestinal tract (due to circadian variations in gastric acid secretion and pH, motility, gastric emptying time, gastrointestinal blood flow), plasma protein binding and drug distribution, drug metabolism (temporal variations in enzyme activity, hepatic blood flow) and in renal drug excretion (due to variation in glomerular filtration, renal blood flow, urinary pH and tubular resorption). Thus, the time of administration of a drug is an important source of variation which must be taken into account in kinetic studies and particular methodological aspects of chronokinetics are needed.

Mechanisms of Chronokinetics

Time-dependent changes in kinetics may result from circadian variations at each step, e.g. absorption, distribution, metabolism and elimination. At each of these steps, biological rhythms may influence the kinetics of a drug, as indicated in figure.

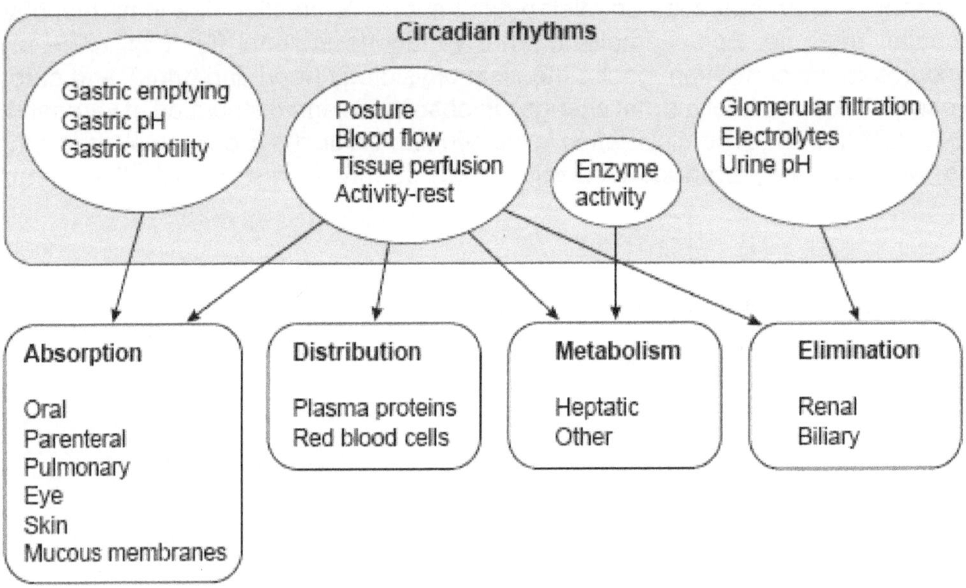

Fig. 9.21 Circadian rhythms of physiological variables involved in chronokinetic mechanisms, i.e. absorption, distribution, metabolism and elimination.

Temporal Variations in Drug Absorption

Several factors, such as the physicochemical properties of the drug, the area and the structure of the biological membrane, gastric emptying rate, gastric pH and motility, and gastrointestinal blood flow, may influence the absorption process after oral drug administration.The influence of posture and the presence of food on bioavailability is well known. In addition, the formulation of a drug may have pronounced effects on drug absorption. Since gastric acid secretion and pH, motility, gastric emptying time and gastrointestinal blood flow vary with the time of day, many studies have reported temporal variations in drug absorption in humans, as well as in rodents.

Most lipophilic drugs seem to be absorbed faster when the drug is taken in the morning compared with the evening, but this has not been reported for highly water-soluble drugs. Meal composition may influence circadian variations and thus affects the kinetics of various drugs including valproic acid (valproate sodium). Significant differences in the kinetics of valproic acid (valproate sodium) depending on morning or evening administration under usual life conditions (i.e. light meal at breakfast and heavy meal at dinner) has been reported. When the same meal conditions (same size and content for breakfast and dinner) were applied, no significant circadian changes were detected between morning and evening administration.

Absorption by other routes of administration may also be influenced by biological rhythms. For instance, in children, the skin penetration of an eutectic mixture of lidocaine (lignocaine) and prilocaine was reported to depend on the time of administration, with a higher rate of penetration occurring in the evening. In addition, circadian dose administration time-dependency in the forearm skin penetration of hydrophilic methylnicotinate and lipophilic hexylnicotinate was recently demonstrated. Circadian variations have also been reported in the ocular absorption of topically applied timolol.

While most chronokinetic studies have been carried out with drugs administered orally, the persistence of significant chronokinetic changes with intravenous, compared with oral, administration suggests that the absorption process does not interfere with chronokinetic changes. Thus, conclusions on whether or not chronokinetic factors are relevant to a particular drug can only be drawn when all variables, including route of administration and galenic formulation, are controlled and taken into consideration.

Temporal Variations in Drug Distribution

Circadian variations in the drug protein binding of acidic and basic drugs have been reported both in human and animal studies. *E.g.* free plasma concentrations for anticonvulsant drugs such as carbamazepine, diazepam, phenytoin and valproic acid, and for antineoplastic drugs such as cisplatin have been documented, These changes are usually reported to be dependent on temporal variations in plasma protein levels, which are circadian-time dependent.

Temporal variations in plasma drug binding may have clinical implications only for drugs that are characterised by a high protein binding (>80%) and a small apparent Vd.

The time-dependency of the passage of drugs into red blood cells also provides a strong argument for the existence of temporal variations in the passage of drugs through biological membranes, for which red blood cells are often used as a model. However, such variations have only been reported for drugs such as local anaesthetics (lidocaine, bupivacaine, etidocaine and mepivacaine), indomethacin and theophylline.

Temporal Variations in Hepatic Drug Metabolism

Hepatic drug metabolism is generally assumed to depend on liver enzyme activity and/or hepatic blood flow: both have been shown to be circadian time-dependent. Circadian variations in enzyme activity were documented in the liver, kidney and brain, however, these data were obtained in animals and no direct data on enzyme activity have been reported in humans.

For drugs with a high extraction ratio, hepatic metabolism depends on hepatic blood flow. Circadian variations in hepatic blood flow induce changes in liver perfusion and, thus, temporal variations in the clearance of such drugs. In one study, estimated hepatic blood flow in supine healthy individuals was greatest at 0800h.

Several experimental and clinical chronopharmacological studies have indirectly investigated temporal variations in hepatic drug metabolism capacity by evaluating the chronokinetics of drugs and their metabolites, even if not pharmacologically active. Thus, conjugation, hydrolysis and oxidation were shown to be circadian time dependent. As far as metabolic phenotype is concerned, the effect of diurnal variation on debrisoquine metabolic phenotyping, with the slowest rate of metabolism occurring during the daytime.

Temporal Variations in Drug Excretion

Most drugs are eliminated via the kidneys. Glomerular filtration, renal blood flow, urinary pH and tubular resorption have all been shown to be circadian time-dependent, with higher values during the daytime in humans. Thus, the urinary excretion of many drugs may depend on these rhythmic variations. In this field, it is particularly important to take into account the physicochemical properties of the drug; daily variations in the renal elimination of hydrophilic drugs (mainly excreted unchanged by the kidneys) are caused by the above-mentioned circadian rhythms in renal functions.

Renal elimination depends partially on the ionisation of drugs, and thus may be modified by temporal changes in urinary pH. This has been described for acidic drugs such as sodium salicylate and sulfasymazine, which are excreted more quickly after evening than morning administration.

Drugs that undergo chronokinetics

Antibiotics: many studies have reported temporal variations in the pharmacokinetics of antimicrobial drugs.Experimental animal models have shown that for Antibiotics such as beta-lactams that have concentration-independent killing effects in vitro, the time that the antibiotic concentration remains greater than the MIC(*T*> MIC) is the most important factor for determining the in vivo efficacy. Therefore, daily Variations in pharmacokinetics may account for impairment in the chemotherapeutic effects. This is of great importance when bacteria with low susceptibility are involved in the infectious processes.

The most important results in chronokinetics studies of antibiotics include:

Aminoglycosides: Peak renal toxicity was observed when aminoglycosides were injected in the middle of the rest period of the experimental animals, while lower toxicity was found when they were treated in the middle of the activity period. Based on many studies and on the evidence available in the current literature, it is quite clear that the renal toxicity of aminoglycosides can be reduced by giving the drug as a single daily injection when patients are active (at day time or in other words in the activity period).The mechanisms responsible for the temporal variation in renal toxicity of aminoglycosides are still unknown.

Gentamicin: both the effectiveness and the toxicity of Gentamicin varied over the 24-h Period and that the efficacy was best at the time when the toxicity of the drug was the lowest. So the administration of gentamicin in the beginning or the middle of the day in humans may reduce renal toxicity and increase the efficacy of these antibiotics.

Tobramycin: Tobramycin was administered at 0200 h (dark period), the CLT was significantly higher and AUC was lower than the values when tobramycin was given at 1400 h (light period).

Amikacin: Amikacin in humans showed higher values for k_{el} in the morning than in the evening.

Ceftriaxone: total clearance of ceftriaxone varies rhythmically during the day, with its maximum during the dark (activity) period and its minimum during the light (rest) period in rats.

Ciprofloxacin: In humans, the amount of ciprofloxacin eliminated in urine was greater when the drug was administered at 1000 h than when it was given at 2200 h.

Ampicillin: Ampicillin biliary and renal clearances were significantly higher during the active cycle of rats than during the sleep cycle.

Antihypertensive drugs: Nearly all physiological functions as well as pathophysiological events display reproducible rhythmic changes within 24 hours of a day, including the cardiovascular system. Clinical chronopharmacological studies with antihypertensive drugs gave evidence that effects on the rhythms in blood pressure and heart rate are also dependent on the time of day. Chronopharmacokinetic studies with propranolol, oxprenolol, nifedipine, verapamil, etc. also revealed daily variations in the drugs' kinetics. In general, C_{max} was higher and/or t_{max} shorter after morning than evening dosing of these rather lipophilic drugs. However, independently of whether or not daily variations in the kinetics were found the dose-response relationship was always dependent on the time of day.

Valporic acid: After oral administration, mean total VPA concentrations in plasma were significantly higher in the morning than in the evening during the absorption phase. Cmax tended to be higher, tmax was shorter and absorption rate constant (ka) tended to be larger for VPA in the morning than in the evening, although no difference was demonstrated in other pharmacokinetic values between morning and evening trials.

Sumatriptan: (drug of choice in migraine treatment) migraine is a disorder that exhibits periodicity in its symptoms and so chronotherapy may be beneficial in treating the problem. The mean peak serum concentration following the 0700 h administration was significantly higher than after the 1900 h administration. The mean area under the serum concentration-time curve from time zero to the last time-point ($AUC_{0\text{-}t}$), the area under the serum concentration-time curve from zero to infinity ($AUC_{0\text{-}\infty}$), and the area under the first moment curve (AUMC) were significantly higher following the 0700 and 0100 h administrations than after the 1900 h administration. Following administration at 0700 h, the mean oral clearance and the apparent volume of distribution were significantly lower than after the 1900 h administration. The variations may be due to the time dependent changes in the extent of absorption and/or circadian variations in hepatic blood flow.

Cyclosporine: one study done on cyclosporine pharmacokinetics in five recipients of pancreatic allografts. Results from these patients demonstrate a slightly increased area under the concentration-time curve resulting from decreased apparent clearance during the resting (PM) versus activity (AM) period. A significant delay in mean residence time was observed after the PM dose, and the PM area under the moment curve was larger than the AM value. Trends and differences suggest that more sophisticated time-dependent cyclosporine dosing methods are needed to balance AM and PM drug exposure and thereby improve immunosuppression.

Methotroxate: in a study involving 6 children with leukemia to methotroxate doses was administered at 10a.m and 9 p.m. the result was a significant decrease in plasma clearance at night. These differences (among other causes) would be mainly linked to variations in passive tubular reabsorption resulting from the rhythm in urine pH. In another study on animals (4 pigs) a significant circadian rhythm of methotroxate serum concentration was found in two pigs at 1:00 p.m.

Time-dependent pharmacokinetics involves an alteration in the biochemistry in an organ or physiologic change in the patient. Repetitive doses of a drug may cause a biochemical change in the levels of biotransformation enzymes. (*autoinduction* or *autoinhibition*). Repeated doses of carbamazepine induce (increase) the enzymes responsible for its elimination, thereby increasing the clearance of the drug. This is called *autoinduction.* This autoinduction is also a dose and concentration dependent, a property common to many time-dependent processes.

Autoinhibition may occur during the course of metabolism of certain drugs. In this case, the metabolites formed increase in concentration and further inhibit metabolism of the parent drug. In biochemistry, this phenomenon is known as *product inhibition.*

Drug	No. and type of participant	Administration regimen	Major significant findings ($p < 0.05$)
Aminosalicylic acid	12 Young healthy males	1.5g × 3 po every 7h, enteric coated tablets immediately after meal or 1h after meal	Diurnal effect: rise of aminosalicylic acid concentrations therefore C_{max} was higher in the morning
Diclofenac	10 Healthy	Single 50mg po 0700, 1900h	Highest peak at 0700h (≠ 30% change), highest AUC (≠ 23% change) No significant difference in t_{max} and $t_{1/2}$
Indomethacin	9 Healthy	Single dose 100mg po at 0700, 1100, 1500, 1900, 2300h	Highest peak at 0700 and 1100h (≠ 52% change), $t_{1/2\beta}$ highest at 1900h
Indomethacin sustained release	16 Patients with osteoarthritis	Single dose 75mg po at 8.00, 12.00, 20.00h	Highest C_{max} at 12.00h (≠ 25% change), highest AUC and highest $t_{1/2}$ at 2000h (≠ 10% change)
Indomethacin sustained release	10 Elderly volunteers	Single dose 75mg po at 0900, 1200, 2100h	t_{max} highest at 2100h (≠ 38% change)
Ketoprofen	8 Healthy	Single dose 100mg po at 0700, 1300, 1900, 0100h	Highest C_{max} (≠ 50% change) and AUC at 0700h (≠ 58% change), highest $t_{1/2}\beta$ at 0100h (≠ 60% change)
Ketoprofen sustained release	10 Healthy	Single dose 200mg po at 0700, 1900h	Shortest t_{max} at 0700 (≠ 24% change)
Ketoprofen constant infusion	8 Patients with sciatics	Constant IV infusion 5 mg/kg/day during 24h, sampling every 2h	Circadian variations of plasma concentrations with a peak at 2100h (≠ 48% change)
Ketorolac	12 Healthy	Single dose 30mg po at 0700, 1300, 1900, 0100h	AUC higher and CL lower at 1900 and 0100h, respectively (≠ 10% change)
Pranoprofen	7 Healthy	Single dose 75mg po at 1000, 2200h	t_{max} shorter at 1000h, no significant difference in AUC, $t_{1/2\beta}$ and CL
Salicylic acid	6 Healthy	Single dose 1h po, 0600, 1000, 1800, 2200h	Highest C_{max} (≠ 20% change), AUC (≠ 17% change) and $t_{1/2\beta}$ (≠ 20% change) at 0600h
Salicylic acid	6 Healthy	Single dose 1g po 0700, 1100, 1500, 1900, 2300h	Urinary elimination longest at 0700h (≠ 22% change)
Sulindac	10 Healthy	400mg/8 days 0800, 2000h	No significant differences in C_{max} and t_{max}. After morning administration, the highest 24h urinary unchanged amount (≠ 76% change)

Likely Questions

1. What are the reasons for a nonlinear behaviour of the drugs?
2. What are the characteristics of an active transport?
3. Derive Michaelis-Menton equation?
4. Give the three linear equations obtained by rearranging the Michaelis-Menten equation.
5. How do you estimate the values of Km and V_{max} in patients by the Direct Method and by a Direct Linear Plot?
6. Develop an equation for the first-order absorption and capacity limited elimination for a drug that follows one a compartment open model.
7. Give an equation for the rate of change in drug concentration in plasma (dC/dt) for:

   (a) Zero-order input and nonlinear elimination,

   (b) Nonlinear absorption and nonlinear elimination.
8. Define dose-dependent and time-dependent pharmacokinetics.
9. A new antibiotic is found to be eliminated from the body by nonlinear pharmacokinetics and has a Km of 100 mg and a V_{max} of 50 mg/hr. If 400 mg and 320 mg are administered to a patient on different occasions, calculate $t_{1/2}$ of the drug at different dose levels. What is your comment on the result?
10. The drug phenytoin is administered to a patient at the dosing rates of 150 mg and 300 mg/day, and the steady-state plasma concentrations found are 8.6 mg/L and 25.1 mg/L, respectively. Find the Km and V_{max} of this patient by Direct method. What would be the dose required to achieve a steady-state concentration of 11.3 mg/L?

Further Readings

1. Anthony Harrison, Alison Betts, Katherine Fenner, Kevin Beaumont, Alan Edgington, Sarah Roffey, John Davis, Pierre Comby and Paul Morgan; *(2004);* Nonlinear Oral Pharmacokinetics Of The '-Antagonist 4-Amino-5-(4-Fluorophenyl)-6,7-Dimethoxy-2-[4-(Morpholinocarbonyl)-Perhydro-1,4-Diazepin-1-Yl]Quinoline In Humans: Use Of Preclinical Data To Rationalize Clinical Observations, DMD vol. 32 no. 2 197-204.
2. Bernard Bruguerolle, (1998) Chronopharmacokinetics: Current StatusClin Pharmacokinet Aug; 35 (2): 83-94.
3. Reza Mehvar; (2001), Principles of Nonlinear Pharmacokinetics American Journal of Pharmaceutical Education, 65, 178-184.
4. Rowland M, Tozet TN. Clinical Pharmacokinetics – Concepts and Applications, 3rd edition, 1995, p. 397.

5. Samir D. Undevia , Gonzalo Gomez-Abuin , Mark J. Ratain; (2005), Pharmacokinetic Variability of Anticancer Agents: Sidebar: Linear Versus Non-Linear Pharmacokinetics Nat Rev Cancer;5(6):447-458.

6. Thomas J. Walsh, Andre J. Jackson, James W. Lee, Michael Amantea, Tin Sein, John Bacher, and Loren Zech, (2000); Dose-Dependent Pharmacokinetics of Amphotericin B Lipid Complex in Rabbits, Antimicrobial Agents and Chemotherapy, 44, 2068-2076.

7. Tozer TN, Winter ME. Phenytoin, In: Evans WE, Schentag JJ, Jusko WJ, Applied Pharmacokinetics – Principles for Therapeutic Drug Monitoring. 3rd edition, 1992, p. 25-12.

10
Noncompartmental Pharmacokinetics

Non Compartmental Pharmacokinetics

So far, the kinetics of drug absorption, distribution, metabolism and elimination are quantitatively evaluated based on compartment models. The concentration of a drug in biological specimen versus time data is used for the estimation of various useful pharmacokinetic parameters based compartment models. Compartment models are developed based on certain set of assumptions regarding the drug movement in the body. The observed data is fitted into an equation that describes a particular compartment model and the parameters are estimated. There exists an inherent variability in these estimated parameters due to variability of the biological system. The magnitude of variability depends on how best the observed data fits into the proposed compartment model. In addition, the number of subjects used in the study are limited, hence, the estimated parameters may not be the representative of the population.

Inspite of inherent variability in the estimated pharmacokinetic parameters based on compartment model, these parameters are useful in describing the drug concentration-time profile of a drug, duration of action of the drug, improving drug therapy and efficacy, therapeutic drug monitoring, minimizing toxicity and adverse reactions, and designing new drug delivery systems.

It is possible to estimate some important parameters that are useful in understanding drug absorption, distribution and elimination in the body without assigning any compartment model to the observed time course of drug levels in biological fluid i.e., non-compartmental pharmacokinetics. An advantage of noncompartmental analysis is that it requires fewer assumptions than that which is necessary with compartmental analysis. Noncompartmental model can be applied to virtually any compartment model, provided that we can assume linear pharmacokinetics. The basic assumption in noncompartmental or model independent approach is that the drug elimination occurs by the first-order process. One of the model independent approaches is based on the statistical moment theory and the other is a physiologic model.

10.1 Statistical Moment Theory

Eventhough, Statistical moment theory is extensively used for data analysis in chemical engineering, but was first applied for pharmacokinetic study in 1979 by Yamaoka et al and Cutler. In 1980, it was applied for evaluation of drug absorption by Riegelman and Collier.

Statistical moment theory is useful in studying the time related changes in macroscopic events. A macroscopic event is considered as the over all event brought about by the constitutive elements involved. The change in plasma concentration of a drug with time is a macroscopic event. This change is because of the elimination of a group of molecules at different time points of measurement. The drug molecules are called constitutive elements.

Let us consider an example to understand the statistical moment theory. 10 milligrams of a drug with a molecular weight of 200g/mole are injected intravenously. The number of molecules injected are equivalent to 3.0115×10^{19} [0.01 g/200 x 6.023×10^{23} (Avogadro's number)]. These drug molecules spend different times within the body. Some are eliminated rapidly, others stay for a long time. Consider the elimination of these molecules from the body in groups from 1 to m, each group containing a different number of molecules, n_i and spending a different residence time, t_i. The *mean residence time* (MRT) is the average time the total number of molecules introduced (N) reside in the body.

$$\text{MRT} = \frac{\text{Total residence time for all drug molecules in the body}}{\text{Total number of drug molecules}} \quad .....(10.1)$$

Therefore,

$$\text{MRT} = \frac{\sum_{i=1}^{m} n_i\, t_i}{\sum_{i=1}^{m} n_i} \quad .....(10.2)$$

or

$$\text{MRT} = \frac{\sum_{i=1}^{m} n_i\, t_i}{N} \quad .....(10.3)$$

Where, n_i is the number of molecules and t_i is the residence time of the ith group of molecules.

The number of molecules eliminated can be expressed in terms of the amount of the drug (mg) eliminated in each group and the following equation may be written,

$$\text{MRT} = \frac{\sum_{i=1}^{m} Xe_i\, t_i}{\sum_{i=1}^{m} Xe_i} \quad .....(10.4)$$

Where Xe_i is the mg of the drug eliminated in i^{th} group. The summation of Xe_i give the I.V. dose (X0). Drug molecules may have a residence time ranging from values near to zero to very large values. The summation approach to calculate the MRT is only an approximation, since the number of groups may be large. Further, in order to get an accurate estimation of the MRT, data must be collected continuously in order not to miss any group. When a data or function needs to be continuously summed over time, integration is an accurate method than a simple summation method. However, nonlinear events cannot be adequately treated by the statistical moment theory.

10.1.1 One Compartment Model - I.V. Bolus

Unchanged Drug in Blood/Plasma: Let us apply this statistical moment theory for a drug that follows a one compartment model. The drug concentration in plasma following an I.V. bolus dose is given by,

$$C = \frac{X0}{Vd} e^{-Kt} \qquad .....(10.5)$$

or

$$X = X0\ e^{-Kt} \qquad .....(10.6)$$

Where, X0 is a I.V. bolus dose, Vd is the volume of distribution of the drug, C0 is the zero time concentration of the drug in plasma, X is the amount of the drug in body at any time t, C is the concentration of the drug in plasma at any time t, and K is the apparent first-order elimination rate constant.

The MRT is determined more rapidly after an I.V. bolus dose than after any other mode of drug administration. Here all the molecules of the dose start their residence in the body at the same time, thus for each group, t_i is the time between drug administration and elimination.

The rate of change in the amount of a drug in the body with respect to time, dX/dt, reflects the rate at which the drug molecules leave the body at any time t. All the molecules are eliminated from the body from t = 0 to infinity. The derivative of Equation 10.6 results in an equation that describes the, dX/dt.

$$dX/dt = -K\ X0\ e^{-Kt} \qquad .....(10.7)$$

Alternatively, the rate of drug molecules exiting at any time t is given by,

$$dXe/dt = -\ dX/dt = K\ X0\ e^{-Kt} \qquad .....(10.8)$$

Rearranging the Equation 10.8 gives,

$$dXe = K\ X0\ e^{-Kt}\ dt \qquad .....(10.9)$$

Wherein, dXe is the amount of the drug (or number of molecules) leaving the body at any time t. Therefore, multiplication of Equation 10.9 by t on both the sides gives the residence of the drug leaving with a residence time of t.

$$dXe\ t = K\ X0\ e^{-Kt}\ t\ dt \qquad ......(10.10)$$

Integration of Equation 10.10 between the limits of t = 0 to ∞ gives the total residence time for all drug molecules in the body and a division by the total number of molecules (I.V. dose), estimates the mean residence time (equation 10.11).

$$\int_0^\infty dXe\ t/X0 = \int_0^\infty (K\ X0e^{-Kt}\ t\ dt)/X0 \qquad .....(10.11)$$

$$MRT = \int_0^\infty K\ e^{-Kt}\ t\ dt \qquad .....(10.12)$$

Division by the dose in Equation 10.11 normalizes the differential function that represents the drug amount (or concentration) in the body. Thus, the MRT is an integrated normalized form of the differential function representing the drug amount (or concentration) in the body. When the function is normalized it becomes dimensionless with regard to unit.

Equation 10.11 is developed in terms of the amount of the drug in the body. An equation that allows a calculation of the MRT with a plasma concentration can be written by substituting C0 Vd for an I.V. dose, X0.

$$\frac{\int_0^\alpha dXe\ t}{X0} = \frac{\int_0^\alpha K\ C0\ Vd\ e^{-Kt}\ t\ dt}{C0\ Vd} \qquad .....(10.13)$$

$$MRT = \frac{\int_0^\alpha K\ C0\ e^{-Kt}\ t\ dt}{C0} \qquad .....(10.14)$$

Equation 10.14 can be used directly to calculate the MRT. It can be modified by dividing the numerator and denominator of Equation 10.14 by K to give,

$$MRT = \frac{\int_0^\alpha C0\ e^{-Kt}\ t\ dt}{C0/K} \qquad .....(10.15)$$

But $\quad C0.\ e^{-Kt} = C$ and $C0/K = [AUC]_0^\infty = \int_0^\infty C.\ dt,$

therefore

$$MRT = \int_0^\infty C.t.dt/ \int_0^\infty C.dt \qquad .....(10.16)$$

The product of t. C is called the *first moment* of the concentration, because concentration is multiplied by time raised to the power 1. Therefore, the numerator is called the area under the (first) moment curve (AUMC), whereas the denominator is the area under the plasma drug concentration-time curve (AUC) and is called *zero moment* curve. The *second moment* of the concentration defines the variation in residence time, VRT (i.e., Variance of the distribution). Higher moments, such as *third* and *fourth moment*, represent skewness and kurtosis of the distribution.

MRT of a drug after an I.V. bolus dose can be measured from plasma drug concentration-time data. AUC from 0 to t is calculated using the trapezoidal rule and the remaining AUC from last time point, t* to infinity is calculated using integration method, as shown below.

$$[AUC]_{t^*}^{\infty} = C^*/K \qquad .....(10.17)$$

Where, t* is the last sampling time and C* is the corresponding drug concentration in plasma. Therefore, $[AUC]_0^{\infty} = [AUC]_0^{t} + [AUC]_t^{\infty}$. The value of AUMC is calculated from the first-moment in a manner similar to that of AUC, but the extrapolated area after the last point (C* at t*) is different. In this case the area remaining can be shown to be:

$$\int_0^{\infty} t^* \cdot C^* \, dt = C^* \, t^*/K + C^*/K^2 \qquad .....(10.18)$$

Where K is the rate constant of the terminal decay of the plasma drug concentration.

When the entire concentration-time profile can be described by a sum of exponentials, the area under the first-moment curve can be determined directly from the coefficients and exponential coefficients defining the equation. For example, for a drug that follows a two compartment model, the concentration of the drug in plasma following an I.V. bolus dose is $C = A \; e^{-\alpha t} + B \; e^{-\beta t}$, then

$$AUMC = \frac{A}{\alpha^2} + \frac{B}{\beta^2} \qquad .....(10.19)$$

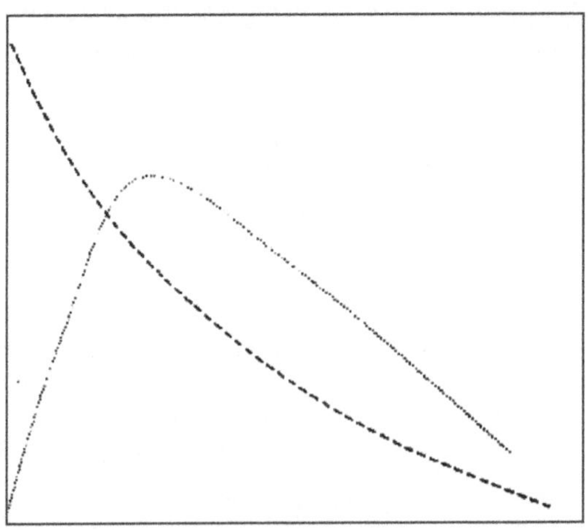

Fig. 10.1 Plasma drug concentration and first-moment versus time curves following I.V. bolus dose.

Figure 10.1 shows the plots of zero-moment and first-moment curves following an I.V. bolus dose of a drug. The drug plasma concentration declines with time but the first-moment, production of time and concentration, rises to a peak and declines with time. The area beyond the last sampling time is greater for the first-moment time curve than for the concentration-time curve.

Urinary Excretion Data

When the fraction of the drug excreted unchanged, fu, remains constant with time, the amount of the drug excreted unchanged in urine in infinite time, $X_u\mu$ = (fu) (X0). Further, the amount of the unchanged drug excreted at any time t is equal to (fu) (Xe) (Xe is the amount of the drug eliminated by all possible pathways including renal at any time t). Therefore, an equation for calculating MRT can be written as given below:

$$MRT = \frac{(X_u^{\alpha} - X_u^{t})\, dt}{Xu^{\alpha}} \quad .....(10.20)$$

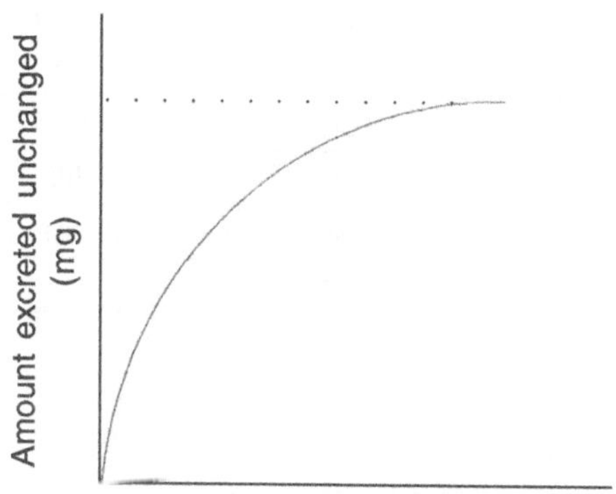

Fig. 10.2 The difference between amount excreted unchanged (solid line) and amount ultimately excreted (dashed line) in the amount to be excreted. The area under the amount remaining to be excreted versus time curve (unshaded), relative to total amount excreted (equation 10.20), is a measure of mean residence time of a drug in the body. Data from Table 10.1.

Fig. 10.2 shows the cumulative amount excreted unchanged, X^t_u, at various times and the amount ultimately excreted unchanged, $X_u\mu$. The area between these curves is the numerator in Equation 10.20. For a given amount excreted unchanged, it is apparent that the area and therefore, the MRT are increased when drug remains longer in the body.

10.1.2 MRT for One Compartment Model

The MRT calculated by either Equation 10.16 or 10.20, is a measure of the average time a drug spends in the body after an I.V. bolus dose. When a drug is given by a constant-rate I.V. infusion or by an extravascular route, the drug spends an additional time in the syringe or at the site of administration (e.g. gastrointestinal tract, muscle or subcutaneous tissues). The observed time, estimated from Equations 10.16 or 10.20, is then the sum of the mean times at these sites and in the body. Table 10.2 shows the *mean input times* (MIT) and observed mean total residence times for three common modes of a drug input.

Table 10.1 Plasma Concentration-Time, and Urinary Excretion-Time Data Following an I.V. Bolus Dose of a Drug (200 mg)

Time (hours)	Plasma drug concentration (mg/L)	First-moment of plasma concentration (mg/hr/L)	Cumulative amount excreted (mg)	Amount remaining to be excreted (mg)
0	10*	0	0	80**
2	6.3	12.6	30	50
4	7.0	16.0	48	32
6	2.5	15.0	60	20
8	1.6	12.8	67	13
10	1.0	10.0	72	8
12	0.63	7.6	75	5
14	0.39	5.5	76.5	3.5
16	0.25	7.0	78	2
20	0.1	2.0	78.6	1.4
24	0.04	0.96	80	0

*Estimated by extrapolation on a semilogarthmic plot to zero time.

**The cumulative amount excreted at infinite time.

10.1.2 MRT for One Compartment Model

The MRT calculated by either Equation 10.16 or 10.20, is a measure of the average time a drug spends in the body after an I.V. bolus dose. When a drug is given by a constant-rate I.V. infusion or by an extravascular route, the drug spends an additional time in the syringe or at the site of administration (e.g. gastrointestinal tract, muscle or subcutaneous tissues). The observed time, estimated from Equations 10.16 or 10.20, is then the sum of the mean times at these sites and in the body. Table 10.2 shows the *mean input times* (MIT) and observed mean total residence times for three common modes of a drug input.

Table 10.2 Mean Residence Times for Selected Modes of Drug Input.

Mode of administration	Model	Mean input time	Observed mean residence time
I.V. Bolus	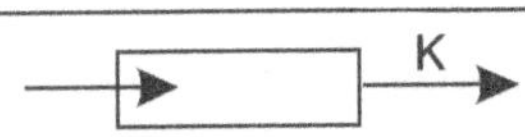	0	1/K
Constant infusion	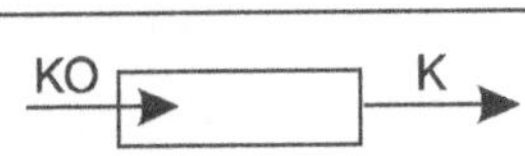	$\tau/2$	$1/K + \tau/2$
Extra vascular dose	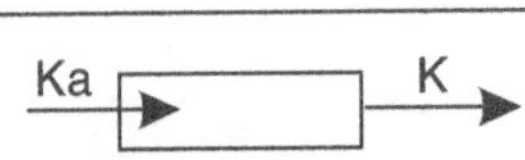	1/Ka	1/K + 1/Ka

10.1.3 MRT for Multicompartment Model

It is possible to calculate the MRT for a drug that has a plasma (central) compartment and one or more tissue or peripheral compartments, using plasma drug concentration-time data. The assumptions made in deriving the MRT of drugs that follow multi-compartment pharmacokinetics are (1) the drug elimination occurs only from the central compartment and (2) the total drug is eliminated by a linear process (constant clearance). The MRT of a drug that follows a multi-compartment model is the summation of the residence time of the drug in each compartment.

$$MRT_{body} = MRTc + MRT_{t1} + MRT_{t2} + ... + MRT_{tn} \quad .....(10.21)$$

Where, MRTc is the mean residence time of the drug in the central compartment and MRTti represents MRT in the tissue compartment. MRT_{body} is the sum of MRTc and MRT in all tissue compartments. The body is treated as a single compartment irrespective of the number of compartments involved with regard to drug distribution. Hence, MRT_{body} is calculated from the plasma drug concentration-time data using AUMC/AUC as explained earlier.

MRT for the Central compartment

Let us develop an equation for the calculation of MRTc based on plasma (Central) drug concentration-time data

Let

X0 = The I.V. bolus dose or drug at time zero.

Xc = Amount of drug in central compartment from which drug is eliminated at time t.

X_e = The amount of drug eliminated to time t.

V_{dc} = Volume of distribution of drug in central compartment.

C = Drug plasma concentration at any time t.

Now, at any time t, the product of the amount of the drug eliminated dXe and the residence time t gives the residence time of that group.

Residence time of a group at

$$t = dXe\ t \quad .....(10.22)$$

Integration of equation 10.22 between the limits of 0 to X_e^{∞} will yield the total residence time.

Total residence time

$$= \int_0^{X_e^{\alpha}} t\ dXe \quad .....(10.23)$$

Integration of dXe from 0 to X_e^{∞} will give the total drug eliminated, which is equal to I.V. dose, X0.

$$\int_0^{X_e^{\alpha}} dXe = X0 \qquad .....(10.24)$$

MRT is obtained by dividing the total residence time (Equation 10.23) by the total drug eliminated (Equation 10.24).

$$MRTc = \frac{\int_0^{X_e^{\alpha}} t\, dXe}{\int_0^{X_e^{\alpha}} dXe} \qquad .....(10.25)$$

The amount of the drug eliminated from the body at any time t is equal to the amount of the drug decreased in the central compartment. Therefore, if elimination occurs only from the central compartment, at any instant dt,

dXe = – dX. Therefore, Equation 10.25 can be written as,

$$MRTc = \frac{\int_0^{X_e^{\alpha}} t\, dXe}{\int_0^{X_e^{\alpha}} dXe} = \frac{\int_o^{XO} t\, dX}{\int_o^{XO} dX} \qquad .....(10.26)$$

Since, dX = dC. Vc, MRT in concentration terms,

$$MRTc = \frac{\int_0^{CO} t\, Vd\, dC}{\int_0^{CO} Vd\, dC} = \frac{\int_0^{CO} t\, dC}{\int_0^{CO} dC} \qquad .....(10.27)$$

Integration of dC with respect to plasma concentration from 0 to C0 is equal to the integration of C with respect to time.

Since $\int_0^{C0} dC = -C0$ and $\int_0^{C0} t\, dC = \int_0^{\alpha} - C.\, dt$

Equation 10.27 can be written as,

$$MRTc = \frac{\int_0^{\alpha} C\, dt}{C0} = \frac{[AUC]_0^{\alpha}}{C0} \qquad .....(10.28)$$

MRTc is known as the *mean residence time or mean transit time* for the central compartment. MRT_{body} is calculated using the equation AUMC/AUC. For a drug that follows two compartment model, the mean residence time for the tissue compartment, MRT_t, can be obtained by subtracting MRTc from MRT_{body}.

$$MRT_t = MRT_{body} - MRTc \qquad .....(10.29)$$

$$MRT_t = \frac{AUMC}{AUC} - \frac{AUC}{C0} \qquad .....(10.30)$$

Another way to calculate MRT_{body} according to statistical moment theory is based on Equation 10.14.

$$MRT = \frac{\int_0^{\alpha} C\,K\,t\,dt}{C0} \qquad .....(10.31)$$

The concentration of drug in plasma (C) at any time t, following an I.V. bolus dose for a two-compartment model is

$$C = [e^{-\alpha t} + e^{-\beta t}]\ \frac{X0}{Vc}\ [\frac{(\alpha - K_{21})}{(\alpha - \beta)}\ e^{-\alpha t} + \frac{(K_{21} - \beta)}{(\alpha - \beta)}\ e^{-\beta t}] \qquad .....(10.32)$$

Therefore,

$$MRT = \frac{\int_0^{\alpha} \frac{X0}{Vc}\ [\frac{(\alpha - K_{21})}{(\alpha - \beta)}\ e^{-\alpha t} + \frac{(K_{21} - \beta)}{(\alpha - \beta)}\ e^{-\beta t}]}{C0}\ K\ t\ dt \qquad .....(10.33)$$

The MRT calculated using 10.33 agrees with the one obtained by AUMC/AUC. However, K (elimination constant from the central compartment) is not known from plasma data and hence equation 10.33 can not be applied directly.

Table 10.3 Shows the Equations for Calculating MRT for Two Compartment Model.

Route	MRT
I.V. Bolus	$(K_{12} + K_{21})/K_{13}\ K_{21}$ or $[(1/\alpha) + (1/\beta)] - (1/K_{21})$
Oral Bolus	$(1/K\alpha) + (K_{12} + K_{21})/K_{13}\ K_{21}$

10.1.4 Steady State Volume of Distribution

MRT is useful in calculating the steady state volume of distribution and probably additional parameters in compartment models. MRT at steady state may be defined as the ratio of the amount of the drug in the body at the steady-state to the clearance rate.

$$MRT = \frac{V_d^{ss}\ C_{ss}}{CL_t\ C_{ss}} = \frac{V_d^{ss}}{CL_t} \qquad .....(10.34)$$

Where V_d^{ss} is the steady-state volume of distribution of the drug, C_{ss} is the steady state drug concentration in plasma and CL_t is the clearance.

Therefore,

$$V_d^{ss} = CL_t \text{ MRT} \qquad .....(10.35)$$

Realizing that CL_t = dose /$[AUC]_0^{\infty}$ following a single dose or Dose/$[AUC]_{t1}^{t2}$, where, $[AUC]_{t1}^{t2}$ is the area under the curve at the steady-state during the dosage interval and MRT = AUMC/AUC, we can write,

$$V_d^{ss} = \frac{\text{Dose}}{[AUC]_0^{\alpha}} \quad \frac{\text{AUMC}}{\text{AUC}} \qquad .....(10.36)$$

Equation 10.36 is useful in estimating V_d^{ss}. MRT values for the central and tissue compartments gives an idea about the drug residence time in the central and tissue compartments that are useful for understanding the duration of the drug action. For example, for drug digoxin, MRT for the body 49.5 hours, for the central and peripheral is 3.68 hours and is 45.8 hours, respectively. The peripheral MRT is the mean total time the drug molecules spend in the peripheral tissue, considering the first as well as possible subsequent entries into the peripheral tissue from the central compartment.

10.1.5 Mean Absorption Time (MAT) and Mean Dissolution Time (MDT)

Following an extravascular administration of a drug solution, the observed total MRT is the sum of MRT in the body due to elimination and the mean absorption time (MAT). Following an I.V. bolus dose of a drug, the observed MRT is only due to the elimination of the drug. Therefore, the mean absorption time can be determined from the difference between MRT values after extravascular and I.V. bolus doses given on separate occasions.

$$MRT_{oral} = MAT + MRT_{iv} \qquad .....(10.37)$$

$$MAT = MRT_{oral} - MRT_{iv} \qquad .....(10.38)$$

Realizing that MRT_{IV} for one compartment model = 1/K,

$$MAT = MRT_{oral} - 1/K \qquad .....(10.39)$$

In some cases, I.V. data are not available or not used as a reference, but data obtained with drug solution may be used to calculate the mean dissolution time (MDT) or mean *in vivo* dissolution time for a solid dosage form. After giving a solid dosage form, the MRT includes time for dissolution of a drug, in addition to the absorption and elimination of drug.

Therefore, the mean dissolution time for a solid product is

$$MDT_{solid} = MRT_{solid} - MRT_{solution} \qquad .....(10.40)$$

Equation 10.40 allows the calculation of *in vivo* dissolution time of a solid dosage form that could not be calculated past. MDT is considered a model independent because MRT is model independent. MDT for drugs that follow one compartment model is readily estimated.

MDT is used to study the comparative bioavailability of generic product and to make *in vitro* dissolution versus *in vivo* bioavailability comparisons. MDT is useful in correlating *in vitro* dissolution results and *in vivo* bioavailability of sustained release-drug products.

10.2 Physiological Pharmacokinetic Model

Physiologic pharmacokinetic models are mathematical models describing drug movement and disposition in the body based on blood flow and the organ spaces penetrated by the drug. In this compartments are chosen to represent physiologiocal compartments of the body. All physiological compartments should be included in the model. The human body is composed of organ systems which are made up of tissues. The blood supplies nutrients and oxygen through the circulatory system, consisting of arteries and veins. The fluid inside the cell is called *intracellular fluid* and the fluid in which they are bathing is called *extracellular fluid*. Hence, the blood capillaries are in direct contact with the extracellular fluid (Fig. 10.3). Once the drug enters the systemic circulation, it is carried to all the tissues. The drug in blood diffuses into and equilibrates with the extracellular fluid rapidly. Some drugs may cross the cell membrane into the interior or fluid (intracellular fluid) of the cell. The drug accumulation in an organ depends on the blood flow rate into the organ and the rate of uptake of the drug. The amount of drug in an organ depends on

1. The size of the organ, into which the drug distributes.
2. The partition coefficient of the drug between the organ and the circulating blood,
3. The blood flow to the organ, and
4. The extent of protein binding of the drug both in plasma and in tissue.

Figure 10.4a shows the concept of drug distribution and elimination as per physiologic model. First, the drug enters the extracellular fluid and rapid equilibrium is achieved between the drug in the blood and the extracellular fluid. Transfer of the drug into the cell depends on the permeability of the cell wall to the drug molecules. The drug that enteres the interior fluid of the cell may bind to the macromolecules present in it leading to high amounts of drug accumulation within the cell. A particular organ in the body may act as a site of distribution or as a site of both distribution and elimination. (Fig.10.4a and10.4b). The relative importance of the various organs as storage and/or elimination sites depend on how fast the drugs get to each organ and how much space or volume is available to hold the drug. Table 10.4 presents a compilation of the tissue weights, rates of blood flow and the weights of blood in an equilibrium with the tissues for a standard man.

Because blood flow, distribution and elimination from individual organs and tissue groups are included, the model is more realistic and meaningful. And hence the prediction of pharmacokinetic parameters is improved. However, the disadvantage is that it is very difficult to determine many of the physiological and anatomical parameters and lot of data is required. In addition to blood and urine data, it is important to know tissue concentrations and organ blood flow rates.

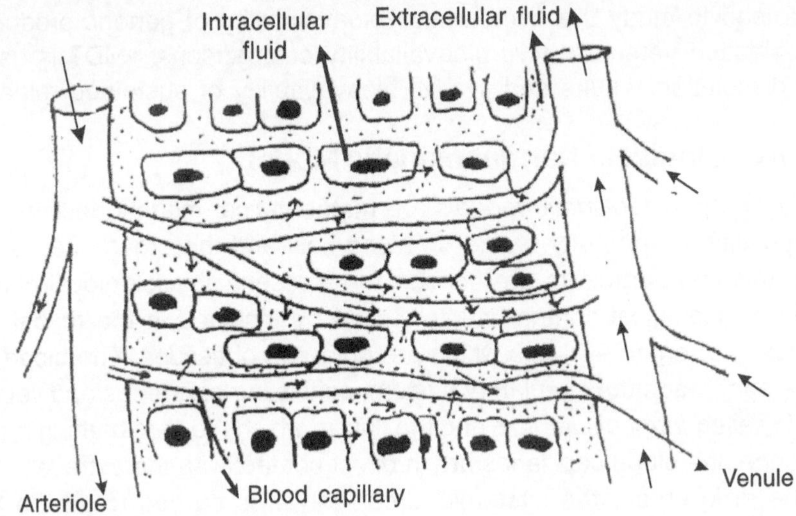

Fig. 10.3 The blood capillaries and tissue cells are in contact with each other.

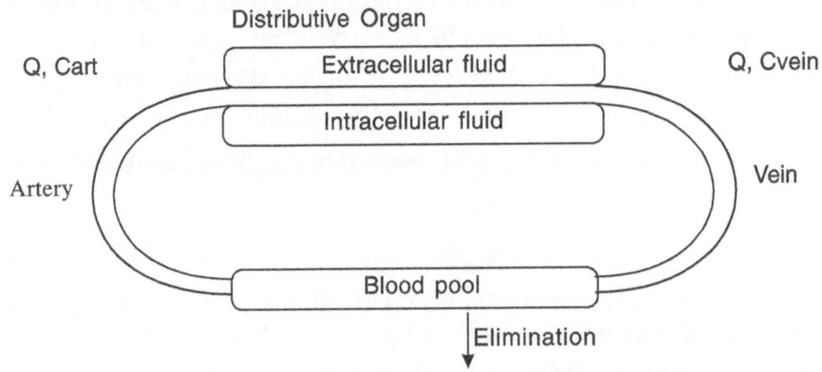

Q = Rate of blood flow; Cart = Drug concentration in artery; Cvein= Drug concentration in vein.

Fig. 10.4 (a) Physiologic pharmacokinetic model - Drug distribution to an organ.

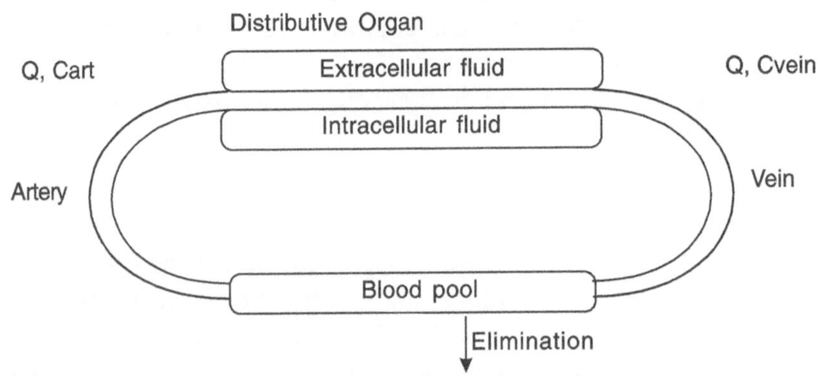

Q = Rate of blood flow; Cart = Drug concentration in artery; Cvein= Drug concentration in vein.

Fig. 10.4 (b) Physiological pharmacokinetic model - Drug distribution to an organ that elimiates the drug.

Table 10.4 Tissue Weights, Rates of Blood Flow, and Weights of Blood Equilibrium With the Tissue for a Standard Man (Body Weight 70.0 kg, Body Surface Area 1.8 m^2, and Cardiac Output 3.5 Liters/min/m^2 (6.3 liters/min)

Tissue	Weight (gm)	Blood flow (mg/100 g/min)	Blood flow (Percent of cardiac output)	Blood in equilibrium (g)
Adrenal glands	20	508.0	1.61	67.5
Thyroid glands	20	500.0	1.59	63.5
Kidneys	300	396.0	18.90	757.3
Heart	300	80.6	3.84	153.5
Brain	1,500	52.9	12.60	503.8
Prostate	20	48.5	0.15	6.2
Red marrow	2,680	39.9	17.00	678.4
Lymphoid tissue Liver + Portal system	3,920	38.6	27.00	960.7
Testes	40	22.8	0.14	5.8
Spinal cord	30	16.2	0.08	3.1
Skin and subcutaneous tissue	6100	5.7	5.52	220.8
Muscle	30,000	2.12	10.10	403.8
Bladder	150	2.12	0.05	2.0
Yellow marrow	1500	2.80	0.67	26.7
Adipose tissue	10,000	2.41	3.83	153.0
Skeleton (less marrow)	7000	0.0**	0.0	0.0
Gastrointestinal* fill	1635*	0.0	0.0	0.0
Teeth	20	0.0**	0.0	0.0
*Not included in 70 Kg total body weight				
**Negligible flow, assumed to be zero for purpose of calculation				

The various regions of the body are listed in decreasing order with respect to the blood flow per unit mass of tissue (adrenal glands highest and bone cortex lowest). The rate of blood flow describes how fast a drug can be delivered to a body region per unit mass of tissue, and reflects the relative rates in which tissues may be expected to come into equilibrium with the blood. How much a drug can be stored or distributed into a tissue will depend on the size of the tissue and the ability of the drug to concentrate in the tissue (i.e. the partition coefficient between the tissue and blood).

Partition coefficient of drug in the tissue (P_{tissue}),

$$= \frac{\text{concentration of drug in tissue, } C_{tissue}}{\text{concentration of drug in blood, } C_{blood}}$$

Therefore, $$P_{tissue} = C_{tissue}/C_{blood} \quad .....(10.41)$$

10.2.1 Blood-Flow Limited Model or Perfusion Model

In its simplest form, a physiological pharmacokinetic model considers that the drug concentration in a tissue depends on the blood flow to the tissue and is called *blood-flow limited* or *perfusion model.* The rate of the blood flow to the tissue is Qt (ml/min), and the rate of change in the drug amount with respect to time is expressed as

$$d\,(V_{tissue}.C_{tissue})/dt = Qt\,(C_{in} - C_{out}) \qquad .....(10.42)$$

$$d\,(V_{tissue}.C_{tissue})/dt = Qt\,(C_{art} - C_{vein}) \qquad .....(10.43)$$

Where, V_{tissue} is the volume of distribution of the drug in the tissue, C_{tissue} is the tissue of the drug concentration, C_{art} is the arterial blood drug concentration and C_{vein} is the venous blood drug concentration (Fig. 10.4 a and b). Qt represents the volume of blood flowing through a typical tissue organ per unit time. If a drug uptake occurs in tissue, the drug concentration in the arterial blood will be greater than the drug concentration in venous blood. The difference in drug concentrations of the arterial and venous blood multiplied by the blood flow gives the amount of the drug taken up by the tissue. In the blood-flow-limited model, the concentration of the drug in the tissue and the drug concentration in the venous blood are in equilibrium. C_{vein} may be calculated from the ratio of the drug in the tissue and blood i.e., $C_{vein} = C_{tissue}/P_{tissue}$ (according to Equatioin 10.41). Substituting C_{vein} value in Equation 10.43,

$$d\,(V_{tissue}.C_{tissue})/dt = Qt\,[C_{art} - (C_{tissue}/P_{tissue})] \qquad .....(10.44)$$

Equation 10.43 describes drug distribution in a distributive (non eliminating) organ or tissue. Drug distribution to the muscle, adipose tissue, and the skin may be written as below

Muscle: $$d\,(V_{muscle}.\,C_{muscle})/dt = Q_{muscle}\,[C_{muscle} - (C_{muscle}/P_{muscle})] \qquad .....(10.45)$$

Adipose tissue: $$d\,(V_{adipose}.\,C_{adipose})/dt = Q_{adipose}\,[C_{adipose} - (C_{adipose}/P_{adipose})] \qquad .....(10.46)$$

Skin: $$d\,(V_{skin}\,.\,C_{skin})/dt = Q_{skin}\,[C_{skin} - (C_{skin}/P_{skin})] \qquad .....(10.47)$$

For tissue organs in which the drug is eliminated (Fig. 10.4b), parameters representing drug elimination from the organs are added to account for drug removal. It is obvious that an organ can not clear the drug from the blood any faster than the drug is delivered to the organ via the blood flow. The drug clearance by an organ or tissue called organ clearance is given by

$$CL_{organ} = Qo\,\frac{C_{art} - C_{vein}}{C_{art}} = Qo\;Eo \qquad .....(10.48)$$

Equation 10.48 indicates that organ clearance may be defined as the product of the blood flow to the organ, Qo, and the extraction ratio, Eo. The blood flow and the extraction ratio appear to be independent parameters controlling drug clearance. However, a good deal of experimental evidence suggests that the extraction ratio decreases with an increasing blood flow. Based on a perfusion model, the extraction ratio of an eliminating organ could be defined as,

$$Eo = CL_{int}/(Qo + CL_{int}) \quad .....(10.49)$$

Where, CL_{int} in the intrinsic clearance of the organ, that is, the maximum ability of the organ to remove the drug from the blood when there are no flow limitations. Substituting Equation 10.49 into Equation 10.48 gives,

$$CL_{organ} = Qo \frac{CL_{int}}{(Qo + C_{int})} \quad .....(10.50)$$

When the intrinsic clearance of an organ is very high compared to the blood flow (i.e., $CL_{int} >> Qo$), the extraction ratio approaches 1 (i.e., Qo in the denominator is negligible) and CLorgan ≈ Qo. Thus, for a drug cleared exclusively in the liver, the maximum blood clearance would be 1580 ml/min. and the maximum renal clearance would be 1240 ml/min.

The total drug taken up by an eliminating organ is not present in the tissue since some fraction of the total drug undergoes elimination either by metabolism (liver) or excretion (kidney). Therefore, the rate of change of drug levels in an organ or tissue which eliminates the drug is given by the following equation,

$$d\,(V_{tissue}.C_{tissue})/dt = Qt\,[C_{art} - (C_{tissue}/P_{tissue})] - C_{tissue}\frac{CL_{tissue}}{P_{tissue}} \quad .....(10.51)$$

The rate of drug elimination by kidneys is

$$d\,(V_{kid}.C_{kid})/dt = Q_{kid}\,[C_{kid} - (C_{kid}/P_{kid})] - C_{kid}\frac{CL_{kid}}{P_{kid}} \quad .....(10.52)$$

In case of the liver blood flows from the G.I. tract, spleen in addition to direct blood flow to liver (Fig. 10.5). Therefore, the rate of drug elimination by the liver may be described as below,

$$d\,(V_{Liv}.C_{liv})/dt = C_{liv}\,(Q_{liv} - Q_{gi} - Q_{sp}) + Q_{gi}\,(C_{gi}/P_{gi}) + Q_{sp}\,(C_{sp}/P_{sp}) - Q_{liv}\,(C_{liv}/P_{liv}) - C_{liv}\,(CL_{int}/P_{Liv}) \quad .....(10.53)$$

The lung is unique because the perfusion from the heart is by the venous blood. The blood from the lungs flows back to the heart through the pulmonary artery. Therefore, the terms in Equation 10.54 describing lung perfusion are reversed compared to those for the perfusion of other tissues.

$$d\,(V_{lung}.C_{lung})/dt = Q_{lung}\,[(C_{lung}/P_{lung}) - C_{lung}] \quad .....(10.54)$$

Since a number of drugs partition readily into the lung, the large blood concentration of the drug entering the lung following an I.V. bolus injected is damped, with the lung serving as a reservoir that releases the drug back into the general circulation, when the drug is cleared from the blood by a hepatic or renal mechanism. It should be remembered that the lung may also serve as a metabolic site for certain drugs and as an excretory route for compounds with a high vapor pressure. Thus, drugs given by the I.V. route may not necessarily be completely available to the sites of action since a certain fraction of the drug could be eliminated by the lung before going into the general circulation. This might be called a lung first-pass effect. In such cases lung clearance term should be included in the equation in addition to lung tissue distribution.

The mass balance equation for the rate of change in drug concentration in the blood pool is as follows.

$$\begin{aligned} d(V_b C_b)/dt &= Q_{muscle} \cdot C_{muscle}/P_{muscle} \\ &+ Q_{adipose}\, C_{adipose}/P_{adipose} \\ &+ Q_{skin}\, C_{skin}/P_{skin} + Q_{liv}\, C_{liv}/P_{liv} \\ &+ Q_{kid}\, C_{kid}/P_{kid} + Q_{lung}\, C_{lung}/P_{lung} \\ &- Q_b\, C_b \text{ (blood)} \end{aligned} \quad .....(10.55)$$

The above differential equation describes the blood-flow limited model as is solved through computer programs. Because of the large number of parameters involved in the mass balance, more than one set of parameters may fit the experimental data.

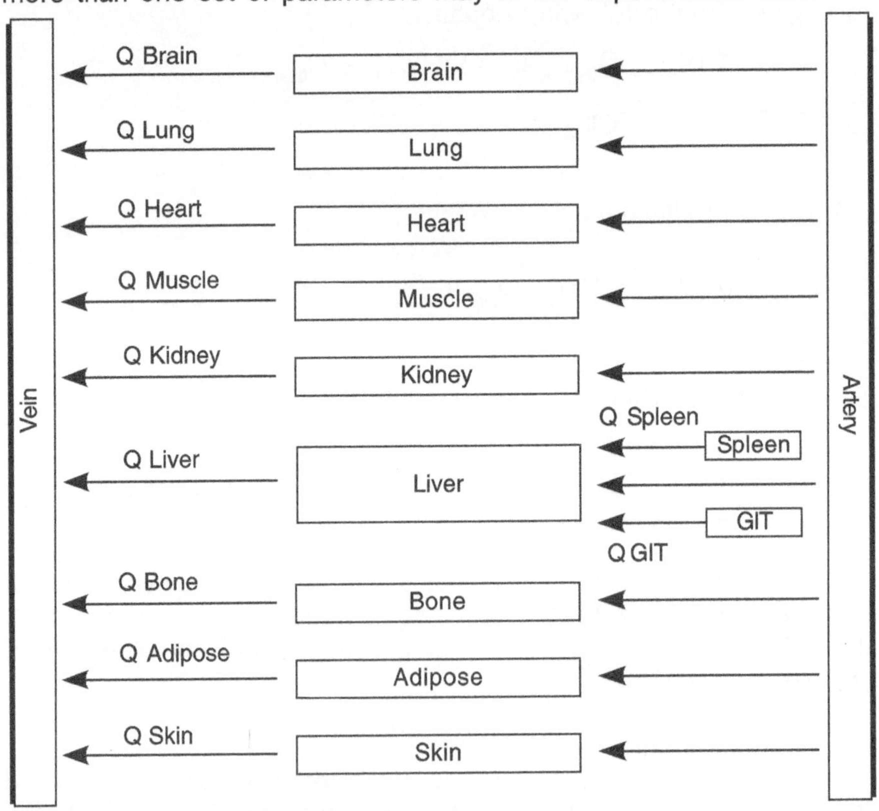

Fig. 10.5 Schematic representation of physiolobical pharmacokinetic model.

Since it is possible to obtain the tissue concentrations of the drug and tissue partition coefficient in animals, physiologic pharmacokinetic models may yield more realistic and reliable information. However, lack of tissue data in human experiments lead to little use of physiologic pharmacokinetic models in human pharmacokinetic studies.

10.2.2 Physiologic Pharmacokinetic Model With Binding

One of the major determinants of drug distribution is the extent of binding of drugs to plasma protein or tissue components. Many drugs, particularly weak acids and bases, bind to the plasma proteins, usually albumin, but some times to globulins as well. Binding of drugs to the plasma proteins has been studied extensively, primarily due to the fact that the experiments can be easily carried out. Tissue binding studies do not have this advantage, and thus knowledge of the qualitative and quantitative aspects of the binding of drugs to tissue components is poorly understood.

The physiologic pharmacokinetic model assumes a flow limited drug distribution without drug binding to either plasma proteins or tissue components. As mentioned above, most drugs show binding to plasma proteins and to some extent to tissue components. Equations describing the rate of change in drug amount can be developed for drugs that show binding, based on following assumptions.

1. Drug binding is linear (i.e., not saturable or concentration dependent).
2. Bound and free drugs in both the tissue and plasma are in equilibrium.
3. The equilibrium between the drug in plasma and tissue attains rapidly.

Figure 10.6 shows the equilibrium conditions in blood and the tissue. The free drug concentration in the tissue. The free drug concentration in emerging blood (venous blood) are equal.

$$[Cb]f = [Ct]f \qquad .....(10.56)$$

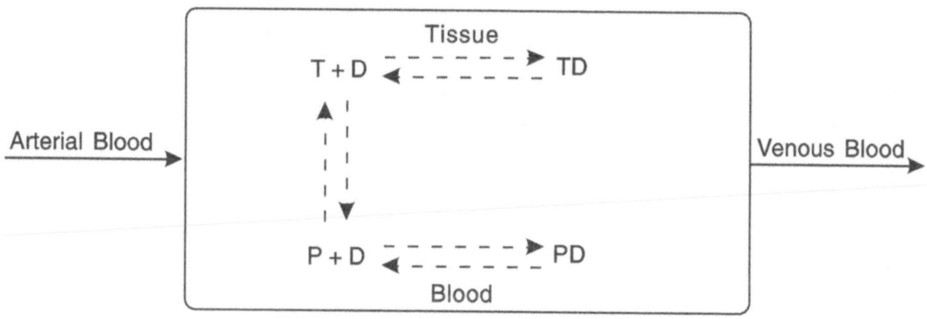

D = free drug; P = free protein; PD = protein-drug complex; T = tissue component; TD = tissue component drug complex

Fig. 10.6 Drug distribution and binding in blood and tissue.

Where, [Cb]f is the free drug in blood and [Ct]f is the free drug in tissue. fb and ft are the blood free drug fraction and the tissue free drug fraction, respectively. Cb and Ct represent the total drug concentration in the blood and the total drug concentration in the tissue respectively. Then,

$$[Cb]f = fb\,[Cb] \;\&\; [Cb] = \frac{[Cb]f}{fb} \qquad .....(10.57)$$

and

$$[Ct]f = ft\,[Ct] \;\&\; [Ct] = \frac{[Ct]f}{ft} \qquad .....(10.58)$$

The tissue partition coefficient of the drug, Pt is the ratio of the concentration of the drug in a tissue to that in the blood.

$$Pt = \frac{[Ct]}{[Cb]} = \frac{fb}{ft} \qquad .....(10.59)$$

Since, $[(Cb)f = [Ct]f$

The tissue partition coefficient, Pt, calculated taking the drug binding into consideration may be incorporated into the equations developed without considering the drug binding. The value of Cb in the new equation is equal to the free drug concentration in the blood. General mass balance of various tissues is given by

$$\begin{aligned} d\,(V_{tissue}\,C_{tissue})/dt &= Qt\,(C_{art} - C_{vein}) \\ &= Qt\,(C_{art} - Ct\,/\,Pt) \\ &= Qt\,(C_{art} - Ct\ ft/fb) \qquad .....(10.60) \end{aligned}$$

Similarly, the rate of drug elimination equations for all tissues can be summed to get the differential equation for the rate of change in the drug levels in the blood.

10.2.3 Diffusion - Limited Model

Perfusion model described earlier, assumes a rapid drug distribution between the tissue and venous blood i.e. a rapid equilibrium between the drug in tissue and the drug in the venous blood is established so that the drug concentration in the venous blood leaving the tissue is equal to that in the tissue. In other words, the cell membrane does not offer any resistance to drug permeation. Hence, drug concentration in the tissue is dependent on rate of blood flow to the tissue. This assumption simplified the mathematics involved in the physiological pharmacokinetic model.

A more complex type of physiologic pharmacokinetic model is called the *diffusion - limited model* or *membrane - limited model*. In the diffusion limited model, the cell membrane acts as a barrier for drug permeation. The drug permeates the cell membrane by diffusion at a slower rate. Because the blood flow is fast and drug permeation is slow, an equilibrium between drug concentration in blood and the tissue is established over time. Therefore, initially the drug concentration in the venous blood leaving the tissue is larger than that of tissue, and an equilibrium is established after some time. The rate-limiting step of drug diffusion into the tissue is dependent on the permeability of the cell membrane rather than the blood flow. Therefore, an equation that describes the rate of change in drug concentration in the blood based on a diffusion limited model is very complex.

10.2.4 Application and Limitations of Physiologic Pharmacokinetic Model

The physiologic pharmacokinetic model relates the drug concentration and tissue distribution based on anatomy and physiology of the organs. Once the physiological pharmacokinetic model is established for a drug, the influence of physiological and anatomic changes in a tissue on drug distribution and kinetics can be predicted and estimated. For example, the influence of a change in blood flow to the liver or an increase in size of an organ, on drug distribution and elimination can be calculated. Since the physiological models are developed based on physiological and anatomical parameters of animal, the pharmacokinetics of a drug in the human body can be predicted from animal data. Changes in drug-protein binding, tissue organ drug partition ratios, and intrinsic hepatic clearance may be inserted into the physiological pharmacokinetic model.

Toxicokinetics is the application of pharmacokinetics to toxicology. Various approaches have been used to compare the toxicity and pharmacokinetics of a drug among different species. *Interspecies scaling* is a method used in toxicokinetics for interpolation and extrapolation based on anatomic, physiological, and biochemical similarities.

Allometry is the study of size. Different animals differ in their size and life span. However, all animals show some common physiological, anatomical and biochemical properties. The assumption in interspecies scaling is that physiologic variables such as clearance, heart rate, organ weight, and biochemical processes are related to the weight or body surface area of the animal species, including human. Therefore, there exists a relation between a physiologic variable (such as heart rate, clearance etc.) and body weight or body surface area of animal. The general allometric equation is,

$$y = -\,b\,w^{a} \quad .....(10.61)$$

Where, 'y' is the physiological or pharmacokinetic property of interest, 'w' is the weight or body surface area of the animal species, 'b' is an allometric coefficient and 'a' is the allometric exponent. Both a and b vary with the drug. Equation 10.61 can be linearized if the data points are plotted on a log-log paper.

Interspecies scaling has been refined by considering the aging rate and life span of the species. In terms of physiological time, each species has a characteristic life span, its *maximum life span potential* (MLP), which is controlled genetically. Because many energy consuming biochemical processes, including drug metabolism, vary inversely with the aging rate or life span of the animal, the allometric approach has been used for drugs that are mainly eliminated by hepatic intrinsic clearance.

The application of MLP to pharmacokinetics is a relatively new concept. Initially, hepatic intrinsic clearance was considered to be related to the volume or body weight. However, a plot of the log drug clearance versus body weight for various animal species resulted in an approximately linear correlation (i.e., a straight line). After correcting intrinsic clearance by MLP, an improved log linear relationship was achieved between free drug CL_{int} and body weight for many drugs. A possible explanation for this relationship is that the biochemical processes, including CL_{int}, in each animal species are related to the animal's normal life expectancy (estimated by MLP) through the evolutionary process. Animals with a shorter

MLP have higher basal metabolic rates, and would tend to have a higher intrinsic hepatic clearance and thus metabolize drugs faster. After correcting for MLP, all species share the same intrinsic clearance for the free drug.

$$(MLP)\ (CL_{int})/B = \text{constant} \quad .....(10.62)$$

$$CL_{int} = a\ B^{x} \quad .....(10.63)$$

Where 'a' is the allometic coefficient, 'x' is the allometric exponent and B is the body weight. The values of a and x depend on the drug. For caffiene, the intrinsic clearance for the free drug is given by

$$CL_{int} = 10.389\ B^{0.225} \quad .....(10.64)$$

Inspite of several advantages, the compartment model is generally regarded as somewhat empirical and lacking physiological relevance. Many disease-related changes in pharmacokinetics are the result of physiological changes, such as impairment of blood flow or a change in organ mass. These pathophysiological changes are better evaluated using a physiologically based pharmacokinetic model. In this regard, the compartment model, owing to its simplicity, often serves as a "first model" that requires further refinement in order to accurately describe the physiological and drug distribution processes in the body. The physiological pharmacokinetic model which accounts for processes of drug distribution, drug binding, metabolism, and blood flow to the body organs is much more realistic. Drug related changes in physiological processes are more readily related to changes in the pharmacokinetics of the drug. Further more, organ mass and volumes and blood perfusion rates are often scaleable based on size, among different individuals, and even among different species. This allows a perturbation in one parameter and the prediction of any change in physiology. The physiological model may also be modified to include the specific feature of a drug. For example, for an anti-tumor agent that penetrates the inside of a cell, both the drug level in the interstitial water and the intracellular water may be considered in the model. Blood flow and tumor size may even be included in the model to study and change in the drug uptake at that site.

The physiological pharmacokinetic model can calculate the amount of the drug in the blood and in the tissue at any time if the initial amount of drug in the blood is known and the dose is given by an I.V. bolus.

Practice Problem

Serum concetrations of a new antibiotic after oral administration in a capsule dosage form are given below. Calculate MRT and MAT for the capsule.

Time (hrs)	0	0.167	0.333	0.50	1.0	1.5	2.0	3.0	4.0	6.0	8.0	10.0	12.0
Serum conc. (ug/ml)	0	0.06	3.59	7.79	13.3	14.5	16.9	16.6	11.9	6.31	3.54	1.36	0.63

Solution: Construct the following table:

Time (hrs)	Serum concentration (ug/ml)	C t	T C dt
0	0	0	–
0.167	0.06	0.010	0.0008
0.333	3.59	1.195	0.100
0.50	7.79	3.895	4.250
1.00	13.3	13.300	4.298
1.50	14.5	21.750	8.762
2.00	16.9	33.800	63.887
3.00	16.6	49.800	41.80
4.00	11.9	47.600	48.70
6.00	6.31	37.860	85.46
8.00	3.54	28.320	66.18
10.00	1.36	13.600	41.92
12.00	0.63	7.56	21.16

Total AUMC = 382.695 (ug/ml)hr2

AUC_0^{12} as determined by the trapezoidal rule = 89.68 ug-hr/ml

K is obtained from the terminal linear portion of the graph obtained by plotting log C versus time. $K = 0.347\ hr^{-1}$

AUC_{12}^{∞} = C*/K = 0.63/0.347 = 1.816 (ug/ml)hr

AUC_0^{∞} = 89.68 + 1.816 = 91.496 (ug/ml)hr

$AUMC_{12}^{\infty}$ = $C^*\ t^*/K + C^*/K^2$ (Equation 10.18)

= $(0.63)(12)/(0.347) + (0.63)/(0.347)^2$

= 27.02 $(ug/ml)hr^2$

$AUMC_0^{\infty}$ = 382.695 + 27.02 = 409.71 $(ug/ml)hr^2$

$MRT_{capsule}$ = $AUMC_0^{\infty}/\ AUC_0^{\infty}$ = 409.71/91.496 = 4.478 hours.

$MAT_{capsule}$ = $MRT_{capsule} - MRT_{IV}$ (Equation 10.38)

But MRT_{IV} = 1/K = 1/0.347 = 2.882 hours.

Therefore, $MAT_{capsule}$ = 4.478 - 2.882 = 1.596 hours.

Likely Questions

1. Write about the Statistical Moment Theory.
2. Derive an equation for MRT from the blood data following an I.V.bolus administration of a drug that eliminates from the body by the first-order process.
3. How do you calculate a steady-state volume of distribuiton from the MRT of a drug?
4. Write a note on the Mean Absorption Time (MAT) and the Mean Dissolution Time (MDT).

5. What is a blood-flow limited model?
6. Give an equaiton for organ clearance (Cl_{organ}).
7. What are the assumptions made in physiological pharmacokinetic model with binding?
8. Write about a diffusion-limited physiological model?
9. What is allometry? How is it useful in understanding physiological variables in different animals?
10. What is MLP? What is the applications of MLP to pharmacokinetics?
11. A drug is administered in capsule and solution forms to a subject on different occations. Serum concentrations of the drug at different time points are given below. Calculate the MRT and MAT for the two products and the MDT for the capsule.

Time (hrs)	Serum concentration of drug Capsule	(ug/ml) Solution
0	0	0
0.167	0.06	17.8
0.333	3.59	29.0
0.50	7.79	29.7
1.00	13.3	25.7
1.50	14.5	19.7
2.00	16.9	17.0
3.00	16.6	11.0
4.00	11.9	7.1
6.00	6.31	3.82
8.00	3.54	1.44
10.00	1.36	0.57
12.00	0.63	0.38

References

1. Cutler DJ, Theory of the mean absorption time, an adjunct to conventional bioavailability studies. Journal of Pharmacy and Pharmacology, 1978 Aug; 30(8):476-8.
2. Gerlowski, LE and jain RK., Physiologically based pharmacokinetic modeling: principles and applications, J. Pharm. Sci., 72 (10): 1103-1127, 1983.
3. "Pharmacokinetics in Drug Discovery and Development", edited by Ronald D. Schoenwald, CRC Press, NY, 2002, pp 283-294.
4. "Pharmacokinetics" 2nd edition, vol 15, Milo Gibaldi and Donald Perrier, Marcel Dekker Inc, NY, pp 409-416.
5. Riegelman, S., Collier, P. The application of statistical momet theory to the evaluation of in vivo dissolution time and absorption time Journal of pharmacokinetics and biopharmaceutics; 8; 509; 1980.
6. Yamaoka, K., Nakagawa, T and Uno, T., Stastical moments in pharmacokinetics. J Pharmacokinetics and Biopharmaceutics, 6; 547; 1978.

11

Bioavailability and Bioequivalence

The ultimate goal of most oral dosage forms is to serve as a vehicle for the delivery of drugs to the blood stream for distribution to the site(s) of action. **Bioavailability** is a measurement of the rate and extent (amount) of drug that reaches the systemic circulation from a drug product or a dosage form. The study of biopharmaceutics gives substantial evidence that the method of manufacture and the final formulation of a drug can markedly affect the bioavailability of the drug. There are two different types of bioavailability studies. **The first type** involves an assessment of the bioavailability of a new drug formulation. That is, pharmacokinetic parameters following different routes of administration of the new drug are obtained and are utilized in developing an optimum dosage regimen. Finally, the new drug is formulated suitably for an intended route of administration and its bioavailability is assessed. **The second type** of bioavailability study involves a comparison of a test formulation with that of a reference standard dosage form that is proved to have therapeutic efficacy and safety. This type of studies are known as **bioequivalence studies**. Laws mandate that new drug products be safe and effective. Therefore, laws allow marketing of the new drug product if it shows bioequivalence, i.e., similar efficacy and safety to that of the innovator product. Two products are considered to be bioequivalent if the drug concentration-time profiles are so similar that they are unlikely to produce differences in their therapeutic or adverse effects. The major concern is **switchability**, i.e., a patient can exchange one product for the other if they are bioequivalent.

11.1 Definitions and Purpose of Bioavaialability Studies

Equivalence: Equivalence is a general term used to compare products taking a specific characteristic or function or a defined set of conditions into consideration. In biopharmaceutics drug products are compared.

Chemical Name: Name used by the organic chemist to indicate the chemical structure of the drug (e.g. 2-(acetyloxy)-benzoic acid).

Generic Name: The established, non-proprietary or common name of the active drug in a drug product (e.g. aspirin).

Drug Product: The finished dosage form (e.g. a tablet or capsule) that contains the active drug ingredient generally but not necessarily in association with inactive ingredients.

Brand Name: Trade name of a drug. The manufacturer or distributor of a drug product assigns a name to distinguish his product from competitors' products (e.g. dispirin, aspro).

Chemical Equivalence: This term implies that two or more drug products contain the same labeled chemical substance as an active ingredient in the same amount.

Pharmaceutical Equivalents: Drug products that contain the same active drug ingredient (same salt, ester or chemical form) and are identical in strength, dosage form and the route of administration.

Therapeutic Equivalents: Therapeutic equivalents are drug products that contain the same therapeutically active drug that should give the same therapeutic effect and have an equal potential for adverse effects under conditions set forth in the labels of these drug products. Therapeutic drug products may differ in certain characteristics, such as color, scoring, flavor, packaging, preservatives, and expiration date. Therapeutic equivalent drug products must be 1. safe and effective, 2. pharmaceutical equivalent, 3. bioequivalent, 4. adequately labeled, and 5. manufactured in compliance with current good manufacturing practices.

Bioequivalence: Bioequivalence is defined in 21 CFR 320.1 as " the absence of a significant difference in the rate and extent to which the active ingredient or active moiety is pharmaceutical equivalents or pharmaceutical alternatives become available at the site of drug action when administered at the same molar dose under similar conditions in an appropriately designed study[1].

Absolute and Relative Bioavailability

Absolute Bioavailability of a drug in a drug product may be measured by comparing the respective bioavailabilities after an oral and intravenous bolus injection. This measurement is valid as long as the volume of distribution (Vd) and elimination rate constant (K) are independent of the route of administration.

The absolute bioavailability of a given drug using blood/plasma data may be calculated by comparing the total areas under the plasma concentration-time curves obtained following the administration of equivalent doses of the drug via an absorption site and via the intravenous route to the same subjects on different occasions.

Typical plasma concentration-time curves obtained by administering equivalent doses of the same drug by the intravenous route (bolus injection) and the extravascular route (oral) are shown in Fig. 11.1.

$$\text{Absolute bioavailability} = \frac{[AUC]_{ev} / (Dose)_{ev}}{[AUC]_{IV} / (Dose)_{IV}} \quad .....(11.1)$$

Cumulative amounts of the unchanged drug or major metabolite excreted in urine are also used to determine the absolute bioavailability.

$$\text{Absolute bioavailability} = \frac{[X_u^{\alpha}]_{ev} / (Dose)_{ev}}{[X_u^{\alpha}]_{IV} / (Dose)_{IV}} \quad .....(11.2)$$

Where, X_u^{∞} is the total amount of the unchanged drug or major metabolite excreted in the urine in infinite time.

The fraction of the dose absorbed (F) is also used to denote absolute bioavailability of a drug product. F value for drugs given by IV bolus injection is equal to unity, since all the drug enters the systemic circulation. F value of drug products may range from zero (where no drug reaches the systemic circulation) to unity (where the total drug reaches the systemic circulation).

Relative Bioavailability is defined as the ratio of bioavailabilities of a drug product and a recognized standard. In general, a recognized standard is either a competitor's marketed drug product or a standard dosage form acceptable Food and Drug by administration or through administration via a different route. When the recognized standard is a competitor's product then it is termed as "bioequivalence". The bioavailability of a test formulation is compared to the availability of the drug in a selected dosage form using a cross-over study.

$$\text{Relative bioavailability} = \frac{[AUC]_{test} / (Dose)_{test}}{[AUC]_{standard} / (Dose)_{standard}} \quad .....(11.3)$$

Percent relative bioavailability is obtained by multiplying this fraction by 100. Percent relative bioavailability can be calculated from the urinary drug excretion data, provided unchanged drug is excreted in the urine.

$$\text{Percent relative bioavailability} = \frac{[X_u^{\alpha}]_{test} / (Dose)_{test}}{[X_u^{\alpha}]_{standard} / (Dose)_{standard}} \quad .....(11.4)$$

Where, $[X_u^{\infty}]$, is the total amount of the unchanged drug or a major metabolite excreted in the urine in infinite time.

The major parameters representing the rate and extent of drug absorption are Discussed in detail later in this chapter Fig. 11.1).

1. Cmax: The peak plasma drug concentration, Cmax is used as a measurement for the drug bioavailability. Cmax has units of mass/volume
2. AUC is the area under the plasma concentration-time curve and is the measurement of extent of bioavailability of the dtug
3. Tmax: is the time of peak plasma concentration (Cmax)

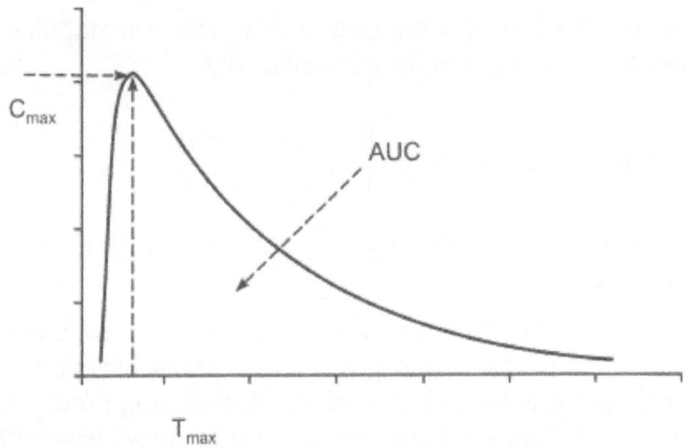

Fig. 11.1 Bioavailability Study Protocol.

11.2 Bioavailability Study

11.2.1 Bioavailability Studies for New Drugs

In vivo bioavailability studies are performed for new drugs to establish essential pharmacokinetic parameters including the rate of absorption, extent of absorption, rates of excretion and metabolism, and elimination half-life after a single and multiple-dose administration. These essential pharmacokinetic parameters are useful in establishing dosage regimens.

Bioavailability studies are also conducted to determine the influence of exipients, manufacturing procedures, packaging materials and patient related factors on the biological performance of a new drug formulation.

11.2.2 Bioavailability Studies for Approved Drugs

Bioavailability studies for approved drugs are performed to develop a new dosage form or to improve on existing dosage form. In approving a drug product for marketing, the FDA must ensure that the drug product is safe and effective for its labeled indications of use. In addition, the drug product must meet all applicable standards of identity, strength, quality and purity. Therefore, a drug product is first subjected to all applicable official laboratory tests. Finally, the FDA requires bioavailability/phamacokinetic studies and where necessary bioequivalence studies to ensure the safety and efficacy of the drug product. In bioequivalence studies, test drug product is compared with a reference standard (generally a FDA approved drug product). Test product is called bioequivalent if it produces a bioavailability equivalent to that of the reference standard.

In certain situations 505(b)(2) is also applied by innovator.

Section 505(b)(2): This provision expressly permits FDA to rely, for approval an NDA, on data not developed by the applicant.

It permits approval of applications other than those for duplicate products and permits reliance for such approvals on literature or on an Agency finding of safety and/or effectiveness for an approved drug product.

Some of the examples of 505(b)(2) applications include

- Change in dosage form, strength, route of administration, dosing regimen,
- Substitution of an active ingredient in a combination product,
- Change in the formulation beyond those considered limited confirmatory studies appropriate to a 505(j) application,
- An application for a not previously approved indication for a listed drug .
- Rx/OTC switch.

11.3 Bioavailability Study Protocol

The assessment of bioavailability of several drug products most often requires the measurement of drug and/or metabolite levels in either the blood or the urine. The bioavailability of a drug from a dosage form depends on the dose and route of administration, time of administration, subjects and dosage form. The aim of bioavailability study is to find out the dosage form influence on the biological performance of the drug. Therefore, the bioavailability study protocol used should be of sufficient sensitivity to detect differences in the rate and extent of absorption that are attributable only to dosage form variability and should avoid variabilities due to other factors. Table 11.1 lists the elements of the bioavailability study protocol.

Sometimes, due to inherent properties of the drug, analytical difficulties are encountered that will preclude the measurement of drug or metabolite levels in body fluids, so other techniques are used to assess bioavailability. The drug may be labeled with a radioactive tag, a pharmacological or clinical response may be measured, or studies may be performed on animals.

Table 11.1 Bioavailability Study Protocol.

A. Study objective
B. Study design
   1. Experimental design
   2. Wash out period
   3. Drug products:
      (a) Test product(s) and (b) Recognized standard
   4. Route of administration
   5. Dosage regimen
   6. Frequency and duration of sampling
   7. Randomization of drug administration
   8. Single-versus multiple-dose study design
   9. Subjects
      (a) Healthy subjects versus patients
      (b) Subject selection
         (i) medical history,
         (ii) Physical examination,
         (iii) Laboratory tests
      (c) Study conditions
   10. Analysis of biological fluids
C. Methods of Assessment of Bioavailablility
   1. Plasma data
   2. Urine data
   3. Acute pharmacological effect
   4. Clinical response
D. Analysis and Presentation of Data
   1. Statistical treatment of data-Analysis of variance (ANOVA)
   2. Format of data

11.3.1 Study Objective

The objective of the bioavailability study decides the study protocol. A study design meant for estimating essential pharmacokinetic parameters differs significantly from a bioequivalence study meant for comparing the test formulation with reference to a standard.

11.3.2 Study Design

Various factors have to be considered in conducting a bioavailability study since the rate and extent of absorption of a drug into the systemic circulation, its distribution and elimination are influenced by a variety of factors. Subject factors such as age, sex, disease state, food habits, general health condition, body weight of subjects, experimental design, time of administration, time of sampling, analytical method used and compartment model used in estimating pharmacokinetic parameters/bioavailability contribute to the observed blood concentration time profile. Therefore, it is necessary to consider all these important factors in a study design.

Selection of study design is based on

- Number of formulations to be compared
- Characteristics of the drug and its disposition
- Study objectives
- Availability of subjects
- Inter- nad intra-subject variabilities
- Duration of the study o rthe number of periods allowed
- Cost of adding a subject relative to that of adding one period
- Dropout rates

For example: If the intra-subject variability is the same as or larger than the inter-subject variability, the inference on the difference in average bioavailability would be the same regardless of which design is used.

Actually, a crossover design in this situation is a poor choice, because blocking results in the loss of some degrees of freedom and will actually lead to a wider confidence interval on the difference between formulations.

In the following sections various factors are discussed keeping the bioequivalence study also in mind. However, they are valid for simple bioavailability studies also.

Parallel Design

The aim of experimental designs is to minimize the experimental variables and to avoid a bias. In a parallel design, two formulations are administered to two groups of volunteers. To avoid a bias, formulations may be administered randomly to the volunteers. The major disadvantage of this design is that the inter-subject variation is not being corrected. It has been proved beyond doubt that most of the times inter-subject variation is greater than the variation between any formulations. Therefore, a cross-over design is preferred in bioavailability/bioequivalence trials to avoid influence of a inter-subject variation.

Parallel design may be considered as an alternative to a crossover design if

- The intersubject variability is relatively small compared with intrasubject variability.
- The drug is potentially toxic or has a very long elimination half-life. For example tamoxifen, triptorelin, toremifene, goserilin acetate, nevirapine.

- The population of interest consisits of very ill patients, and
- The cost for increasing the number of subjects is much less than that of adding additional treatment period.

Other examples include bioequivalence study of topical antifungals like ketoconazole, clotrimazole.

Cross-over Design

Usually, a substantial inter-subject variability exists in the drug levels achieved from any given dose of medication in a panel of subjects. The cross-over design minimizes the effect of inter-subject variability in the study by using each subject as his or her own control. Generally, two types of cross-over designs are used in bioavailability trails. They are, 1. Latin Square cross-over design and 2. Balanced Incomplete Block Design (BIBD).

Latin Square Cross-Over Design

A standard approach for conducting a comparative bioavailability study is to use a randomized, balanced, cross-over design called a Latin square or complete cross-over design. In this design, 1. each subject receives just once each formulation, and 2. each formulation is administered just once in each study period. The basic elements of this design are shown in Table 11.2, where the first design is a two-way cross-over design. The three- and four-way cross-over designs shown in the table 11.2 represent one of the several possible combinations.

In a two-way cross-over study, 12 subjects are used to study the bioequivalencies of two formulations, treatment A and treatment B. During the first study period, subjects 1 to 6 receive treatment A, while subjects 7 to 12 receive treatment B. A second study period is initiated after the washout period, during which a complete elimination of the drug and its major metabolites takes place. In the second study period, subjects 1 to 6 now receive treatment B and subjects 7 to 12 receive treatment A. Therefore, each subject acts as his own control. This design has several advantages, listed under,

1. It minimizes the effect of inter-subject variability in the study by using each subject as his or her own control.
2. It minimizes the carry-over effects which could occur when a given dosage form influences the bioavailability of a subsequently administered dosage form since each formulation is preceded and succeeded by other formulations or dosage forms.
3. It minimizes the time effect on bioavailabilty since each dosage form is administered in each study period.
4. It requires less number of subjects to get meaningful results.

Table 11.2 Latin Square Designs.

Two-Way Crossover					
Group No.	*Subjects in Group*	*Treatment for Period No.*			
		I	II		
1.	1,2,3,4,5,6	A	B		
2.	7,8,9,10,11,12	B	A		
Three-Way Crossover					
Group No.	*Subjects in Group*	*Treatment for Period No.*			
		I	II	III	
1.	1,2,3,4,5,6	A	C	B	
2.	7,8,9,10,11,12	B	A	C	
3.	13,14,15,16,17,18	C	B	A	
Four-Way Crossover					
Group No.	*Subjects in Group*	*Treatment for Period No.*			
		I	II	III	IV
1.	1,2,3,4,5,6	A	B	C	D
2.	7,8,9,10,11,12	B	D	A	C
3.	13,14,15,16,17,18	C	A	D	B
	19,20,21,22,23,24	D	C	B	A

The major disadvantages of the Latin-square design (Table 11.2) are the following :

1. It requires longer time to complete the study since a washout period exists between two study periods. The higher the biological half-life of drug, the longer will be the time required for completing the study.
2. The time to complete the trial depends on the number formulations evaluated in the study. It takes a longer time to complete the study as the number of formulations increases.
3. Increased number of study periods leads to high subject dropouts and the study becomes difficult.
4. Medical ethics does not allow too many trials on a subject continuously for a longer time.

These disadvantages can be overcome by use of a balanced incomplete block design.

Balanced Incomplete Block Design

A balanced Incomplete Block Design (BIBD) eliminates many of the difficulties encountered with the Latin square design (Table 11.3 & 11.4). The salient features of this design are:

1. Each subject receives not more than two formulations.
2. Each formulation is administered the same number of times.
3. Each pair of formulations occurs together in the same number of subjects.

Table 11.3 shows BIBD for four formulations A, B, C and D. In this design, as discussed above, each subject receives two formulations, each formulation is administered six times and each pair of formulations occurs together in two subjects (the pairs are AB, AC, AD, BC, BD and CD).

Table 11.3 Balanced Incomplete Block Design (BIBD) for Four Formulations.

Subject	Treatment	for Period No.
	I	II
1	A	B
2	B	A
3	A	C
4	C	A
5	A	D
6	D	A
7	B	C
8	C	B
9	B	D
10	D	B
11	C	D
12	D	C

Table 11.4 Randomization Scheme Used in a Bioavailability Study.

Group No.	Subjects in Group	Treatment for Period No.		
		I	II	III
1.	1,2,3,4,5,6	A	C	B
2.	7,8,9,10,11,12	B	A	C
3.	13,14,15,16,17,18	C	B	A

Replicated Crossover design

Replicated crossover designs are critical when an individual BE approach is used to allow estimation of within-subject variances for the T and R measures and the subject-by-formulation interaction variance component

Following is the four-period, two-sequence, two-formulation design recommended for replicated BE studies

		Period			
		1	2	3	4
Sequence	1	**T**	**R**	**T**	**R**
	2	**R**	**T**	**R**	**T**

For this design, the same lots of the T and R formulations should be used for the replicated administration. Each period should be separated by an adequate washout period.

Other replicated crossover designs are possible. For example, a three-period design, as shown below, could be used.

<table>
<tr><td colspan="5">Period</td></tr>
<tr><td rowspan="3">Sequence</td><td></td><td>1</td><td>2</td><td>3</td></tr>
<tr><td>1</td><td>T</td><td>R</td><td>T</td></tr>
<tr><td>2</td><td>R</td><td>T</td><td>R</td></tr>
</table>

A greater number of subjects would be encouraged for the three-period design compared to the recommended four-period design to achieve the same statistical power to conclude BE.

Other Designs

For the highly variable drugs(HVD) and highly variable drug products (HVDP) having within subject variability of more than 30%, FDA has recommended "reference scaled average bioequivalence approach" where the bioequivalence limits are not determined by the sample size. Rather, they are scaled based on the within-subject variability of the reference product. For drugs with an expected within-subject variability of 30% or greater, a BE study with three-period, reference- replicated, crossover design with sequences of TRR, RTR, and RRT is proposed. Specifically, subjects receive a single dose of the test product once and reference product twice on separate occasions with random assignment to the three possible sequences of product administration. This partial replicate design allows for the estimation of withinsubject variability for the reference product. Treatments should be separated by a washout period of adequate duration such that the drug of interest can no longer be detected in plasma. that would be acceptable is 24. The three-period design was selected over a four-period design because of efficiency. The only advantage of the four period design is that it allows the calculation of the variability of the test product. The test product variability is not used in the proposed statistical method.

11.3.3 Washout Period

In a Latin Square cross-over study design each subject receives each formulation and even in BIBD each subject receives two formulations at different occasions. The time interval between the two treatments is called "washout period". Washout period is required for the elimination of the administered dose of a drug so as to avoid the carryover. A guideline, which has come into use for a crossover design for most drugs is that a period of at least 10 half-lives should be allowed between treatments. This should ensure an elimination of 99.9% of the administered dose and a maximum carryover of less than 0.1% from the first treatment. Washout period is a function of the half-life and the dose of the drug administered. The number of washout periods in a study depends upon the type of crossover design used and the number of formulations to be evaluated. In the case of digitoxin, which has a half-life of 6 to 9 days, the total study period exceeds one year if four formulations have to be evaluated using the Latin Square design. Because a very large number of drugs have been found to have a half-life between 1 and 10 hours, a washout period of 1 week was usually found suitable in most of the reported studies.

It should be noted that the metabolites of the drug should also be eliminated from the body before the commencement of next treatment. Unfortunately, the exact metabolic scheme of all drugs is not known. Whether all the metabolites of the drug are eliminated or not is unknown. However, as most of the metabolites are more water-soluble than the parent drug and have a shorter residence time in the body than the parent drug molecule, it is assumed that their elimination occurs well before the elimination of the parent compounds.

11.3.4 Drug Products

Test Products: Test product(s) may be new drug formulations developed by a pharmaceutical technologist or new dosage forms of an existing drug. A test product may be compared to a reference standard recognized by the Food and Drug Administration for getting approval for marketing the drug product. Test products are generally evaluated for following reasons.

1. To select best dosage form of a new drug or existing drug among different dosage forms (e.g. Tablet, capsule, emulsion, and suspension).
2. To select the best formulation of a new drug or existing drug among different formulations that have shown equal performance in in-vitro tests.
3. To compare biological performance of a test product to that of a recognized standard (i.e. bioequivalence studies).

Reference Standard

A chemical or generic product has to be compared with some standard dosage form to verify its in-vivo performance. In general, the Food and Drug Administration (FDA) accepts any innovator's drug product as a reference standard. The innovator is the one who originally received approval from the FDA to market the product in the country. Some times, several manufacturers may hold approval for certain drugs. Therefore, any one of the permitted drug products can be used as a reference standard.

In many of these instances, the FDA would request that only one of these products be used as a reference product in order to obtain a more easily comparable data.

Generally highest dose is the reference listed drug. There are some exceptions in case where the safety of the volunteer is a concern.

For example, atomoxetine Hcl(60mg), glimiperide (1mg), risperidone (1mg), terazocin (2mg), Lamotrigine (2×25mg), olanzepine(5mg).

Route of Administration

Most of the times, orally administered dosage forms are subjected for bioavailability studies. However, dosage forms administered by other routes such as buccal, transdermal, intramascular should also be evaluated for their biological performance. The therapeutic utility of these dosage forms depends on the rate and extent of absorption of the drug form these dosage forms.

In general, orally administered dosage forms show a much variation in their performance because of inter-subject and intra-subject variations. All the dosage forms administered by an extravascular route do require a bioavailability assessment.

11.3.5 Single- Versus Multiple- Dose Study Design

Whether a single dose studies are better or multiple-dose studies are better for the assessment of the bioavailability of a drug product? It is always difficult to give a single answer. However, it is possible to discuss the issue thoroughly so as to understand the concepts involved in deciding the dosage regimen for a bioavailability study. If the dosage forms are to be evaluated only for bioequivalence purposes, single-dose studies are usually sufficient. This is because the relative bioavailability of most tablets and capsules can be determined on a single-dose basis, and usually, this is predictive of multiple-dose levels. Dosage forms meant for a single dose administration for a therapeutic benefit such as analgesics for the relief of head ache need only single-dose studies. However, certain dosage forms designed to achieve special release profiles of drugs may require multiple-dose studies. For example, time-release products, enteric-coated preparations, some intramuscular injections. Even the drugs that undergo the first-pass metabolism do need a multiple-dose study. Use of an improper study design leads to the collection of insufficient and/or inappropriate data. Further, if special dosage regimens such as loading dose or twice-a-day dosing are to be used, a multiple-dose study design may also be necessary.

11.3.6 Administration of Drug Products

Administration of drug products to the subjects should be based on randomization. After the administration of the drug products, blood samples are withdrawn from the subjects at fixed time points. It takes some time to take a sample from each subject, and the total time difference between first subject and the last subject may range from 10 to 20 minutes depending upon the number of subjects and technicians in the study. If the sampling schedule is not followed rigorously in the same sequential manner, significant differences can conceivably exist in the actual duration of the drug in the body and the stated sampling time given for each subject. This 10 to 20 minutes' difference would represent a substantial change in the drug concentrations observed in the blood. If under these conditions treatments are administered to the subjects in a sequential manner (such as treatment A to the first 6 volunteers, treatment B to volunteers 7 to 12, and treatment C to volunteers 13 to 18, as shown in table 11.4), the error between the time of administration and sampling will gradually increase from treatment group to treatment group. This is because of sequential administration of drug products to different treatments. To avoid this type of effect, randomized administration of drug products is used. The order of dosing is not sequential but a part of each treatment is given first, a part in the middle and a part in the last.

Multiple-dose study

Multiple-dose study may be required to determine the bioavailability of a drug product in the following circumstances.

- There is a difference in the rate of absorption but not in the extent of absorption.
- There is excessive variability in bioavailability from subject to subject.
- The concentration of the active drug ingredient or therapeutic moiety, or its metabolite(s), in the blood resulting from a single dose is too low for accurate determination by analytical method.
- The drug product is an extended release dosage form.

Examples for the drugs for which multiple-dose study is performed are rivastigmine tartarate(oral capsules), quatiapine fumerate (tablets oral).

11.3.7 Sampling

The biological sample to be used in the study has to be decided before the commencement of a bioavailability study. If the bioavailability of a given dosage form is to be evaluated by a blood level study, some estimate of the area under the serum concentration versus time curve, peak serum concentration, and time of peak serum concentration must be obtained from the study. Therefore, the frequency of sampling and the duration of sampling are very important since these factors can markedly influence the "apparent" results obtained in a given study. While the blood sampling schedule required to evaluate bioavailablity will vary with the drug, it is possible to list a few factors that will ensure a satisfactory determination of the blood-level profile. The sampling scheme should be frequent enough to define the absorption phase, the peak, and the elimination phase during a drug's time course in the body.

In order to estimate the rate of absorption it is necessary to have enough data points in the absorption phase and hence, the frequency of sampling is more in this phase. Even though the frequency of collection of samples is monitored, it may not be possible to get the time of peak serum concentration directly from the data and is generally estimated from the data. Since the relative amount of the drug absorbed is determined from the AUC parameter, there must be sufficient sampling points to allow for proper evaluation of the area under the blood-level curve. The absorption rate, volume of distribution, and elimination rate, all influence the apparent drug concentration one obtains in a given sample. It is necessary to see that all these factors influence each dosage form equally. To estimate the AUC from the data, sampling has to be carried out till the concentration of the drug reaches the linear elimination phase. For first-order process, the time necessary for a complete elimination would be infinity. However, for all practical purposes it is a period of 10 half-lives for any given drug. A rule of thumb sampling in a blood-level study is to sample for three to five half-lives of the drug. If the half-life is not known, sampling should proceed until 1/10 or 1/20 of the peak levels are reached.

In the case of urinary excretion studies, the same principles apply. Generally, urinary excretion studies are used when it is either not possible to measure a given drug in the blood, plasma, or serum or when ethical considerations do not allow the collection of samples over a period of time (e.g. subjects such as patients, children). The advantages of urinary excretion studies are: 1. it involves non-invasive method of sampling, 2. the concentration of the drug in the urine is often greater than that in blood/serum allowing easy estimation of the drug, and 3. the amount of the drug excreted in urine is obtained directly. In the case of a blood-level study, the amount of the drug in the body is estimated using pharmacokinetic parameters. On the other hand, urinary excretion method has several disadvantages as well. 1. urinary excretion studies are not useful in estimating the absorption rate of a rapidly absorbing drug. This is because it is difficult to obtain many samples during the absorption phase to define the absorption rate accurately. Subjects feel difficulty in emptying the urinary bladder frequently and it leads to a carryover effect on the next sample. 2. In some cases, the metabolites of the drug are also concentrated in the sample that interferes with the estimation of the unchanged drug in the urine sample.

However, in order to obtain useful data, it is necessary to plan the frequency and duration of sampling carefully. If possible, urine samples should be collected for 10 half-lives of the drug to ensure a 99.9% of elimination of the drug in urine. If the elimination half-life is not known, a plot of the cumulative amount of drug excreted over time will reach a plateau at some point in time consistent with a complete elimination of the drug.

11.3.8 Selection of Subjects

Healthy Subjects Versus Patients: Bioavailability studies are designed to find out the dosage form biological performance. Hence, it is necessary to minimize all possible variations if it is not possible to eliminate them. Use of healthy volunteers avoids much of variations that are possible with patients. However, it is true to say that the conditions should mimic as much as possible the actual conditions of usage for patients. The variables associated with most disease states make it impossible to design a meaningful bioequivalence test. Some of the specific problems associated with testing in patients are given below:

1. It is difficult to obtain many patients in a given place.
2. The severity of a disease varies from one patient to another.
3. Ethical considerations do not allow withdrawal of many blood samples from the patients for a longer time.
4. It is not ethical to administer a dosage form to a patient whose therapeutic efficacy is unknown.
5. Since treatment of a disease involves use of several drugs simultaneously, the effect of these drugs on the bioavailability of the drug to be tested should be known before the interpretation of the bioavailability test results.

   Therefore, normal subjects are preferred in the bioavailability studies over patients.

   Examples for the drugs for which patients are used in bioavailability studies include

   Anticancer drugs like azacitine, nabilone, temozolomide, capaecitabine, leuprolide acetate.

Selection of Subjects

If it is accepted that healthy volunteers should be used in bioavailability studies, the next question one faces is, what is meant by "healthy" volunteers? Healthy means a person having an overall good state of physical health. It is ascertained by vital signs such as temperature, pulse, respiration, blood pressure, and laboratory tests on blood (RBC count, WBC count, hemoglobin, blood sugar, etc.), urine (pH, albumin, sugar etc.) and also by liver function tests such as serum alkaline phosphatase and serum glutamic-oxaloaceticransaminase. Depending upon the drug products used in the study, certain tests may be included or excluded.

Age, sex and body weight also influence the blood level profile of a drug product. In general 21-year old, male subjects weighing 150-lb are ideal to act as volunteers in the study. It is difficult to obtain a sufficient number of subjects with these specifications and hence acceptable normal ranges are 20-50 years of age and 120 to 200 lb of body weight. Males are preferred over females because menstrual cycle, pregnancy, lactation and menopause stages that occur in females may affect the blood level profiles of the drug. However, females are also included in the bioavailability study taking above points into consideration.

Medical history of the subjects has to reviewed critically by a panel of experts. For example, a person who has undergone gastrectomy shows normal values for the general screening tests used, but he may not absorb certain drugs like normal volunteers because of difference in the gastric pH.

The selected subjects should be distributed randomly to different groups in order to achieve a uniform distribution of the available volunteers with respect to age, sex, and body weight and to avoid bias.

11.3.9 Study Conditions

The selected subjects should be maintained on a uniform diet and none of them should have taken any drug at least one week prior to the study. Before the commencement of the study it is necessary to define the study conditions such as the fasting period before the administration, time period after drug product administration during which fasting is continued, standard diet to be given after fasting, fluid intake and volume to be allowed, etc. The quality and quantity of food intake drastically affects the bioavailability of some drugs. In general, bioavailability trails are conducted on subjected that has fasted overnight.

11.3.10 Analysis of Biological Samples

Ideally, the biological samples collected as per the sampling procedure have to be analyzed immediately after the study. But most of the times, the samples are stored for several days before they are subjected to a chemical analysis. The storage of biological samples is an important aspect in a bioavailability study, since, during storage the sample may undergo a chemical degradation, adsorption on to the walls of the container, etc. The analytical method used for the estimation of the active ingredient responsible for the therapeutic efficacy must be selective and sensitive. Nonspecific analytical methods measuring a mixture of the unchanged drug and metabolites are less desirable even in well-controlled cross-over studies. Drugs that undergo the first-pass effect exhibit different unchanged drug/metabolite ratio depending on the rate of absorption. If the analytical method used is nonspecific, then the results of the study may not reveal the difference in therapeutic efficacy that exists between drug products. Most of the manufacturers use the latest analytical technique for the analysis of the samples. Only one analytical method should be used for the analysis of all the samples of a study. There may be more than one selective and sensitive methods for the analysis of the given chemical moiety. Any one of them may be used for the analysis but the results obtained with one analytical method in one study should not be compared with those obtained in a other study with a different analytical method. In summary, the analytical method used must be specific to the active chemical moiety and should exhibit high sensitivity.

11.3.11 Estimation of Drugs and/or its Metabolites in Biological Fluids

Since bioequivalence testing is based on the premise that equivalent blood levels produce equivalent pharmacological responses, it is obvious that one must be certain that equivalent components are measured in the biological fluids after administration of chemical equivalent products. The development of highly sensitive and specific instrumental techniques, coupled with advances in selective extraction and separation procedures, has enabled a residue analysis of drugs and their metabolites in biological fluids with a high degree of precision and accuracy. In most analytical problems, the final quantitative analytical step is the least difficult part of the entire procedure. In the analysis of blood or urine, the most easily obtainable and useful biological fluids, the major problem is to extract quantitatively and then separate the intact drug from its major metabolites or even to separate a mixture of two or more drugs from their metabolites.

Ideally, the pharmacologically active component should be measured in the biological sample. The analytical method used must be specific to the active component and should show good sensitivity. Since usually there are several potential methods of analysis that are usable, the type of procedure employed should be mentioned and also, a concise statement as to whether the unchanged drug, metabolite, or some other combination of products measured should be included with the bioavailability data.

11.4 Methods of Assessment of Bioavailability

There are several methods of assessing bioavailability in humans and the selection of a method depends on the purpose of the study, nature of the dosage form, and the analytical method of drug measurement. The methods available are classified as pharmacokinetic methods and pharmacodynamic methods.

The assumption in using pharmacokinetic methods for the assessment of bioavailability of drug products is that there exist a linear relation between the drug level in the a biological fluid and therapeutic response. Therefore, these methods are also known as **indirect methods**. Because the free or therapeutically active drug can be accurately measured in biological fluids, plasma and urine data give the most objective information on bioavailability.

11.4.1 Indirect Methods or Pharmacokinetic Methods

The parameters that are useful in determining the bioavailability of a drug from a drug product based on indirect methods are:

1. Plasma Data
   (a) The time of peak plasma concentration (t_{max})
   (b) The peak plasma concentration (C_{max})
   (c) The area under the plasma concentration-time curve (AUC)
2. Urine Data
   (a) The rate of drug excretion in the urine (dXu/dt)
   (b) The cumulative amount of drug excreted in the urine (X_u^{∞})
   (c) The time for maximum urinary excretion (t_u^{∞})

11.4.1.1 Plasma Data

This is the most widely used and accepted method for the assessment of bioavailability of drug products. For some drugs like sirolimus, indapamide, tacrolimus, whole blood and for some drugs like triptorelin, aminosalicylic acid, serum is used for assessing bioavailability.

The basic assumption in this method is that drug products that are bioequivalent produce superimposable plasma level-time curves. By definition, bioavailability is a measure of the rate and extent of absorption of a drug from a drug product. The parameters t_p and C_{max} are the measures of the rate of absorption of the drug while the parameter AUC is a measure of the extent of absorption.

(a) The time of peak plasma concentration (t_{max}): The time required to reach the maximum drug concentration in plasma after drug administration is known as the time of peak plasma concentration (t_{max}) (Fig. 11.2). It indicates the time at which the rate of absorption is maximum following drug administration. At t_{max}, the rate of drug absorption exactly equals the rate of drug elimination. Therefore, when comparing drug products, t_{max} can be used as an approximate indicator of the drug absorption rate. Small t_{max} value indicate that less time is required to reach peak plasma concentration. In other words, small t_{max} means a more rapid absorption. Units for t_{max} are units of time (e.g. hours, minutes).

Mathematiacally, t_{max} is a function of both absorption and elimination rate constants.

It is highly dependent on the sampling scheme, and it is therefore difficult to use it to detect differences between two products, especially when t_{max} values are less than 2 hrs.

In contrast, for slow-reeleasing dosage forms, plasma concentrations are maintained at a plateau for long time and t_{max} does not reflect the rate of bioavailability.

Statistical comparisions of t_{max} for the innovator and generic products are usually only undertaken for rapid reelase compounds and/or when t_{max} is known to have some clinical relevance.

(because t_{max} is not normally distributed, a distribution free, non parametric approach is recommended).

(b) The peak plasma concentration (C_{max}): The peak plasma concentration represents the maximum plasma drug concentration obtained following an extravascular administration of the drug (Fig. 11.2). C_{max} provides an indication that the drug is sufficiently absorbed to elicit a response. It also indicates whether the drug level in plasma is within therapeutic levels or reaching toxic levels. C_{max} is expressed as ug/ml or ng/ml.

Because Cmax reflects extent of absorption, there is strong correlation between AUC and C_{max}.

It should be recognized that C_{max} is only an indirect measure of the rate of drug absorption and is influenced by extent of absorption.

Based on its clinical applicability [it reflects the highest drug exposure (e.g. concentration) in the body and may relate to patients risk for toxicity and/or efficacy] a strong case can be made that (although C_{max} is a poor measure, it is the most clinically appropriate one for assessing rate of absorption[9].

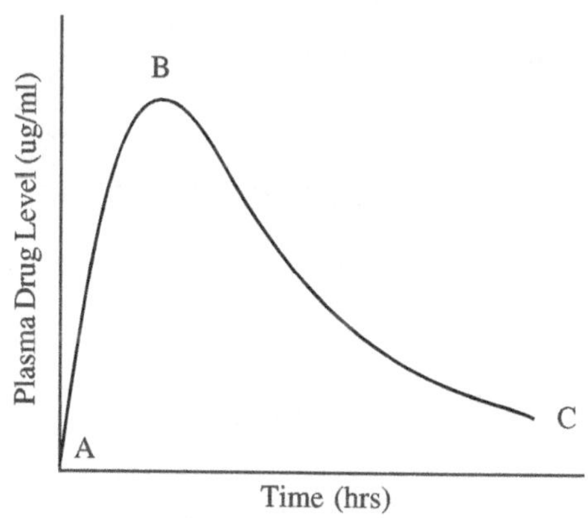

Fig. 11.2 Plasma drug level versus time curves following oral administration.

(c) The area under the plasma concentration-time curve (AUC): The area under the plasma concentration-time curve, AUC, is a measure of the extent of drug absorption from a dosage form or the fraction of the dose that reaches the systemic circulation. The $[AUC]_0^\infty$ is the sum of $[AUC]_0^t$ and $[AUC]_t^\infty$, where 't' is the last time point of plasma sample collection. $[AUC]_0^t$ is calculated by the Trapezoidal rule and the $[AUC]_t\mu$ is obtained from the Equation 11. 6.

$$[AUC]_0^\infty = [AUC]_0^t + [AUC]_t^\infty \quad .....(11.5)$$

$$[AUC]_t^\infty = C^*/K \quad .....(11.6)$$

Where, C* is the concentration of the drug in the last plasma sample and K is the overall elimination rate constant. AUC is independent of the route of administration and processes of drug elimination as long as the elimination process do as not change. The units for AUC are concentration-time/volume (e.g. μg-hr/ml).

For many drugs, AUC is directly proportional to the administered dose. Nonlinearity between the administered dose and AUC, in general, indicates the existence of a saturable kinetics of absorption and/or elimination. When the AUC is not directly proportional to the dose, bioavailability of the drug is difficult to evaluate.

In the case of multiple dose studies, AUC for one dosing interval at the steady-state level is a measure of the extent of drug absorption from the dosage form. The following equations are used to estimate the fraction of the dose absorbed, F (i.e., the bioavailability of the drug product).

$$F = \frac{[AUC]oral \times [Dose]iv}{[AUC]iv \times [Dose]oral} \quad .....(11.7)$$

If doses are equal, then

$$F = \frac{[AUC]oral}{[AUC]iv} \quad .....(11.8)$$

Where F = Absolute bioavailability

$$Fr = \frac{[AUC]text \times [Dose]\ standard}{[AUC]\ standard \times [Dose]test} \quad .....(11.9)$$

If doses are equal, then

$$Fr = \quad .....(11.10)$$

Where, Fr = Relative bioavailability.

Truncated AUC

The common measures used in bioequivalence study are AUC and Cmax.

Estimation of AUC requires frequent blood samples. For long half-life drugs, sampling for long periods of time may become cumbersome. To resolve this issue some investigators have suggested the use of truncated AUC in bioequivalence studies for long half-life drugs.

For example, pimozide, sirolimus, entacavir, salefivacin succinate, atavaquone, apriprazole, anastrazole.

Partial AUC

Here AUC is truncated at tmax for the innovator compound.

For orally administered immediate release products, measures of peak and total exposure may be sufficient. However, in situations in which clinical safety and/or efficacy trials or pharmacokinetic-pharmacodynamic studies indicate that bettet control of drug absorption into systemic circulation may be warranted, assessment of early exposure via use of partial AUCs may be indicated.

For example zolpidem extended release tablets.

11.4.1.2 Urine Data

Urinary excretion of the unchanged drug versus time data can be used to estimate the bioavailability of a drug product. This method is based on the general observation that the rate of urinary excretion of a drug is directly proportional to the concentration of the drug in the blood. In other words, the same fraction of absorbed drug always reaches the urine unchanged. Therefore, the bioavailability can be calculated as the ratio of the total amount of the unchanged drug recovered in urine following the administration of test and standard formulations. Example for which urine data is used to assess bioavalability is alandronate.

In order to obtain valid estimates, the drug must be excreted in significant quantities in urine and urine samples must be collected for at least 7 half-lives. This method is useful for all the drugs that are excreted in urine unchanged in significant quantities. Urinary metabolite excretion data is not used for the estimation of bioavailability since the drug can undergo metabolism at different sites including the gut and liver and the rates of metabolism may vary because of various factors.

(a) **The average rate of drug excretion in urine (ΔXu/Δt):** The rate of excretion of the unchanged drug in urine generally follows first order process, since, it depends on the blood concentration of the drug. Therefore, a plot of ΔXu/Δt versus time at the mid point of urine collection (t') is a mirror image of the plasma drug concentration versus time curve (compare Figures 11.2 and 11.3). In Fig. 11.3, the maximum rate of drug excretion would be at point B, (ΔXu/Δt)max, and it corresponds to the time at which C_{max} occurs. Hence, (ΔXu/Δt)max is used to estimate the bioavailability of drug products.

(b) **The cumulative amount of drug excreted in the urine in infinite time (X_u^∞) :**

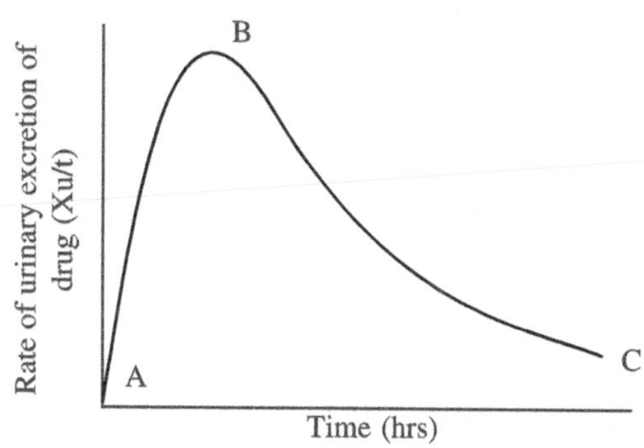

Fig. 11.3 Rate of urinary excretion of drug versus time plot.

The cumulative amount of the drug excreted in the urine is directly related to the amount of the drug absorbed. The drug excretion into urine continues till the drug level in blood falls to zero. Therefore, urine samples must be collected for a longer time (at least for 7 half-lives) in order to get a better estimate of X_u^{∞}. A graph of cumulative amount of the unchanged drug excreted into the urine versus time is shown in Fig. 11.4. The cumulative amount of the drug excreted up to point C corresponds to X_u^{∞}. This value is used for the estimation of bioavailability.

Absolute bioavailability,

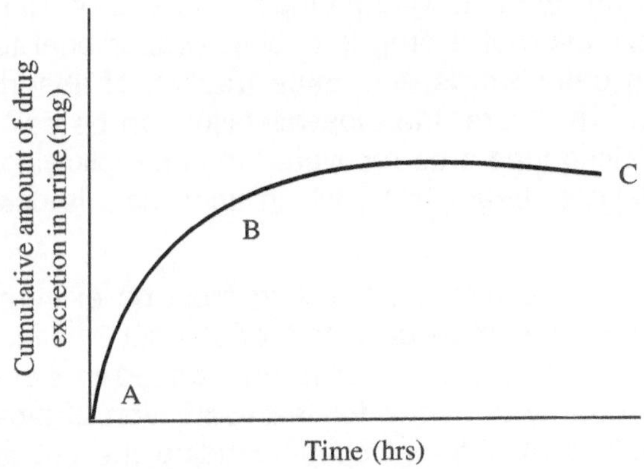

Fig. 11.4 Cumulative amount of unchanged drug excreted in urine versus time following oral administration.

$$F = \frac{[X_u^{\alpha}]\text{oral} \times [\text{Dose}]\text{iv}}{[X_u^{\alpha}]\text{iv} \times [\text{Dose}]\text{oral}} \quad \text{.....(11.11)}$$

Relative bioavailability,

$$Fr = \frac{[X_u^{\alpha}]\text{test} \times [\text{Dose}]}{[X_u^{\alpha}]\text{standard} \times [\text{Dose}]\text{test}} \quad \text{.....(11.12)}$$

When doses administered are equal,

Absolute bioavailability,

$$F = \frac{[X_u^{\alpha}]\text{oral}}{[X_u^{\alpha}]\text{iv}} \quad \text{.....(11.13)}$$

and Relative bioavailability,

$$Fr = \frac{[X_u^{\alpha}]\text{test}}{[X_u^{\alpha}]\text{standard}} \quad \text{.....(11.14)}$$

(c) **The time for maximum urinary excretion (t_u^∞):** The time at point C in Fig. 11.4, is nothing but t_u^∞. It is the time required for the absorption and a complete elimination of the drug following the administration of a drug product. t_u^∞ is a useful parameter in bioequivalence studies comparing several drug products, since, it is a measure of both the rate and extent of drug absorption from a drug product.

Steady state: For studies at steady state, the following characteristics should be calculated during one dosing interval or cycle, Ô,at steady state: AUC(0-T): Cmin; and peak-trough fluctuation, PTF = (Cmax-Cmin)/Cav, where Cav= AUC (0-T/T) denotes the average steady state concentration.

For confirmative bioequivalence assessment. Primary characteristics for the rate and extent of absorption should be stipulated prospectively in the study protocol[11].

11.4.2 Direct Methods or Pharmacodynamic Methods

The pharmacokinetic methods are based on the assumption that the drug concentration in blood or the drug excretion in the urine are related to the observed therapeutic effect. Pharmacodynamic methods are used when the assessment of bioavailability by pharmacokinetic methods is not possible due to non-availability of a sensitive analytical method for the measurement of the drug or the analytical method lacks sufficient accuracy and/or reproducibility. The two pharmcodynamic methods used for the estimation of bioavailability are based on the measurement of:

1. Acute pharmacological effect
2. Clinical response

11.4.2.1 Measurement of Acute Pharmacological Effect

In order to estimate the bioavailability of a drug product accurately by this method, the following criteria should be met.

1. An established dose-related response curve.
2. An easily measurable pharmacological response such as heart rate, ECG, blood pressure, pupil diameter, etc.

Experimentally, the pharmacological effect is measured at different time intervals following the administration of a drug product. A plot of observed pharmacological effect versus time is made in order to get a smooth curve. The area under this curve is a measure of the performance of the drug product and is used for the estimation of the bioavailability. The frequency of measurement of the pharmacological effect and the total duration of the study affect the results. The study should be conducted for at least three times the half-life of the drug and a measurement of the pharmacological response should be made with sufficient frequency to permit a reasonable estimate of the total area under the curve. The main drawback of this method is that an accurate linear relationship between the drug level and observed pharmacological response is difficult to obtain.

11.4.2.2 Clinical Response

Theoretically, this method seems to be the best among the methods discussed so far. But, practically, it is not. This is because of the fact that observed differences in therapeutic response following different formulations can not be attributed only to the formulation. Differences in the clinical response may be due to differences both in the pharmacokinetic and pharmacodynamic behavior of the drug among individuals. The drug may be available to the systemic circulation from a drug product at a sufficient rate and extent, but may not elicit a clinical response in an individual because his receptors are less sensitive to the drug compared to others. This is because of differences in pharmacodynamics of the drug in a particular patient. Various factors affecting a pharmacodynamic drug behavior may include age, drug tolerance, drug interactions and unknown pathophysiological factors. In addition, quantification of clinical response is too inaccurate to be useful in the assessment of bioavailability of drug products. Examples mesalamine, ketoconazole, clotrimazole.

In vitro studies: In some cases in vitro studies are recommended for bioequivalence studies.

Binding studies: in case of sevelamer carbonate and sevelamer Hcl tablets two in vitro teste are suggested by FDA.

(i) in vitro equilibrium binding which is considered as a pivotal bioequivalence study and

(ii) in vitro kinetic binding which is used to support the pivotal equilibrium binding study.

The bioequivalence is based on Langmuir binding consatant k_2 from the equilibrium binding study.

Similarly in vitro studies are also recommended for calcium acaetate (in vitro phosphate binding), colesevelam hydrochloride and cholestyramine powder.

11.5 Statistical Analysis of the Data

The purpose of a bioavailability test is to find out whether the test formulation gives a blood-level profile identical (i.e., superimposable) to that observed for a reference standard product or not. Due to the limitation in sampling techniques the resultant blood-level curve is influenced by both the number and duration of blood samples obtained in any study. Unfortunately, due to biological and experimental variations, some differences always exist and it is necessary to ascertain whether these differences are simply chance occurrences or are due to actual differences in treatment administered to the subjects. By conevention, all bioequivalence data are expressed as a ratio of the average response (AUC nad C_{max}) for Test/Reference. The statistical criteria for acceptance of a generic product (test) are based on 90% confidence intervals (CIs) and not based upon differences in average values for AUC and C_{max}. The 90% cis for the test product must fall within 80% to 120% of the Reference product based on nonlog transformed data. The use of log-transformed data tends to normalize the statistical distribution of the data. Therefore, based on log-transformed data, the 90% CIs for the tets product must fall within 80% to 125% of the Reference product.

The U.S. Food and Drug Administration (FDA) currently uses bioequivalence(BE) limits for fasting state be studies that are based on 90% confidence interval for ratio of difference of the test and reference products C_{max} and AUC falling within 80% to 125%. The FDA has also proposed that BE limits be used similarly for AUC and C_{max} measurements for fed state BE studies.

In some cases, regulatory agencies has considered a wider BE limit for Cmax, because of the typically higher variability of Cmax compared to AUC (Canada regulatory).

The 2003 FDA guidance requires that the evaluation of ABE (average bioequivalence) should be based on the exposure measures AUC(0-t), AUC(0-"), and C_{max}. There fore, for these three measures of systemic exposure, geometric average, arithemetic averages, ratio of the averages, and 90% confidence intervals should be provided. In addition, ABE between the test and reference formulations is concluded at the 0.05 significance level if the 90% confidence intervals for the ratios of the population averages for the three measures of the systemic exposure are completely within 80% and 125%. In addition, the traditional limits of 80% and 125% for the non-narrow therapeutic range drugs remained unchanged for the three exposure measures of narrow therapeutic range drugs. Furthermore, the 2003 FDA guidance does not allow the rounding off of the lower and upper limits of the 90% confidence intervals. In other words, to conclude ABE at the 5% significance level, the lower limit should be at least 80% an dthe upper limit should be no more than 125%.

Statistical methods are used to evaluate the data in order to identify the different sources of variation and, if possible, to measure the contribution of each identified variable and isolate the specific observation of primary interest. The analysis of variance (ANOVA), a statistical procedure used for a crossover design, is used widely in bioavailability testing and is the procedure that will be encountered most frequently by the health scientist. In order to understand the application of ANOVA in bioavailability testing, the following example is used.

11.5.1 Analysis of Variance (ANOVA)

Purpose of Bioavailability Study: To find out whether the test product (tablet) is bioequivalent to the standard product or not.

Study Design: Latin Square cross-over design and randomized drug administration.

Wash out Period: One week (half-life of drug is 2 hours).

Recognized standard: Marketed Tablets

Frequency and Duration of Sampling: Blood samples were collected at 0.0, 0.25, 0.5,1.0, 2.0, 3.0, 5.0, 7.0, 10.0, 12.0, 16.0, 20.0 and 24.0 hours.

Single or Multiple Dose Study Design: Single dose study design.

Subjects: Twelve healthy adult male volunteers between the ages of 20 to 35 (mean 25 years) and weighing between 62 to 90 kg (mean 72 kg) were selected for the study. The subjects are randomly assigned to 2 groups of 6 each and two formulations are administered randomly according to a 2 × 2 Latin Square design.

Study Conditions: All subjects fasted overnight prior to receiving the test tablet or standard tablet the following morning. The tablet is administered with 200 ml of water. Fasting of subjects is continued for 6 hours after the administration of tablets. Blood samples are taken just prior to the dose and at specified time points as per schedule into heparinized tubes. The plasma fraction is separated from the blood and analyzed for the drug content by HPLC.

Assessment of Bioavailability

Plasma data were used to estimate the **area under the curve** by the Trapezoidal rule up to the last time point and the remaining AUC is obtained by integration method. The total AUC for each treatment in each volunteer is presented in Table 11.5.

Table 11.5 The AUC's Obtained in the Bioavailability Study

Subject	1st week Test	2nd week Standard	Ri	$(Ri)^2$
1	76	83	159	25281
2	59	54	113	12769
3	96	81	177	31329
4	68	61	129	16641
5	86	79	165	27225
6	57	68	125	15625
	Standard	Test		
7	98	84	179	32041
8	64	50	114	12996
9	66	61	127	16129
10	57	48	105	11025
11	70	74	144	20736
12	88	91	179	32041
	Oi = 882	Oi = 834		= 253838
Average AUC Test = 70.83 and Standard = 72.17; Ft = s850 and Fs = 866 and x = 1716				

Differences in the estimated values of AUC for test and standard arise because of the order of administration, subjects, formulations and error. The total sum of squares observed is due to all the sources of variation just mentioned. The error sum of squares is the total sum of squares minus the sum of squares due to order, subjects, and formulations.

Order sum of squares

$$= \frac{\Sigma Oi^2 - C.F}{n_s} \qquad .....(11.15)$$

Where Oi = order and C.F = correction factor and n_s = number of determinations in each order (subjects)

$$C.F = \frac{(\Sigma x)^2}{N} = \frac{(\text{sum of all values})^2}{\text{total no. of determinations}} = \frac{(1716)^2}{24} = 122694$$

ΣOi is the summation of 1st week and 2nd week values. Hence,

Order sum of squares

$$= \frac{(882)^2 + (834)^2}{12} - 122694 = 96$$

Between Subject sum of squares

$$= \frac{\Sigma Ri^2 - C.F}{n_i} \quad .....(11.16)$$

Where ΣRi^2 = sum of squares of values in each row and n_i = number of treatments (i.e., 2).

Between subjects sum of squares

$$= \frac{(159^2 + 113^2 + ... + 179^2)}{2} - 122694$$

$$= \frac{253838}{2} - 122694 = 4225$$

Between Formulations sum of squares

$$= \frac{\Sigma Fi^2}{n_s} - C.F \quad .....(11.17)$$

Where ΣFi = sum of all values of each formulation i.e., sum of the test and sum of the standard AUC values in individuals. In this the case, sum of the test (SFt = 850) and the sum of the standard (SFs = 866) and n_s = 12.

Between Formulations sum of squares

$$= \frac{(850^2 + 866^2)}{12} - 122694 = 10.67$$

Total sum of squares

$$= \Sigma xi^2 - C.F \quad .....(11.18)$$

Where Σxi^2 = sum of squares of individual AUC values in the table 11. 5.

Total sum of squares

$$= (76^2 + 83^2 + 59^2 + ... + 91^2) - 122694 = 4708$$

Now, error sum of squares can be calculated.

Error sum of squares

$$= \text{Total SS} - \text{Order SS} - \text{Subject SS} - \text{Formulation SS} \quad .....(11.19)$$

$$= 4708\text{-}96 - 4225\text{-}10.67 = 376.33$$

Now, we can construct an ANOVA table using the above values and realizing that degrees of freedom, DF = N-1. Mean sum of squares (MS) is obtained by dividing the sum of squares with DF. F ratios are calculated by dividing the MS by error MS.

Therefore, $$MS = \frac{\text{Sum of squares (SS)}}{\text{Degrees of Freedom (DF)}} \quad .....(11.20)$$

$$\text{MS of parameter F ratio} = \frac{\text{MS of parameter}}{\text{Error MS}} \quad .....(11.21)$$

The $F_{1,10}$ means, we have to see F value under f1=1 and f2=10. For most of the bioavailability studies the level of significance accepted is 95% confidence limits (p>0.05). Therefore, we have to look for a tabled value under f1=1 and f2=10 at 95% confidence level to obtain the $F_{1,10}$ value ($F_{1,10}$ value is 4.96 at p>0.05). **The calculated value is less than table value**. Therefore, the F test for formulations and order of administration are not significant, suggesting that the values of total absorption from both the formulations are similar.

ANOVA

Source	DF	SS	MS	F ratio
Subjects	11	4225	384.1	$F_{11,10} = 10.2$
Formulations	1	10.67	10.67	$F_{1,10} = 0.28$
Order	1	96	96	$F_{1,10} = 2.55$
Error	10	376.33	37.63	–
Total	23	4708		

Conclusion: The test tablet is bioequivalent to the standard tablet used in the study.

For the example shown in Table 11.5, 95% confidence limits on the difference between the formulations for "area under the curve" can be constructed as per the procedure given below.

Find the "t" value from t-table for DF=10 at p>0.05 (t with DF=10 at p>0.05 is 2.23).

The 95% confidence limits

$$= \text{(average of standard - average of test)}$$

$$\pm \text{ t EMS } \sqrt{(1/n_i + 1/n_j)} \qquad \text{.....(11.22)}$$

Where,

t = 't' value from t-table for given degrees of freedom at p>0.05

EMS = error mean square

n_i = number of subjects in ith group

n_j = number of subjects in jth group

The 95% confidence limits

$$= (72.17\text{-}70.83) \pm 2.23\ 37.63\ (1/12 + 1/12)$$

$$= 1.34 \pm 5.58$$

$$= (-4.24 \text{ to } 6.92)$$

The true difference between the AUCs for the formulations lies between -4.24 and 6.92 with a probability of 95%.

11.5.2 ANOVA for Multiple Comparisons

Many times a bioavailability study involves more than two formulations. In such cases, the conclusion by the above method will be either the formulations are same or different. If the conclusion drawn out of a bioavailability study involving four formulations (labeled as A,B,C and D) is that they are different, then, whether all the formulations are different from one another or a particular formulation is different from the other formulations is unknown. In other words, out of the four formulations, which are bioequivalent, which are not can not be identified by the F value only. For this purpose, it is necessary to use tests like Newman-Kuels Test.

In order to understand the significance of these statistical tests, let us consider one example. A bioavailability trail is conducted using 4 x 4 Latin Square design for the assessment of bioequivalence of four formulations labeled as A, B, C and B. The AUCs of plasma versus time data are used to assess the bioequivalence. The data is presented in Table 11.6. It is desired to know whether the formulaitons A, B, C, and D are bioequivalent or not. If it is found that there is a significant difference in means of the treatments, it may be desired to find *which pairs*, among all possible pairs of means, are different. Analysis of variance table can be constructed as per the procedure described for repeated measures and the F ratio can be used to find out whether there is a siginificant difference between the means of treatments or not. Table 11.7 shows the procedure to be followed in constructing the ANOVA table for calculating the F ratio. The following equations may be used for calculating the sum of squares of various sources of variation.

Table 11.6 AUC's of Formulations Used in the Bioavailability Study.

		Formulation			
Subjects	A	B	C	D	Total
1	42	35.6	39.6	35.3	152.5
2	41	34.0	40.2	33.9	149.1
3	39	33.2	38.9	34.3	145.4
4	36	34.9	37.0	33.8	141.7
Total	158	137.7	155.7	137.3	588.7

$$C.F = (588.7)^2/16 = 21660.48$$

Total sum of squares (S.S)

$$= (42.0^2 + 35.6^2 + ...+ 33.8^2) - C.F$$

$$= 21786.25 - 21660.48 = 125.77$$

Treatment sum of squares (Between formulations) (T.S.S)

$$= (158.0^2 + 137.7^2 +... + 137.3^2)/4 - C.F$$

$$= 21754.77 - 21660.48 = 94.29$$

Between subjects sum of squares (S..S.S)

$$= (152.5^2 + 149.1^2 +...+ 141.7^2)/4 - C.F$$

$$= 21676.78 - 21660.48 = 16.23$$

Within Subject sum of squares or Error sum of squares or a residual sum of squares

$$(E.S.S) = S.S - S.S.S\text{-}T.S.S = 125.77 - 16.23 - 94.29 = 15.19$$

Now, the ANOVA table can be constructed using the formulae given in the Table 11.7. From the ANOVA Table 11.8, it is evident that the calculated F value (18.60) is greater than the critical value of 3.86 ($F_{3,9}$ at p >0.05). Therfore, it can be concluded that the means of the treatments differ significantly. Now, we are interested to find which pairs, among all possible pairs of means, are different. For this purpose **Newman-Keuls Test** is quite useful.

Table 11.7 Formulae Used for the Construction of ANOVA Table for Repeated Measures.

Sources of variation	Sum of Squares	Degrees of Freedom	Mean Square	F
Total sum of Squares	S.S	nk–1 (4 × 4 – 1 = 15)		
Between Treatment sum of Squares	T.S.S	K – 1 (4 – 1 = 3)	$S_t^2 = \frac{T.S.S}{k-1}$	S_t^2 / S_t^2
Between Subjects sum of Squares	S.S.S	n – 1 (4 – 1 = 3)	$S_s^2 = \frac{S.S.S}{n-1}$	S_s^2 / S_s^2
Within Subjects or Error Sum of Squares	E.S.S.	(n – 1) (k – 1) = 9	$S_p^2 = \frac{E.S.S}{(n-1)(k-1)}$	

Table 11.8 Analysis of Variance of the Data (ANOVA).

Sources of variation	Sum of Squares	Degrees of Freedom	Mean Square	F
Total sum of Squares	125.77	15		
Between Treatment sum of Squares	94.23	3	31.41	18.60
Between Subjects sum of Squares	16.30	3	5.43	3.213
Within Subjects or Error Sum of Squares	15.19	9	1.69	

In Newman-Keuls test, for k treatments (formulations) the number of pairs is k(k-1)/2. The k treatment means are first arranged in order of increasing magnitude.

Accordingly, in this case, 34.33 (**D**), 34.43 (**B**), 38.93 (**C**), 39.50 (**A**)

Consider the pair means of A versus D; for these a standrad error (SE) is computed using the respective samples sizes n_a and n_d and the value of S_p^2 (mean square of error or within subjects), see Table 11.8.

Standard error (SE)

$$= [(S_p^2 /2)(1/n_a + 1/n_d)]^{1/2}$$
$$= [(1.69/2)\ (1/4+1/4)]^{1/2}$$
$$= 0.65 \qquad .....(11.23)$$

Also needed is the value of the "studentized range" denoted by q:

$$Q = \frac{\text{Mean of A - Mean of D}}{\text{SE}} \qquad .....(11.24)$$

$$q = \frac{39.50 - 34.33}{0.65} = 7.953$$

And the value, w, equal to the number of means in the range of the pair being tested. (for the pair A,D, the value w = k = 4; for the pair A, B, the value w = k-1 = 3 etc.,). The calculated value of q from equation 11.24 is then compared with the critical value of $qa_{,v,w}$ from the 'q' table, using a desired confidence value α (usually 0.05 or 0.01), the "within sample" degrees of freedom, v, and the value of w previously defined. If the calculated $q > q\mu_{,v,w}$, then the pair of means differ significantly at the α level. For example, the calculated q for A, D pair is 7.953 which is larger than the table value of q = 5.91 at α = 0.05, for 3 degrees of freedom (v) and w = 3. A similar test is made on each pair of the means.

The order of comparison of means is "largest" against "smallest" (k vs 1), then "largest" against "second-smallest" (k vs 2), etc; then "second-largest" against "smallest" (k-1 vs 1), and "second-largest" against "second-smallest" (k-1 vs 2). Table 11.9 shows the results of Newman-Keuls test on the above data.

Conclusions:

1. Formulations A & C and B&D are bioequivalent.
2. Formulations A&C showe a higher bioavailability and they differ significantly from B&D.

Table 11.9 Results of Newman-Keuls Test on the Data Presented in table 11.5.

Comparison	Difference of Means	SE	w	q	P<0.05
A versus D	39.50 – 34.33 = 5.18	0.65	4	7.968	YES
A versus B	39.50 – 34.33 = 5.08	0.65	3	7.814	YES
A versus C	39.50 – 38.93 = 0.58	0.65	2	0.885	NO
C versus D	38.93 – 34.33 = 4.60	0.62	3	7.083	YES
C versus B	38.93 – 34.43 = 4.50	0.65	2	6.929	YES
B versus D	34.43 – 34.34 = 0.10	0.65	2	0.154	NO
Degrees of freedom = 9					

Likely Questions

1. Define the following
   (a) Generic name
   (b) Brand name,
   (c) Pharmaceutical equivalents,
   (d) Therapeutic equivalent.
2. How do you estimate the absolute bioavailability and relative bioavailability ?
3. What are the two types bioavailability studies ?
4. Give the table showing bioavailability protocol.
5. What are the advantages and disadvantages of a parallel design over a cross-over design?
6. What are the merits and demerits of a Latin-Square design?
7. What are the salient features of a Balanced Incomplete Block Design (BIBD) ?
8. Give a four-way cross-over design for four products A, B, C and D.
9. Why a washout period has to be given in a bioavailability study ?
10. What are the difficulties encountered in using patients as subjects in bioavailability study ?
11. Write a noted on the analysis of biological samples.
12. What are the different methods available for the assessment of bioavailability ?
13. What are the important pharmacokinetic parameters calculated from the plasma data for the assessment of bioavailability ? What is their significance ?
14. How do you assess the bioavailability of a product using the cumulative amount of a drug excreted in urine in infinite time (X_u^{∞}) data ?
15. Write about the pharmacodynamic methods used for the assessment of bioavailability.

References

1. 21 Code of Federal Regulations Part 320, Section 320.27.. Guidelines on Design of Multiple-dose In Vivo Bioavailability Study. Food and Drug Administration, Department Of Health and Human Services, April 2009.

   http://www.accessdata.fda.gov/scripts/cdrh/cfdocs/cfcfr/CFRSearch.cfm?fr=320.27
2. Bioequivalence Approaches for Highly Variable Drugs and Drug Products, By Sam H. Haidar, Barbara Davit, Mei-Ling Chen, Dale Conner, LaiMing Lee, Qian H. Li,Robert Lionberger, Fairouz Makhlouf, Devvrat Patel, Donald J. Schuirmann, and Lawrence X. Yu, Pharmaceutical Research, Vol. 25, No. 1, January 2008.
3. Bioequivalence studies in Drug Development methods and applications, by Dieter Hauschke, Volker Steinijans and Iris Pigeot, Page NO: 7.

4. Chen ML, Shah V, Patnaik R, Adams W, Hussain A, Conner D, Mehta M, Malinowski H, Lazor J, Muang SM, Mare D, Lesko L, Spron D, Williams R. Bioavailability and bioequivalence: an FBA regulatory overview Pharm Res. 2001, 12; 1645 - 50.

5. Design and Analysis of Bioavailability and Bioequivalence Studies, 3rd edition, by Shein-Chin Chow, Jen-pei Liu, page no-35-36.

6. Generic Drug Product Development- Bioequivalenece Issues , Edited By Isadore Kanfer, Leon Shargel.

7. Guidance for Industry: Bioavailability and Bioequivalence Studies fir Orally Administered Drug Products- General Considerations, Center for Drug Evaluation and research(CDER), FDA 2003.

8. Guidance for Industry: Statistical Approaches to Establish Bioequivalence, U.S. Department of Health and Human Services, Food and Drug Adiminstration, Center for Drug Evaluation and Research, January 2003.

9. Guidance for the industry: Applications covered by section 505(b)(2),U.S. Department of Health and Human Services, Food and Drug Administration, Center for Drug Evaluation and Research, October 1999.

   http://www.fda.gov/downloads/Drugs/GuidanceComplianceRegulatoryInformation/Guidances/UCM079345.pdf

10. Impact of truncated area under the curve on failed bioequivalence studies: A computer simulation analysis, mahmood Iftekhar, journal:Drug metabolism and drug interactions, volume 20; 2004; no 1-2; pp 77-83.

11. Individual product bioequivalence recommendations, guidances (drugs).

    http://www.fda.gov/Drugs/GuidanceComplianceRegulatoryInformation/Guidances/ucm081327.htm

12. Limits for the scaled Average Bioequivalence of Highly Variable Drugs and Drug Products, by Laszlo Tothfalusi and Laszlo Endrenyi, Pharmaceutical Research, Vol 20, No 3, March 2003.

13. Meyer MC, Straughn AB, Mhatre Am, Shah VP, Chen ML, Williams RL, Lesko LJ. Variability of the Phenytoin Capsules use males and females. Pharm Res. 2001; (3); 394 - 7.

14. Scientific issues Embeded in the Generic Drug Approval process: Assessment of in Vivo Bioequivalence: Key issues.

    www.medscape.com/viewarticle/421495_4

15. www.fda.gov/downloads/drugs/GuidanceComplianceRegulatoryInformation

12

Biostatistics

Statistics is the science of collecting, summarizing, presenting and interpreting data, and of using them to test hypothesis. One scientist wants to study the effect of a drug on the blood pressure. The blood pressure of human beings shows intrinsic variation. Blood pressure not only differs from person to person, but it varies in the same person from day to day and from hour to hour. Statistical methods would be needed to assess whether an observed average blood pressure above that of the general population could simply be due to chance variations or whether it represents a real indication of the effect of drug.

The objectives of statistics are two folds: 1. to organize and summarize data and 2. to reach decisions about a large body of data by examining only a small part of the data. The concepts and methods necessary for achieving the first objective are studies under the heading of *descriptive statistics*, and the second objective is reached through the study of what is called *inferential statistics*.

Like al fields of learning, statistics has its own vocabulary. The following are some terms that are used frequently in statistics.

Statistics is a field of study concerned with 1. the collection, organization, summarization, and analysis of data, and 2. drawing of inferences about a body of data when only a part of the data is observed.

Biostatistics: When the data being analyzed are derived from the biological sciences and medicine, the term biostatistics is used to distinguish this particular application of statistical tools and concepts.

Population

A population may consist of animals, machines, places or cells. Population means the total number of entities or units with a desired character at a particular time. For example, one scientist wishes to study the quality life of diabetic patients in a particular city, then all the diabetic patients of that city constitutes the population for his study.

Sample

A part of population collected scientifically from the population is called a *sample*. The sample from a population is supposed to possess all the characters of population i.e., it is a true representative of a population. The scientist in the above example can select some diabetic patients randomly. The selected diabetic patients constitute the sample.

In daily life also we observe the sample before we purchase rice, wheat grapes etc. When some characters of a population have to be determined, strictly speaking, all the units in the population are to be evaluated. This is not only impractical if not impossible in some cases, but also impossible in some cases. Therefore, samples are evaluated to find out the characters of the population that they represent.

Data: the raw material of statistics is *data*. Data contains numbers obtained either by *measurement* or by *counting*. For example, the body weight of patients is measured while the number of patients admitted into a hospital per day is counted. The singular of data is *datum*.

Sources of Data

The performance of statistical activities is motivated by the need to answer a question. For example, what is the percent of occurrence of malaria in a particular area? To answer this question, we have to get data. Such data are usually available from one or more of the following sources.

1. *Routinely Kept Records*: Hospital medical records contain immense amount of information of the patients admitted into the hospital. This type of records that are routinely maintained can be used as a source of data.
2. *Surveys*: If the data needed to answer a question are not available from routinely kept records, we may have to conduct a survey to get data. For example, research personnel visit the houses in that area and gather information about the people suffered from malaria.
3. *Experiments*: The question raised may require an experimentation to get the data. For example, it is desired to know whether the patients like the newly developed syrup or the capsule of a drug. Then, an experiment has to be conducted by giving two formulations to the patients on different occasions and getting information about their preference.
4. *External Sources*: The data needed to answer a question may already exist in the form of published reports, commercially available data banks, or the research literature. In other words, some one else has already asked the same question, and the answer they obtained may be applicable to our present situation.

Variables

A characteristic take on different values in different persons, places, or things is called a *variable*. Some examples of variables include diastolic blood pressure, heart rate, the heights of adult males, and the number of patients visiting a government hospital. Variables may be divided as quantitative variables, qualitative variables, and random variables.

1. *Quantitative Variables:* A *quantitative variable* is one that can be measured in the usual sense. Measurement of heights of adult males, weights of pre-school children, and ages of patients seen in a dental clinic. These are examples of quantitative variables. Measurements made on quantitative variables convey information regarding amount.
2. *Qualitative Variables:* Some characters can not be measured but can be categorized. In such cases, measurement consists of categorizing the population, for example, based on sex, ethnic group etc. Measurements made on qualitative variables convey information regarding attribute. In the case of qualitative variables we can count the number of persons, places, or things belonging to various categories.
3. *Random Variables:* Measurement of the height, weight or age of an individual result a *value* of the respective variable. When the values obtained arise as result of chance factors, so that they can not be exactly predicted in advance, the variable is called a *random variable.* For example, attained adult height is the result of numerous genetic and environmental factors. Values resulting from measurement procedures are often referred to as *observed* or *measurements.* Random variables are further studied under the heading of discrete random variables and continuous random variables.
   (a) *Discrete Random Variables*: Gaps or interruptions in the values that it can assume characterize discrete random variables. These gaps or interruptions indicate the absence of values between particular values that the variable can assume. For example, the number of patients admitted into a general hospital per day is a discrete random variable since the number of admissions each day must be represented by a whole number such as 0,1,2 or 3. The number of admissions on a given day can not be a number such as 1.6, 3.987, or 4.444.
   (b) *Continuous Random Variables*: A continuous random variable does not possess the gaps or interruptions characteristic of a discrete random variable. A continuous random variable can assume any value within a specified relevant interval of values assumed by the variable. Examples of continuous variables include the various measurements that can be made on individuals such as height, weight, and skull circumference. The instrument used decides the precision of the measurement.

Descriptive Statistics

The data may be summarized in to a single number called *descriptive measure.* Descriptive measures may be computed from data of a sample or the data of a population. To distinguish between them the following definitions are used.

1. A descriptive measure computed from the data of a sample is called *statistic.*
2. A descriptive measure computed from the data of a population is called *parameter.*

Several types of descriptive measures can be computed from a set of data but many of the time's measures of central tendency and measures of dispersion are considered.

Measures of Central Tendency

In each of the measures of central tendency, there is a single value that is considered to be typical of the set of data as a whole. The three most commonly used measures of central tendency are *the mean, the median,* and *the mode.*

Mean: Suppose from a population or universe a sample of 'n' observations is taken as usual in order to determine some characteristics of the population. A chemist chosen 9 tablets from a batch and analyzed for their drug content. The following amounts were found in the tablets.

4.1, 4.4, 4.0, 4.3, 4.2, 4.7, 4.9, 4.6, and 4.4 mg. The total number of tablets is 9 (n). The sum of the 9 values is 39.6. If the sample of 'n' determinations can be designated by X_1, X_2, X_3, ...X_n. The sample mean, X, can be determined by

$$\bar{X} = \frac{X_1 + X_2 + X_3 + ... + X_n}{n} = \frac{\Sigma Xi}{n} \qquad .....(12.1)$$

Where, i goes from 1 to n. Therefore, the average or mean of the above data is,

$$X = \frac{4.1 + 4.4 + 4.0 + ...4.4}{9} = \frac{39.6}{9}\ 4.4 \text{ mg}$$

The mean simply reflects the arithmetic average of the values. Extreme values in the data seriously affect the mean.

Median: Median is the central value of the data when the data is arranged in ascending order.

4.0, 4.1, 4.2, 4.3, 4.4, 4.4, 4.6, 4.7, 4.9

The median is the central value of the data. If the number of values in a sample, "n", is an odd number, the median is given by,

$$\text{Median} = (n+1)/2 = (9+1)/2 = 5 \qquad .....(11.2)$$

When the number of values, n, is an even number, then there is no single value in the middle of the data. In this case, the median is the average of the two values in the middle, when the values have been arranged in ascending order. For example, if the number of values is 12, then the median of the data is (12+1)/2=6.5. It means, the average of the 6th and 7th value of the data that has been arranged in ascending order is the median of the data.

Mode: The mode of a set of values is that value which occurs most frequently. If all the values are different there is no mode; on the other hand, a set of values may have more than one mode, if more values occur in similar frequency. In our example, the mode is 4.4 which occurred more number of times than any other value.

The mode may be used for describing qualitative data. For example, the number of patients suffering form a particular disease admitted into a hospital in a year may be more than any other disease. The disease occurring most frequently in the patients is called the modal disease.

Measures of Dispersion

The *dispersion* of a set of observations refers to the variety that they exhibit. A measure of dispersion conveys information regarding the amount of variability present in a set of data. Other terms used synonymously with dispersion include variation, spread and scatter. Range, standard deviation, and variance are generally determined to measure the dispersion of a data.

Range: The simplest measure of variation is *range* (R). It is the difference between the largest value (X_l) and the smallest value (X_s) in a series of observations. In our example, the range would be ($X_l - X_s$)= 4.9-4.0 = 0.9. The range is most valuable in small series of observations, usually for n less than 10.

Standard Deviation: The standard deviation is the measure of variation most commonly used. When n=2, the range and standard deviation are equal. These two are quite closely related for sample sizes less than ten. For n greater than ten, the standard deviation gives a much better estimate of the variation than the range.

The standard deviation of the population is usually designated by 'σ', and the standard deviation of the sample by 's'. The standard deviation of a sample is calculated by getting the differences of each observation from the mean and putting them in the following formula.

$$s = \sqrt{(X_1 - \bar{X})^2 + (X_2 - \bar{X})^2 + (X_3 - \bar{X})^2 + ...(X_n - \bar{X})^2 / (n - l)} \qquad .....(12.3)$$

In simplified form,

$$s = \sqrt{\Sigma(X_i - \bar{X})^2 / (n - 1)}$$

or

$$s = \sqrt{[\Sigma(X_i)^2 - (\Sigma X_i)^2 / n](n - 1)} \qquad .....(12.4)$$

The standard deviation of the example cited above can be calculated using above equations. For our example, n = 9, the sum of the 9 observations (ΣX_i) is 39.6. The sum of the squares of the observations

$$\Sigma(X_i)^2 = (4.1)^2 + (4.3)^2 +...+ (4.4)^2 = 174.92.$$

Putting these values in the formula:

$$s = \sqrt{[174.92 - (39.6)^2]/(9 - 1)} = \sqrt{[174.92 - 174.24]/8} = 0.29$$

The n-1 in the denominator of the formula for the calculation of standard deviation is called the *degrees of freedom.* The standard deviation gives a measure of the variation of individual observations around the average. A comparable measure of variation of average of samples about their average is called the *standard error of an average.* It can be calculated from the standard deviation, s, and the number of observations, n.

Standard error of the average =

$$S_x = s/\sqrt{n} \quad .....(12.5)$$

For our example, $S_x = 0.20/\sqrt{9} = 0.29/3 = 0.0966$

A short cut (and only approximate) method of estimating the standard error of the average is to divide the range by the number of observations. This method can be used only if 'n' is less than ten.

$$S_{\overline{X}} = \text{range}/n \quad .....(12.6)$$

$$S_{\overline{X}} = 0.9/9 = 0.1$$

Coefficint of variation: The coefficient of variation expresses the standard deviation of a percentage of the sample mean. This is useful when interest is in the size of the variation relative to the size of the observation, and it has the advantage that the coefficient of variation is independent of the units of observation. For example, the value of the standard deviation of a set of weights will be different depending on whether they are measured in kilograms or pounds. The coefficient of variation, however, will be the same in the two units.

$$\text{Coefficient of variation, c. v.} = \frac{s}{\overline{X}} \times 100$$

Where s is the standard deviation and $\overline{x}$ is the mean of the data.

Variance: Variance is the square of the standard deviation and the variance of an average is the square of the standard error of the average. In our example, variance $(s^2) = (0.20)^2 = 0.0841$ and variance of an average $= (S_x)^2 = (0.0966)^2 = 0.00093$.

Bias, Precision, and Accuracy

The bias or systematic error **:** It is indicative of the tendency to measure something other than what was intended. For example, a 10ml pipette may not measure exactly if it has a manufacturing defect. Suppose, the 10ml pipette actually measures 10.5ml but labeled as 10ml by the manufacturer, then every time it measures 10.5ml than desired volume (10ml).

Precision or Reproducibility **:** It denotes the agreement among repeated measurements. For example, you are determining the volume of acid required to neutralize 10ml base for five times. If your determinations are constant or nearly constant, then you are precise. The method is reproducible. One important point to be remembered is that the determinations may not be correct.

Accuracy**:** Accuracy refers to the closeness of the measurements to the "true" values. For example, a tablet contains 100mg of a drug and the drug content was found to be 100mg by an analytical method. The method is said to be an accurate method. In other words, accuracy shows how closely a method measure what it is supposed to measure.

The interrelations of bias, precision, and accuracy are clearly illustrated in Fig. 12.1.

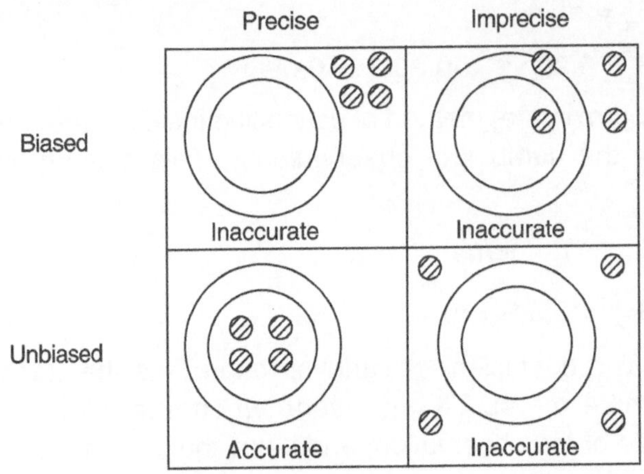

Fig. 12.1 Diagram illustrating bias, precision, and accuracy. The shots on targets (1) and (2) are biased; in both cases the shots cluster away from bull's eye. The clusters on targets (3) and (4) are both unbiased; the center of each cluster is on bull's eye. The shots on targets (1) and (3) are precise; both sets are bunched together. The shots on targets (2) and (4) are widely scattered, hence imprecise. Only the shots on target (3) are accurate, i.e., precise and unbiased.

The Theory of Probability

Probability refers to the possibility of occurrence of an event out of different events that can occur. Probability is calculated from the data that shows the occurrence of a particular characteristic and the total number of trials.

***Classical Probability*:** If an event can occur in N mutually exclusive and equally likely ways, and if "m" of these possess a characteristic, E, the probability of the occurrence of E is equal to m/N.

$$\text{Probability of E, P (E)} = m/N \qquad .....(12.7)$$

For example, if a fair six-sided die is labeled as 1 to 6 and rolled, the probability that side 1 is up is 1/6 and is the same for other faces. The process of abstract reasoning calculates probabilities such as these. Similarly, the probability of a getting a tail when a coin is tossed is ½.

***Relative Frequency Probability*:** If some process is repeated a large number of times n, and if some resulting event with the characteristic, E occurs 'm' times, the relative frequency of occurrence of E, m/n, will be approximately equal to the probability of E.

$$P(E) = m/n \qquad .....(12.8)$$

m/n is only an estimate of P (E).

In this case, we are not aware of possibilities of occurrence like in classic probability. The occurrence of a specific character out of the several events is used for the calculation of probability. For example, probability of rain in the third week of June in a city can be computed from the data of previous years.

Elementary Properties of Probability

The three basic properties from which a whole system of probability theory is constructed through the use of mathematical logic are:

1. Given some process (or experiment) with n mutually exclusive out comes (called events), E_1, E_2,....E_n, the probability of any event, E_i, is assigned a non-negative number. That is ,

$$P(E_i) \geq 0 \qquad .....(12.9)$$

Two events are said to be *mutually exclusive* if they can not occur simultaneously. For example, if a coin is tossed, it will result either head or tail. The head and tail are mutually exclusive and can not occur simultaneously.

2. The sum of the probabilities of all mutually exclusive out comes is equal to 1.

$$P(E_1) + P(E_2) + ... + P(E_n) = 1 \qquad .....(12.10)$$

This is the property of *exhaustiveness* and refers to the fact that the observer of a probabilistic process must allow for all possible events, and when all are taken together, their probability is 1. The requirement that the events be mutually exclusive is specifying that the events E_1, E_2,....E_n, do not overlap.

3. If E_i and E_j are two mutually exclusive events, the probability of the occurrence of either E_i or E_j is equal to the sum of their individual probabilities.

$$P(E_i \text{ or } E_j) = P(E_i) + P(E_j) \qquad .....(12.11)$$

If the two events E_i and E_j are not mutually exclusive, then the overlapping of the events has to be found to estimate the probability of occurrence of either E_i or E_j. The system becomes much complicated.

Calculation of the Probability of an Event

Scientists were interested to find out the frequency of use of a habit-forming drug (cocaine) by the drug addicts in their lifetime. The following data were obtained (Table 12.1).

Table 12.1 The data obtained in a study.

Life-time Frequency of cocaine use		Male (M)	Female (F)	Total
1-19 times	(A)	32	07	39s
20-99 times	(B)	18	20	38
100 + times	(C)	25	09	34
Total		75	36	111

Suppose, we pick a person at random from this sample, what is the probability this person to be a male ?

Answer : We assume that male and female are mutually exclusive categories and that the likelihood of selecting any one person is equal to the likelihood of selecting any other person. The desired probability may be defined as the ration of the number of subjects with the characteristic of interest (male) to the total number of subjects.

$$P\ (M) = \text{number of males/total number of subjects} \quad .....(12.12)$$

$$P\ (M) = 75/111 = 0.6757$$

Conditional Probability: On occasion, the set of "all possible out comes" may constitute a subset of the total group. In other words, the size of the group of interest may be reduced by conditions not applicable to the total group. When the probabilities are calculated with a subset of the total group as the denominator, the result is a *conditional probability*. The probability obtained when no conditions were imposed to restrict the size of denominator is known as *marginal probability*.

Question: Suppose we pick a subject at random from the 111 subjects and found that the subject is male (M). What is the probability that this male will be one who has used cocaine 100 times or more during his life-time (C)?

Answer: With the selection of male, the females are eliminated and hence we have no interest in total number of subjects. Therefore, given that the selected subject is a male (M), what is the probability that the subject has used cocaine 100 times or more during his life-time (C)? This is a conditional probability and is written as P (C|M) in which the vertical line is read "given". The number of males (75) becomes the denominator of this conditional probability, and 25, the number of males who have used cocaine 100 times or more during their life-time, becomes the numerator. Our desired probability, then, is

$$P\ (C|M) = C/M = 25/75 = 0.33 \quad .....(12.13)$$

Joint Probability: Some times it may be required to find the probability that a subject picked at random from a group of subjects possess two characteristics at the same time. Such probability is referred to as a *joint probability*.

Question: What is the probability that a person picked at random from the 111 subjects will be a male (M) and be a person who has used cocaine 100 times or more during his life-time (C)?

Answer: The desired probability may be written in symbolic notation as $P\ (M \cap C)$ in which the symbol $\cap$ is read either as "intersection" or "and". The statement $M \cap C$ indicates the joint occurrence of conditions M and C. The number of subjects satisfying both of the desired conditions is found in the table at the intersection of the column labeled M and the row labeled C and is seen to be 25. Since, the selection will be made from the total set of subjects the denominator is 111. Thus, the joint probability is,

$$P\ (M \cap C) = C/\ \text{total} = 25/111 = 0.2252 \quad .....(12.14)$$

The Multiplication Rule: A probability may be computed from other probabilities. For example, a joint probability may be computed as the product of an appropriate marginal probability and an appropriate conditional probability. This is the *multiplication rule* of probability.

Question: Compute the joint probability of male (M) and a life-time frequency of cocaine use of 100 times or more from a knowledge of an appropriate marginal probability and an appropriate conditional probability.

Answer: The marginal probability of males, P (M) = 75/111 = 0.6757 and the conditional probability, P (C|M) = 25/75 = 0.333.

Therefore, the joint probability

$$P\ (M \cap C) = P\ (M) \times P\ (M) \qquad .....(12.15)$$

$$= (0.6757)\ (0.333) = 0.2252$$

Therefore, multiplication rule can be expressed in general terms for any two events A and B,

$$P\ (A \cap B) = P\ (B) \times P\ (A|B),\ \text{if } P\ (B) \neq) = 0 \qquad .....(12.16)$$

or $$P\ (A \cap B) = P\ (A) \times P\ (B|A),\ \text{if } P\ (A) \neq) = 0 \qquad .....(12.17)$$

Other equations can be developed from the above equations.

$$P\ (A|B) = [P\ (A \cap B)]/\ P\ (B) \text{ if } P\ (B) \neq) = 0 \qquad .....(12.18)$$

$$P\ (B|A) = [P\ (A \cap B)]/\ P\ (A) \text{ if } P\ (A) \neq) = 0 \qquad .....(12.19)$$

The Additional Rule: The third property of probability given previously states that the probability of the occurrence of either one or the other two mutually exclusive events is equal to the sum of their individual probabilities. When a person picked at random from the 111 represented in table, what is the probability that this person will be a male (M) or a female (F)? This probability is written in symbolic from as P ($M \cup F$) where the symbol "$\cup$" is read either as "union" or "or". Since the two genders are mutually exclusive,

$$P\ (M \cup F) = P\ (M) + P\ (F)$$

$$= (75/111) + (25/111)$$

$$= 0.6757 + 0.3243 = 1.$$

What happens if two events are not mutually exclusive? This case is covered by what is known as the *additional rule*. Given two events A and B, the possibility that event A or event B, or Both occur is equal to the probability that A occurs, plus the probability that event B occurs, minus the probability that both the events occur simultaneously.

The additional rule may be written as,

$$P\ (A \cup B) = P\ (A) + P\ (B) - P\ (A \cap B) \qquad .....(12.20)$$

Question: When a person is picked at random from the 111 subjects represented in table, what is the probability that this person will be a male (M) or will have used cocaine 100 times or more during his life-time (C) or both ?

Answer: $$P\ (M \cup C) = P\ (M) + P\ (C) - P\ (M \cap C)$$

$$P\ (M \cup C) = (75/111) + (34/111) - (25/111)$$

$$= 0.6757 + 0.3063 - 0.2252 = 0.7568$$

The Binomial Distribution

This is applicable to data, where one of two mutually exclusive and independent out comes are possible as result of a single observation or experimental trail. Independent means the out come in one experimental unit does not influence the out come of another. For example, when a coin is tossed the result may be either tail or head. The out comes, tail and head, are mutually exclusive and independent. In a trail when the out come is head, it automatically excludes the possibility of getting the tail. The out come of the next trial is not influenced by the previous result. Another examples are survived or dead, yes or no, success or failure, etc.

In case of binomial distributions, the probability of "x" out comes of one kind (e.g., success), in "n" binomial trials is given by,

$$P(x) = \binom{n}{x} p^x q^{n-x}$$

Where, P (x) is the probability of exactly 'x' successes.

Where $$\binom{n}{x} = (n!)/(x!)\,(n-x)! \qquad .....(12.22)$$

Probability of failure

$$q = 1 - p \qquad .....(12.23)$$

And $$p + q = 1 \qquad .....(12.24)$$

An antibiotic cures 80% of the patients. It means, the general probability of the curing rate of the antibiotic, p=0.8. What is the probability of exactly 3 successes (cures) in 6 patients ?

$$P(3) = \binom{6}{3} 0.8^3\, 0.2^{6-3} = \frac{6.5.4.3.2.1}{(3.2.1)\,(3.2.1)}\; 0.512 \times 0.008 = 0.082$$

Therefore, the probability of exactly 3 cures in 6 patients with p=0.80 is approximately 8 in 100. It means if 6 patients are treated in-groups for 100 times, the probability of observing 3 cures in 6 patients is 8 times.

Interpretation of Experimental Results

The results of an experiment have to be interpreted and the out come of the experiment has to be understood. The large amount of numerical data has to be analyzed with appropriate statistical tests to find out whether the experimentally determined out come is significant or not. There are three types of significance tests that are quite generally used: the t-test, chi-square (χ^2) test, and F-test or analysis of variance (ANOVA). The very purpose of these tests is to find out whether the observed out come of an experiment is attributable to the study conditions or the observed out come has occurred by chance. For example, a newly developed diuretic drug was administered to group of rats (drug treated group) as an aqueous solution and another group of rats (control group) was given distilled water. The urine volume of the rats in both the groups is recorded for 24 hours. There is difference in the urine volumes between the two groups. Now, the question is whether the observed difference is significant or not. In other words, the difference in urine volume observed between the two groups is a natural random difference or due to the drug effect is assessed with the help of these tests.

The t-test of Significance

In general two types of t-test are used to find out the significance of difference observed between the results obtained with experimental conditions and control. They are 1) Two independent sample t-test and 2) Paired t-test.

Two Independent Sample t-test

If two samples are to be compared to see if they are drawn from the same population, i.e., whether they are samples of the same thing or whether they are significantly different, the t-test may be used as a means of comparison. The t-test is also applied to the example cited above.

The formula used to calculate the 't' value of the data is given by,

$$t = (\text{difference})/(\text{standard error of difference}) \quad .....(12.25)$$

$$t = \frac{\bar{X}_1 - \bar{X}_2}{s}\sqrt{\frac{n_1 n_2}{n_1 + n_2}} \quad .....(12.26)$$

$$s^2 = \frac{[\Sigma X_{li}^2 - (\Sigma X_{li})^2/n_1] + [\Sigma X_{21}^2 - (\Sigma X_{21})^2/n_2]}{n_1 + n_2 - 2} \quad .....(12.27)$$

Where s^2 is called pooled variance.

Practice Problem: Two samples of tablets were submitted for analysis in a chemical laboratory to find out whether they are different or same. The amount of drug present in each tablet was determined. The following data were obtained.

Sample 1 : 10.1, 13.6, 12.5, and 11.4 mg
Sample 2 : 9.8, 9.6, 10.1, 11.4, and 9,1 mg

The data has to be processed to calculate the t-value (Table 12.2)

Table 12.2 Processing of data to calculate the t-value.

Parameter	Sample 1	Sample 2
	10.1	9.8
	13.6	9.6
	12.5	10.1
	11.4	11.4
	—	9.1
ΣX_i	47.6	50.0
ΣX_i^2	573.18	502.98
$\bar{X}$	11.90	10.00
n	4	5

$$s^2 = [573.18 - (47.6)^2/4 + 502.98 - (50)^2/5]/(4+5-2) = 1.3886$$

The square root of the pooled variance is,

$$s = \sqrt{1.3886} = 1.18$$

Therefore, t value is,

$$t = \frac{11.90 - 10.00}{1.18} \sqrt{\frac{(4)(5)}{4+5}} = 1.61\ (1.49) = 2.40$$

The degrees of freedom (DF) for this case is given by,

$$DF = (n_1 - 1) + (n_2 - 1) \qquad 12.28$$

$$= (4 - 1) + (5 - 1) = 7$$

In order to interpret the results of the test it is necessary to find out the natural variance possible for the experimental conditions. A t-table (Table 12.3) is used to get the possible natural values under the experimental conditions. In the t-table columns represent the t-values against the DF values in the rows. There are two types of t-values called one-tail and two-tail. When the measured value from an experimental unit can take both directions from the control value, then the two-tail should be used. When the effect of the experimental conditions on the experimental unit is unknown then also the two-tails should be preferred. For example, a newly developed drug is tested for its diuretic activity, then it can increase or decrease the urine volume from the experimental animals. In this case, two-tail should be used. In another case, protein is added to a standard diet of the rats to find out the effect of amount of the protein on the weight gain. In this case, the protein will increase the weight of the animal or at the most doesn't affect the weight of the animal. Therefore, the one-tail t-values should be used. Further, The t-values have to be looked under a particular probability value. For majority of the scientific studies the probability of 0.05 is used. It means, the results of a study will occur 95 times out of 100 times.

In our example, we have to look for the t-value at P=0.05 under the two-tail for DF of 7. The t-value from the table is 2.365.

Conclusion: Since the calculated t-value (2.40) is greater than the tabled t-value (2.365), the means are significantly different at P=0.05.

The Paired t-test

Paired t-test is applied when two different treatments are given to a single group of experimental units. For example, in a bioavailability study the test formulation and reference formulation are given to the same subjects on different occasions. Another example is the comparison of a new analytical method with already existing method by analyzing the equal parts of a sample.

In independent sample data the variability is due to intra-subject and inter-subject variation whereas in paired data only intra-subject variation exists. Therefore less variation is observed in paired data compared to independent sample data. The paired design can be used only when there is natural or easy way of pairing the experimental units. For example, there is no obvious way of pairing the dissolution of tablets in different dissolution media, because the unit is destroyed in the test.

Table 12.3 The t table

Distribution of t Giving Both the Two-Sided or Two-Tailed Probability and the One-Sided or One-tailed Probability According to Degee of Freedom

				One Tail				
	p 0.4	*p* 0.3	*p* 0.2	*p* 0.1	05	*p* 0.025	*p* 0.01	*p* 0.005
				Two Tails				
DF	*p* 0.8	*p* 0.6	*p* 0.4	*p* 0.2	*p* 0.1	*p* 0.025	*p* 0.02	*p* 0.01
1	0.325	0.727	1.376	3.078	6.314	12.706	31.821	63.657
2	0.289	0.617	1.061	1.886	2.920	4.303	6.695	9.925
3	0.277	0.584	0.978	1.638	2.538	3.182	4.541	5.841
4	0.271	0.569	0.941	1.533	2.132	2.776	3.747	4.604
5	0.267	0.559	0.920	1.476	2.015	2.571	3.365	4.032
6	0.265	0.553	0.906	1.140	1.943	2.447	3.143	3.707
7	0.263	0.549	0.896	1.415	1.895	2.365	2.998	3.499
8	0.262	0.546	0.889	1.397	1.860	2.306	2.896	3.355
9	0.261	0.543	0.883	1.383	1.833	2.262	2.821	3.250
10	0.260	0.542	0.879	1.372	1.812	2.228	2.764	3.169
11	0.260	0.540	0.876	1.363	1.796	2.201	2.718	3.106
12	0.259	0.539	0.873	1.356	1.782	2.179	2.681	3.055
13	0.259	0.538	0.870	1.350	1.771	2.160	2.650	3.012
14	0.258	0.537	0.868	1.345	1.761	2.145	2.624	2.977
15	0.258	0.537	0.866	1.341	1.753	2.131	2.602	2.947
16	0.258	0.535	0.865	1.337	1.746	2.120	2.583	2.921
17	0.257	0.534	0.863	1.333	1.740	2.110	2.567	2.898
18	0.257	0.534	0.862	1.330	1.734	2.101	2.552	2.878
19	0.257	0.533	0.861	1.328	1.729	2.093	2.539	2.845
20	0.257	0.533	0.860	1.325	1.725	2.086	2.528	2.845
21	0.257	0.532	0.859	1.323	1.721	2.080	2.518	2.831
22	0.256	0.532	0.858	1.321	1.717	2.074	2.508	2.819
23	0.256	0.532	0.858	1.319	1.714	2.069	2.500	2.807
24	0.256	0.531	0.857	1.318	1.711	2.064	2.492	2.797
25	0.256	0.531	0.856	1.316	1.708	2.060	2.485	2.787
26	0.256	0.531	0.856	1.315	1.706	2.056	2.479	2.779
27	0.256	0.531	0.855	1.314	1.703	2.052	2.473	2.771
28	0.256	0.531	0.855	1.313	1.701	2.048	2.467	2.763
29	0.256	0.530	0.854	1.311	1.699	2.045	2.462	2.756
30	0.256	0.530	0.854	1.310	1.697	2.042	2.457	2.750
40	0.255	0.529	0.851	1.303	1.684	2.021	2.423	2.704
60	0.254	0.527	0.848	1.296	1.671	2.000	2.390	2.660
120	0.254	0.526	0.845	1.289	1.658	1.980	2.358	2.617
∞	0.253	0.524	0.842	1.282	1.645	1.960	2.326	2.576

Computation:

The following equations are used to calculate the variance and the t-value of the paired data.

$$s^2 = \frac{\Sigma d_i^2 - (\Sigma d_i^2)/n}{(n-1)} \tag{12.29}$$

$$t = (\overline{d}/s)\ \sqrt{n} \tag{12.30}$$

Where, s^2 is the variance of the data, 'd_i' is the difference between two observations in an experimental unit, '$\overline{d}$' is the mean of the differences between the two observations in an experimental unit and 'n' is the number of units in the experiment.

Practice problem: The duration of loss of righting reflex, (When the animal is kept on its supine position, it tries to come to its normal position. This reflex is called righting reflex.), was measured in 16 mice following treatment with a barbiturate administered in the morning and the afternoon. It is desired to find out whether time of administration has influence on the duration of loss of righting reflex or not.

Process the data as shown in Table 12.4.

Table 12.4 Processing of the data for the estimation of t-value

Mouse Number	Loss of righting reflex (minutes)		Difference, $d=(X_1-X_2)$
	Morning	Afternoon	
1	75	73	2
2	86	89	-3
3	93	89	4
4	87	79	8
5	91	95	-4
6	87	81	6
7	76	77	-1
8	83	89	-6
9	87	82	5
10	95	91	4
11	91	87	4
12	86	86	0
13	83	78	5
14	76	69	7
15	82	78	4
16	93	88	5

$\Sigma d_i = 40$, $\Sigma d_i^2 = 354$, $\overline{d} = 2.5$ and $n = 16$.

$$s^2 = \frac{354 - (40)^2/16}{15} = 16.9333$$

$$s = \sqrt{16.9333} = 4.11$$

$$t = (d/s)\ \sqrt{n} = (2.5/4.11)\ \sqrt{16} = 2.43$$

The degrees of freedom (DF) = (n-1) = 16-1 = 15. The t-value under two-tail for DF=15 and P=0.05 is 2.131(see Table 12.3).

Conclusion: Since the calculated t-value (2.43) is greater than the tabled t-value (2.131), the two treatments are different. It means the loss of righting reflex in the morning in mice is significantly more than that of afternoon.

The Chi-Squared Tests of Significance

The chi-square test can assume many different forms. In one form it test agreement between expected frequencies and frequencies observed. Chi-square (χ^2) is a probability distribution derived from the sum of squares of a chi-square statistic, and if the calculated value exceeds the tabled value (chi-square table), a significant difference is declared.

$$\text{Chi-square } (\chi^2) = \frac{(\text{Observed frequency - expected frequency})^2}{\text{Expected frequency}} \qquad 12.31$$

Practice problem: Suppose that a coin is tossed 50 times and 31 times heads and 19 times tails were obtained, where as 25 heads and 25 tails are expected. Is the coin biased or weighted in some way?

$$\chi^2 = [(31\text{-}25)^2/25] + [(19\text{-}25)^2/25] = 2.88$$

The degrees of freedom

$$(\text{DF}) = (\text{number of categories} - 1) \qquad 12.32$$

In this example, DF = 2 - 1 = 1. The χ^2 value for DF = 1 at P = 0.05 is 3.84 (Table 12.5).

Table 12.5 The CHI-Square Table

Probability

d.t.	p = 0.20	p = 0.10	p = 0.05	p = 0.01
1	1.64	2.71	3.84	6.64
2	3.22	4.61	5.99	9.21
3	4.64	6.25	7.82	11.34
4	5.99	7.78	9.49	13.28
5	7.29	9.24	11.07	15.09
6	8.56	10.61	12.59	16.81
7	9.80	12.02	14.07	18.48
8	11.03	13.36	15.51	20.09
9	12.24	14.68	16.92	21.67
10	13.44	15.99	18.31	23.21
20	25.04	28.41	31.41	37.57
30	36.25	40.26	43.77	50.89

Conclusion: Since the calculated χ^2 value (2.88) is less than the tabled value (3.84), the coin is not biased.

The Chi-Squared Test for Contingency Tables

When there are two qualitative variables, the data are arranged in a *contingency table.* The categories for one variable define the rows, and the categories for the other variable define the columns. For example, it is desired to find out whether a newly developed drug prevents death of animals suffering from a disease or not. Drug treated and control groups define the rows and the survived and dead define the columns.

Practice Problem: A drug is tested for its efficacy to treat a dreadful disease in cows. In the drug treated group, 25 cows were survived out of 39 while 21 survived in control group out of 43. Whether the drug under test is having significant effect or not?

The data has to be arranged as a contingency table as shown in Table 12.6.

Table 12.6 Contingency table for c2 test.

Treatment	Survived	Died	Total
Drug	A = 25	B = 14	A + B = 39
Control	C = 21	D = 22	C + D = 43
Total	A + C = 46	B + D = 36	N = 82

Calculate the c2 value of the data using the following equation.

$$\chi^2 = \frac{(|AD - BC| - N/2)^2 N}{(A+B)(C+D)(A+C)(B+D)} \qquad 12.33$$

$$\chi^2 = \frac{(|25 \times 22 - 14 \times 21| - 82/2)^2\, 82}{(25+14)(21+22)(25+21)(14+22)}$$

$$\chi^2 = 3790450/2777112 = 1.365$$

The degree of freedom (DF) for R x C

contingency table = (R-1) (C-1) 12.34

Therefore for 2 x 2 contingency table, the DF =1. The χ^2 value for DF = 1 at P = 0.05 is 3.84 (Table 12.5)

Conclusion: The calculated χ^2 value (1.365) is less than the tabled value (3.84), hence, the two groups are not different. It means, the drug under investigation is not significantly effective.

Analysis of Variance (ANOVA)

Analysis of variance (ANOVA) is a statistical test used in many of the bioavailability studies. It is useful to interpret the data from several groups and also to rank them. It is dealt in detail in chapter 11. The reader is advised to read this topic in chapter 11.

STATISTICS OF STRAIGHT LINE (LINEAR REGRESSION)

Straight lines are found in many theoretical relationships in physical and biological chemistry. First order and zero order kinetics can be expressed in a linear form. Michaelis-Menton's equation for enzyme kinetics and Arrhenius relationship used in stability studies can be transformed into linear forms. The reasons for the desirability of straight-line relationships include the ease of extrapolation and interpolation as well as simplification of the determination of the parameters of the line, the slope and the intercept. The straight line is defined by these parameters and these parameters often have biological and/or physical significance.

One of the problems in estimating the slope and intercept from practical data is the variability and a plot does not clearly define a straight line. If the variability is large, it may be very difficult to decide how to draw the line (Fig.12.2). Lack of an exact fit will be considered due to variability (error) in 'Y' (the dependent variable). In most cases, which are encountered, the 'X' variable (independent variable) tends to have little error relative to the 'Y' variable. In pharmacokinetic study, the X variable (time) can be measured with great accuracy. The dependent variable (concentration), is variable due to biological system, analytical error etc. The practical data can be fit into a line, using the statistical equations given below.

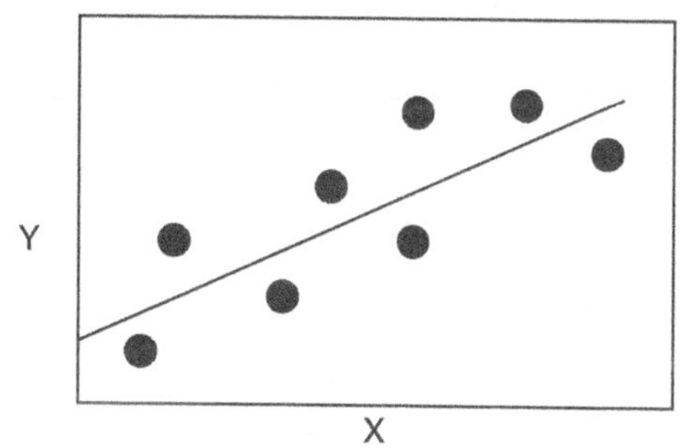

Fig. 12.2 Scattered data showing positive correlation.

$$\text{Slope} = m = \frac{\Sigma(X - \bar{X})(Y - \bar{Y})}{\Sigma(X - \bar{X})^2} \qquad 12.35$$

or

$$\text{Slope} = m = \frac{\Sigma X_i Y_i - (\Sigma X_i \Sigma Y_i)/n}{\Sigma (X_i - \bar{X})^2} \qquad 12.36$$

$$\text{Intercept} = c = \bar{Y} - m\bar{X} \qquad 12.37$$

Using 'm' and 'c' values, Y values can be calculated with the equation Y = m X + c. The calculated Y values for different X values can be compared and deviation can be estimated. The line obtained with best fit is called Least Square Line.

In order to apply the statistical inference procedures to the data, certain assumptions are necessary.

1. The X variable is measured without error. In practical situations, the error in X should be small compared to the error in the Y variable.
2. The Y variable is distributed normally with a true mean equal to M x + C (M and C are true values of the slope and intercept) and with the same variance, at all values of X.

Practice Problem: The reaction rate of a drug was measured at different temperatures. The following data were obtained. Using linear regression of the data, find out the parameters governing the straight-line relationship.

Temperature, X (°C)	10	20	30	40
Reaction rate, Y (mg/hr)	0.241	0.492	0.710	0.978

According to the equations mentioned above,

$$\text{Slope} = m = \frac{\Sigma X_i Y_i - (\Sigma X_i \Sigma Y_i)/n}{\Sigma (X_i - \bar{X})^2}$$

$$\text{Intercept} = c = \bar{Y} - m\,\bar{X}$$

$$m = \frac{7267 - (100 \times 2.421)/4}{500} = 0.02429$$

$$c = 0.6052 - 0.02429\,(25) = -0.002$$

Fitting a Line without Intercept

In some cases a straight-line relation exists between the dependent and the independent variables in such a way that the value of dependent variable is zero when the value of independent variable is zero. In such cases the intercept is zero. The slope of such line is given by,

$$m = \Sigma X_i\, Y_i / \Sigma X_i^2 \qquad 12.38$$

And $Y = m\,X$ is the straight-line equation for this case.

Correlation Coefficient

Correlation is a measure of the linear relationship between two variables. Correlation is used when both the variables are subject to error. The correlation coefficient (r) is calculated to know whether a linear relationship really exists between the two variables or not. Linear regression of the data forcibly fits the data into a straight-line equation even if the two variables are not related linearly.

The measure of association is the correlation coefficient, r. If X and Y are variables,

$$r = \frac{\Sigma X_i Y_i - (\Sigma X_i \Sigma Y_i)/n}{\Sigma (X_i - \bar{X})^2\, \Sigma (Y_i - \bar{Y})^2} \qquad 12.39$$

The correlation coefficient can vary between +1 and −1. A correlation coefficient of +1 would result if all points fall exactly on a single line with positive slope; this is a perfect positive correlation (Fig.12.3). Similarly, if all points fall on a line with negative slope, r = -1, a perfect negative correlation is observed (Fig.12.4). If r = 0, the variables are not correlated (Fig.12.5). In real situations, these extreme results are seen rarely, but rather some intermediate value of 'r' is observed (Fig.12.6 & 12.7). The statistical question of interest usually is concerned with the significance of the correlation, i.e. a test of r versus 0. In order to find out the significance of the correlation a null hypothesis is tested with the help of t-test.

$$t = \frac{r\sqrt{n-2}}{\sqrt{1-r^2}} \qquad 12.40$$

The degrees of freedom (DF) = n - 2

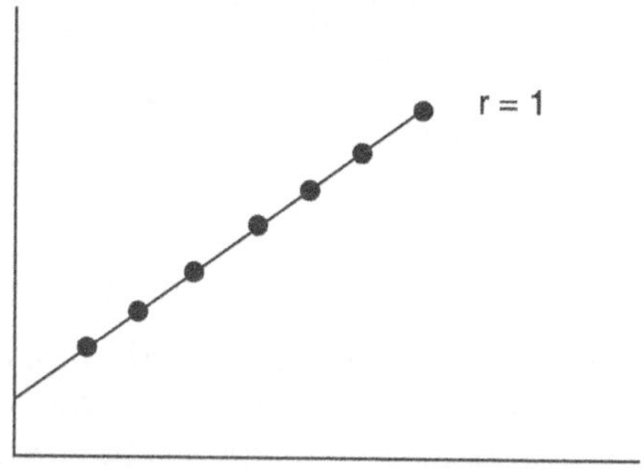

Fig. 12.3 Perfect positive correlation.

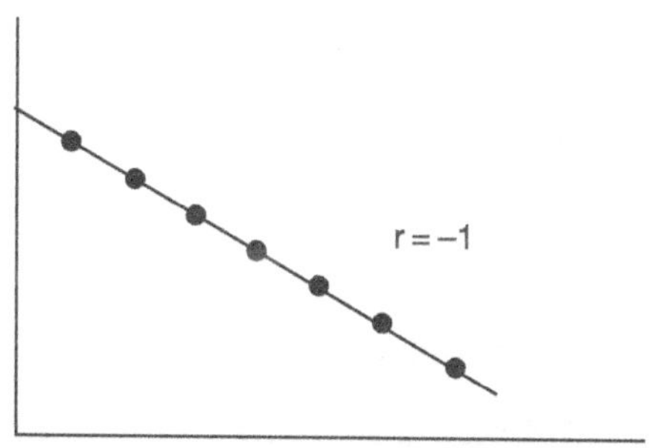

Fig. 12.4 Perfect negative correlation.

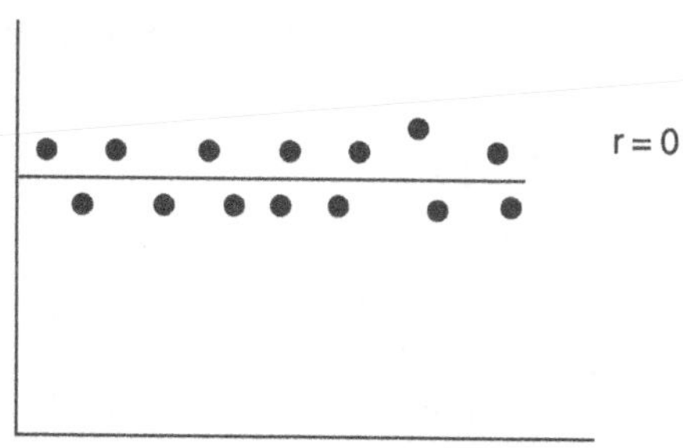

Fig. 12.5 Data showing no correlation.

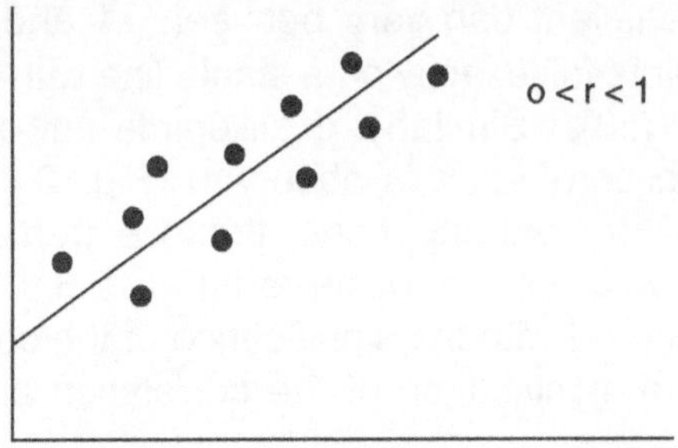

Fig. 12.6 Imperfect positive correlation.

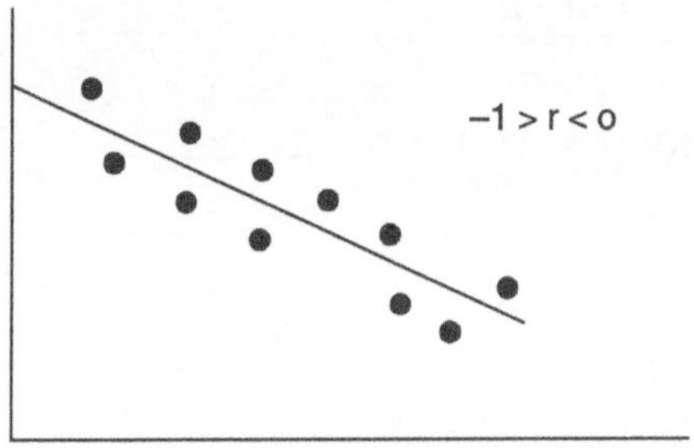

Fig. 12.7 Imperfect negative correlation.

Practice Problem: An experiment was performed to examine the relationship of tablet hardness to tablet dissolution. Dissolution was measured as the time (min) for 50% for the drug to dissolve in USP dissolution test apparatus. Hardness was measured in kg per square inch with the help of Monsanto Hardness Tester. The data are given below. Is there any correlation between the hardness and time required for the dissolution of 50% of drug from the tablet?

Time for 50% dissolution (min.)	18	17	21	26	28	20	25	29	31	18
Hardness (kg/square inch)	6.8	5.3	5.8	7.2	6.9	6.0	6.8	8.1	7.5	6.3

Calculate the correlation coefficient, r.

$$r = \frac{1585.5 - (233 \times 66.7)/10}{\sqrt{(236.1)(6.321)}} = 0.81$$

Now, calculate the t-value in order to find out the significance of the correlation between the two variables.

$$t = \frac{0.81\sqrt{10-2}}{\sqrt{1-(0.81)^2}} = 3.94$$

The DF = n-2 = 10-2 =8. The tabled t-vale for DF = 8 and P=0.05 is 2.228. Since the calculated value is greater than the table valued of t, the null hypothesis is rejected. A correlation exists between the dissolution time for 50% of drug release and hardness of the tablet.

Likely questions

1. Define the terms biostatistics, statistics and data.
2. What is a population in statistical terms?
3. Write about variables.
4. What are descriptive statistics? Write about median.
5. What are measures of dispersion? Write about standard deviation.
6. With the help of a diagram, explain the interrelationship between bias, precision, and accuracy.
7. What is the difference between classical probability and relative frequency probability?
8. Write about the elementary properties of probability.
9. What do you mean by conditional probability, marginal probability, and joint probability?
10. Write a note on multiplication and additional rules in probability.
11. Explain the concept of binomial distribution.
12. What is the significance of inferential statistics?
13. What is the difference between paired t-test and two independent sample t-test?
14. Write a note on the use of chi-square test in inference statistics.
15. Write a note on linear regression.
16. What is the significance of correlation coefficient?
17. The concentration of a biological marker was measured in 8 cancer patients and the following data were obtained. Calculate mean, median, mode, standard deviation, standard error of the average, variance and coefficient of variation. Concentration of the marker (ug/ml) 2.86, 2.75, 2.62, 3.37, 3.49, 2.76, 3.05 and 3.12.
18. An examination was conducted to the students of a college to find out their intelligence quotient. The following data were obtained.

Marks	Boys (X)	Girls (Y)	Total
0-20 (A)	1	2	3
21-40 (B)	3	2	5
41-60 ©	10	12	22
61-80 (D)	8	3	11
81-100 (E)	4	3	7
Total	26	22	48

Suppose we pick a student at random from this sample, (a) what is the probability this student to be girl? And (b) what is the probability that this girl will be one who got marks between 61-80.

19. The success rate of a drug to treat a disease is 84%. What is the probability of exactly 7successes in 9 patients?

20. A drug was tested for its efficacy to prevent the death of chicken suffering from a disease. 20 chickens were survived in drug treated group out of 28 whereas 28 survived in the control group out of 36. Whether the drug under test is having significant effect are not?

21. A survey was carried out to find out the influencing of smoking on the weight of the baby at birth. The following data was obtained. Is really smoking has influence on the weight of the baby at birth?

    NS = non-smoker and S = Smoker

	Weight in kgs.														
NS	3.99	3.79	3.60	3.73	3.21	3.60	4.08	3.61	3.83	3.31	4.13	3.26	3.54	3.51	2.71
S	3.18	2.84	2.90	3.27	3.85	3.52	3.23	2.76	3.60	3.75	3.59	3.63	2.38	2.34	---

22. In a study, subject weight (kg) and plasma volume (l) were measured. It is interested to know whether there exists a linear relation between these two parameters or not?

Subject	1	2	3	4	5	6	7	8
Weight	58.0	70.0	74.0	63.5	62.0	70.5	71.0	66.0
Plasma volume	2.75	2.86	3.37	2.76	2.62	3.49	3.05	3.12

13

In-vitro Dissolution Testing

Ample oral bioavailability is a key pre-requisite for any orally administered drug to be systemically effective. Dissolution is of prime importance for all conventionally constructed solid oral dosage form in general and for modified release in particular and can be a rate limiting step in for the drug administered orally.

Physicochemically dissolution can be defined as "Process by which a solid substance enters the solvent phase to yield a solution". In general dissolution refers to the process through which a solid phase (tablet or powder) goes into a solution phase such as water or GIT fluid. Dissolution of the drug substance is a multistep process involving heterogeneous reactions/interactions (this includes 1. removal of solute from solid phase 2. accommodation of solute in liquid phase and 3. diffusive and/or convective transport of solute away from solid/liquid interface to bulk phase) between different phases of solute-solute and solvent-solvent phase and also at solute-solvent interface. From dosage form perspective, it can be defined as the process by which drug molecules are liberated from solid phase and enter in solution phase.

When a solid dosage form (*e.g.* tablet) is introduced in to a beaker of water or into gastrointestinal tract, the drug begins to pass into solution from the intact solid. Unless the tablet is a polymeric device, the solid matrix also breaks or disintegrates into granules and these granules deaggregate in turn into fine particle which get dissolved to form the solution. Thus disintegration, deaggregation and dissolution are the processes that occur simultaneously with the release.

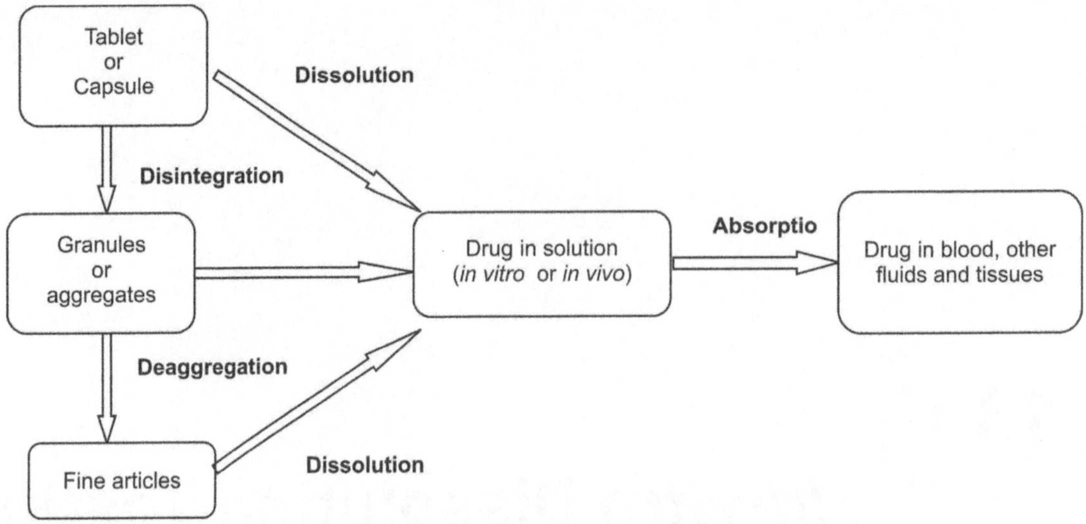

Fig 13.1 Disintegration, deaggregation and dissolution stages of drug release.

The drug in solution form is available for absorption as soon as it uniformly distributes in fluid of the stomach. Some times a drug in solution when administered may precipitate in the fluids of the stomach due to a change in pH; in that case the precipitated fine precipitate should dissolve again in GIT fluids in order to get absorbed. The drug particles of a suspension must undergo dissolution so that the drug is in solution for absorption. In case of tablet or capsule dosage forms, they should first undergo disintegration to release aggregates or granules and then deaggregation into fine particles. The dissolution of a drug takes place from a dosage form as such, aggregates or granules and fine particles. A drug in solution is absorbed through the gastric mucosa and reaches systemic circulation. Stomach emptying causes the emptying of the drug in solution, fine particles, aggregates and even the dosage form into the small intestine which undergo dissolution as explained above.

Mechanisms of Dissolution

Dissolution is nothing but the rate of solution of a solid in a solvent; that is, it is the transfer of solute molecules from the surface of solid into the bulk of a solvent. In order for the dissolution of a solid to occur, solute molecules must first escape from the surface of the solid and then undergo some form of transport process away from the surface into the bulk of the solvent. Three types of dissolution models are proposed depending on the relative significance of two processes mentioned above and the means by which the transport is affected. These three models which, either alone or in combination, can be used to describe the dissolution rate mechanisms. The three models are:

1. Diffusion Layer Model or Film Theory
2. Interfacial Barrier Model or Limited Solvation Theory and
3. Danckwerts' Model or Surface Renewal Theory

(a) Diffusion Layer Model or Film Theory

According to this there is a static liquid film adjacent to the solid surface. The reaction at the solid/liquid film interface is assumed to be rapid and the rate of dissolution is governed entirely by the diffusional transport of the solute molecules through the liquid film. Once the solute molecules pass the liquid film/bulk film interface, rapid mixing occurs and the concentration gradient is destroyed. The model is depicted in the rate at which the dissolution of a drug takes place from a particle into its surrounding fluid according to this model can be assessed by the Noyes-Whitney equation. The assumptions made in developing the Noyes-Whitney equation are:

1. Drug particles are spherical in shape and equal in size,
2. The dissolution process is controlled by diffusion of molecules or ions,
3. There is no chemical reaction between the drug and the components of the fluid in which the drug is present, and
4. The thickness of the diffusion layer (h) and the saturation solubility of drug in diffusion layer (Cs) are constant irrespective of the particle size.

According to Noyes and Whitney, the rate of dissolution (dm/dt) is given by,

$$\frac{dM}{dt} = \frac{DA(CS - Cg)}{h} \quad .....(13.1)$$

Where:

dm/dt	=	rate of the dissolution of the particles
D	=	diffusion coefficient of the drug in solution in the GI fluids (greater the value, faster the dissolution. But is inversely proportional to viscosity of the medium)
A	=	effective surface area of the drug particles (greater the surface area, faster the dissolution and can be increased by micronization)
h	=	the thickness of the diffusion layer (stationary layer of the solvent) around the drug particles (more the thickness, lesser is the diffusion and dissolution, can be reduced by agitation)
Cs	=	saturation solubility of the drug in the diffusion layer
Cg	=	concentration of the drug in solution in the bulk of GI fluids
(Cs-cg)	=	concentration gradient (greater the concentration gradient faster is the dissolution)

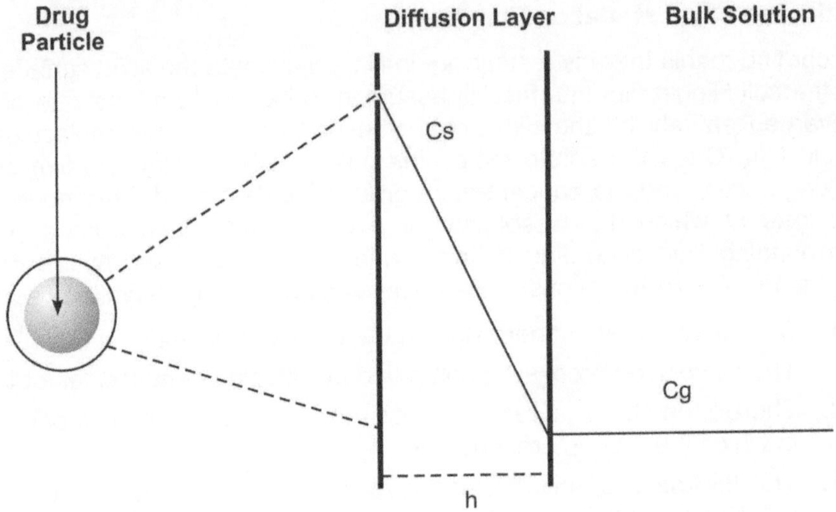

Fig. 13.2 Dissolution of drug particles according to diffusion layer model.

Equation 13.1 represents a first order dissolution process, where the driving force is the concentration gradient (Cs-Cg) and dissolution is said to be under non-sink condition which is true in case of in–vitro dissolution (where dissolution is done in limited dissolution medium). During such dissolution, after sometimes, the dissolution slows down because of drug concentration but *in-vivo* dissolution (dissolution in human stomach) is always rapid than in-vitro because of the moment of dissolved drug (from dissolution site to blood) resulting in Cg=0, thus dissolution will be at its max as sink condition is maintained.

Since during sink condition (keeping the volume and surface area constant),

$$dC/Dt = K$$

where K = constant

For our purposes, we consider a cell membrane that is composed of phospholipids and proteins. Absorption of drugs across the stomach lining/mucosa and the blood/brain barrier are two representative examples and important for understanding drug transport into the circulation and CNS, respectively. Skin is another great example of a membrane for the entry of drugs. The transport of drug molecules through a non-porous membrane occurs by diffusion. Transport through porous membranes occurs by diffusion and convection (not covered here). Similar to dissolution, the diffusion equation is…

$$\frac{dM}{dt} = \frac{DAK(C_1 - C_2)}{h}$$

M = amount of drug (material) dissolved (usually mg or mmol)

t = time (seconds)

D = diffusion coefficient of the drug (cm^2/s)

A = surface area of membrane (cm2)

K = oil/water partition coefficient

h = thickness of the liquid film

$C_1 - C_2$ = concentration gradient where C_1 is the concentration of drug at donor side of membrane and C_2 is the concentration of drug in the membrane at receptor side.

However, C_1 and C_2 are not measured since these are values within the membrane. Typically, the gradient is measured as C_d - C_r, representing the partition at each phase, namely Ko/w = C_1/C_d and Ko/w = C_2/C_r. The Integrated Studies uses C_1 and C_2 where C_d and C_r should be used, but it doesn't really matter for the calculation so long as you know what the gradient is. The rate of drug transport into diffusional system is predominantly dependent upon the magnitude of the concentration gradient – the other parameters are constant. $C_1C_rC_2C_d$hdonor compartment (high drug concentration) receptor compartment (low drug concentration)

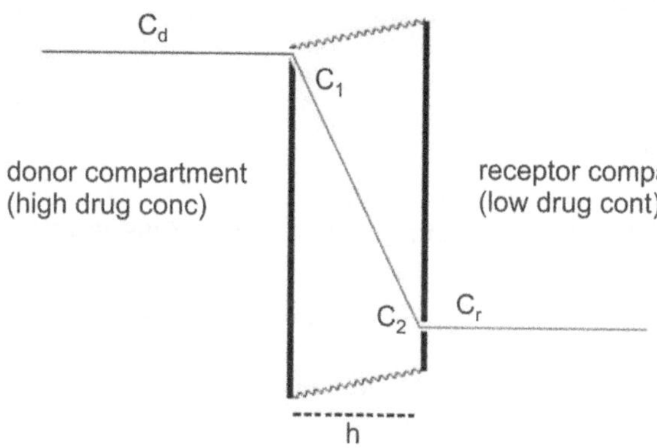

Fig 13.3 Fick's law of diffusion.

Fig 13.4 schematically illustrates the relationship of the terms in equation 13.10a to the dissolution process. It should be emphasized that this crude model does not completely describe the dissolution process. The model has, however, helped to explain many experimental results. Each term in the equation influences the rate of dissolution of a drug in GI fluids.

As the dissolution of drug particles take place, the particle size and surface area are also changed. Hixon and Crowell developed an equation to account for these changes during dissolution and is known as *Hixon and Crowell's Cube Root Law of dissolution.*

$$W_o{}^{y3} - W_t{}^{y3} = k\,t \qquad .....(13.2)$$

Where, W_o = original mass of the drug

W_t = mass of the drug remained at time t

K = dissolution rate constant

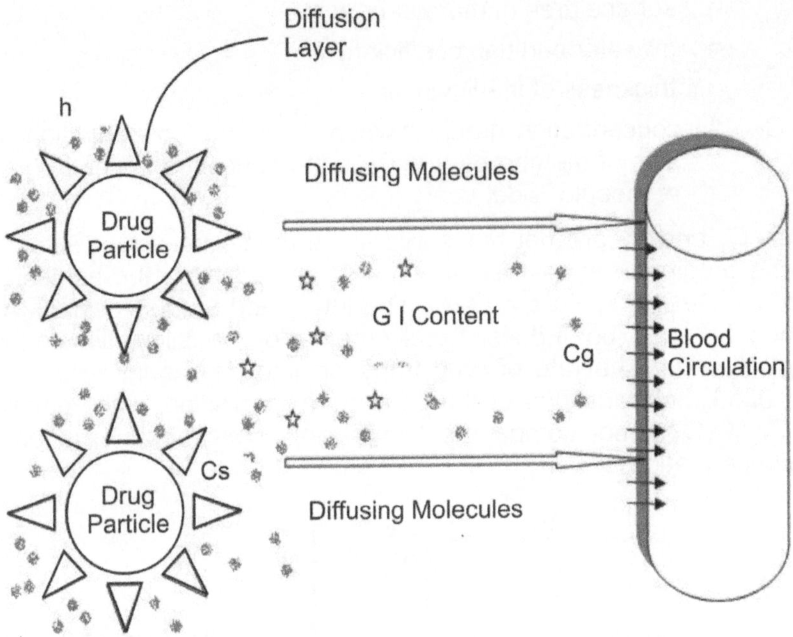

Fig 13.4 Schematic diagram of dissolution.

(b) Interfacial Barrier Model or Limited Solvation Theory

In the interfacial barrier model, it is assumed that the reaction at the solid/liquid interface is not instantaneous due to a high activation free energy barrier which has to be surmounted before the solid can dissolve. Therefore, the rate of solubility of solid in the liquid film becomes rate limiting rather than diffusion of dissolved molecules. The situation is illustrated in Fig. X 5 for the case where the now relatively rapid transport process occurs by diffusion through a static liquid film.

Equation for describing the dissolution rate of a solid by this model is,

$$dm/dt = Ki\ (Cs - Cg)$$

Where,

dm/dt = dissolution rate per unit area

Ki = Effective interfacial transport constant

Cs and Cg are as defined previously and Ki is the effective interfacial transport rate constant.

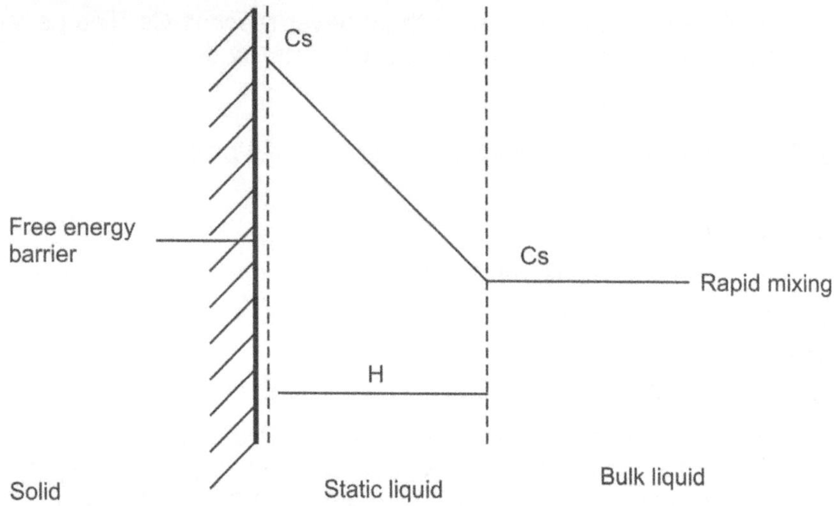

Fig 13.5 Diagrammatic representation of the free energy barrier to dissolution.

(c) Danckwerts'Model or Surface Renewal Theory

Dankwerts' never agreed for the existence of a saturated diffusion layer and proposed that the transport of a solute away from the solid surface is achieved by means of macroscopic packets of solvent which attach themselves to the surface, absorb the solute by normal diffusion, and are then replaced by fresh packets of solvent. Since fresh solvent packets attack the new solid surface each time to effect dissolution, the theory is also known as *Surface Renewal Theory*.

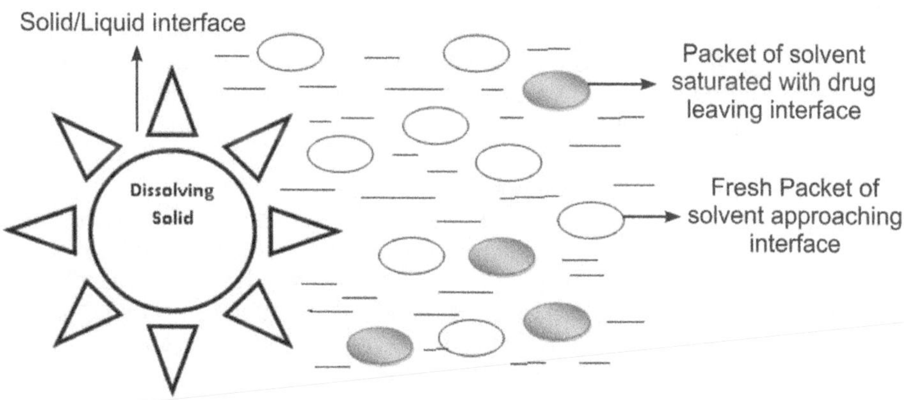

Fig. 13.6 Surface renewal theory.

The turbulence present in the dissolution medium at the solid/liquid interface is responsible for the rapid movement of solvent packets or macroscopic mass of eddies that reach the solid/liquid interface in random manner. Because of the rapid movement of these solvent packets, the drug concentration in them never reaches Cs. The general expression used for the rate of dissolution of a solid by Danckwerts' model is,

$$dm/dt = S^{1/2} D^{1/2} (Cs - Cg)$$

Where, S is the mean rate at which a fresh surface is produced and all other terms are as defined previously.

Factors affecting Dissolution

Factors that can affect the dissolution can be characterized in following categories

1. Physical properties of the drug
2. Dosage form factors
3. Dissolution conditions

The various physicochemical properties of drug that affect dissolution and its rate are solubility, particle size, polymorphism, salt-form, pseudo polymorphism, complexation, wettability etc and dosage form factors including formulation factors and excipients incorporated has already been discussed in chapter 2.

Factors related to the dissolution conditions

Generally dissolution testing is conducted using a dissolution apparatus that conforms to the specifications outlined in the United States Pharmacopeia. There are seven types of dissolution apparatus; the apparatus chosen to perform dissolution testing depends primarily on the drug dosage form.

Methods of dissolution testing

Official Methods of Dissolution

This test is provided to determine compliance with the dissolution requirements where stated in the individual monograph for a tablet or capsule dosage form, except where the label states that the tablets are to be chewed. Requirements for dissolution do not apply to liquid-filled soft gelatin capsules. Of the types of apparatus described herein, use the one specified in the individual monograph.

Rotating Basket Method (Apparatus 1)

The assembly consists of the following: a covered vessel made of glass or other inert, transparent material; a motor; a metallic drive shaft; and a cylindrical basket made up of a stainless steel mesh of No.40 and attached to a motor through a shaft. The vessel is partially immersed in a suitable water bath of any convenient size or placed in a heating jacket. The water bath or heating jacket permits holding the temperature inside the vessel at 37 ± 0.5 during the test and keeping the bath fluid in constant, smooth motion. No part of the assembly, including the environment in which the assembly is placed, contributes significant motion, agitation, or vibration beyond that due to the smoothly rotating stirring element. Apparatus that permits observation of the specimen and stirring element during the test is preferable. A speed-regulator is used to allow the shaft rotational speed to be selected and maintained at the rate specified in the individual monograph. The basket holds the sample and rotates in the vessel containing the dissolution medium.

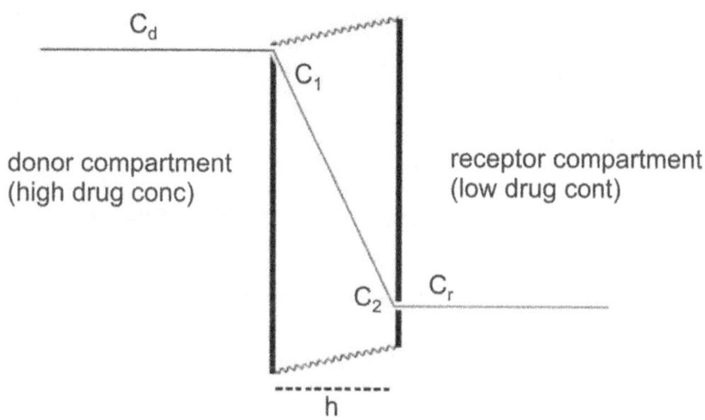

The vessel is cylindrical, with a hemispherical bottom and with one of the following dimensions and capacities: for a nominal capacity of 1 L, the height is 160 mm to 210 mm and its inside diameter is 98 mm to 106 mm; for a nominal capacity of 2 L, the height is 280 mm to 300 mm and its inside diameter is 98 mm to 106 mm; and for a nominal capacity of 4 L, the height is 280 mm to 300 mm and its inside diameter is 145 mm to 155 mm. Its sides are flanged at the top. A fitted cover may be used to retard evaporation. The shaft is positioned so that its axis is not more than 2 mm at any point from the vertical axis of the vessel and rotates smoothly and without significant wobble. A speed-regulating device is used that allows the shaft rotation speed to be selected and maintained at the rate specified in the individual monograph, within ±4%. Shaft and basket components of the stirring element are fabricated of stainless steel, type 316 or equivalent, to the specifications shown in Figure.

The rotational speed and the position of the basket must meet specific requirements set forth in the current pharmacopoeia. The position and alignment of the stirrer are specified in the pharmacopoeia. Dissolution calibration standards are available to make sure that these mechanical and operating requirements are met. Individually test 1 tablet of the *USP Dissolution Calibrator, Non-disintegrating type*, according to the operating conditions specified. The apparatus is suitable if the results obtained are within the acceptable range stated in the certificate for that calibrator in the apparatus tested.

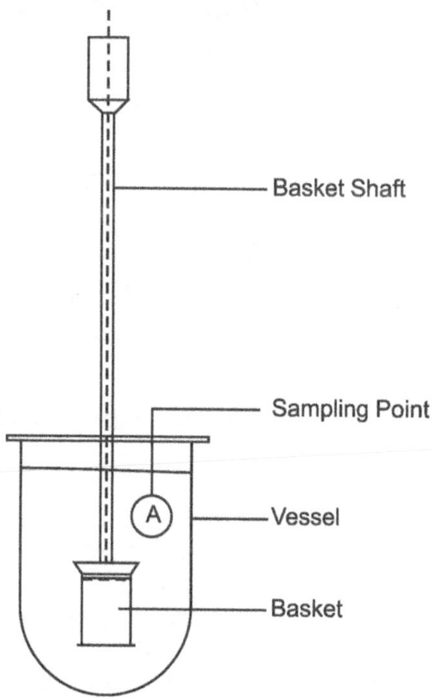

Fig. 13.7 Basic design of apparatus I.

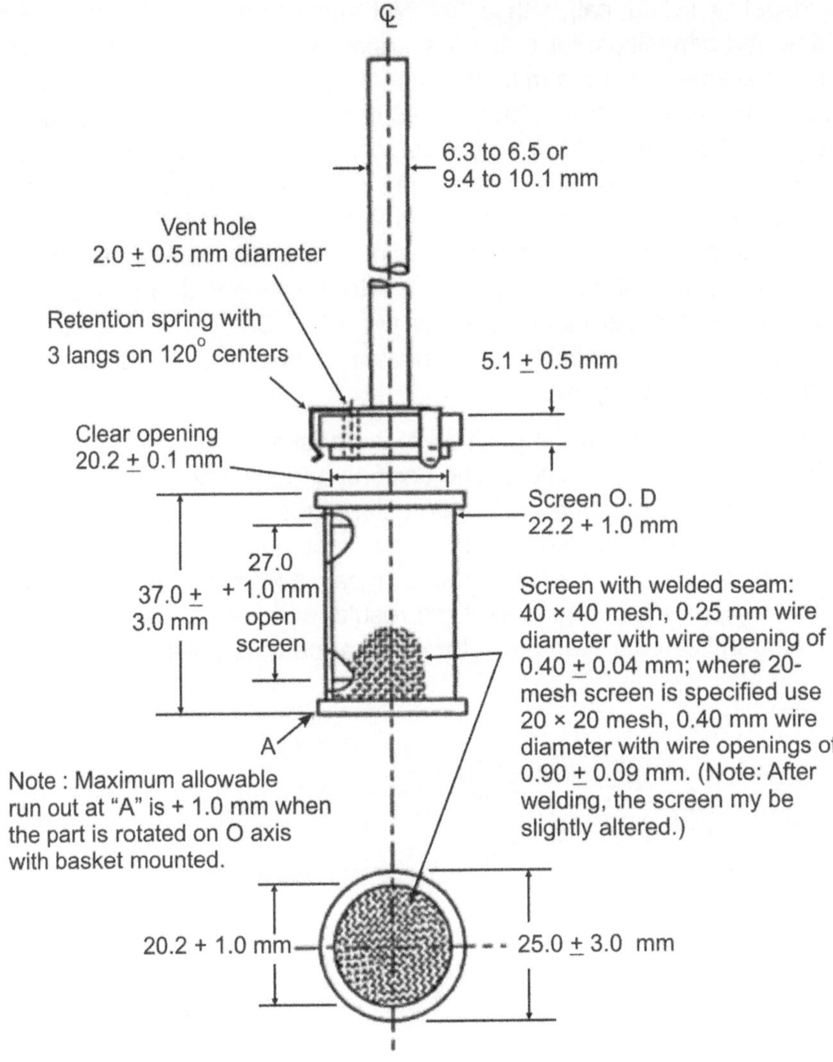

Fig. 13.8 Dimensions of the apparatus I.

Paddle Method (Apparatus 2)

Apparatus 2 is the same as Apparatus 1, except that a paddle formed from a blade and a shaft is used as the stirring element. The metallic blade and shaft comprise a single entity that may be coated with a suitable inert coating. The paddle is vertically attached to a variable-speed motor that rotates at a controlled speed and creates minimum turbulence due to stirring. The tablet or capsule is placed into a round-bottomed dissolution flask. The dissolution flask is immersed in a water-bath maintained at 37 °C. The position and alignment of the paddle are specified in the USP. The paddle method is sensitive to tilting than the basket method, therefore, improper alignment may drastically affect the dissolution results with some drug products. Calibration of the apparatus is carried out using official dissolution calibration tablets.

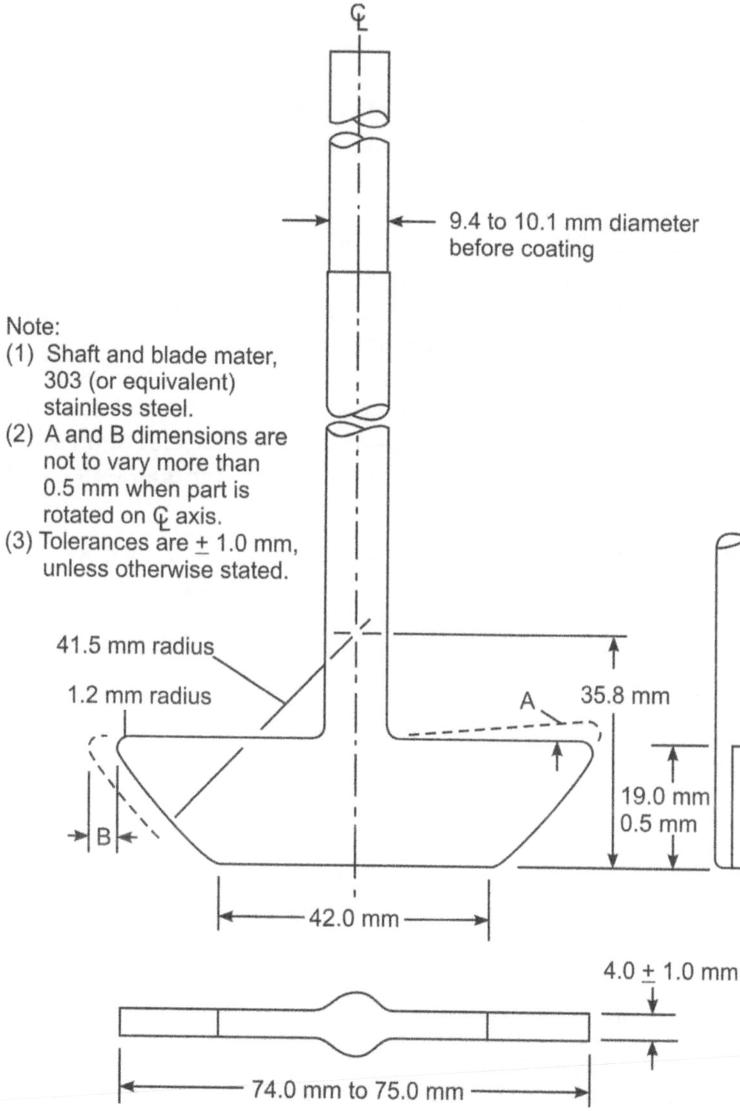

Fig. 13.9 Dimensions of the apparatus II.

The distance of 25 ± 2 mm between the blade and the inside bottom of the vessel is maintained during the test. The metallic or suitably inert, rigid blade and shaft comprise a single entity. A suitable two-part detachable design may be used provided the assembly remains firmly engaged during the test. The paddle blade and shaft may be coated with a suitable inert coating. The dosage unit is allowed to sink to the bottom of the vessel before rotation of the blade is started. A small, loose piece of nonreactive material such as not more than a few turns of wire helix may be attached to dosage units that would otherwise float. Other validated sinker devices may be used.

Methods for Capsules, Uncoated Tablets, and Plain Coated Tablets

(Apparatus I and II): Place the stated volume of the Dissolution Medium (±1%) in the vessel of the apparatus specified in the individual monograph, assemble the apparatus, equilibrate the Dissolution Medium to 37 ± 0.5, and remove the thermometer. Place 1 tablet or 1 capsule in the apparatus, taking care to exclude air bubbles from the surface of the dosage-form unit, and immediately operate the apparatus at the rate specified in the individual monograph. Within the time interval specified, or at each of the times stated, withdraw a specimen from a zone midway between the surface of the Dissolution Medium and the top of the rotating basket or blade, not less than 1 cm from the vessel wall. [NOTE: Replace the aliquots withdrawn for analysis with equal volumes of fresh Dissolution Medium at 37 or, where it can be shown that replacement of the medium is not necessary, correct for the volume change in the calculation. Keep the vessel covered for the duration of the test, and verify the temperature of the mixture under test at suitable times.] Perform the analysis as directed in the individual monograph4. Repeat the test with additional dosage form units.

Dissolution Medium: A suitable dissolution medium is used. Use the solvent specified in the individual monograph. The volume specified refers to measurements made between 20 and 25. If the Dissolution Medium is a buffered solution, adjust the solution so that its pH is within 0.05 unit of the specified pH given in the individual monograph. [NOTE—Dissolved gases can cause bubbles to form, which may change the results of the test. If dissolved gases influence the dissolution results, dissolved gases should be removed prior to testing.

If automated equipment is used for sampling and the apparatus is modified, validation of the modified apparatus is needed to show that there is no change in the agitation characteristics of the test.

Where capsule shells interfere with the analysis, remove the contents of not fewer than 6 capsules as completely as possible, and dissolve the empty capsule shells in the specified volume of Dissolution Medium. Perform the analysis as directed in the individual monograph. Make any necessary correction. Correction factors greater than 25% of the labeled content are unacceptable.

Method for a Pooled Sample for Capsules, Uncoated Tablets, and

Plain Coated Tablets: Use this procedure where Procedure for a Pooled Sample is specified in the individual monograph. Proceed as directed under Procedure for Capsules, Uncoated Tablets, and Plain Coated Tablets. Combine equal volumes of the filtered solutions of the six or twelve individual specimens withdrawn, and use the pooled sample as the test solution. Determine the average amount of the active ingredient dissolved in the pooled sample.

Methods for Testing Enteric-Coated Products

The USP provides two methods for testing enteric-coated products.

Method A

The apparatus type to be used for testing a particular drug product is specified in the drug monograph. The product is first tested in 0.1 N HCl for 2 hours, and then changed to pH 6.8 by adding 0.2 M tribasic sodium phosphate. Final adjustment of the pH of dissolution medium can be made either with 2N NaOH or HCl if necessary. The test is then generally carried for 45 minutes. No significant dissolution should occur in an acidic medium (less than 10% for any specific sample unit), and a specified percent of the drug must be released in the buffer medium. Specifications are set in the individual drug monographs.

Method B

Dissolution is carried out in the apparatus specified in the individual drug monograph (usually apparatus 1 or 2). This method involves testing the drug product in 0.1 N HCl for 2 hours, and then draining the acidic medium and replacing it with a pH 6.8 buffer medium prepared by mixing 0.2 M tribasic sodium phosphate with 0.1N HCl. The temperature of the buffer medium must be at 37° C before replacement. The acceptance criteria are the similar to those for method A.

Apparatus 3 (Reciprocating Cylinder): (Not accepted by The Japanese Pharmacopoeia) The assembly consists of a set of cylindrical, flat-bottomed glass vessels; a set of glass reciprocating cylinders; inert fittings (stainless steel type 316 or other suitable material), and screens that are made of suitable nonsorbing and nonreactive material and that are designed to fit the tops and bottoms of the reciprocating cylinders; and a motor and drive assembly to reciprocate the cylinders vertically inside the vessels and, if desired, index the reciprocating cylinders horizontally to a different row of vessels. The vessels are partially immersed in a suitable water bath of any convenient size that permits holding the temperature at 37 ± 0.5 during the test. No part of the assembly, including the environment in which the assembly is placed, contributes significant motion, agitation, or vibration beyond that due to the smooth, vertically reciprocating cylinder. A device is used that allows the reciprocation rate to be selected and maintained at the specified dip rate given in the individual monograph within ±5%. An apparatus that permits observation of the specimens and reciprocating cylinders is preferable. The vessels are provided with an evaporation cap that remains in place for the duration of the test. The components conform to the dimensions shown in Figure unless otherwise specified in the individual monograph.

Method

Immediate-Release Dosage Forms

Place the stated volume of the Dissolution Medium in each vessel of the apparatus, assemble the apparatus, equilibrate the Dissolution Medium to 37 ± 0.5, and remove the thermometer. Place 1 dosage-form unit in each of the six reciprocating cylinders, taking care to exclude air bubbles from the surface of each dosage unit, and immediately operate the apparatus as specified in the individual monograph. During the upward and downward stroke, the reciprocating cylinder moves through a total distance of 9.9 to 10.1 cm. Within the time interval specified, or at each of the times stated, raise the reciprocating cylinders and withdraw a portion of the solution under test from a zone midway between the surface of the Dissolution Medium and the bottom of each vessel. Perform the analysis as directed in the individual monograph. If necessary, repeat the test with additional dosage-form units.

Dissolution Medium: Proceed as directed for Immediate-Release Dosage Forms under Apparatus 1 and Apparatus 2.

Time: Proceed as directed for Immediate-Release Dosage Forms under Apparatus 1 and Apparatus 2.

Extended-Release Dosage Forms

Proceed as directed for Immediate-Release Dosage Forms under Apparatus 3.

Dissolution Medium: Proceed as directed for Extended-Release Dosage Forms under Apparatus 1 and Apparatus 2.

Time: Proceed as directed for Extended-Release Dosage Forms under Apparatus 1 and Apparatus 2.

Delayed-Release Dosage Forms

Proceed as described for Delayed-Release Dosage Forms, Method B under Apparatus 1 and Apparatus 2 using one row of vessels for the acid stage media and the following row of vessels for the buffer stage media and using the volume of medium specified (usually 300 mL).

Time: Proceed as directed for Immediate-Release Dosage Forms under Apparatus 1 and Apparatus 2.

Apparatus 4 (Flow-Through Cell)

The assembly consists of a reservoir and a pump for the Dissolution Medium; a flow-through cell; and a water bath that maintains the Dissolution Medium at 37 ± 0.5. Use the specified cell size as given in the individual monograph.

The pump forces the Dissolution Medium upwards through the flow-through cell. The pump has a delivery range between 240 and 960 mL per hour, with standard flow rates of 4, 8, and 16 mL per minute. It must deliver a constant flow (±5% of the nominal flow rate); the flow profile is sinusoidal with a pulsation of 120 ± 10 pulses per minute.

The flow-through cell (see Figures 4 and 5), of transparent and inert material, is mounted vertically with a filter system (specified in the individual monograph) that prevents escape of undissolved particles from the top of the cell; standard cell diameters are 12 and 22.6 mm; the bottom cone is usually filled with small glass beads of about 1-mm diameter with one bead of about 5 mm positioned at the apex to protect the fluid entry tube; and a tablet holder (see Figures 4 and 5) is available for positioning of special dosage forms, for example, inlay tablets. The cell is immersed in a water bath, and the temperature is maintained at 37 ± 0.5.

Method

Immediate-Release Dosage Forms

Place the glass beads into the cell specified in the monograph. Place 1 dosage unit on top of the beads or, if specified in the monograph, on a wire carrier. Assemble the filter head, and fix the parts together by means of a suitable clamping device. Introduce by the pump the Dissolution Medium warmed to 37 ± 0.5 through the bottom of the cell to obtain the flow rate specified in the individual monograph and measured with an accuracy of 5%. Collect the eluate by fractions at each of the times stated. Perform the analysis as directed in the individual monograph. Repeat the test with additional dosage-form units.

Dissolution Medium: Proceed as directed for Immediate-Release Dosage Forms under Apparatus 1 and Apparatus 2.

Time: Proceed as directed for Immediate-Release Dosage Forms under Apparatus 1 and Apparatus 2.

Extended-Release Dosage Forms

Proceed as directed for Immediate-Release Dosage Forms under Apparatus 4.

Dissolution Medium: Proceed as directed for Immediate-Release Dosage Forms under Apparatus 4.

Time: Proceed as directed for Immediate-Release Dosage Forms under Apparatus 4.

Delayed-Release Dosage Forms

Proceed as directed for Delayed-Release Dosage Forms under Apparatus 1 and Apparatus 2, using the specified media.

Time: Proceed as directed for Delayed-Release Dosage Forms under Apparatus 1 and Apparatus 2.

Interpretation of Results of Dissolution Test

Unless otherwise specified in the individual monograph, the requirements are met if the quantities of an active ingredient dissolved from the units tested conform to the accompanying acceptance table (Table 2.2). Continue testing through the three stages unless the results conform to either S1 or S2. The quantity, Q, is the amount of the dissolved active ingredient specified in the individual monograph, expressed as a percentage of the labeled content; both 5% and 15% values in the acceptance table are percentages of the labeled content so that these values and Q are in the same terms.

Dissolution Acceptance Table 1

Stage	Number	Acceptance Criteria
S1	6	Each unit release not less than Q+5%
S2	6	Average of 12 units (S1+S2) is equal to or greater than Q, and no unit is less than Q-15%
S3	12	Average of 24 units (S1 + S2 + S3) is equal to or greater Q, not more than 2 units are less than (Q-15%), and no unit is less than (Q-25%)

For Pooled Sample: Unless otherwise specified in the individual monograph, the requirements are met if the quantities of active ingredient dissolved from the pooled sample conform to the accompanying Acceptance Table for a Pooled Sample. Continue testing through the three stages unless the results conform at either S1 or S2. The quantity, Q, is the amount of dissolved active ingredient specified in the individual monograph, expressed as a percentage of the labeled content.

Acceptance Table for a Pooled Sample 2

Stage	Number Tested	Acceptance Criteria
S1	6	Average amount dissolved is not less than Q + 10%.
S2	6	Average amount dissolved (S1 + S2) is equal to or greater than Q + 5%.
S3	12	Average amount dissolved (S1 + S2 + S3) is equal to or greater than Q

Extended-Release Dosage Forms

Unless otherwise specified in the individual monograph, the requirements are met if the quantities of active ingredient dissolved from the dosage units tested conform to Acceptance Table 2. Continue testing through the three levels unless the results conform at either L1 or L2. Limits on the amounts of active ingredient dissolved are expressed in terms of the percentage of labeled content. The limits embrace each value of Qi, the amount dissolved at each specified fractional dosing interval. Where more than one range is specified in the individual monograph, the acceptance criteria apply individually to each range.

Acceptance Table 3

Level	Number Tested	Criteria
L1	6	No individual value lies outside each of the stated ranges and no individual value is less than the stated amount at the final test time.
L2	6	The average value of the 12 units (L1 + L2) lies within each of the stated ranges and is not less than the stated amount at the final test time; none is more than 10% of labeled content outside each of the stated ranges; and none is more than 10% of labeled content below the stated amount at the final test time.
L3	12	The average value of the 24 units (L1 + L2 + L3) lies within each of the stated ranges, and is not less than the stated amount at the final test time; not more than 2 of the 24 units are more than 10% of labeled content outside each of the time.

Delayed-Release Dosage Forms

Acid Stage: Unless otherwise specified in the individual monograph, the requirements of this portion of the test are met if the quantities, based on the percentage of the labeled content, of active ingredient dissolved from the units tested conform to Acceptance Table 4 Continue testing through all levels unless the results of both acid and buffer stages conform at an earlier level.

Acceptance Table 4

Level	Number Tested	Criteria
A1	6	No individual value exceeds 10% dissolved.
A2	6	Average of the 12 units (A1 + A2) is not more than 10% dissolved, and no individual unit is greater than 25% dissolved.
A3	12	Average of the 24 units (A1 + A2 + A3) is not more than 10% dissolved, and no individual unit is greater than 25% dissolved.

Buffer Stage: Unless otherwise specified in the individual monograph, the requirements are met if the quantities of active ingredient dissolved from the units tested conform to Acceptance Table 4. Continue testing through the three levels unless the results of both stages conform at an earlier level. The value of Q in Acceptance Table 4 is 75% dissolved unless otherwise specified in the individual monograph. The quantity, Q,specified in the individual monograph is the total amount of active ingredient dissolved in both the Acid and Buffer Stages, expressed as a percentage of the labeled content. The 5%, 15%, and 25% values in Acceptance Table 5 are percentages of the labeled content so that these values and Q are in the same terms.

Acceptance Table 5

Level	Number Tested	Criteria
B1	6	Each unit is not less than Q + 5%.
B2	6	Average of 12 units (B1 + B2) is equal to or greater than Q, and no unit is less than Q 15%.
B3	12	Average of 24 units (B1 + B2 + B3) is equal to or greater than Q, not more than 2 units are less than Q – 15%, and no unit is less than Q – 25%.

For many drug products, the passing of Q is set at about 75% in 45 min. and this standard has been proposed for all drug products. Setting the dissolution specification for a new drug product requires a thorough consideration of the physical and chemical properties of the drug. However, the dissolution test must ensure consistent bioavailability of the product. Further the test must provide for variations in manufacturing and testing variables so that a product may not be improperly rejected.

The USP monograph for aspirin tablets contains a dissolution test requiring the use of Apparatus 1 at 50 rpm with 500 ml of 0.05M acetate buffer (pH 4.5). Not less than about 80% of the aspirin in each tablet must dissolve in 30 minutes. In the case of the digoxin tablets dissolution test, Apparatus 1 is specified. The test has to be carried out at 120 rpm and the dissolution medium is diluted hydrochloric acid. Not less than 65% of the labeled amount of digoxin must dissolve in 60 minuets. Other tablets for which a dissolution requirement is provided include nitrofurantoin, phenylbutazone, hydrochlorthiazide, quinine sulfate and prednisone.

Unofficial Methods of Dissolution

Beaker Method

Levy and Hayes in 1960 described this method. In their original work, they used a 400 cm^3 beaker containing 250 cm^3 of dissolution medium, which was agitated by means of a three-bladed polyethylene stirrer with a diameter of 50 mm. The stirrer was immersed to a depth of 27 mm into the dissolution medium and rotated at 60 rpm. Tablets were placed in the beaker and the test was carried out by collecting samples of the dissolution medium at different time intervals. The samples were filtered and analyzed for drug content. The major disadvantages of this method are: 1. a tablet can take different positions on the bottom of the beaker, and 2. the formation of 'mounds' of particles in different positions on the flat bottom of the beaker.

Flask-Stirrer Method

This method was developed by Poole in 1969. The apparatus includes a round-bottomed flask and a stirring element similar to that used in the beaker method. The use of round-bottomed flask helps to avoid the problems that may arise from the formation of 'mounds' of particles in different positions on the flat bottom of a beaker.

Rotating Bottle Method

The equipment consists of a rotating rack that holds bottles in which the products are tested for dissolution. The dissolution medium and drug product are placed in the bottles, the bottles are capped tightly and rotated in a water-bath maintained at 37 °C. At selected time intervals the samples are removed from the bottles, filtered through a 40-mesh screen, and the samples are assayed for drug content. Equal volumes of a fresh dissolution medium are added into the bottles and the dissolution test is continued. A dissolution test with a pH 1.2 medium for 1 hour, pH 2.5 medium for the next 1 hour, followed by pH 4.5 medium for 1.5 hours, a pH 7.0 medium for 1.5 hours, and pH 7.5 medium for 2 hours are recommended to simulate the condition of the GIT.

This method was suggested in NF-XIII and has become less popular. The rotating bottle method is used mainly for controlled release beads. For this purpose the dissolution media may be changed, such as from gastric juice to artificial intestinal juice. The main disadvantage is that this procedure is manual and tedious.

Flow-Through Dissolution Method

In this method, a tablet or capsule is placed in dissolution chamber and the dissolution medium is pumped through the dissolution chamber. The flow rate is usually maintained between 10 and 100 ml/min. Laminar flow of the medium is maintained by using a pulseless pump. The dissolution medium may be fresh or recirculated. In the case, where fresh dissolution medium is pumped continuously, the dissolution rate at any time point can be obtained, whereas in the official basket or paddle methods cumulative dissolution rates are obtained. When the dissolution medium is recirculated, cumulative dissolution rates are obtained. A major advantage of the flow through method is the easy maintenance of a sink condition for dissolution. A large volume of dissolution medium may also be used, and the mode of operation is easily adopted to automated equipment.

Rotating and Static Disc Methods (Intrinsic Dissolution Method)

In these methods, the drug that is to be assessed for the rate of dissolution is compressed into a non-disintegrating disc without excipients. The disc is mounted in a holder so that only one face of the disc is exposed to the dissolution medium. The holder and the disc are immersed in the dissolution medium and either held in a fixed position in the static disc method or rotated at a given speed in the rotating disc method. Samples of dissolution medium are collected at predetermined times, filtered and analyzed for drug content.

In both the methods discussed above, the surface area through which the dissolution of the drug takes place is assumed to be constant. Therefore, the dissolution rate of the drug obtained from these methods is expressed as $mg/cm^2.min$. *i.e.* the amount of the drug dissolved per unit of time and unit of the surface area. This is referred to as intrinsic dissolution rate and is different from the dissolution rates estimated by using other methods in which the surface area for dissolution is not constant.

Factors affecting Dissolution

Many experiments proved that the disintegration time of a solid dosage form is unable to predict the bioavailability of drug from the dosage form. From the basic principles one can expect a linear relationship between drug absorption and dissolution rather than disintegration, particularly for poorly water-soluble drugs. Dissolution tests *in-vitro* measures the rate and extent of dissolution of a drug in an aqueous medium from a dosage form. Extensive research work on *in-vitro* dissolution and in-vivo availability of drugs revealed the fact that *in-vitro* dissolution test can be used to predict the in-vivo performance of the dosage form. There are a number of factors that must be considered when performing a dissolution test.

Factors related to apparatus

1. ***Size and shape:*** The size and shape of the dissolution vessel may affect the rate and extent of dissolution. For example, the vessel may range in size from several milliliters to several liters. The shape may be flat or round bottomed so that in one case the tablet may lie in a different position in different experiments and in other case it may be in one position in all the experiments. The flow pattern of fluids and the degree of turbulence created may also be influenced by the shape.
2. **Eccentricity of the stirring device:** According to USP, stirring shaft must rotate smoothly without significant wobbling as it may lead to uneven distribution of medium. An eccentricity of 0.005 in (0.11 mm) at a distance of inch from the chuck will be barely perceptible but at 6 in will amount to 0.3 in (o.75mm) which is maximum that can be tolerated.
3. **Vibrations:** Vibration can lead to variable flow patterns of the liquid and introducing unwanted energy to the dynamic system which may significantly change the dissolution rate. The speeds of rotational device in official compendium are 50 or 100 rpm.
4. **Alignment of the stirring elements:** Tilt and Agitation intensity are two important parameters to control as Increase in tilt increases dissolution rate (Tilt ecess in 1.5 degree may increase dissolution rate from 2% to 25% in USP II) and change in agitation condition markedly affects the diffusion controlled dissolution as it affects the thickness of diffusion layer.
5. **Temperature:** Since drug solubility is a temperature dependent so a careful temperature control during the dissolution process is very important.

Factors related to dissolution media

1. **pH of dissolution media:** The acidic solution tends to disintegrate the tablets slightly faster than the water or buffers of natural pH and thus can increase the dissolution by enhancing the effective surface area. Thus proper media should be selected on the basis of the pH dependent solubility and release pattern. Various investigators have used dilute gastric juice, 0.1 N HCl, phosphate buffer, acetate buffer, simulated

gastric juice, water, and simulated intestinal juice, depending on the nature of the drug product and the location in the GIT where the drug is expected to dissolve.

2. **Surface tension:** Surfactants and wetting agents have shown a significant effect on the dissolution rate of drugs and their release from dosage form by lowering the contact angle and increasing penetration.
3. **Viscosity:** For diffusion controlled dissolution process, dissolution rate decreases with increase in viscosity due to lesser flow and low permeability in the formulation.
4. **Nature of medium:** The nature and the quantity of the dissolution medium will also affect the dissolution test. Which medium is best is a matter of considerable controversy. However, the medium selected for the study must be able to show the in-vitro and in-vivo correlation. In selecting the volume of dissolution medium, the solubility as well as the amount of drug in the dosage form must be considered. Usually, a volume of medium larger than the amount of solvent needed to completely dissolve the drug is used in such test.

The design of the dissolution test apparatus must consider all the factors discussed above. To-date there is no single apparatus and test that can be used for all drug products. Each drug product must be evaluated with a dissolution test that best correlates to its in-vivo bioavailability. The United States Pharmacopoeia has played an important role in the development of dissolution standards for many drug products.

The pharmacopoeia specifies the conditions under which a dissolution test should be carried out for a specific drug product. The specifications include the apparatus, volume and nature of dissolution medium, stirring speed, temperature of dissolution medium, and the time periods after which samples have to be collected for analysis.

Usually, the report on a dissolution test will state that a certain percentage of the labeled amount of the drug product must dissolve within a specified period of time. In practice, the absolute amount of a drug in a drug product may vary from tablet to tablet. Therefore, a number of tablets from each lot are usually tested to get a representative dissolution rate for the product.

Control of Variables in Dissolution Testing

There are a number of methods and equipment for the assessment of dissolution rate of drug products. There are several equipment and operating variables associated with dissolution testing. Even if the discussion is restricted to the official methods, the problems of variable control in dissolution testing still exist. Variation of about 25% or more occurs with the same type of equipment and procedure. The variables may or may not exert a profound effect on the dissolution rate of the drug, depending upon the particular dosage form.

The basket method is more sensitive to clogging due to gummy materials. Fine drug particles and sticky materials can clog up the basket screen and decrease the dissolution rate by creating a local non-sink condition for dissolution. The centering and alignment of the paddle is critical in the paddle method. Turbulence can create an increased agitation, resulting in a higher dissolution rate. Wobbling and tilting due to worn equipment should be avoided. The basket method is relatively insensitive to the tilting effect. Degassing of the dissolution medium is to be carried out before testing, since the dissolved gases may form air bubbles on the surface of the dosage form and can affect dissolution in both the basket and paddle methods.

For many drug products, the dissolution rates are higher with the paddle method than the basket method. Dissolution rates obtained at 50 rpm with the paddle method may be comparable with the dissolution rates obtained at 100 rpm with the basket method. It was observed that the dissolution rates obtained with the paddle method from theophylline tablets of 4.0 kg hardness at 50 rpm were higher than that of basket method. This difference in the dissolution rates was not observed when the tablets of 6.8 kg hardness were tested at 125 rpm by both the methods. However, the dissolution rates were increased with increase in stirring rate. No simple correlation can be made for dissolution results obtained with different methods.

It is generally impossible to make meaningful conclusions about bioavailability from dissolution data alone, unless an in-vitro and in-vivo correlation has been well established. The use of various testing methods makes it even more difficult to interpret dissolution results, because there is no simple correlation among dissolution results obtained with various methods. In the absence of in-vivo data, the selection of the dissolution method is based on the type of drug product to be tested. For example, a gummy preparation may clog up the basket screen, a low-density preparation may be poorly wetted in the basket method, and therefore the paddle method is preferred.

In-vitro and *In-vivo* Correlations

Bioavailability testing is a complicated and expensive way to ensure the proper performance of drug products. Great economies in time, labor, and money would be possible if in-vitro tests could be developed that would predict bioavailability. Such in-vitro tests, if available, could be used as quality control tests and compendial standards and would help to ensure that every drug product performs as expected. It is not that simple to predict the biological performance of a drug product based on in-vitro test results alone. Bioavailability problems have arisen with tetracycline tablets, nitrofurantoin tablets and digoxin tablets in products that meet all compendial tests and have similar in-vitro performance.

Development and optimization of formulation is an integral part of manufacturing and marketing of any therapeutic agent which is indeed a time consuming and costly process. Optimization process may require alteration in formulation composition, manufacturing process, equipment and batch sizes. If these types of changes are applied to a formulation, studies in human healthy volunteers may be required to prove that the new formulation is bioequivalent with the old one. Certainly, implementation of these requirements not only halts the marketing of the new formulation but also increases the cost of the optimization processes. It would be, desirable, therefore, to develop *in vitro* tests that reflect bioavailability data.

Several research publications describe a good correlation between the in-vitro dissolution profile and bioavailability of the dosage form. Quantitative linear correlations between in-vivo data and dissolution data have been found with different brands of prolonged released amphetamine, aspirin tablets, and different esters of erythromycin and different salts of penicillin V. An excellent correlation was observed between the dissolution rate of oxazepam tablet and the peak concentration of oxazepam in the blood following oral administration of the tablet. In another study, it was found that the percent of salicylamide in solution and the mean percentage of the dose excreted in urine were linearly correlated.

The term correlation is frequently employed within the pharmaceutical and related sciences to describe the relationship that exists between variables. Mathematically, the term correlation means interdependence between quantitative or qualitative data or relationship between measurable variables and ranks. From biopharmaceutical standpoint, correlation could be referred to as the relationship between appropriate *in vitro* release characteristics and *in vivo* bioavailability parameters. Two definitions of IVIVC have been proposed by the USP and by the FDA.

United State Pharmacopoeia (USP) definition: The establishment of a rational relationship *between* a biological property, and a parameter derived from a biological property produced by a dosage form, and a physicochemical property or characteristic of the same dosage form.

Food and Drug Administration (FDA) definition: IVIVC is a predictive mathematical model describing the relationship between an *in vitro* property of a dosage form and a relevant *in vivo* response. Generally, the *in vitro* property is the rate or extent of drug dissolution or release while the *in vivo* response is the plasma drug concentration or amount of drug absorbed.

Correlation Levels

Five correlation levels have been defined in the IVIVC FDA guidance (3). The concept of correlation level is based upon the ability of the correlation to reflect the complete plasma drug level-time profile which will result from administration of the given dosage form.

Level A Correlation

A correlation of this type is generally linear and represents a point-to-point relationship between *in vitro* dissolution and the *in vivo* input rate (e.g., the *in vivo* dissolution of the drug from the dosage form). In a linear correlation, the *in vitro* dissolution and *in vivo* input curves may be directly super imposable or may be made to be superimposable by the use of a scaling factor. Nonlinear correlations, while uncommon, may also be appropriate. Alternative approaches to developing a Level A IVIVC are possible....Whatever the method used to establish a Level A IVIVC, the model should predict the entire *in vivo* time course from the *in vitro* data. In this context, the model refers to the relationship between *in vitro* dissolution of an ER dosage form and an *in vivo* response such as plasma drug concentration or amount of drug absorbed.

Generally, percent of drug absorbed may be calculated by means of model dependent techniques such as Wagner-Nelson procedure or Loo-Riegelman method or by model-independent numerical deconvolution. These techniques represent a major advance over the single-point approach in that these methodologies utilize all of the dissolution and plasma level data available to develop the correlations.

The purpose of Level A correlation is to define a direct relationship between *in vivo* data such that measurement of *in vitro* dissolution rate alone is sufficient to determine the biopharmaceutical rate of the dosage form. In the case of a level A correlation, an *in vitro* dissolution curve can serve as a surrogate for *in vivo* performance. Therefore, a change in manufacturing site, method of manufacture, raw material supplies, minor formulation modification, and even product strength using the same formulation can be justified without the need for additional human studies. It is an excellent quality control procedure since it is predictive of the dosage form's *in vivo* performance.

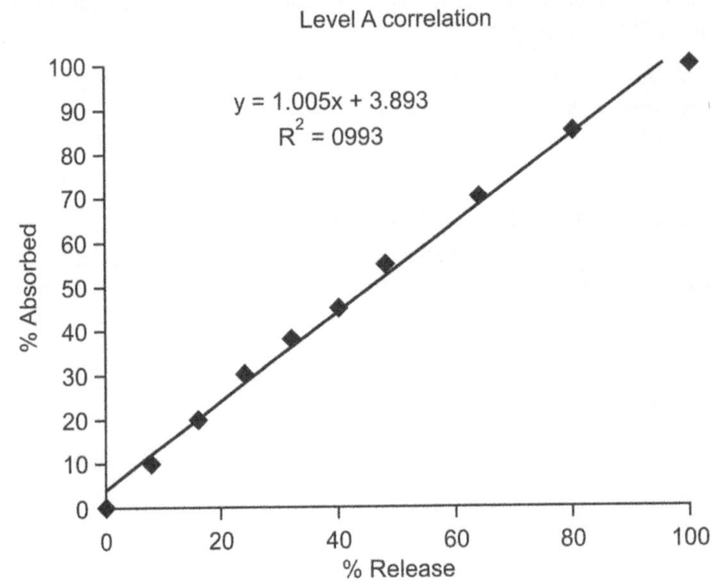

Fig. 13.10 Level A correlation.

Level B Correlation

A level B IVIVC utilizes the principles of statistical moment analysis. In this level of correlation, the mean *in vitro* dissolution time (MDT_{vitro}) of the product is compared to either mean *in vivo* residence time (MRT) or the mean *in vivo* dissolution time (MDT_{vivo}). MRT, MDT_{vitro} and MDT_{vivo} will be defined throughout the manuscript where appropriate. Although a level B correlation uses all of the *in vitro* and *in vivo* data, it is not considered to be a point-to point correlation, since there are a number of different *in vivo* curves that will produce similar mean residence time values.

Drawbacks: A level B correlation does not uniquely reflect the actual *in vivo* plasma level curves. Therefore, one can not rely upon a level B correlation alone to justify formulation modification, manufacturing site change, excipients source change, etc. In addition *in vitro* data from such a correlation could not be used to justify the extremes of quality control standards.

Level C Correlation

In this level of correlation, one dissolution time point (t50%, t90%, etc.) is compared to one mean pharmacokinetic parameter such as AUC, tmax or Cmax. Therefore, it represents a single point correlation and doses not reflect the entire shape of the plasma drug concentration curve, which is indeed a crucial factor that is a good indicative of the performance of modified-release products.

Drawbacks: This is the weakest level of correlation as partial relationship between absorption and dissolution is established. Due to its obvious limitations, the usefulness of a Level C correlation is limited in predicting *in vivo* drug performance.

The usefulness of this correlation level is subject to the same caveats as a Level B correlation in its ability to support product and site changes as well as justification of quality control standard extremes. Level C correlations can be useful in the early stages of formulation development when pilot formulations are being selected. While the information may be useful in formulation development, waiver of an *in vivo* bioequivalence study (bio-waiver) is generally not possible.

Multiple-level C correlation

A multiple level C correlation relates one or several pharmacokinetic parameters of interest (Cmax, AUC, or any other suitable parameters) to the amount of drug dissolved at several time points of the dissolution profile. A multiple point level C correlation may be used to justify a bio-waiver, provided that the correlation has been established over the entire dissolution profile with one or more pharmacokinetic parameters of interest.

A relationship should be demonstrated at each time point at the same parameter such that the effect on the *in vivo* performance of any change in dissolution can be assessed. If such a multiple level C correlation is achievable, then the development of a level A correlation is also likely. A multiple Level C correlation should be based on at least three dissolution time points covering the early, middle, and late stages of the dissolution profile.

Level D correlation

Level D correlation is a rank order and qualitative analysis and is not considered useful for regulatory purposes. It is not a formal correlation but serves as an aid in the development of a formulation or processing procedure.

Various parameters used in IVIVC depending on the level

Level	In vitro	In vivo
A	Dissolution curve	Input (absorption) curves
B	Statistical moments: MDT	Statistical moments: MRT, MAT, etc
C	Disintegration time, Time to have 10, 50, 90% dissolved, Dissolution rate, Dissolution efficiency	Cmax, Tmax, Ka, Time to have 10, 50, 90% absorbed, AUC (total cumulative)

Fig. 13.10 Parameters used for IVIVC calculations.

Methodology

Establishing an IVIVC is nothing more complicated than trying to reproduce all the complex phenomena that lead to the *in vivo* release and solubilization of the API in the gut in a "simple" *in vitro* system like a vessel agitated with a paddle! In contrast to *in vivo* studies, *in vitro* methods are less "standardized," as USP Apparatus 1 to 4 could be used with various media (HCl, simple buffer, addition of surfactant or enzymes, etc.) and various technical parameters (e.g. volume, rate).

***In vivo* Data**

The *in vivo* data are derived from the plasma concentration curve. Various phenomena can occur after administration of drug depending of the route of administration. The plasma concentration curve is a global representation; it depends on drug input within the blood, which depends on the dosage form and the properties of the drug, and thereafter its pharmacokinetic input processes.

The disposition of the drug afterwards depends only on the drug and patient. As stated by the FDA, absorption curves can be calculated by various methods by estimating "the *in vivo* absorption or dissolution time course using an appropriate deconvolution technique for each formulation and subject (e.g.,Wagner-Nelson, numerical deconvolution)."After the calculations are performed, the input curve, known as "absorption" curve, is presented as the percentage of the fraction of dose (%FD:0–100%) absorbed versus time. This absorption curve represents the sum of all the phenomena such as release or dissolution but also the permeability through the intestinal membranes. To obtain a good estimation of the absorption curves, a sufficient number of well-positioned samples are required.

***In vitro* Data**

In the case of oral administration of a solid dosage form, the limiting factor for the appearance of the drug in the blood could be the release from the drug dosage form, or the solubility of the active ingredient or the pure permeability through the intestinal membrane (mainly for Class III and IV of the BCS). In case of solubility-limited product (Class II and IV of BCS), the absorption could be governed by physicochemical characteristics of the API (such as solubility, dissolution rate, particle size, crystal shape, polymorphism, pKa, stability in GIT) and not by its permeability or formulation.

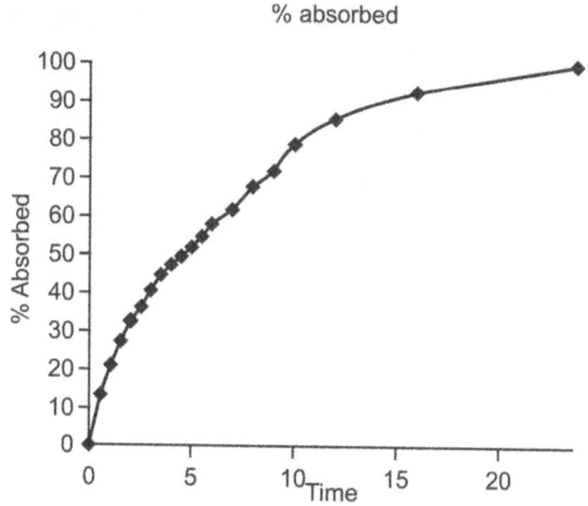

Fig. 13.11 % Absorbed vs. time Graph.

In the case of release-limited formulations, the absorption is limited by the drug release from the drug dosage form. As described above, to establish IVIVC, the release must be the limiting factor; in this case, solubility (or dissolution rate) and permeability must be faster than the release. Correlations are always possible with Class I drugs and depend on the relative magnitude of the various factors versus the release rate for the other classes. The active substance is the core of any formulation; the physico-chemical characteristics and the stability of the API are the main points to be considered first. In the case of oral products, there are two types of formulations. The first is an immediate-release (IR) product that disintegrates and disperses rapidly after administration. The second is an extended-release (ER) formulation, which keeps its integrity throughout much of the GIT.

Various dissolution tests exist and can be used to generate the *in vitro* data. In order to compare the results, the same method must be used for all the formulations. The *in vitro* dissolution curves depend on the release characteristics of the formulation and manufacturing process, the characteristics of the API such as the solubility and dissolution rate, and the apparatus, method parameters, dissolution medium. The dissolution curves are expressed as the percentage dissolved versus time and should usually reach 100% at infinity (or in practice at the end of dissolution).

The best dissolution method for *in vivo—in vitro* correlation is, obviously, the method that describes what happens *in vivo*. The main factors that can influence drug release *in vivo* includes pH, surfactant, enzyme, movement and ionic strength etc). All of these factors cannot be easily reproduced *in vitro* by a simple dissolution method. In addition, the relative importance of these factors is not similar if the subject is in fed or fasted state; in the fed state, food also has a direct influence on the API or formulation behavior.

In vitro Media

Usually, aqueous based media are used, most of them being described in pharmacopeias. To simulate gastric media, the simplest one is composed of 0.1 N/0.01 HCl. A more complicated medium called simulated intestine fluid (SIF) can also be used. For other pHs, acetate or phosphate buffers are usually used (or sometime TRIS). For specific applications (e.g. poorly soluble drugs), the pharmacopeias recommend the addition of either enzymes or surfactant. Noncompendial media are also described to simulate the fasted and fed states *in vivo*: fasted state simulated intestinal fluid (FaSSIF) and fed state simulated intestinal fluid (FeSSIF). These media try to reproduce, not the direct food influence on the formulations, but rather the secretions occurring in either fasted or fed state in the small intestine.

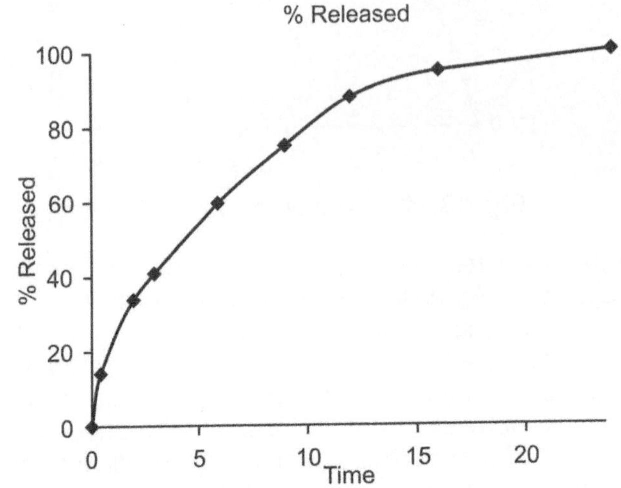

Fig. 13.12 % Release vs. time Graph.

Calculation of IVIVC: After calculating % absorbed and % release, both are plotted on a graph and a regression line is draw to tell the significance of correlation

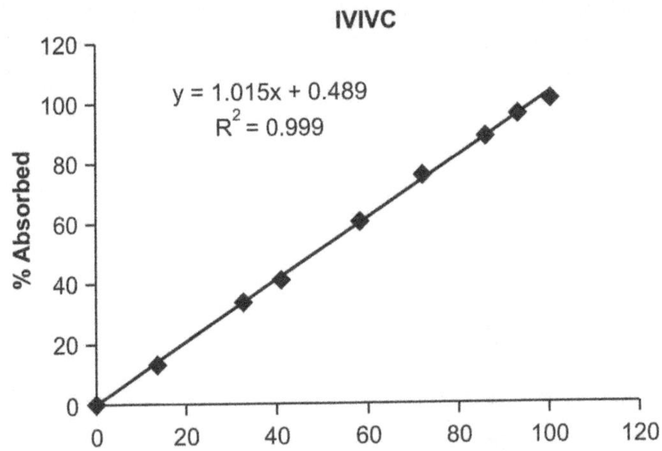

Fig. 13.13 % Absorbed vs. % Release plot.

Developing the Correlation

The most commonly seen process for developing a Level A IVIVC is to (1) develop formulations with different release rates, such as slow, medium, fast, or a single release rate if dissolution is condition independent; obtain *in vitro* dissolution profiles and *in vivo* plasma concentration profiles for these formulations; (3) estimate the *in vivo* absorption or dissolution time course using an appropriate deconvolution technique for each formulation and subject (e.g., Wagner-Nelson, numerical deconvolution). These three steps establish the IVIVC model. Alternative approaches to developing Level A IVIVCs are possible. Further general information follows:

- The IVIVC relationship should be demonstrated consistently with two or more formulations with different release rates to result in corresponding differences in absorption profiles. Although an IVIVC can be defined with a minimum of two formulations with different release rates, three or more formulations with different release rates are recommended. Exceptions to this approach (i.e., use of only one formulation) may be considered for formulations for which *in vitro* dissolution is independent of the dissolution test conditions (e.g., medium, agitation, pH).
- Ideally, formulations should be compared in a single study with a crossover design.
- If one or more of the formulations (highest or lowest release rate formulations) does not show the same relationship between *in vitro* dissolution and *in vivo* performance compared with the other formulations, the correlation may still be used within the range of release rates encompassed by the remaining formulations.
- The *in vitro* dissolution methodology should adequately discriminate among formulations. Dissolution testing can be carried out during the formulation screening stage using several methods. Once a discriminating system is developed, dissolution conditions should be the same for all formulations tested in the biostudy for development of the correlation and should be fixed before further steps towards correlation evaluation are undertaken.
- During the early stages of correlation development, dissolution conditions may be altered to attempt to develop a 1-to-1 correlation between the *in vitro* dissolution profile and the *in vivo* dissolution profile.
- Time scaling may be used as long as the time scaling factor is the same for all formulations. Different time scales for each formulation indicate absence of an IVIVC.

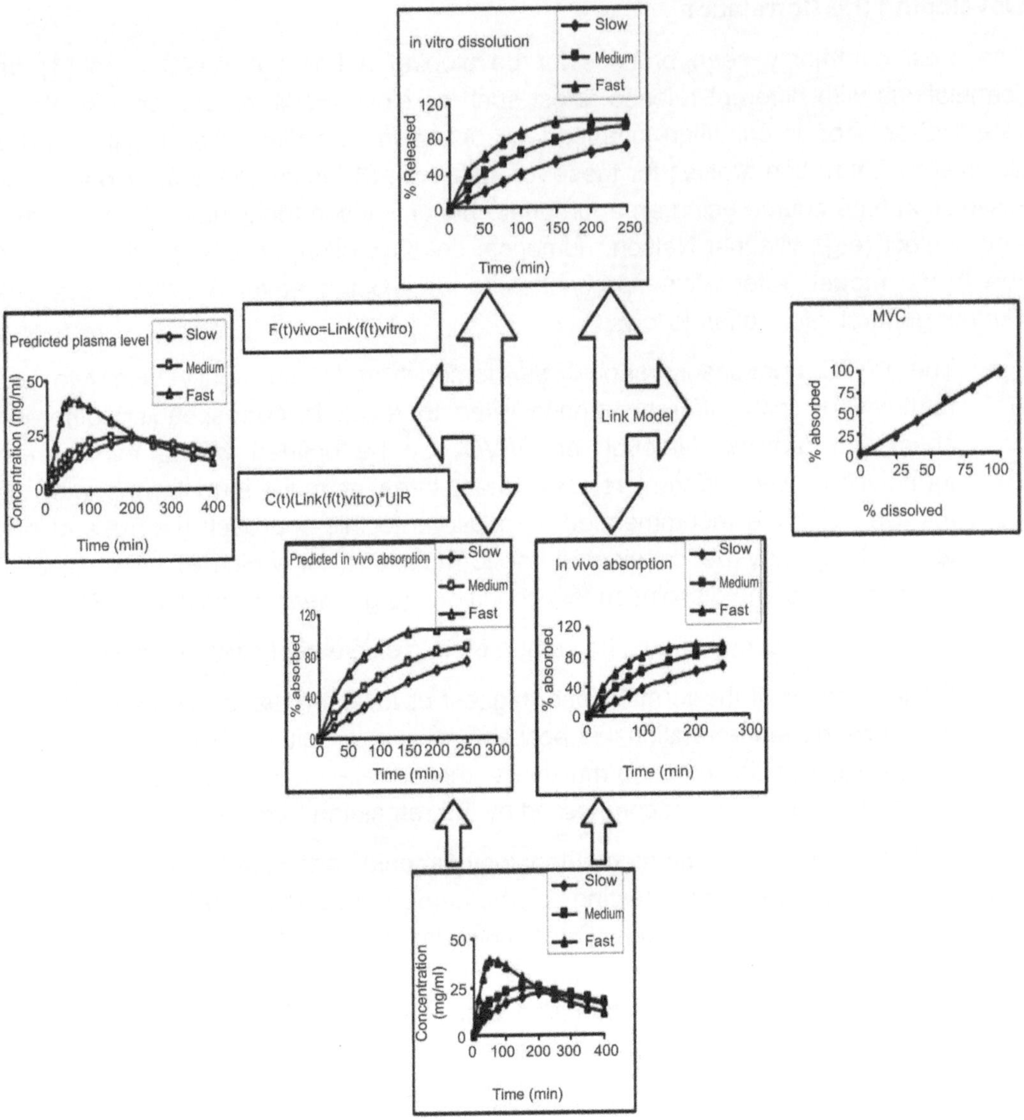

Fig. 13.14 Steps Involved in IVIVC.

IVIVC and BCS

As the drug dissolution and intestinal permeability are the fundamental parameters governing rate and extent of drug absorption, drugs could be categorized into high/low solubility and permeability classes. Thus, the expectations regarding IVIVC could be stated more clearly as are summarized.

IVIVC expectations for immediate release products based on BCS

Class	Solubility	Permeability	Absorption rate control	IVIVC expectations for Immediate release product
I	High	High	Gastric emptying	IVIVC expected, if dissolution rate is slower than gastric emptying rate, otherwise limited or no correlations
II	Low	High	Dissolution	IVIVC expected, if *in vitro* dissolution rate is similar to *in vivo* dissolution rate, unless dose is very high.
III	High	Low	Permeability	Absorption (permeability) is rate determining and limited or no IVIVC with dissolution
IV	Low	Low	Case by Case	Limited or no IVIVC is expected

Fig. 13.15 IVIVC and BCS relationship.

The FDA ranked the levels as follows: A Level A IVIVC is considered the most informative and is recommended, if possible. Multiple Level C correlations can be as useful as Level A correlations. However, if a multiple Level C correlation is possible, and then a Level A correlation is also likely and is preferred. Level C correlations can be useful in the early stages of formulation development when pilot formulations are being selected. Level B correlations are least useful for regulatory purposes.

Further Reading

1. Aristides Dokoumetzidis, Panos Macheras, (2006); Historical Perspectives A century of dissolution research: From Noyes and Whitney to the Biopharmaceutics Classification System. International Journal of Pharmaceutics, 321, 1–11.
2. Blanquet,S.;Zeijdner,E.;Beyssac,E.;Meunier, J-P.;Denis, S.;Havenaar, R.;Alric,M. (2004); A dynamic artificial gastrointestinal system for studying the behavior of orally administered drug dosage forms under various physiological conditions. Pharm.Res.,21,37–49.
3. Deirdre M. D'Arcy, Owen I. Corrigan, Anne Marie Healy, (2006); Evaluation of hydrodynamics in the basket dissolution apparatus using computational fluid dynamics—Dissolution rate implications. European journal of pharmaceutical sciences, 27, 259–267.
4. Ekarat Jantratid, Vincenzo De Maio, Emanuela Ronda, Valentina Mattavelli, Maria Vertzoni, Jennifer B. Dressman, (2009) Application of biorelevant dissolution tests to the prediction of in vivo performance of diclofenac sodium from an oral modified-release pellet dosage form. European Journal of Pharmaceutical Sciences, 37 ,434–441.

5. Galia,E.; Nicolaides,E.;Hörter,D.;Löbenberg, R.;Reppas C.;Dressman J. B. (1998); Evaluation of various dissolution media for predicting in vivo performance of Class I and II drugs. Pharm.Res.,15,698–705.
6. Jaber Emami, (2006);In vitro - In vivo Correlation: From Theory to Applications J Pharm Pharmaceut Sci, 9 (2): 169-189.
7. Jantratid, E., Janssen, N., Reppas, C., Dressman, J.B., (2008). Dissolution media simulating conditions in the proximal human gastrointestinal tract: an update. Pharm. Res. 25, 1663–1676.
8. Jelena Paroj˘ci´c, Dragana Vasiljevi´c, Svetlana Ibri´c, Zorica Djuri, (2008) Tablet disintegration and drug dissolution in viscous media: Paracetamol IR tablets, International Journal of Pharmaceutics, 355, 93-99.
9. J-M. Cardot, E. Beyssac, and M.Alric; (2007); In Vitro–In Vivo Correlation: Importance of Dissolution in IVIVC, Dissolution Technologies, Feb, 15-19
10. Klein, S., Rudolph, M.W., Skalsky, B., Petereit, H.U., Dressman, J.B., 2008. Use of the BioDis to generate a physiologically relevant IVIVC. J. Control. Release 130, 216–219.
11. Klein, S., Wunderlich, M., Dressman, J., 2005. Development of dissolution tests on the basis of gastrointestinal physiology. In: Dressman, J., Krämer, J. (Eds.), Pharmaceutical Dissolution Testing. Taylor & Francis Group, LLC, Boca Raton, FL.
12. Kortejärvi, H., Mikkola, J., Bäckman, M., Antila, S., Marvola, M., 2002. Development of level A, B and C in vitro-in vivo correlations for modified-release levosimendan capsules. Int. J. Pharm. 241, 87–95.
13. Lue BM, Nielsen FS, Magnussen T, Schou HM, Kristensen K, Jacobsen LO, Müllertz A., (2008); Using biorelevant dissolution to obtain IVIVC of solid dosage forms containing a poorly-soluble model compound. Eur J Pharm Biopharm. 69(2):648-57.
14. McCarthy, L.G., Kosiol, C., Healy, A.M., Bradley, G., Sexton, J.C., Corrigan, O.I., (2003), Simulating the hydrodynamic conditions in the United States Pharmacopeia paddle dissolution apparatus. AAPS PharmSciTech. 4 (Article 22).
15. Persson, E.M., Gustafsson, A.S., Carlsson, A.S., Nilsson, R.G., Knutson, L., Forsell, P., Hanisch, G., Lennernas, H., Abrahamsson, B., (2005). The effects of food on the dissolution of poorly soluble drugs in human and in model small intestinal fluids. Pharm. Res. 22, 2141–2151.
16. Saccone C D, Tessore J, Olivera Silvino A., and Nora S. Meneces,(2004) Statistical Properties of the Dissolution Test of USP, Dissolution Technologies, 25-29.
17. Saccone CD, Meneces NS, Tessore J. (2005); Statistical properties of the USP dissolution test with pooled samples. J Pharm Sci Technol. 59(5):310-9.
18. Souliman,S.;Blanquet,S.;Beyssac,E.;Cardot, J-M. (2006); A level A in vitro/in vivo correlation in fasted and fed states using different methods:Applied to solid immediate release oral dosage form. Eur.J.Pharm.Sci., 27,72–79.

19. Vertzoni M, Dressman J, Butler J, Hempenstall J, Reppas C. (2005), Simulation of fasting gastric conditions and its importance for the in vivo dissolution of lipophilic compounds. Eur J Pharm Biopharm. 60(3):413-7.

20. Vinod P. Shah a, Assad Noory, Carol Noory, Bruce McCullough , Sanford Clarke, Richard Everett, Helen Naviasky, B.N. Srinivasan, Don Fortman, Jerome P. Skelly, (1995); vitro dissolution of sparingly water-soluble drug dosage forms., International Journal of Pharmaceutics 125 99-106.

Appendix-I

Estimation of Area Under the Curve

There are several methods for estimating the area under a drug concentration-time curve. The most common method of estimating the area is the use of the trapezoidal rule. The plasma drug concentration versus time plot is made first on an ordinary Cartensian graph paper (Figs A.1 and A.2). It is divided into several trapezoids at the sampling time points. The areas of individual trapezoids are calculated and summed to get the area under the curve.

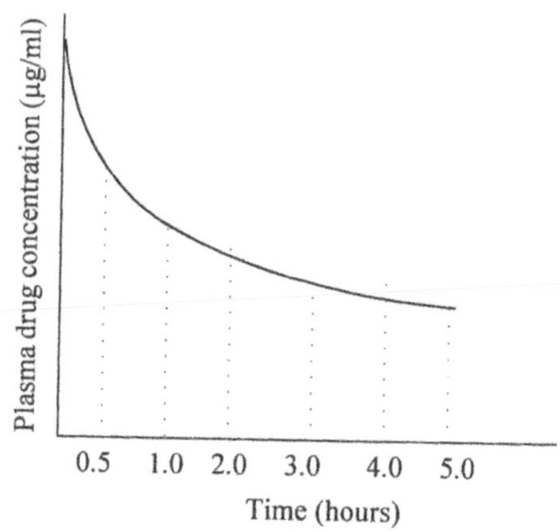

Fig. A.1 Drug concentration (μg/ml) versus time (hours) plot of data presented in Table A.1. Trapezoids are made by joining data points.

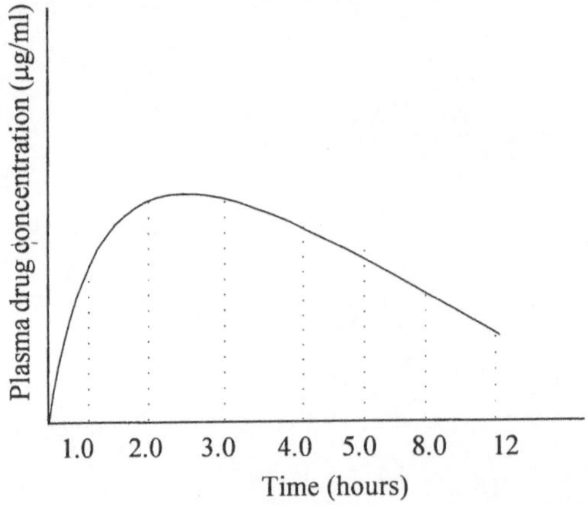

Fig. A.2 Drug concentration (μg/ml) as a function of time (hours) after an oral adminstration. The data points are connected by straight line segments, to apply trapezoidal rule. (data from Table A.2).

The area bounded by the trapezoids approximates the area under the curve. The assumption is that the trapezoid side (curve) is straight and is valid when the number of data points is more and closer.

The area of a trapezoid is equal to the product of one half of the sum of heights, and width. The area under the plasma drug levels versus time curve is approximated by the following equation

$$\text{Area} = (1/2)(C_1 + C_2)(t_2 - t_1) + (1/2)(C_2 + C_3)(t_3 - t_2) + (1/2)(C_3 + C_4)(t_4 - t_3) \ldots\ldots + (1/2)(C_{n-1} + C_n)(t_n - t_{n-1})$$

Where C and t represent plasma drug concentration and time, respectively. The subscripts refer to the sample numbers.

Table A.1 Drug concentration as a function of time after I.V. injection (bolus)

Sample	Time (hr)	Concentration (μg/ml)	Area
1	0	10.0*	4.27
2	0.5	7.07	3.02
3	1.0	5.0	3.75
4	2.0	2.5	1.86
5	3.0	1.25	0.94
6	4.0	0.625	0.47
7	5.0	0.313	–
		Total	14.31 μg-hr/ml

* Estimated by extrapolating the semi-logarithmic plot of the data

Table A.2 Drug Concentration as a Function of Time after oral Administration

Sample	Time (hr)	Concentration (μg/ml)	Area
1	0	0.0	2.90
2	1.0	5.8	6.45
3	2	7.1	7.00
4	3	6.9	6.55
5	4	6.2	2.75
6	6	4.8	2.08
7	8	3.5	0.68
8	12	19	–
		Total	28.41 μg-hr/ml.

If the sampling time intervals are equal, then

$$AUC = \frac{C_1 + C_2}{2}\,\Delta t + \frac{C_2 + C_3}{2}\,\Delta t + \frac{C_3 + C_4}{2}\,\Delta t + \frac{(C_{n-1} + C_n)}{2}\,\Delta t$$

$$AUC = \frac{\Delta t}{2}\,(C_1 + 2C_2 + 2C_3 \ldots\ldots + 2C_{n-1} + C_n)$$

A general form for the calculation AUC is given by the following equation

$$AUC = \sum_{i=0}^{i=n} \frac{C_{n-1} + C_n}{2}\,(t_n - t_{n-1})$$

The application of the trapezoidal rule in the estimation of AUC is illustrated in Tables A.1 and A.2.

Area under the curve of the first, second and fifth trapezoids of data shown in Table A.1 are calculated as follows

$$\text{Area (1)} = (1/2)\ (10.0 + 7.07)\ (0.5 - 0)$$
$$= 4.27\ \mu g - hr/ml$$

$$\text{Area (2)} = (1/2)\ (7.07 + 5.0)\ (1 - 0.5)$$
$$= 3.02\ \mu g - hr/ml$$

$$\text{Area (5)} = (1/2)\ (1.25 + 0.625)\ (4.0 - 3.0)$$
$$= 0.94\ \mu g - hr/ml$$

Appendix-II

Integration Method for the Estimation of AUC

The AUC calculated using the trapezoidal rule is the area under the curve from t = 0 to the last sampling time. In order to calculate the AUC from t = 0 to t = $\propto$, an integration of the equation $C = Co.e^{-kt}$ with respect to time is carried.

$$\int_0^{\alpha} C.dt = \int_0^{\alpha} C0.e^{-Kt}.dt \qquad \text{A1}$$

The term C. dt is nothing but AUC_0^{α}

$$\therefore \quad AUC_0^{\propto} = \int_0^{\alpha} C0\ e^{-Kt}.dt \qquad \text{A2}$$

$$= C0 \left| \frac{e^{-K\alpha}}{-K} + \frac{e^{-K.0}}{K} \right|$$

$$AUC_0^{\propto} = C0 \left| \frac{e^{-\alpha}}{-K} + \frac{e^{0}}{K} \right|$$

Since $e^{-\propto} = 0$ and $e^0 = 1$

$$AUC_0^{\propto} = C0 \left| O + \frac{1}{K} \right|$$

$$AUC_0^{\alpha} = C0/K \qquad \text{A.3}$$

Where, C0 is extrapolated concentration at time zero and K is the first order elimination rate constant.

At times, the area under the plasma level time curve is extrapolated to $t = \infty$. In this case, the residual area AUC_t^∞ is calculated as follows.

$$AUC_0^\infty = C^* / K \qquad A.4$$

Where C^* is the last observed plasma concentration at t and K = first order elimination rate constant.

Equation A.4 is also used to estimate $[AUC]_t^\infty$ from oral data, provided that C^* is on the terminal linear portion of the graph.

Appendix-III

The Method of Residuals

The method of residuals, also known as a feathering or peeling technique, is useful in the pharmacokinetic analysis of the data that can be described by a biexponential equation. For example, 1. the time course of the metabolite levels in plasma following an I.V bolus administration of a drug that follows one compartment open model, 2. unchanged drug levels in plasma versus time data following oral administration of a drug that follows a one component open model and 3. unchanged drug levels in plasma versus time data following an I.V. bolus of a drug that follows two-compartment model, etc.

Let us apply the method of residuals to plasma concentration versus time data obtained following oral administration of a drug that follows one compartment open model. The data presented in Table A3 is used to explain the method.

Table A.3 Plasma concentrations and "Residuals" versus time

Time (hr)	Observed drug conc. C (μg/ml)	Extrapolated C (μg/ml)	Residual Conc. μg/ml
0.25	2.2	11.4	9.2
0.50	3.8	10.9	7.1
0.75	5.0	10.6	5.6
1.0	5.8	10.1	4.3

Table A.3 *Contd...*

1.5	6.8	9.4	2.6
2.0	7.1	8.7	1.6
2.5	7.1	8.1	1.0
3.0	6.9	7.5	0.6
4.0	6.2	6.4	0.2
6.0	4.8	4.8	—
8.0	3.5	3.5	—
12.0	1.9	1.9	—
18.0	0.8	0.8	—
24.0	0.3	0.3	—

The equation that describes plasma drug level versus time data is given by

$$C = \frac{KaFX0}{Vd\,(Ka - K)}\,(e^{-Kt} - e^{-Kat}) \qquad A.5$$

Equation A5 is a biexponential equation. The concentration of the drug in plasma (C) is influenced by both the absorption process and elimination process. However, after some time t, the absorption of drug will be completed and elimination of the drug still continues. Further, in general the value of absorption rate constant, Ka is several times more than the elimination rate constant, K. As a result, after the post absorptive phase, the plasma drug level versus time data can be explained by a mono-exponential equation, given below.

$$C = \frac{KaFX0}{Vd\,(Ka - K)}\,e^{-Kt} \qquad A.6$$

or

$$\log C = \log \frac{KaFX0}{Vd\,(Ka - K)} - Kt/2.303 \qquad A.7$$

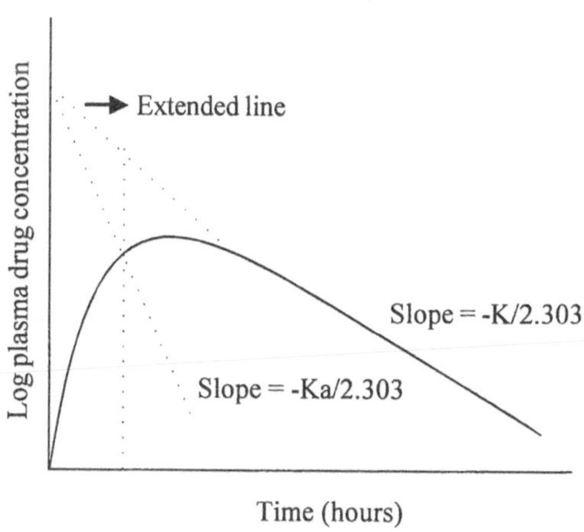

Fig. A.3 Plot of log of observed plasma drug concentration and 'residuals' versus time for an orally administered drug absorbed by a first-order process.

Hence, a plot of log plasma concentration of drug versus time is a curve initially and becomes a straight line after some time (Fig. A.3). The terminal linear portion can be described by the Equation A.7 and the slope of the line is equal to -K/2.303. The elimination half-life is equal to 0.693/K. This straight line can be extended to cut Y-axis to get a intercept = log [(KaFX0)/ Vd (Ka-K)]. The exptrapolated line (dashed line) and the terminal linear portion is governed by Equation A.6.

Now, the method of residuals is applied by subtracting the actual plasma concentration of drug at a time point from plasma concentration of drug on extended line (dashed line) at the same point.

Residual conc. = Drug conc. on extended line - Drug conc. on the curve. A.8

$$Cr = \frac{KaFX0}{Vd\,(Ka-K)}\, e^{-Kt} - \frac{KaFX0}{Vd\,(Ka-K)}\,(e^{-Kt} - e^{-Kat}) \qquad A.9$$

Therefore,

$$Cr = \frac{KaFX0}{Vd\,(Ka-K)}\, e^{-Kat} \qquad A.10$$

or

$$\log Cr = \log \frac{KaFX0}{Vd\,(Ka-K)} - Kat/2.303 \qquad A.11$$

Therefore, a plot of log Cr versus time gives a straight line with a slope = -Ka / 2.303 and the intercept of log [KaFX0 / Vd (Ka-K)]. From the slope, the absorption rate constant, Ka, can be estimated. The absorption half-life is equal to 0.693 / Ka. In this method of calculation it is important to remember that the following assumptions are made:

1. It is assumed that Ka is at least five times larger than K, if not neither constant can be determined accurately.
2. It is assumed that the absorption and elimination processes both follow the first order; if not the residual line and, perhaps, the elimination line will not be straight.
3. It is assumed that the absorption is complete; if not the estimate of Vd will be erroneously high. If the fraction of the dose absorbed, (F) is known, then Vd can be estimated.

Answers to the Problems

CHAPTER 2

Answers to 59

The equations govering the degree of ionization of the drugs are given below:

For weak acids

$$\text{pH} = \text{pKa} + \log \frac{[\text{ionized}]}{[\text{unionized}]}$$

and

Percent of drug ionized

$$= \frac{10^{(\text{pH - pKa})}}{1+10^{(\text{pH - pKa})}} \times 100$$

For weak bases

$$\text{pH} = \text{pKa} + \log \frac{[\text{ionized}]}{[\text{unionized}]} \text{ and}$$

Percent of drug ionized

$$= \frac{10^{(pKa-pH)}}{1+10^{(pKa-pH)}} \times 100$$

Using the above equations, the table given below can be constructed.

Drug	Stomach		Intestine		Blood	
	% ionized	% unionized	% ionized	% unionized	% ionized	% unionized
Ibuprofen	3.83	96.17	96.17	3.87	99.9	0.1
Diazepam	83.36	16.64	0.788	99.212	0.001	99.999

It can be concluded from the table that Ibuprofen is better absorbed from the stomach and diazepam from the small intestine, since the percent of unionized forms of the drugs are higher in the stomach and small intestine respectively.

CHAPTER 3

Answers to 35

Construct the following table

Drug	Before displacement	After displacement	% increase in free drug
Chloremphenicol			
Percent bound	53	45	
Percent unbound	47	55	+17
Phenytoin			
Percent bound	93	85	
Percent unbound	7	15	+114
Erythromycin			
Percent bound	75	67	
Percent unbound	25	33	+32
Morphine			
Percent bound	35	27	
Percent unbound	65	73	+12

It can be concluded from the table that the displacement of phenytoin from its binding sites caused a 114% increase in the free drug level and hence it will lead to the precipitation of toxic effects of phynytoin.

In case of erythromycin, a 32% increase may effect the bacteria and hence may be useful in the therapy provided that this will not affect the host. Other drugs may not show a recognizable change in their therapeutic effect.

Answers to 36

The liver is an important organ for the synthesis of the plasma proteins. In chronic alcoholic liver diseases or cirrhosis, less plasma proteins are synthesized in the liver, resulting in a lower plasma protein concentration. Thus, for a given dose of naproxen, less drug is bound to the plasma proteins and the total plasma drug concentration in smaller. Any decreased plasma protein binding leads to an increase in free drug concentration of naproxen.

Answers to 37

Percent unbound drug outside plasma

$$= \frac{Vd - 3}{Vd} \times 100$$

Therefore, the percent of the bound drug present outside plasma for drug A = 70, B = 92.5 and C = 99.

CHAPTER 4

Answers to 34

The equation for a weak acid for the estimation of saliva/plasma drug concentration ratio is the following.

$$\frac{Cs}{Cp} = \frac{1+10^{(pHs - pKa)}}{1+10^{(pHp - pKa)}} \times \frac{fup}{fus}$$

$$\frac{Cs}{Cp} = \frac{1+10^{(6.5 - 5.4)}}{1+10^{(7.4 - 5.4)}} \times \frac{0.09}{1.0}$$

Saliva/plasma drug concentration ratio (Cs/Cp) = 0.012

CHAPTER 6

Answers to 31

1. Slope = 0.125

$$K = 0.125 \times 2.303 = 0.288\ hr^{-1}$$

$$t_{1/2} = 2.41\ hrs.$$

2. C0 = intercept of semilogarthmic plot = 31.3 μg/ml
3. Vd = X0/C0 = 325 mg/31.3 ug/ml = 10383.38 ml = 10.38 L
4. AUC_0^{∞} = C0/K = (31.3 μg/ml)/(0.288 hr^{-1}) = 108.68 μg-hr/ml
5. Total body clearance, CL_t = Vd. K = 10.38 x 0.288 hr^{-1} = 2.99 L/hr

Answer to 32

(a) Prepare a semilogarithmic plot of plasma concentration of the drug versus time. Estimate the half-life of the drug from the slope of the line.

Slope = 0.01146

K = (2.303) (0.01146) = 0.02567 hr^{-1}

Biological half-life = 0.693/K = 0.693/0.02567 = 28 hours

(b) Estimate the total AUC of the drug.

(i) $AUC_0^{\infty} = C0/K = \frac{141.2}{0.02567} = 5500$ mg-hr/L

(ii) AUC calculated using traperzoidal rule = 5700 mg-hr/L

Clearance = 33 ml/L

(c) Calculate the volume of distribution

$$Vd = \frac{184 mg}{141.2 mg/L} = 1.3\ L$$

(d) Clearance, CL_t = Vd K = (1.3 L) (0.02467 hr^{-1}) = 0.0335 L/hr = 33.5 ml/hr

Answers to 33

1. Slope = 0.4299

K = 0.4299 x 2.303 = 0.99 hr^{-1}

$t_{1/2}$ = 0.693/K = 0.693/.99 = 0.7 hours

2. C0 = 233.35 μg/L

Vd = X0/C0 = 33mg/233.35 μg/L = 141.4 liters

volume of distribution per kg of body weight = 141.4/75 = 1.885 L

3. AUC_0^{∞} = C0/K = 235.7 μg-hr/L

4. Clearance, Cl_t = Vd K = 139.986 L/hr

Answers to 34

Construct the following table : X_u^{∞} = 984 mg

Time	Cumulative amount (Xu)	ΔXu	Δt	ΔXu/Δt	t'	$(X_u^{\infty}-X_u^{t})$
0	0	-	-	-	-	984
0.25	160	160	0.25	640	0.125	824
0.50	300	140	0.25	560	0.375	684
1.0	500	200	0.5	400	0.75	484
2.0	750	250	1.0	250	1.5	234
4.0	938	188	2.0	94	3.0	46
6.0	984	46	2.0	23	5.0	0

I. **Rate Excretion Method:** Construct a graph of log ($\Delta Xu/\Delta t$) versus t'. Calculate the slope.

Slope = 0.3009

$K = 0.3009 \times 2.303 = 0.693\ hr^{-1}$

Biological half-life,

$t_{1/2} = 0.693/K = 0.693/0.693 = 1hour$

Intercept = log Ke X0 = 2.8337

Therefore, Ke X0 = antilog 2.337 = 681.912

$Ke = 681.912/X0 = 681.912/1000 = 0.6819\ hr^{-1}$

II. **Sigma-Minus Method:** A plot of log ($X_u^{\infty} - X_u^{t}$) versus time gives a straight line with a slope = 0.3009 and hence $K = 0.693\ hr^{-1}$ and $t_{1/2}$ = 1 hour and $Ke = 0.681\ hr^{-1}$

Answers to 35

(a) 16.7 hrs estimated from the slope of the semilogarithmic plot of data following I.V. administration (not shown). $K = 0.0415\ hr^{-1}$.

(b) $AUC_{I.V.}$ = 217 mg-hr/L ; AUC_{oral} = 191 mg-hr/L. Estimated by the traperzoidal rule upto 48 hrs and using the equation C*/K.

(c) CL_t = 2.3 L/hr; V_d = 55 L.

$CL_t = Dose/AUC_{I.V.}$ = 500 mg/217 mg-hr/L = 2.3 L/hr

$V_d = Cl_t/K = (2.3\ L/hr)/(0.0415\ hr^{-1}) = 55\ L.$

(d) F = 0.88. Since, I.V. dose = Oral dose,

$$F = \frac{AUC_{oral}}{AUC_{I.V}} = \frac{191}{217} = 0.88$$

Answers to 36

(a) Absorption rate limits griseofulvin elimination for 24 to 40 hrs. This time corresponds to the normal transit time of food in the gut. Thereafter, unabsorbed drug is expelled from the gut, and the plasma concentration of griseofulvin then falls parallel to that following the I.V. dose.

(b) Griseofulvin is incompletely absorbed in this subject: A cursory examination of the data plotted on a regular graph paper indicates that based on the AUC corrected for the dose, griseofulvin is poorly bioavailable (F approximately 0.4). Griseofulvin, sparingly soluble in water (10 mg/L), is difficult to dissolve.

Answers to 37

(a) Bioavailability = 1.01

The AUC is calculated using the trapezoidal rule

$$F = \frac{[AUC/Dose]_{I.M}}{[AUC/Dose]_{I.V.}} = \frac{[(75.8\,mg\text{-}hr/L)/500mg]}{[(136.3\,mg\text{-}hr/L)/250mg]} =$$

$$= \frac{0.5516}{0.5452} = 1.01$$

(b) A semilogarthmic plot shows that a decline in plasma concentration after I.M. administration is slower than that following I.V. administration, indicating that absorption from the I.M. site rate-limits the elimination of phenytoin from the body.

Answers to 38

Dose (I.V. bdus) = 6 mg/kg x 50 kg = 300 mg.

(a) $$Vd. = \frac{I.V.\,dose}{C0} = \frac{300}{8.4\,\mu g/ml} = 35.7\ L$$

1. Plot the data on semilog graph paper and find out the slope.
   Intercept = C0 = 8.4 mg/ml Slope = 0.075
   K = 0.075 x 2.303 = 0.173 hr^{-1}
2. $t_{1/2}$ = 0.693/0.173 = 4 hours

(b) C0 = 8.4 mg/ml; C = 2.5 mg/ml; K = 0.173 hr^{-1}

log C = log C0 - Kt/2.303

$$\log 2.5 = \log 8.4 - \frac{0.173\,t}{2.303}$$

t = 7 hrs

The duration of action of the drug is 7 hours.

Alternatively, the duration of action may be found from a graph of C versus t.

(c) Time required for a 99% of the drug to be eliminated : **26.67 hours**

Initial concentration is 100% = 8.4 μg/ml

Final concentration is (100% - 99%) = 1% of 8.4 μg/ml

$$\log 0.084 = \log 8.4 - \frac{0.173\,t}{2.303}$$

t = 26.67 hr.

(d) If the dose is doubled, then C0 will also be doubled. However, the elimination half-life or first-order rate constant will remain the same. Therefore,

C0 = 16.8 mg/ml, C = 2.5 mg/ml, K = 0.173 hr^{-1}

$$\log 2.5 = \log 16.8 - \frac{0.703 \times t}{2.303}$$

$$t = 11.03 \text{ hrs}$$

The duration of action of the drug is 11.03 hours.

Notice that a doubling of the dose does not double the duration of activity.

Answers to 39

Dose = X_υ = 300 mg

V_d = 12% of body weight = (0.12) (80 kg) = 96 L = 9600 ml.

At 4 hrs,

C = 1.52 mg/100 ml

Vd = X/C

9600 ml = X/(1.52mg/100ml)

Therefore, X = 145.92 mg.

Amount of the drug in the body at 4 hrs = 145.92mg.

$$\log X = \log X_0 - Kt/2.303$$

$$\log 145.92 = \log 300 - \frac{K(4)}{2.303}$$

$$K = \frac{(\log 300 - \log 145.92)}{4} \times 2.303.$$

$$K = 0.18 \text{ hr}^{-1}$$

$$\text{Biological half-life} = \frac{0.693}{K} = \frac{0.693}{0.18} = 3.85 \text{ hrs.}$$

Answers to 40

The equation that describes the time course of the drug concentration in the blood following an I.V. bolus injection for a drug that follows one compartment open model is the following:

$$C = C0.e^{-Kt}$$

The given data fits into $C = 78\ e^{-0.46\ t}$

It means C0 = 78 mg/ml and K = 0.46 hr^{-1}

(a) $t_{1/2}$ = 0.693/K = 0.693/0.46 = 1.5 hrs

(b) V_d = I.V.dose/C0

I.V. dose = (4 mg/kg) (75 kg) = 300 mg

V_d = 300 000 ug/78 ug/ml = 3846 ml

(c) 1. $C = C0.e^{-Kt}$ at 4 hrs

$C = 78\ e^{-(0.46)(4)}$ = (78) (0.1588) = 12.4 mg/ml.

2. $\log C = \log C0 - Kt/2.303$

$$\log C = \log 78 - \frac{(0.46)(4)}{2.303} = 1.892 - 0.7986$$

$\log C = 1.093$

$C = \text{antilog } 1.093 = 12.4\ \mu g/ml.$

(d) At 4 hrs.

1. $X = C.Vd = (12.4 \text{ mg/ml})\ (3846 \text{ ml}) = 47690 \text{ mg} = 47.69 \text{ mg}$
2. $X = X0\ e^{-Kt} = (300)(e^{-(0.46) \times (4)}) = 47.64 \text{ mg}.$

(e) $V_d = 3846$ ml.

Average weight = 75kg

Percent body weight = (3. 864 L/75 kg) (100) = 5.1%

The apparent V_d approximates the plasma volume.

(f) C = 2 mg/ml find t

$1.2 \text{ mg/ml} = 78 \text{ mg/ml} \times e^{-0.46 \times t}$

$$e^{-0.46t} = \frac{2}{78} = 0.02564$$

$-0.46\ t = \ln 0.02564 = -3.7$

$$-t = \frac{-3.7}{0.46} = 8 \text{ hrs.}$$

t = 8 hrs

2. $$\log 2 = \log 78 - \frac{0.46 \times t}{2.303}$$

$$\frac{-0.46\ t}{2.303} = \log 2 - \log 78$$

$-0.1997\ t = -1.59106$

$$t = \frac{+1.59106}{+0.1997} = 7.967 = 8 \text{ hrs.}$$

Next dose will be administered 8 hrs. after the first dose.

Answers to 41

(a) $C0 = \text{I.V.dose}/V_d = 400 \text{ mg}/(0.15 \text{L/kg})(52 \text{ kg}) = 51.28 \text{ mg/L}$

(b) At t = 6 hrs.

1. $\log X = \log X0 - Kt/2.303$

$$\log X = \log 400 - \frac{(0.576)(6)}{2.303}$$

$\log X = 1.1$

$X = \text{antilog } 1.1 = 12.58 \text{ mg}$

2. $X = X0\ e^{-Kt} = 400\ mg \times e^{-0.576 \times 6} = 12.62\ mg$

Drug in the body after 6 hrs = 12.62 mg.

(c) C0 = 51.28 mg/L or C = 1.8 mg/ml or 1.8 mg/L.

log(1.8 mg/L) = log(51.28 mg/L) - (0.576)(t)/(2.303)

-0.25 t = log(1.8) - log(51.28) = -1.455

t = 1.455/0.25 = 5.82 hrs.

Answers to 42

For the first-order elimination kinetics, one-half of the initial quantity is lost in each $t_{1/2}$. The following table may be developed.

Time (hrs)	Number of $t_{1/2}$	Amount of Drug in body (mg)	Percent of Drug in body	Percent of Drug lost
0	0	300	100	0
4	1	150	50	50
8	2	75	25	75
12	3	37.50	12.5	87.50
16	4	18.750	6.25	93.75
20	5	9.375	3.13	96.87
24	6	4.688	1.56	98.44

Method 1

From the Table the percent of the drug remaining in the body after each $t_{1/2}$ is equal to 100% time $(1/2)^n$, where n is the number of half-lives.

$$\text{Percent of drug remaining} = \frac{100}{2^n}$$

where n = number of $t_{1/2}$

$$\text{Percent of drug eliminated} = 100 - \frac{100}{2^n}$$

At 24 hrs, n = 6 since $t_{1/2}$ = 4 hrs

$$\text{Percent drug lost} = 100 - \frac{100}{2^6} = 100 - 1.56 = 98.43.$$

Method 2

The equation for a first-order elimination after an I.V. bolus injection is log X = log X0 - Kt/2.303.

$$\log X = \log 300 - \frac{(0.173)(24)}{2.303}$$

Where :

X0 = Dose = 300 mg

X = amount of drug in the body at any time t.

t = 24 hrs

$$K = \frac{0.693}{t1/2} = 0.173$$

X = 4.72 mg

Amount lost = X0 - X = 300 - 4.72 = 295.28 mg.

$$\text{Percent lost} = \frac{295.28\,\text{mg}}{300\text{mg}} \times 100 = 98.43.$$

Answers to 43

log X = log X0 - Kt/2.303

X0 = 600 mg

$K = 0.693/t_{1/2} = 0.693/8 = 0.0866\ hr^{-1}$

t = 24 hrs.

$$\log X = \log 600 - \frac{(0.0866)(24)}{2.303}$$

log X = 1.875

X = antilog 1.875 = 74.99 mg.

$$\text{The percent lost in 24 hrs} = \frac{600 - 74.99}{600} \times 100 = 87.5.$$

$$\text{Plasma drug conc. at 24 hrs} = \frac{74.99}{Vd} = \frac{74.99}{(0.4\ L/kg) \times 62\ kg} = 3.02\ mg/L$$

Answers to 44

Set up the following Table

t' (hrs)	Xu (mg)	Δ Xu/Δ t (mg/hr)	T'
0	0		
4	100	100/4 = 25	2
8	26	26/4 = 6.5	6

The elimination the half-life may be obtained graphically after plotting ΔXu/Δt versus t' (mid point of urine collection). The $t_{1/2}$ obtained graphically is approximately 2 hrs.

$$\log \frac{\Delta Xu}{\Delta t} = \log Ke\,Xo - Kt'/2.303$$

$$\text{Slope} = \frac{-K}{2.303} = \frac{\log(6.5) - \log(25)}{6 - 2} = -0.146$$

$K = (0.146)(2.303) = 0.337\ hr^{-1}$

$t_{1/2} = 0.693/K = 0.693/0.337\ hr^{-1} = 2.06$ hrs.

CHAPTER 6

Answers to 10

(a) A, B, α and β

$A = 67$; $B = 33$; $\alpha = 14$ and $\beta = 3$

(b) The volume of the central compartment (V_c).

$V_c = 6.5$ liters

(c) The volume of the peripheral compartment.

$V_p = 3.95$ liters

(d) The apparent volume of distribution at steady-state (V_d^{ss}).

$V_d^{ss} = 10.45$ liters

(e) The volume of distribution by area (V_d^{area}).

$V_d^{area} = 13.7$ liters

(f) The volume of distribution using b.

$V_d\beta = 13.715$ liters

(g) The microconstants K_{12} and K_{21}.

$K_{12} = 4.035\ hr^{-1}$; $K_{21} = 6.63\ hr^{-1}$

(h) Elimination rate constant (K_{13}).

$K_{13} = 6.33\ hr^{-1}$

(I) The biological half-life ($t_{1/2}$).

$t_{1/2} = 0.231$ hrs

(j) The total body clearance (Cl_t).

$Cl_t = 682.6$ ml/min.

CHAPTER 8

Answers to 6

V_d = 20% of the body weight = (0.20) (50-kg) = 10L or 10,000 ml

$K = 0.693/t_{1/2} = 0.693/2 = 0.3465\ hr^{-1}$, $\tau = 8$ hours

I.V. Dose = (1 mg/kg) (50-kg) = 50 mg

$R = e^{-k\tau} = e^{-(0.3465)(8)} = 0.0625$

C_1^0 = I.V.dose/V_d = 50 mg/10L = 5 mg/L or 5 ug/ml

$C_{max} = C_1^0/(1-R) = 5/(1 - 0.0625) = 5.33$ ug/ml
$C_{min} = C_{max}\ R = (5.33)\ (0.0625) = 0.33\ \mu g/ml$
C_{ave} = I.V.Dose/$V_d\ K\ \tau = 50/(10)(0.3465)(8) = 1.8$ ug/ml

Answers to 7

$V_d = (0.20)(82\text{-kg}) = 16.4$ L

$K = 0.693/t_{1/2} = 0.693/3 = 0.231\ hr^{-1}$ and $\tau = 8$ hours and $R = e^{-K\tau} = e^{-(0.231)(8)} =$ 0.15755

(a) I.V.dose = $C_1^0\ V_d$; $C_1^0 = C_{max}\ (1 - R)$. According to the problem, the maximum safe level is 10 μg/ml. Therefore, $C_{max} = 10\ \mu g/ml$

I.V. dose (X0) = $16.4 \times 10\ (1 - e^{-Kt}) = 16.4 \times 10\ (1 - 0.15755) = 138.16$ mg to be given every 8 hours.

(b) $C_{min} = C_{max}\ R = (10)\ (0.15755) = 1.58$ ug/ml.
$C_{ave} = X0/V_d\ K\ t = 138.16\text{mg}/\ (16.4)(0.231)(8) = 4.56\ \mu g/ml$.

(c) In the above dosage regimen, the C_{min} of 1.58 μg/ml is below the desired C_{min} of 2 μg/ml. Therefore, the dosage regimen has to be changed from $\tau = 8$ hours to $\tau = 6$ hours.

Then, the I.V.dose = $(16.4)(10)\ (1-e^{-(0.231)\ (6)}) = 123$ mg to be given every 6 hours.

Now, $C_{min} = C_{max}\ R = (10)\ (0.25) = 2.5\ \mu g/ml$.

$C_{ave} = 123/(16.4)(0.231)(6) = 5.41\ \mu g/ml$.

Answers to 8

Maintenance dose = $X^*\ (1-e^{-K\tau})$

Loading dose, X^* = Maintenance dose/$(1 - e^{-K\tau}) = 200/(1 - e^{-0.(23)(3)}) = 401.26$ mg.

CHAPTER 9

Answers to 9

According to equation 9.20,

$t = 1/V_{max}\ (D_0 - D_t + Km\ \ln D_0/D_t)$
$D_0 = 400$ mg ; D_t = 50% of 400 = 200 mg; $V_{max} = 50$ mg/hr; Km = 100 mg
$t = 1/50\ (400 - 200 + 100\ \ln 400/200) = 5.39$ hours

Similarly, for a dose of 320 mg,

t = 1/50 (320 -160 + 100 ln 320/160) = 4.59 hours.

For a capacity-limted elimination, the $t_{1/2}$ is dose-dependent because the drug elimination process is partially saturated. Therefore, small changes in the dose will produce large differences in the time for 50% of drug elimination. The parameters Km and V_{max} determine the dose required to saturate the system.

Answers to 10

According to Equation 9.17,

$$Km = \frac{D_2 - D_1}{(D_1 / C_1) - (D_2 / C_2)}$$

$$Km = \frac{300 - 150}{(150 / 86) - (300 / 25.1)}$$

$$Km = 27.3 \text{ mg/L}$$

$$v = \frac{V_{max}\, C}{Km + C}$$

$$V_{max} = v(Km+C)/C = 150(27.3+8.6)/8.6 = 626 \text{ mg/day}$$

CHAPTER 10

Answers to 11

1. Capsule : The overall elimination rate constant, K= 0.347 hr^{-1}(calculated from terminal linear portion of the graph of log C versus time).

   $AUC_0^{\infty} = AUC_0^{12} + AUC_{12}^{\infty} = 89.68 + 1.816 = 91.496$ (μg/ml)hr

   $AUMC_0^{\infty} = AUMC_0^{12} + AUMC_{12}^{\infty} = 382.695 + 27.71 = 409.71$ (μg/ml)hr^2

   $MRT_{capsule} = 409.71/91.496 = 4.478$ hours

   $MAT = MRT_{capsule} - MRT_{IV}$, but $MRT_{IV} = 1/K = 1/0.347 = 2.882$ hours

   MAT = 4.478 - 2.882 = 1.596 hours.

2. Solution :

   K = 0.455 hr^{-1} (Obtained from the terminal linear portion of the graph of log C versus time).

   $AUC_0^{\infty} = AUC_0^{12} + AUC_{12}^{\infty} = 87.665 + 0.835 = 88.5$ (μg/ml)hr

   $AUMC_0^{\infty} = AUMC_0^{12} + AUMC_{12}^{\infty} = 220.64 + 11.86 = 232.50$ (μg/ml)hr^2

   $MRT_{solution} = 232.50/88.5 = 2.63$ hours

   $MAT = MRT_{solution} - MRT_{IV}$, but $MRT_{IV} = 1/K = 1/0.455 = 2.20$ hours

   $MAT_{solution} = 2.63 - 2.2 = 0.43$ hours.

   Now, $MDT_{capsule} = MRT_{capsule} - MRT_{solution} = 4.478 - 2.63 = 1.848$ hours.

CHAPTER 12

Answers to 17

1. Mean: Number of observations, n is 8. The mean = $\sum X_i^2/n$

   $= (2.86+2.75+.....+3.12)/8 = 3.001$ ug/ml

2. Median: Rearranging the measurements in increasing order gives:

   2.62, 2.75, 2.76, 2.86, 3.05, 3.12, 3.37, 3.49

   Median = (n+1)/2 = (8+1)/ = 4.5. It mean the average of the 4th and 5th values.

   Median = (2.86+3.05)/2 = 2.961

3. Mode: There is no mode to this data because no value is having highest frequency.

4. Standard deviation:

   $$s = \sqrt{[\Sigma(X_i)^2-(\Sigma X_i)^2/n]/(n-1)}$$

   $$= \sqrt{[72.798 - (24.02)^2/8]/8-1} = \sqrt{09685} = 0.3112$$

5. Standard error of the average = $s/\sqrt{n} = 0.3112/\sqrt{8} = 0.11$

6. Variance = $s^2 = (0.3112)^2 = 0.09685$

7. Coefficient of variation, c.v. = $(s/\bar{X})100 = (0.3112/3.001)100 = 10.36$

Answers to 18

(a) The probability of the student picked from the sample to be a girl = (number of girls)/(total number of students) = 22/48 = 0.4583

(b) This is the conditional probability, P (D|Y) = 3/22 =0.136

Answers to 19

The probability of 7 successes out of 9, $P(7) = \binom{9}{3} 0.84^7\, 0.16^{9-7}$

$$= \frac{9!}{7!(9-7)} 0.84^7\, 0.16^2$$

$$P(7) = \frac{362880}{10080} (0.295)(0.0256) = 0.2718$$

Answers to 20

Arrange the data as a contingency table.

Treatment	Survived	Dead	Total
Drug	20 (A)	8 (B) 28	
Control	28 ©	8 (D) 36	
Total	A + C = 48	B + D =16	N = 64

$$\chi^2 = \frac{(|AD - BC| - N/2)^2 N}{(A+B)(C+D)(A+C)(B+D)}$$

$$\chi^2 = \frac{(|20x8 - 8x28| - 64/2)^2 64}{(20+8)(28+8)(20+28)(8+8)} = 0.7619$$

The degrees of freedom (DF) = 1. The χ^2 value for DF=1 at P=0.05 is 3.84. Since the calculated χ^2 value (0.7619) is less than the tabled value, the drug is not having significant effect in treating the disease.

Answers to 21

	Weight in kgs.														
NS	3.99	3.79	3.60	3.73	3.21	3.60	4.08	3.61	3.83	3.31	4.13	3.26	3.54	3.51	2.71
S	3.18	2.84	2.90	3.27	3.85	3.52	3.23	2.76	3.60	3.75	3.59	3.63	2.38	2.34	---

The following values have to be calculated to estimate the t-value. This example comes under the category of two independent sample t-test.

$$t = \frac{\bar{X}_1 - \bar{X}_2}{s}\sqrt{\frac{n_1 n_2}{n_1 + n_2}} \qquad 26$$

$$s^2 = \frac{\left[\Sigma X_{1i}^2 - (\Sigma X_{1i}^2)^2/n_1\right] + \left[\Sigma X_{2i}^{\;2} - (\Sigma X_{2i})^2/n_2\right]}{n_1 + n_2 - 2}$$

$$s^2 = \frac{\left[195.6 - (53.8995)^2/15\right] + \left[146.77 - (44.8406)^2/14\right]}{15+14-2} = 0.1878 \qquad 27$$

$$s = \sqrt{\;}\ 0.1878 = 0.4335$$

$$t = \frac{3.5933 - 3.2029}{0.4335}\sqrt{\frac{15 \times 14}{15 + 14}} = 2.42$$

DF= 15 + 14 – 2 = 27. The t-value for DF = 27 at P = 0.05 (two-tail) is 2.052. Since the calculated t-value is greater than the table value, it is concluded that smoking influences the weight of the child at birth.

Answers to 22

Subject	1	2	3	4	5	6	7	8
Weight	58.0	70.0	74.0	63.5	62.0	70.5	71.0	66.0
Plasma volume	2.75	2.86	3.37	2.76	2.62	3.49	3.05	3.12

The following equations are used to calculate the correlation coefficient.

$$t = \frac{\Sigma X_i Y_i - (\Sigma X_i \Sigma Y_i)/n}{\sqrt{\Sigma(X_i - \bar{X})^2 \, \Sigma(Y_i - \bar{Y})^2}}$$

$$t = r\sqrt{\frac{n-2}{1-r^2}}$$

$n = 8$

$\Sigma X_i = 535$ $X = 66.875$ $\Sigma X_i^2 = 35983.5$ $\Sigma(X\text{-}Y)^2 = 205.38$

$\Sigma Y_i = 24.05$ $Y = 3.0025$ $\Sigma Y_i^2 = 72.7980$ $\Sigma(X\text{-}Y)^2 = 0.6780$

$(\Sigma X_i \, \Sigma Y_i) = 1615.295$

$$r = \frac{161.5295 - (535 \times 24.02/8)}{\sqrt{(205.38)(0.678)}} = 0.759$$

$$t = 0.759\sqrt{\frac{8-2}{1-(0.759)^2}} = 2.855$$

The DF = n-2 = 6. The tabled t-value for DF = 6 at P = 0.05 (two-tail) is 2.447. Since the calculated t-value (2.855) is greater than the table value (2.447), there exists a linear relation between the body weight of the subject and plasma volume.

Index

A

B

C

D

E

F

G

H

I

K

L

M

N

O

P

R

S

T

U

V

W

9 789352 30053